Practical Diagnosis
of
Hematologic Disorders

Authors

Carl R. Kjeldsberg, MD
Professor of Pathology and Medicine
Chairman of Pathology
University of Utah Health Sciences Center
President, ARUP Inc
Salt Lake City, Utah

Kathryn Foucar, MD
Director, Pathology Services
Professor of Pathology
University of New Mexico School of Medicine
Albuquerque, New Mexico

Robert W. McKenna, MD
John Childers Professor and Vice-Chair of Pathology
University of Texas Southwestern Medical Center
Dallas, Texas

Sherrie L. Perkins, MD, PhD
Assistant Professor of Pathology
Director, Hematopathology
University of Utah Health Sciences Center
ARUP Inc
Salt Lake City, Utah

LoAnn C. Peterson, MD
Professor of Pathology
Northwestern University Medical School
Chicago, Illinois

Powers Peterson, MD
Associate Professor of Pathology
Cornell University Medical College
New York, New York
Director, Laboratory of Clinical Hematology
The New York Hospital
New York, New York
Director, Clinical Laboratories
The New York Hospital Westchester Division
White Plains, New York

George M. Rodgers, MD, PhD
Associate Professor of Medicine and Pathology
Medical Director, Coagulation Laboratory
University of Utah Health Sciences Center and Veterans Affairs Medical Center
ARUP Inc
Salt Lake City, Utah

Practical Diagnosis
of
Hematologic Disorders

Second Edition

Carl R. Kjeldsberg, MD, Editor

ASCP Press
American Society of Clinical Pathologists
Chicago, Illinois

Printed in Canada

ISBN 0-89189-401-2

Library of Congress Cataloging-in-Publication Data
Practical diagnosis of hematologic disorders / [edited by] Carl Kjeldsberg. —
  2nd ed.
    p. 834 cm.
  Includes bibliographical references and index.
  ISBN 0-89189-401-2
  1. Blood—Diseases—Diagnosis. I. Kjeldsberg, Carl R., 1938-
  [DNLM: 1. Hematologic Diseases—diagnosis. 2. Hematologic Diseases
therapy—handbooks. WH 39 P895 1995]
RC636.P72 1995
616. 1'5075—dc20
DNLM/DLC   95-15075
for Library of Congress   CIP

99 98 97 96 95   5 4 3 2 1

Contents

Preface

The excellent response and positive feedback that we received following publication of the first edition of *Practical Diagnosis of Hematologic Disorders* encouraged us to write a second edition. Our goal in the new edition remains the same as that for the first: to provide an up-to-date, concise source of guidelines to the selection, use, and interpretation of laboratory tests, while at the same time providing an overview of the pathogenesis, clinical features, and treatment of the most common hematologic disorders. To ensure that we have met that goal, the entire text has been revised, reworked, rephotographed, or rewritten. Substantial new material has been added, including nearly twice as many tables and twice as many photomicrographs, all of which are in color.

A unique strength of the book has always been its consistent organization of presentation and devotion to inclusion of practical information. Each chapter defines a disorder, discusses the relevant pathophysiology, clinical findings, approach to diagnosis, hematologic findings, other laboratory tests, and clinical course and treatment. To each chapter is appended a thoughtfully considered set of up-to-date references. Chapters are heavily complemented with useful tables, work-up algorithms, and brilliant color images. Because most chapters discuss primarily one disorder, information on each disease is easy to find. Finally, an appendix of reference values for various hematologic parameters, which lists both conventional and SI units for laboratory values, completes the volume.

We hope that this nonspecialist book will continue to interest a broad audience, including medical students, residents and fellows in pathology and medicine, pathologists, internists, pediatricians, and medical technologists. Naturally, we would expect such a practical, easy-to-use volume to be particularly helpful to those preparing for boards in pathology and internal medicine, and also for those hematologists/oncologists who need a quick source for review of particular information. In any event, the book remains easier to heft and handle than a standard textbook, which alone ought to recommend it to busy, burdened clinicians.

Acknowledgments

I gratefully acknowledge the excellent work and support of my coauthors, M. Kathryn Foucar, MD, Robert W. McKenna, MD, Sherrie L. Perkins, MD, PhD, LoAnn C. Peterson, MD, Powers Peterson, MD, and George M. Rodgers, MD, PhD. I also wish to express my sincere appreciation to Joshua Weikersheimer, Director of the ASCP Press, for help and guidance with this project.

Carl R. Kjeldsberg, MD

PART
1

Anemias

1

Diagnosis of Anemia

The bone marrow contains pluripotential stem cells that have the capacity to self-renew as well as to differentiate into mature blood cells. Under the influence of cytokines such as erythropoietin (for the production of red blood cells), this primitive stem cell undergoes cellular division and differentiation to form pronormoblasts and normoblasts. This process requires 6 to 7 days and four rounds of cellular division within the bone marrow. During the final step of differentiation, the nucleus is extruded to form a reticulocyte, which still contains cytoplasmic RNA. Reticulocytes may enter the peripheral blood circulation, where they appear as faintly blue-gray polychromatophilic cells, which may persist for about 24 hours. On loss of the cytoplasmic RNA, a mature red blood cell is formed. The mature red blood cell will remain in the peripheral blood circulation for 120 days before being removed by the spleen and reticuloendothelial system.

Normal and Pathologic Red Blood Cells

The normal red blood cell is a biconcave disk, 6 to 9 μm in diameter and 1.5- to 2.5-μm thick. In a peripheral smear, red blood cells are anucleate with a dense outer rim and a clearer center that occupies approximately one third of the diameter of the red blood cell. The cytoplasm is uniformly pink without inclusions. Pathologic red blood cells can be larger or smaller than normal red blood cells, are often abnormally shaped, and may contain inclusions. Variation in size is referred to as "anisocytosis"; variation in shape is termed "poikilocytosis." Some pathologic red blood cell forms are associated with specific diseases. Table 1-1 presents a summary of the names and morphologic abnormalities in red blood cells that may be seen on blood smears.

Automated Hematology

In both the office and hospital settings, most patients' blood is evaluated with an electronic blood cell counter. The two principal mechanisms used to analyze samples are voltage pulse-impedance analysis and low- or high-angle light scatter from a coherent light source, such as a laser. In an impedance counter, such as those first developed by Coulter Electronics (Hialeah, Fla), the passage of a particle through an orifice of standard size and volume displaces conductive electrolyte solution within the orifice. If an electric current is applied across the orifice, a change in resistivity and conductivity of the electrolyte solution occurs as the particle passes through it. A detector notes a pulse when a particle passes through the orifice, which is proportional to the volume of the electrolyte solution displaced by the particle. Thus, the counter is capable of counting and sizing particles simultaneously. In a light scatter counter, such as the Technicon H*1 (Technicon, Tarrytown, NY), interruption of the laser beam by a particle produces a pulse, and the angle of light scatter and the intensity of the light scattered at particular angles is proportional to several physical properties of the cell, especially size.

With these data, the instrument can generate a histogram of size distribution on the x axis and relative number of particles on the y axis. From these data, the red blood cell number and mean corpuscular volume (MCV) can be determined, and the other indices, such as mean corpuscular hemoglobin concentration (MCHC), can be calculated. In addition, the newer instruments generate an index that provides the degree of dispersion of red blood cell sizes (anisocytosis) compared with a "normal" size distribution histogram. On the Coulter and Technicon instruments, this index of average size dispersion, or degree of anisocytosis, is referred to as a red cell distribution width (RDW).

Evaluation of the Peripheral Blood Smear

Examination of the peripheral blood smear by a physician who is aware of the patient's clinical condition is extremely useful in the total evaluation of the anemic patient. Highly skilled laboratory personnel may occasionally overlook subtle changes, such as minimal hypersegmentation of neutrophils in cases of combined folate and iron deficiency (so-called masked macrocytosis), or basophilic stippling in a patient with thalassemia and complicating causes of anemia. These signs may be useful in the differential diagnosis if they are noted by a physician familiar with the patient. Electronically derived red and white blood cell indices, although useful, are simply representations of the mean and overall degree of dispersion of the cell distribution and give little information concerning other parameters, especially the shape of the red blood cells (poikilocytosis), the presence or absence of minor populations of abnormal red blood cells, and subtle changes in white blood cells. Examination of the blood smear for specific shape variations, such as those listed in Table 1-1, can provide valuable information in the diagnosis of the patient's underlying disease.

Anemia

The primary function of the red blood cell is to deliver oxygen to the tissues. Anemia is defined as a reduction in the total number of red blood cells, amount of hemoglobin in the circulation, or circulating red blood cell mass. This results in impaired oxygen delivery, giving rise to physiologic consequences secondary to tissue hypoxia and the compensatory mechanisms initiated by the organism to correct anoxia. These signs and symptoms include fatigue, syncope, dyspnea, and impairment of organ function due to

Table 1-1   Pathologic Red Blood Cells in Blood Smears

Red Blood Cell Type	Description
Acanthocyte (spur cell)	Irregularly spiculated cells with projections of varying length and dense center
Basophilic stippling	Punctuate basophilic inclusions
Bite cell (degmacyte)	Smooth semicircle taken from one edge
Burr cell (echinocyte), or crenated cell	Cells with short, evenly spaced spicules and preserved central pallor
Cabot's rings	Circular blue thread-like inclusion with dots
Ovalocyte (elliptocyte)	Elliptically shaped cell
Howell-Jolly bodies	Small, discrete basophilic dense inclusions; usually single
Hypochromic cell	Prominent central pallor
Leptocyte	Flat, wafer-like, thin, hypochromic cell
Macrocyte	Cells larger than normal (>8.5 μm), well-filled with hemoglobin
Microcyte	Cells smaller than normal (<7 μm)
Pappenheimer bodies	Small, dense basophilic granules
Polychromatophilia	Gray or blue hue frequently seen in macrocytes
Rouleaux	Cell aggregates resembling stack of coins
Schistocyte (helmet cell)	Distorted, fragmented cell, two or three pointed ends
Sickle cell (drepanocyte)	Bipolar, spiculated forms, sickle-shaped, pointed at both ends
Spherocyte	Spherical cell with dense appearance and absent central pallor; usually decreased in diameter
Stomatocyte	Mouth- or cup-like deformity
Target cell (codocyte)	Target-like appearance, often hypochromic
Teardrop cell (dacrocyte)	Distorted, drop-shaped cell

Abbreviations: G6PD = glucose-6-phosphate dehydrogenase; DIC = disseminated intravascular coagulation; TTP = thrombotic thrombocytopenic purpura.

Table 1-1 *Continued*

Underlying Change	Disease States
Altered cell membrane lipids	Abetalipoproteinemia, parenchymal liver disease, postsplenectomy
Precipitated ribosomes (RNA)	Coarse stippling: lead intoxication, thalassemia; fine stippling: a variety of anemias
Heinz body "pitting" by spleen	G6PD deficiency, drug-induced oxidant hemolysis
May be associated with altered membrane lipids	Usually artifactual: seen in uremia, bleeding ulcers, gastric carcinoma
Nuclear remnant	Postsplenectomy, hemolytic anemia, megaloblastic anemia
Abnormal cytoskeletal proteins	Hereditary elliptocytosis
Nuclear remnant (DNA)	Postsplenectomy, hemolytic anemia, megaloblastic anemia
Diminished hemoglobin synthesis	Iron deficiency anemia, thalassemia, sideroblastic anemia
	Obstructive liver disease, thalassemia
Young cells, abnormal cell maturation	Increased erythropoiesis, oval macrocytes in megaloblastic anemia, round macrocytes in liver disease
	See hypochromic cell
Iron-containing siderosome or mitochondrial remnant	Sideroblastic anemia; postsplenectomy
Ribosomal material	Reticulocytosis, premature marrow release of red blood cells
Cell clumping by circulating paraprotein	Paraproteinemia
Mechanical distortion in microvasculature by fibrin strands, disruption by prosthetic heart valve	Microangiopathic hemolytic anemia (DIC, TTP), prosthetic heart valves, severe burns
Molecular aggregation of hemoglobin S	Sickle cell disorders (not including S trait)
Decreased membrane redundancy	Hereditary spherocytosis, immunohemolytic anemia
Membrane defect with abnormal cation permeability	Hereditary stomatocytosis, immunohemolytic anemia
Increased redundancy of cell membrane	Liver disease, postsplenectomy, thalassemia, hemoglobin C disease
	Myelofibrosis, myelophthistic anemia

Table 1-2 Patient History in the Diagnosis of Anemia

Historical Information	Possible Causes of Anemia
Age of onset	Inherited or acquired disorder, continuous or recent onset
Duration of illness	Results of previous examinations, blood counts
Prior therapy for anemia	Vitamin B_{12}, iron supplementation, and how long ago
Suddenness or severity of anemia	Symptoms of dyspnea, palpitations, dizziness, fatigue, postural hypotension
Chronic blood loss	Menstrual and pregnancy history, gastrointestinal symptoms, black or bloody stools
Hemolytic episodes	Episodic weakness with icterus and dark urine
Toxic exposures	Drugs, hobbies, and occupational exposures
Dietary history	Alcohol use, unusual diet, prolonged milk ingestion in infants
Family history and racial background	Possible inherited disorder: anemia, gallbladder disease, splenomegaly, splenectomy
Underlying diseases	Uremia, chronic liver disease, hypothyroidism

decreased oxygen; pallor and postural hypotension due to decreased blood volume; and palpitations, onset of heart murmurs, and congestive heart failure due to increased cardiac output. One should always remember that anemia is not a diagnosis, but a sign of underlying disease. Hence, the workup of an anemic patient is directed at elucidating the causes for a patient's decreased red blood cell mass. A thorough history and physical examination are crucial for an intelligent, directed approach to the differential diagnosis of anemia. Tables 1-2 and 1-3 show important features in a patient's history and physical examination that can yield diagnostic clues as to the cause of the anemia, hence reducing the laboratory tests that need to be performed.

Examination of the Blood.   Anemias have been classified under a number of different schemes, none of which is completely satisfactory. For practical purposes, an initial morphologic classification of anemia with examination of red blood cell indices

Table 1-3   Physical Signs in the Diagnosis of Anemia

Physical Sign	Associated Disease
Skin and mucous membranes	
Pallor	Nonhemolytic anemia
Scleral icterus	Hemolytic anemia
Smooth tongue	Pernicious anemia, severe iron deficiency
Petechiae	Thrombocytopenia and bone marrow replacement
Gum hyperplasia	Acute monocytic leukemia
Lymph nodes	
Lymphadenopathy	Infectious mononucleosis, lymphoma, leukemia
Heart	
Cardiac dilatation, tachycardia, loud murmur	Severe anemia
Soft murmurs	Anemia, usually mild
Abdomen	
Splenomegaly	Infectious mononucleosis, leukemia, lymphoma
Massive splenomegaly	Chronic myelogenous leukemia, myelofibrosis
Hepatosplenomegaly with ascites	Liver disease
Central nervous system	
Subacute combined degeneration of spinal cord	Pernicious anemia (vitamin B_{12} deficiency)
Delayed Achilles' tendon reflex	Hypothyroidism

and the peripheral blood smear is probably most useful. With use of the MCV and the RDW or red blood cell morphologic index (RCMI), anemias may be classified into six categories (Table 1-4). The anemia may be characterized by cell size as microcytic, normocytic, or macrocytic. The absence or presence of anisocytosis (as measured by RDW) further subdivides these three size categories. In general, anemias caused by deficiency states (such as iron, folate, or vitamin B_{12}) tend to have a greater degree of anisocytosis than anemias caused by genetic defects or primary bone marrow disorders. However, it should be noted that difficulties in

Table 1-4   Classification of Anemia Based on Red Blood Cell Size and Distribution Width

Cell Size	Normal RDW	High RDW
Microcytosis (MCV <70 μm^3 [70 fL])	Thalassemia minor, anemia of chronic disease, hemoglobinopathy traits	Iron deficiency, hemoglobin H disease, some anemia of chronic disease, some thalassemia minor, fragmentation hemolysis
Normocytosis	Anemia of chronic disease, hereditary spherocytosis, some hemoglobinopathy traits	Early iron or vitamin deficiency, sickle cell anemia or sickle cell disease
Macrocytosis (MCV >100 μm^3 [100 fL])	Aplastic anemia, some myelodysplasias	Vitamin B_{12} or folate deficiency, autoimmune hemolytic anemia, cold agglutinin disease

Abbreviations: RDW = red cell distribution width; MCV = mean corpuscular volume.

classification using this scheme arise, particularly with regard to the anemia of chronic disease.

In addition to pure morphologic criteria, anemias may also be classified by the degree of bone marrow response or peripheral blood reticulocytosis as hyperproliferative, normoproliferative, or hypoproliferative. This often provides insights into the pathogenesis of the process. Thus, defects in red blood cell proliferation or maturation would tend to have little or no increase in reticulocytes, reflecting the inability of the bone marrow to increase red blood cell production in response to the anemia (hypoproliferative). In contrast, anemias caused by decreased survival of the red blood cell with a normal bone marrow proliferative response would show increased peripheral blood reticulocytes (normoproliferative or hyperproliferative; Figure 1-1). If the degree of reticulocytosis is adequate to correct the loss of red blood cells, the anemia is said to be "compensated." If the bone marrow response is not adequate, the anemia is likely to worsen.

Finally, anemias due to decreased red blood cell survival are often subdivided by pathogenetic mechanism into those caused by intrinsic or inherited defects, or anemias that are acquired or caused by extrinsic factors. This classification is often useful in understanding the underlying disease process and may facilitate the workup of anemias that arise secondary to survival defects.

Differential Diagnosis of Anemia. Anemia may be either relative (due to increased plasma volume with a normal red blood cell mass) or absolute (due to a decreased red blood cell mass). It is important to rule out causes of relative anemia, such as pregnancy or macroglobulinemia, since they represent disturbances in plasma volume rather than red blood cell mass. Decreased plasma volume, caused by dehydration, may mask a real decrease in circulating red blood cell mass.

Use of the morphologic classification scheme with red blood cell indices data and the reticulocyte count allows for practical classification of anemias into broad groups. This may facilitate intelligent selection of other laboratory tests to determine the underlying cause of the anemia.

Macrocytic Anemia. Macrocytic anemias (MCV >100 μm^3 [100 fL]) are less common than normocytic or microcytic anemias. The macrocytic anemias may be subdivided into those with normal RDW (principally those caused by bone marrow failure, such as aplastic anemia and myelodysplasia), and those with a high RDW (caused by deficiencies of vitamin B_{12} or folic acid, or caused by autoimmune hemolysis or cold agglutinins). However, many exceptions to this general scheme of classification exist. For example, a mild degree of macrocytosis (MCV in the range of 102-105 μm^3 [102-105 fL]) with a normal RDW is relatively common as a direct effect of alcohol. Similarly, some cases of myelodysplasia may have a high RDW.

Further classification of a macrocytic anemia based on the presence or absence of a reticulocyte response is often helpful (Figure 1-1). Hemolytic anemias, blood loss, and partially treated vitamin B_{12} or folic acid deficiencies will show an increased reticulocyte count. If not present, autoimmune hemolysis, disorders of membrane structural proteins (eg, elliptocytosis), paroxysmal nocturnal hemoglobinuria, and fragmentation hemolysis should be suspected (Figure 1-2). For those patients with a normal or decreased corrected reticulocyte count, disorders associated with

Figure 1-1 Classification of macrocytic anemias by reticulocyte count.

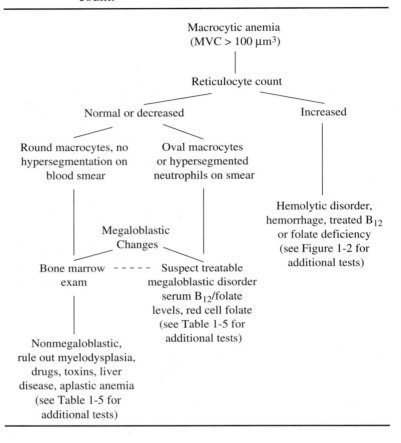

decreased bone marrow function, including untreated vitamin deficiency, drugs or toxins, liver or thyroid disease, or primary bone marrow, failure should be suspected. Blood smears that show morphologic features compatible with megaloblastic anemia (oval macrocytes and hypersegmented neutrophils) may warrant further evaluation with vitamin assays without a need for bone marrow examination. When megaloblastic changes are present without signs to suggest vitamin B_{12} or folate deficiency, bone marrow examination and additional testing (Table 1-5) may be needed. A more detailed and extensive consideration of macrocytic anemia is found in Chapter 5.

Figure 1-2 Classification of normocytic or megaloblastic anemias with elevated reticulocyte counts.

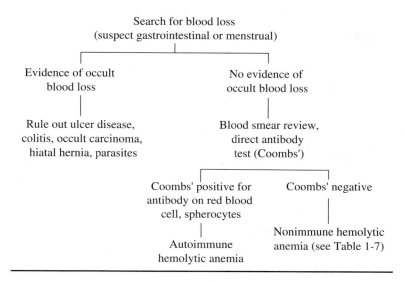

Table 1-5 Ancillary Tests for Macrocytic Anemia Without Increased Reticulocyte Response

No megaloblastic bone marrow changes present:
    Thyroid function tests
    Assess iron stores—serum iron, iron-binding capacity, ferritin
    Cytogenetic analysis—evaluate for myelodysplasia

Megaloblastic bone marrow changes present:
    Dietary and drug history
    Malabsorption studies
    Schilling test if vitamin B_{12} deficiency

Microcytic Anemia.   The three most common causes of microcytic anemias (MCV<75 μm^3 [75 fL]) are iron deficiency, thalassemia minor, and anemia of chronic disease (ACD) (Figure 1-3). The RDW is useful in distinguishing thalassemia, which generally (but not invariably) has elevated red blood cell counts and lower RDWs than would be expected for the MCV and the degree of anemia. Iron deficiencies are almost always associated with a high RDW. The values seen in ACD are extremely variable. Some ACDs may be normocytic. Other ACDs, particularly in patients with renal disease, are microcytic, but are associated with normal to high serum ferritin levels. Thus, by using serum iron and total iron-binding studies, iron deficiency anemia and ACD can usually be distinguished without a bone marrow examination (Figure 1-4). A more detailed consideration of the microcytic anemias may be found in Chapter 2.

Normocytic, Normochromic Anemia. Patients with normal or hypoproliferative reticulocyte counts and normocytic, normochromic anemias generally require bone marrow evaluation. A peripheral blood smear may provide valuable clues for the differential diagnosis (Table 1-6). Patients with normocytic anemia and an elevated reticulocyte count undergo the same general evaluation as patients with macrocytosis and an elevated reticulocyte count (Figure 1-2). Normocytic, normochromic anemias with elevated reticulocyte counts can be divided into those with positive direct antiglobulin test results (Coombs' test) and those lacking evidence of red blood cell bound antibodies. Coombs'-negative hemolytic anemias are quite heterogeneous. The peripheral blood smear and the history often suggest possible causes for the anemia (Table 1-7). More detailed discussion of nonhemolytic normocytic anemia may be found in Chapter 3, and the hemolytic anemias are presented in Chapters 6 to 15.

The differential diagnosis of anemia is often tempered or modified by knowledge of other patient data. All algorithmic classification schemes should be tempered by the pragmatic knowledge of the physician considering the probable causes for anemia in an individual patient or patient group. For example, because 98% or more of the anemias in children under the age of 4 years are caused by iron deficiency, many pediatricians simply treat all anemic children in this group with iron supplementation and work up only those failing to respond to iron therapy. In many situations, clinical knowledge can suggest several possible causes of anemia. Thus, classification algorithms are suggested paths for physicians to follow in test utilization and should not be considered required routes.

Table 1-6 Normochromic, Normocytic Anemia Without High
Reticulocyte Response

Findings on Peripheral Blood Smear	Further Workup
Leukoerythroblastosis	Suspect myelophthistic process—bone marrow examination for space-occupying lesion (metastatic tumor, lymphoma, myelofibrosis)
Abnormal white blood cells	Suspect leukemia, lymphoma—bone marrow examination
Rouleaux	Suspect myeloma—serum and urine electrophoresis, radiographs to look for lytic lesions, bone marrow examination
No abnormal cells	Suspect anemia of chronic disease or sideroblastic anemia—bone marrow examination; rule out chronic disease processes

Table 1-7 Workup of Coombs'-Negative Anemia

Feature of Anemia	Possible Processes	Tests
Episodic anemia	Enzyme deficiency	G6PD, other enzymes
	Paroxysmal nocturnal hemoglobinuria	Sucrose hemolysis, Ham's test
Red blood cell fragmentation	Disseminated intravascular coagulation or thrombotic thrombocytopenic purpura	Coagulation tests, serum haptoglobin levels
Abnormal red blood cells		
Stippling	Lead poisoning	Lead levels
	Thalassemia	Hemoglobin electrophoresis
Abnormal shapes or increased target cells	Hemoglobinopathy or thalassemia	Hemoglobin electrophoresis
Spherocytes	Hereditary spherocytosis	Osmotic fragility test

Abbreviation: G6PD = glucose-6-phosphate dehydrogenase.

Figure 1-3 Classification of microcytic anemias.

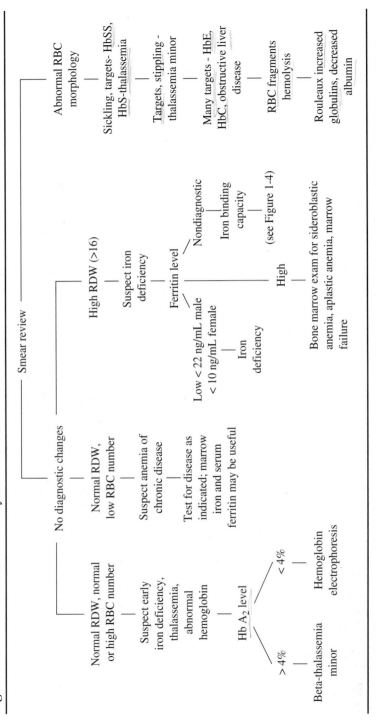

Figure 1-4 Iron deficiency vs anemia of chronic disease.

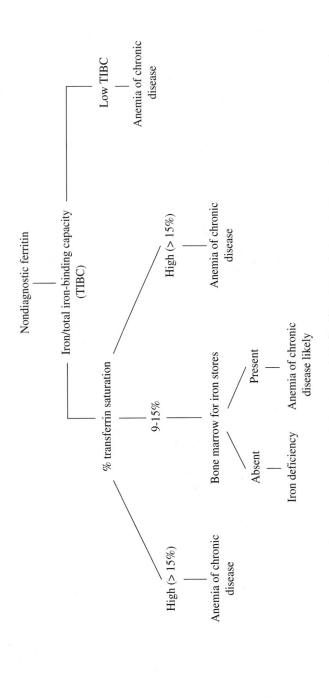

Other Laboratory Tests

1.1 The Reticulocyte Count

Purpose. To enumerate the number of reticulocytes, indicating bone marrow production of new red blood cells.

Principle. Residual RNA in immature red blood cells is precipitated and stained with a supravital dye.

Specimen. Venous or capillary blood.

Procedure. Blood is stained with brilliant cresyl blue or methylene blue. A blood smear is made, and the red blood cells containing stained reticular material are counted per 1,000 red blood cells and expressed as percent reticulocytes (absolute number per 100 red blood cells).

Interpretation. Reticulocytes are defined as immature red blood cells seen in the peripheral blood that contain at least two dots of stained reticulin material in their cytoplasm. More immature forms have multiple dots and small networks or skeins of bluish material. Intraobserver variation and uneven distribution of reticulocytes introduces a high analytic variation in reticulocyte counting, with interlaboratory coefficients of variation in the 20% range. Duplicate reticulocyte counts or 3-day average values may help to reduce the imprecision of the raw reticulocyte count.

Effective red blood cell production is a dynamic process and the number of reticulocytes should be compared with the number released in a patient without anemia who produces 1% of $5 \times 10^6/\text{mm}^3$ ($5 \times 10^{12}/\text{L}$) red blood cells daily for an absolute reticulocyte production of $50 \times 10^3/\text{mm}^3$ ($50 \times 10^9/\text{L}$). The corrected reticulocyte count takes into account normal red blood cell proliferation for the hematocrit and may be calculated with the following formula:

$$\text{Corrected Reticulocyte Count} = [\text{Percent Observed Reticulocytes} \times \text{Patient's Hematocrit Value}] \div 45$$

Another complicating factor in reticulocyte count correction is that an anemic patient may release reticulocytes prematurely into the circulation. Reticulocytes are usually present for 1 day in the blood before they extrude the residual RNA and become erythrocytes. However, if they are released early from the bone marrow, they may be present in the reticulocyte form in peripheral blood for 2 or 3 days. The situation is most likely to occur in those patients whose severe anemia causes a marked acceleration in erythropoiesis and release. Some authors have advocated correction of the reticulocyte count for "shift" reticulocytes, called the reticulocyte production index (RPI):

$$\text{RPI} = [(\text{Percent Reticulocyte x Patient's Hematocrit Value}) \div 45] \text{ x } [1 \div \text{Correction Factor}]$$

The correction factor calculation is shown in Table 1-8.

In cases of low erythropoietin (often seen in patients with renal or hepatic disease), application of an RPI correction may hide bone marrow response failure, since the shift does not take place fully or at all. In general, however, RPI values less than 2 indicate failure of bone marrow red blood cell production or a hypoproliferative anemia. RPIs of 3 or greater indicate marrow hyperproliferation or an appropriate response.

New automated tests for reticulocyte counts using flow cytometric analysis or Coulter automated hematology counters are becoming available. These provide intralaboratory consistency of results due to automation and counting of large numbers of cells.

1.2   Bone Marrow Examination

Purpose.   Bone marrow examination allows assessment of the cellularity, maturation, and composition of the hematopoietic elements in the bone marrow as well as allowing evaluation of iron stores. Some infections may also be cultured from the bone marrow when all other workup has been negative for infections.

Table 1-8 Correction Factor Calculation

Patient's Hematocrit Value, %	Correction Factor
40-45	1.0
35-39	1.5
25-34	2.0
15-24	2.5
<15	3.0

Principle. The cortical bone is penetrated and a sample of the bone marrow is aspirated. In most cases, a small biopsy specimen of the medullary bone and marrow is obtained. The most common sites for the procedure are the posterior iliac crest and the sternum.

Specimen. Bone marrow aspiration and biopsy samples.

Procedure. Bone marrow aspiration and biopsy are innocuous procedures in expert hands. Several sites in the skeleton have been used for bone marrow sampling. Since active hematopoiesis occurs in the long bones of the arms and legs in infants under the age of 8 months, aspiration from the anterior aspect of the tibial tuberosity is useful. For adults, the posterior iliac crest is the recommended site. The sternum is aspirated relatively easily, but its structure does not allow biopsy. The occasional dramatic fatal laceration of the heart or internal mammary arteries and the psychologic effect on the patient produced by insertion of the sternal needle render sternal aspiration a relatively poor choice for bone marrow sampling in all but the very elderly. In these patients, sternal bone marrow may be most representative of the patient's hematopoiesis and superior to that of the acellular iliac crest. Sternal aspiration may also be most appropriate for patients who have lesions in the sternum or ribs.

Processing and interpretation have significant technical variables and require experienced personnel. Bone marrow examination should be limited to situations where noninvasive procedures do not yield clear answers. Table 1-9 illustrates the most common indications for bone marrow examination.

Table 1-9   Indications for Bone Marrow Examination

Abnormalities in blood counts and/or peripheral blood smear
    Unexplained cytopenias
    Unexplained leukocytosis or abnormal white blood cells
    Teardrop cells or leukoerythroblastosis
    Rouleaux
    No or low reticulocyte response with anemia

Possible systemic disease evaluation
    Unexplained splenomegaly, hepatomegaly, lymphadenopathy
    Tumor staging: solid tumors, lymphomas
    Monitoring of chemotherapy effect
    Fever of unknown origin (with bone marrow cultures)
    Evaluation of trabecular bone in metabolic bone disease
      (use undecalcified bone)

Interpretation.   When both a Wright-stained aspirate preparation and a histologic core needle biopsy are available, optimal evaluation may be performed. The false-negative rate for metastatic carcinoma using aspiration alone is about 25%; for lymphomas it seems to be somewhat higher—30% to 40%—depending on the cell type. However, because of the small nature of the biopsy specimen, sampling error may still be a problem, causing false-negative results. Additional testing, such as iron stains to evaluate iron stores, immunohistochemical staining, flow cytometric analysis, and cytogenetic analysis, may also be performed on aspirated bone marrow specimens to provide additional information about the disease process.

Treatment

Anemia is a symptom rather than a disease, so treatment of anemia is usually aimed at correcting the abnormality that leads to anemia. This may involve identification of a source of blood loss, iron or vitamin supplementation, or discontinuing a drug that is predisposing a patient to hemolysis. The acquired anemias that are associated with hematopoietic diseases, such as myelodysplasia or aplastic anemia, and the inherited anemias may require the use of transfusions when symptoms arise due to the decreased oxygen delivery to the tissues. The benefit of transfusion therapy must be carefully balanced against the risks of disease transmission. Usually, transfusions are not required unless the hemoglobin concentration falls below 7 g/dL (70 g/L), unless significant cardiac or pulmonary disease is present where hypoxia would be exacerbated by even modest decreases in oxygen delivery. In addition, long-term transfusion therapy may lead to iron overload and subsequent organ failure.

In some patients, such as those who have hereditary hemochromatosis, transfusions can exacerbate iron overload, as these patients are unable to decrease gut mucosal iron absorption when iron loading occurs via transfusion. Patients with homozygous hereditary hemochromatosis are found at a frequency of 0.1% to 0.2%; many patients have clinically silent disease. Patients with homozygous hemochromatosis may be identified by screening tests for transferrin saturation, which is considered suspicious if greater than 60% saturation is found in a man and greater than 50% in a woman. When follow-up testing of serum ferritin finds levels above normal for age and sex in addition to elevated transferrin saturation, it strongly suggests that a patient has clinically silent hemochromatosis, and iron overload due to transfusion therapy may present significant problems.

References

Bains BJ. *Blood Cells: A Practical Guide.* Philadelphia, Pa: JB Lippincott Co; 1989.

Bessman JD, Gilmer PR, Gardener FH. Improved classification of anemia by MCV and RDW. *Am J Clin Pathol.* 1983;80:322-326.

Edwards CQ, Kushner JP. Screening for hemochromatosis. *N Engl J Med.* 1993; 328:1616-1620.

Erslev AJ. Clinical manifestations and classification of erythrocyte disorders. In: Williams WJ, Beutler E, Erslev AJ, et al, eds. *Hematology.* 4th ed. New York, NY: McGraw International Book Co; 1990:423-429.

Erslev AJ. Production of erythrocytes. In: Williams WJ, Beutler E, Erslev AJ, et al, eds. *Hematology.* 4th ed. New York, NY: McGraw International Book Co; 1990:389-398.

Heckner F, Lehmann HP, Kao YS. *Practical Microscopic Hematology.* Baltimore, Md: Urban and Schwarzenberg; 1988.

Hyun BH, Gulati GL, Ashton JK. *Color Atlas of Clinical Hematology.* New York, NY: Igaku-Shoin Medical Publishers Inc; 1986.

Wintrobe MM, Lee GR, Boggs DR, et al, eds. The approach to the patient with anemia. In: *Clinical Hematology.* 9th ed. Philadelphia, Pa: Lea & Febiger; 1993:715-744.

2

Hypochromic Microcytic Anemias

Decreased rates of hemoglobin synthesis give rise to a hypochromic microcytic anemia. Such a synthetic defect may arise due to insufficient amounts of iron or abnormal iron metabolism, as a result of heme synthesis inhibition due to acquired or hereditary sideroblastic disorders, or due to hereditary abnormalities in globin synthesis (such as the thalassemias or the unstable hemoglobins). The most common causes of hypochromic anemia are listed in Table 2-1.

Pathophysiology

Hypochromic anemias are characterized by normal proliferation and DNA synthesis, but decreased hemoglobin production. The red blood cell precursors continue to divide, but the lack of hemoglobin leads to formation of hypochromic cells that are smaller than a normal red blood cell. The principal causes of hypochromic anemias include defective synthesis of heme secondary to abnormal iron metabolism or metabolic abnormalities (sideroblastic anemias), and disorders of globin synthesis in the form of the thalassemic disorders.

Table 2-1   Causes of Hypochromic Anemia

Disorders of iron metabolism
    Iron deficiency
    Chronic infections
    Neoplasia
Disorders of heme synthesis
    Sideroblastic anemias
        Hereditary (X-linked or autosomal)
        Acquired idiopathic (myelodysplasia)
        Acquired toxic (lead, drugs, alcohol)
Disorders of globin synthesis
    Thalassemic syndromes
        Alpha-thalassemia
        Beta-thalassemia

The primary cause of defective heme synthesis is iron deficiency. Iron deficiency is the most common cause of anemia and ranks among the most common of all diseases in humans. In infants and children, a negative iron balance may occur because the dietary intake of iron is inadequate to meet the requirements for growth. In adults, iron deficiency is usually the result of pregnancy or blood loss. Normal daily losses of iron are very small, so that decreased dietary intake plays, at most, a contributory role in the etiology of the disease. Physicians must identify the underlying cause of iron deficiency to treat the anemia. It should be kept in mind that the first sign of a malignant lesion of the gastrointestinal or genitourinary tract is often occult blood loss and resultant hypochromic, microcytic anemia (Image 2-1).

Iron metabolism may also be deranged in many people who have chronic inflammatory diseases or malignancies that are not causing overt blood loss. This derangement in iron metabolism is characterized by defective iron cycling between macrophages and developing red blood cells, so that iron becomes trapped within the macrophage and is unavailable for heme synthesis. This, so-called "anemia of chronic disease," is discussed further in Chapter 3.

Another group of disorders, the sideroblastic anemias, are characterized by abnormal iron metabolism within the red blood cell itself. In these disorders, iron accumulates in the developing red blood cell mitochondria and is unavailable for heme synthesis. The iron swells and distorts the mitochondria. Since the mitochondria in a developing normoblast are found in a perinuclear distribution, iron stains in these disorders show a characteristic pattern of iron around the nucleus forming a ringed sideroblast (Image 2-2). Sideroblastic anemias may be hereditary (either X-linked or autosomal), idiopathic (usually as a part of a myelodysplastic disorder), or secondary to a toxic insult (drugs, lead, or alcohol). The hereditary sideroblastic anemias are extremely rare in comparison to the acquired forms.

Hereditary disorders of globin synthesis, or the thalassemic syndromes, are also very common in Asian, Mediterranean, and black populations. They may rival iron deficiency as a cause of microcytic, hypochromic anemia in these groups. The thalassemias are discussed in further detail in Chapter 10.

Clinical Findings

The clinical findings of hypochromic anemias depend on the severity of the anemia and its underlying cause. Severe anemia is associated with pallor, weakness, palpitations, and even dyspnea. These symptoms may be more prominent in iron deficiency anemia, where the deficiency state contributes to the symptoms, than they are in mild thalassemia with the same degree of anemia. Mild to moderate chronic anemia is well tolerated by most patients, particularly those in the younger age groups.

Approach to Diagnosis

Following a clinical history and physical examination, the evaluation of hypochromic anemias may be undertaken as follows:

1. Examination of red blood cell morphology, indices, and size distribution.
2. Estimation of serum iron levels and total iron-binding capacity or ferritin levels. These measurements reflect iron stores and help to distinguish iron deficiency from other causes of microcytic, hypochromic anemia.
3. Measurement of free erythrocyte protoporphyrin, which is of particular value as a screening test for distinguishing iron deficiency from thalassemia minor.

4. Examination of aspirated bone marrow for stainable iron, the most direct assessment of iron stores. Associated dysplasia or the presence of ringed sideroblasts may reflect a sideroblastic anemia.
5. Hemoglobin electrophoresis, particularly to determine levels of hemoglobin A_2, which are increased in most patients with beta-thalassemia.
6. Determination of globin chain synthetic ratios, which is often the only means of making a positive diagnosis of mild forms of alpha-thalassemia.
7. Cytogenetic analysis to document a myelodysplastic syndrome, which shows cytogenetic abnormalities in up to 80% of cases. Cytogenetic abnormalities associated with myelodysplasia include complex chromosomal defects, monosomy 7, deletion of 5q, and trisomy 8.
8. Documentation of the hematologic response to iron supplementation therapy, which confirms the diagnosis of iron deficiency.

Hematologic Findings

Hypochromia, microcytosis, and anisocytosis are usually present in well-developed iron deficiency anemia. However, in early or mild iron deficiency no morphologic abnormalities of the red blood cells may be present. Hypochromia and microcytosis are found uniformly in the thalassemic syndromes, and the reductions in mean corpuscular volume (MCV) and mean corpuscular hemoglobin concentration (MCHC) are generally greater than those observed in iron deficiency anemia of the same degree. Microcytosis with significant elevations of the red blood cell count to greater than $6 \times 10^6/mm^3$ ($6 \times 10^{12}/L$) are common in thalassemia minor. Basophilic stippling of red blood cells is commonly seen in thalassemia, but is unusual in iron deficiency anemia. Hypochromia is often present in patients with sideroblastic anemia, but it is by no means a universal finding. It also occurs in patients with chronic inflammatory or neoplastic disorders and the associated "anemia of chronic disease." Changes in the size distribution of the red blood cells are determined best with automated cell-counting equipment. Characteristically, the variability of red blood cell size is increased in iron deficiency, but is much less so in thalassemia. The size distribution in sideroblastic anemias is variable, but a characteristic dimorphic population of normocytic or microcytic cells and macrocytes is seen in the acquired types.

Blood Cell Measurements. The MCV is decreased in severe iron deficiency anemia and thalassemias. The MCV may be increased in many of the sideroblastic anemias, although microcytosis is more common in the hereditary types. The reticulocyte count may be modestly decreased, normal, or modestly increased. Indices are often normal in patients with hemoglobin levels greater than 10 g/dL (100 g/L). The red blood cell number is often not decreased or may be significantly increased in patients with thalassemia, and is not proportional to the low hemoglobin level or degree of microcytosis. In contrast, iron deficiency anemia usually shows concordant decreases in red blood cell number, hemoglobin levels, and MCV.

Peripheral Blood Smear Morphology. Hypochromia and microcytosis are present in severe iron deficiency anemia, but may be lacking in less severe cases of iron depletion (Image 2-1). When hypochromia and microcytosis are present, differentiating iron deficiency anemia from a thalassemic syndrome may become necessary. Important features in distinguishing these two entities are noted in Table 2-2. Sideroblastic anemias usually have notable anisocytosis and poikilocytosis in addition to hypochromia. Occasionally, dysplastic features may be noted in the white blood cells in idiopathic cases.

Bone Marrow Examination. Bone marrow examination is usually not required for the diagnosis of iron deficiency anemia or thalassemia, but may be important in documenting a sideroblastic anemia. Erythroid hyperplasia is often present in all of the microcytic anemias, but it is not as prominent as it is in the hemolytic anemias. The only specific findings in this group are decreased or absent stainable storage iron in iron deficiency anemia, increased reticuloendothelial iron with decreased sideroblastic iron in anemias of chronic disease, and the presence of ring sideroblasts in sideroblastic anemias. Iron stores are often increased in thalassemias.

Table 2-2   Blood Smear Findings in Hypochromic Anemia

Cause of Hypochromic Anemia	Anisopoikilocytosis	Basophilic Stippling
Iron deficiency	Yes	No
Thalassemia minor	No	Yes
Sideroblastic anemias		
Hereditary	Yes	Yes
Acquired	Variable	Yes
Chronic disease	No	No

Other Laboratory Tests

2.1   Serum Iron Quantitation and Total Iron-Binding Capacity

Purpose.   Serum iron and total iron-binding capacity (TIBC) determinations are particularly useful in distinguishing iron deficiency anemia from other microcytic hypochromic anemias. In mild iron deficiency anemia, decreased serum iron levels may precede changes in red blood cell morphology or in red blood cell indices.

Principle.   All iron transported in the plasma is bound in the ferric form to the specific iron-binding protein, transferrin. Serum iron measures the transferrin-bound iron. TIBC, the concentration iron necessary to saturate the iron-binding sites of transferrin, is a measure of transferrin concentration. Saturation of transferrin is calculated by the following formula:

$$\% \text{ Transferrin Saturation} = [\text{Serum Iron (mol/L)} \div \text{TIBC (}\mu\text{mol/L)}] \times 100$$

Normal mean transferrin saturation is approximately 30%. Unsaturated iron-binding capacity (UIBC) is the difference between TIBC and serum iron.

Specimen.   A specimen of blood should be drawn in the morning due to diurnal variations in serum iron levels. Serum is used for the determination.

Procedure.   Serum iron is freed from transferrin by acidification of the serum and is reduced to the ferrous form. After the protein has been precipitated out, the iron in the filtrate is detected spectrophotometrically after reaction with a chromogen, such as bathophenanthroline sulfonate. TIBC is measured by adding iron to serum followed by removal of excess, unbound iron by magnesium carbonate absorption. The bound iron is then released from transferrin and reduced, and its concentration is measured as in the serum iron test. The TIBC also can be determined by measuring transferrin with immunodiffusion.

Interpretation.   The representative normal range of values for serum iron is 60 to 180 μg/dL (12.7-35.9 μmol/L); for TIBC, the range is 250 to 410 μg/dL (45.2-77.7 μmol/L); and for percent saturation, the range is 20% to 50%. The serum iron level and percent saturation is low in both iron deficiency anemia and the anemia of chronic disease. Although the value for percent saturation is often reduced to levels below 16% in iron deficiency anemia and is frequently more than 16% in anemia of chronic disease, values overlap in the two conditions. The TIBC is uniformly increased in severe uncomplicated iron deficiency anemias and is decreased or normal in the microcytic anemia of chronic disease. In mild iron deficiency anemia, both the serum iron and TIBC may be normal. Serum iron concentration is increased in the sideroblastic anemias and in some cases of thalassemia (Table 2-3).

Notes and Precautions.   Serum iron concentrations show wide diurnal variations, with highest levels in the morning. Thus, specimens should be collected in the morning and oral iron therapy should be withdrawn 24 hours before the blood sample is drawn. Iron dextran administration causes plasma iron levels to be elevated for several weeks. A normal plasma iron level and iron-binding capacity do not rule out the diagnosis of iron deficiency when the hemoglobin level of the blood is above 9 g/dL (90 g/L) (women) and 11 g/dL (110 g/L) (men).

Table 2-3 Serum Iron, Iron-Binding Capacity, and Storage Iron in Hypochromic Anemia

Cause of Hypochromic Anemia	Serum Iron	TIBC	Percent Saturation	Bone Marrow Storage Iron
Iron deficiency	Decreased[*]	Increased[*]	Decreased[*]	Decreased
Thalassemias	Increased or normal	Decreased or normal	Increased or normal	Increased or normal
Sideroblastic anemias	Increased	Decreased or normal	Increased	Increased
Chronic disease	Decreased	Decreased	Decreased	Increased

Abbreviation: TIBC = total iron-binding capacity.
[*]Serum iron and TIBC are occasionally normal in iron deficiency.

2.2 Stainable Bone Marrow Iron

Purpose. The most direct means for assessing body iron stores is by histochemical examination of aspirated bone marrow for storage iron.

Principle. Iron is stored in reticuloendothelial cells, and iron granules are formed in developing normoblasts. Normoblasts that contain one or more particles of stainable iron are known as sideroblasts. Iron is stored as ferritin (iron is complexed to the apoferritin protein) and hemosiderin (iron-protein complexes with a high iron content and denatured ferritin aggregates). Hemosiderin is the stainable form of storage iron that appears blue when treated with an acid potassium ferrocyanide solution used in the Prussian blue reaction.

Specimen. Either sectioned bone marrow aspirate fragments (clot section) or particle smears are used for the assessment of reticuloendothelial iron, but bone marrow aspirate films must be used to detect sideroblasts.

Procedure. The bone marrow aspirate is stained with the Prussian blue reaction. Heating the staining mixture to 56°C increases its sensitivity. The search for sideroblasts is aided by a counterstain, such as basic fuchsin.

Interpretation. Normally, hemosiderin granules are seen in reticuloendothelial cells in every third or fourth oil immersion field. With reduced iron stores, either no or only a few hemosiderin granules are seen in the entire preparation. With increased iron stores, hemosiderin granules are seen in every oil immersion field, often deposited in clumps.

    The appraisal of reticuloendothelial iron is extremely helpful in the differential diagnosis of anemia (Table 2-3). Since iron from breakdown of red blood cell heme cannot be excreted, it is diverted to the storage compartment. Thus, increased iron is generally present in the marrow of anemic patients who are not iron-deficient. An exception may exist in myeloproliferative disorders in which bone marrow iron stores may be absent without other evidence of iron deficiency, perhaps resulting from impaired storage function. When storage iron is present in the bone marrow, anemia cannot be a result of iron deficiency, unless the patient has been treated with parenterally administered iron.

    Normally, 20% to 40% of red blood cell precursors are sideroblasts. Although a sideroblast count is not ordinarily necessary for the diagnosis of iron deficiency anemia, it may be useful when an inadequate number of bone marrow particles were obtained and in patients who have received parenterally administered iron. Loss of sideroblasts from the bone marrow is seen in iron deficiency anemia, after acute blood loss when reticuloendothelial stores have not yet been depleted, and in anemia of chronic disease. Sideroblastic anemia is characterized by the presence of ring sideroblasts. These are normoblasts that contain iron granules surrounding at least three fourths of the nuclear circumference (Image 2-2).

Notes and Precautions. Some practice is required to distinguish stainable reticuloendothelial iron from artifacts. When a patient has received iron by the parenteral route, either as iron dextran or in the form of blood transfusions, histochemically stainable iron stores may be seen in the bone marrow in the presence of iron deficiency anemia. A well-prepared bone marrow aspirate film is essential for the detection of iron granules in normoblasts, and appropriate positive control slides should also be performed simultaneously.

2.3 Serum Ferritin Quantitation

Purpose. Small amounts of ferritin or the antigenically equivalent apoferritin normally circulate in the plasma. Estimating serum ferritin levels provides a semiquantitative, less invasive test for iron store determination than the histochemical examination of aspirated bone marrow.

Principle. Ferritin is a storage complex of the protein apoferritin and iron. The largest quantities of ferritin are found in the liver and reticuloendothelial cells. Ordinarily, serum ferritin concentration reflects the amount of stored iron.

Specimen. Serum is obtained.

Procedure. Reliable estimation of serum ferritin levels has been achieved with a sensitive radioimmune method using a sandwich technique. Ferritin is removed from the serum by solid phase antiferritin antibodies, and radioactively labeled antiferritin antibodies are then permitted to bind to the removed ferritin.

Interpretation. The normal concentration of serum ferritin varies from 10 to 500 ng/mL (10-500 µg/L). In iron deficiency anemia, serum ferritin level is diminished and appears to be a relatively sensitive and reliable indicator of the presence of iron deficiency. Serum ferritin levels may be low in iron deficiency that is not associated with overt anemia. Elevated ferritin levels are common in iron overload states, including sideroblastic anemia and hemochromatosis. Serum ferritin levels are also elevated in patients with inflammatory diseases and, for poorly understood reasons, in patients with Gaucher's disease.

Notes and Precautions. When iron deficiency and inflammatory disease coexist, serum ferritin levels may be in the normal range.

2.4   Free Erythrocyte Protoporphyrin

Purpose. Free erythrocyte protoporphyrin (FEP) levels are elevated in anemias associated with failure of iron incorporation into heme.

Principle. When insufficient iron is available for developing erythroblasts, excess protoporphyrin that was destined to be converted to heme accumulates as FEP. This substance is elevated both in iron deficiency and in conditions associated with an internal block in iron utilization, such as anemia of chronic disease, lead poisoning, and sideroblastic anemias.

Specimen. Whole anticoagulated blood is collected. There is also a spot test for blood specimens collected on filter paper.

Procedure. FEP is extracted from red blood cells with ethyl acetate/acetic acid and is quantitated fluorometrically.

Interpretation. FEP is normally less than 100 µg/dL (1.7 µmol/L) packed red blood cells. Elevated levels are seen in iron deficiency, in chronic disease states associated with decreased transferrin saturation, and in acquired idiopathic sideroblastic anemia. Marked elevation of FEP is seen in sideroblastic anemia secondary to lead intoxication with FEP values of about 1,000 µg/dL (17 µmol/L) packed red blood cells. In microcytic anemias associated with abnormal globin synthesis rather than abnormal heme synthesis, such as thalassemia minor, FEP levels are normal. Because iron deficiency anemia and thalassemia minor are the first and second most common causes, respectively, of hypochromic, microcytic anemia, measurement of FEP may be particularly useful as a screening test to distinguish these two disorders.

Test Selection

Examination of the peripheral blood smear and red blood cell indices is essential for determining the etiology of a microcytic anemia. The red blood cell number, hemoglobin content, MCV, and RDW provide important clues as to the cause of anemia. If iron deficiency is suspected on the basis of a high RDW, iron studies may be ordered. If a thalassemia is suspected on the basis of a high red blood cell count for the degree of microcytosis and a normal RDW or the presence of target cells, then testing can be aimed at determination of the hemoglobin A_2 level and possible hemoglobin electrophoresis. If a dimorphic population of red blood cells or dysplastic changes are seen in the other blood cells, then a bone marrow examination will probably be required.

Course and Treatment

Ultimately, the diagnosis of iron deficiency depends on demonstration of an adequate response to iron therapy. Treatment usually consists of the oral administration of a ferrous iron salt, such as ferrous sulfate, in a dosage providing 0.06 to 0.12 g of iron three times a day. Under some circumstances, the parenteral administration of iron may be preferred. Reticulocytosis and a significant rise in blood hemoglobin concentration may occur as early as the third or fourth day after treatment, particularly in children, but is more usually seen after 7 or 8 days. The hemoglobin concentration in the blood may not rise significantly until 10 days of treatment. Thereafter, complete restoration of the hemoglobin level to normal should be rapid (essentially complete by the sixth week after institution of therapy) regardless of the initial severity of the anemia. Infection, inflammatory disease, or neoplastic disease may prevent an adequate response, and continued bleeding may blunt the apparent therapeutic effect. The most common cause of failure of a hypochromic, microcytic anemia to respond to iron therapy is an incorrect diagnosis. It is important to identify the cause of the iron deficiency (almost always blood loss or pregnancy in adults) and to correct it, if possible. It should be kept in mind that iron deficiency can be an early warning of gastrointestinal or genitourinary tract cancer.

The sideroblastic anemias, other than the idiopathic forms, may respond to treatment with pyridoxine. Many of the drugs that cause toxic sideroblastic anemias are pyridoxine antagonists. If a toxic etiology is suspected, discontinuing the drug or alcohol will often lead to rapid improvement in the anemia. Some of the hereditary sideroblastic anemias are pyridoxine-resistant, indicating heterogeneous metabolic abnormalities in these patients. In both the acquired idiopathic form of the disease and hereditary forms, repeated transfusions may be required to treat severe anemia. Iron overload, due to long-standing transfusion therapy, may become a problem and require chelation therapy. The acquired idiopathic form of the disease is a myelodysplastic syndrome, and small numbers of the patients will develop progressive bone marrow failure, cytopenias, or overt acute myelogenous leukemia. However, most patients will have stable anemia and associated symptoms over many years.

References

Bessman JD, Gilmer PR, Gardener FH. Improved classification of anemias by MCV and RDW. *Am J Clin Pathol.* 1983;80:322-329.

Beutler E. Hereditary and secondary acquired sideroblastic anemias. In: Williams WJ, Beutler E, Erslev A, et al, eds. *Hematology.* 4th ed. New York, NY: McGraw-Hill International Book Co; 1990:554-557.

Fairbanks VF, Beutler E. Iron in medicine and nutrition. In: Shils ME, Young VR, eds. *Modern Nutrition in Health and Disease.* Philadelphia, Pa: Lea & Febiger; 1988:193-226.

Fairbanks VF, Beutler E. Iron deficiency. In: Williams WJ, Beutler E, Erslev A, et al, eds. *Hematology.* 4th ed. New York, NY: McGraw-Hill International Book Co; 1990:482-505.

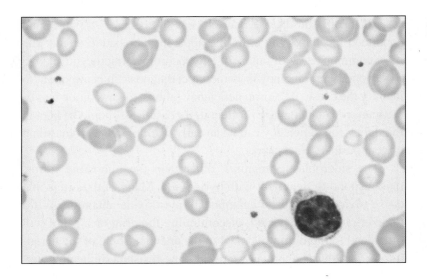

Image 2-1 Iron deficiency anemia. The red blood cells are hypochromic and microcytic.

Image 2-2 Ringed sideroblast. Iron stains show a bone marrow normoblast with coarse iron granules extending completely around the nucleus.

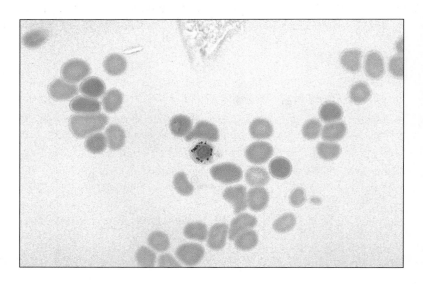

3

Anemia of Chronic Disease and Normochromic, Normocytic Nonhemolytic Anemias

Anemia occurring in patients with chronic diseases is often caused by multiple simultaneously acting mechanisms, including nutritional deficiencies, blood loss, and anemia of chronic disease (ACD). ACD is defined by a constellation of clinical, morphologic, and laboratory features (Table 3-1) and is second only to iron deficiency anemia in incidence. In a tertiary care setting, chronic disease may be the most frequently encountered cause of anemia. Affected patients usually develop normocytic, normochromic anemia that is mild and nonprogressive 1 to 2 months after the onset of chronic disease. This anemia is associated with multiple iron-related abnormalities, including decreased serum iron level, decreased transferrin level, decreased transferrin saturation, and normal to increased storage iron (ferritin). The bone marrow examination reveals that erythroid precursors are generally present in normal numbers, but the erythroid iron is decreased while the storage iron is increased.

A variety of inflammatory, infectious, and neoplastic disorders (Table 3-2) are associated with ACD. Because the etiologies of anemias are considerably more complex in patients with renal, endocrine, and hepatic disorders and AIDS, these will be discussed separately at the end of the chapter.

Table 3-1   Characteristics of Anemia of Chronic Disease

Clinical
  Development of anemia 1-2 months after onset of chronic disease
Blood
  Usually normocytic, normochromic anemia with normal mean corpuscular
    volume, mean corpuscular hemoglobin concentration, and red cell
    distribution width
  Inappropriately low reticulocyte count
Iron studies
  Decreased serum/plasma iron
  Decreased transferrin (total iron-binding capacity)
  Decreased transferrin saturation
  Normal to increased ferritin
Bone marrow
  Normal numbers of erythroid precursors
  Decreased sideroblasts (decreased iron-containing erythroid cells)
  Increased storage iron

Pathophysiology

Three separate pathophysiologic defects together produce ACD: failure of erythropoiesis, lack of iron for hemoglobin synthesis, and decreased red blood cell (RBC) survival. The major defect is thought to be a failure of sufficient erythropoiesis to compensate for the decreased RBC survival, although erythroid precursors are present in the bone marrow. The decreased availability of iron for hemoglobin synthesis further aggravates this inadequate erythropoiesis. Erythroid precursors normally acquire from transferrin the iron necessary for hemoglobin synthesis. The decrease in serum iron level, serum transferrin level, and stainable iron in erythroid precursors indicates that insufficient iron is available for hemoglobin synthesis. The mildly decreased RBC survival is caused by extracorpuscular abnormalities rather than any intrinsic RBC defect; in patients with ACD, the marrow is unable to compensate for this survival defect.

Current evidence suggests that the three pathophysiologic defects responsible for the development of ACD can be attributed largely to sustained secretion of one or more cytokines, notably interleukin-1 and tumor necrosis factor. In response to a chronic inflammatory process, levels of secretion of tumor necrosis factor are high. This factor induces sustained secretion of interleukin-1 by

Table 3-2   Diseases Commonly Associated With Anemia of Chronic Disease

Chronic inflammatory disorders
Rheumatoid arthritis
Systemic lupus erythematosus
Sarcoidosis
Trauma
Chronic infections
Tuberculosis
Pyelonephritis
Osteomyelitis
Chronic fungal infections
Subacute bacterial endocarditis
Neoplasms
Malignant lymphoma
Carcinoma

a variety of cells, including monocytes and macrophages. Both tumor necrosis factor and interleukin-1 have overlapping broad multiorgan and multisystem effects that result in neutrophilia, decreased plasma iron, shunting of iron to macrophages via lactoferrin, decreased transferrin, and lymphocyte activation (Table 3-3). Once iron has bound to lactoferrin, it is delivered exclusively to macrophages and is therefore not available for erythropoiesis.

Clinical Findings

Because ACD is generally mild, the patient's symptoms are related largely to the underlying disease. There are no physical examination findings unique to ACD.

Approach to Diagnosis

In a patient with anemia and a chronic illness, the contribution of ACD to this anemia can vary from major to insignificant. Because multiple underlying causes of anemia in such a patient population are the rule rather than the exception, the patient's evaluation should also establish the diagnosis of other types of anemia. For

Table 3-3   Mechanisms by Which Interleukin-1 May Cause
Anemia of Chronic Disease

Indirect suppression of erythropoiesis

    Interleukin-1 regulates lymphoid cells and monocytes, which in turn
    regulate hematopoiesis

Lactoferrin release from secondary granules of neutrophils

    Lactoferrin competes with transferrin for iron

    Lactoferrin delivers iron exclusively to macrophages, rendering it
    unavailable for erythropoiesis

Indirect responsibility for the mild red blood cell survival defect

    Fever may cause shortened red blood cell survival

    Activated macrophages more readily ingest erythrocytes

---

example, a patient with a neoplasm may suffer from iron deficiency anemia secondary to chronic blood loss, myelophthistic anemia secondary to bone marrow replacement by tumor, hypoplastic anemia secondary to bone marrow suppression by chemotherapeutic agents, or even microangiopathic hemolytic anemia secondary to drug treatment or mucin production by the tumor. Table 3-4 lists these and other possible factors that contribute to the anemias that occur in patients with neoplasms. During the course of the clinical and hematologic evaluation of the patient, it is often readily apparent that one or more of these additional causes of anemia is present. In clinical practice, the distinction between ACD and iron deficiency anemia is the most frequent diagnostic dilemma.

The laboratory evaluation of patients for ACD usually includes the following:

1. Measurement of standard hematologic parameters with reticulocyte count

2. Evaluation of peripheral blood smear for "clues" suggesting other types of anemia

3. Iron studies, including assays of serum iron, transferrin, and iron stores

4. Appropriate laboratory testing to establish or exclude diagnoses of other types of anemia

Table 3-4 Causes of Anemia in Patients With Nonhematologic Malignancies

Anemia of chronic disease
Blood loss
Bone marrow replacement by tumor
Bone marrow suppression by chemotherapy
Chemotherapy-related myelodysplasia
Hypersplenism
Microangiopathic hemolytic anemia secondary to drug treatment
  (eg, mitomycin C)
Microangiopathic hemolytic anemia secondary to intravascular mucin
  released from certain widespread adenocarcinomas
Immune-mediated hemolysis (autoantibody produced by certain
  B-cell neoplasms)

5. Bone marrow aspiration, with iron stains, and biopsy in selected cases that are not clear-cut after other studies

The laboratory approach to the evaluation of these patients must always be correlated with the patient's clinical findings. The approach should be tailored to each case using clues from the patient's history and physical examination to direct the sequence of tests utilized.

Hematologic Findings

There are no pathognomonic findings in the peripheral blood in patients with ACD. These patients generally have a mild to moderate anemia that is not associated with an increase in the reticulocyte count.

Blood Cell Measurements. In ACD, the hemoglobin level ranges from 7.0 to 11.0 g/dL (70-110 g/L). These cells vary little in size, as indicated by their normal or near-normal red cell distribution width (RDW). The mean corpuscular volume (MCV), mean corpuscular hemoglobin (MCH), and mean corpuscular hemoglobin concentration (MCHC) are generally normal, although the MCV and MCHC may be mildly decreased. Although the reticulocyte count is usually within the normal range, it is decreased when corrected for the degree of anemia. White blood cell and platelet counts are usually normal.

Peripheral Blood Smear Morphology. Erythrocytes are generally normocytic and normochromic without significant anisopoikilocytosis or polychromasia. These cells occasionally are mildly hypochromic, and there are usually no abnormalities of white blood cells or platelets.

Bone Marrow Examination. Erythroid elements in the bone marrow are generally morphologically normal and present in normal numbers. Sideroblasts are decreased, while the storage iron is increased substantially. Myeloid and megakaryocytic elements are usually unremarkable. Depending on the underlying chronic disease, a variety of other bone marrow abnormalities may be detected.

Other Laboratory Tests

While no single laboratory test is specific for ACD, a well-established laboratory profile includes serum iron, iron transport protein, and storage iron measurements that can aid in this diagnosis.

3.1   Serum Iron Quantitation

Purpose.   The determination of serum iron, in conjunction with other iron studies described below, is important in distinguishing ACD from other types that may develop in these patients.

Principle, Specimen, Procedure, Notes, and Precautions. See Test 2.1.

Interpretation.   A prompt decline in serum iron level is associated with infection and other types of tissue injury. This decrease precedes the development of anemia, which occurs only if the infection or injury is sustained. Low serum iron level is seen also in iron deficiency anemia.

3.2 Transferrin Measurement (Total Iron-Binding Capacity)

Purpose, Principle, Specimen, Procedure, Notes, and Precautions. See Test 2.1.

Interpretation. Transferrin is characteristically decreased in patients with ACD in contrast to the substantial elevation of this protein level that occurs in patients with iron deficiency anemia. This test, however, is neither specific nor sensitive enough to consistently distinguish between these two types of anemia.

3.3 Transferrin Saturation

Purpose. The percent saturation of transferrin reflects the availability of iron for erythropoiesis and can be calculated by dividing the serum iron level by the transferrin level.

Interpretation. The percent saturation of transferrin is generally decreased in patients with ACD, in whom a range of 10% to 25% saturation is usually found. Although in iron deficiency anemia the percent saturation of transferrin is usually less than 15%, there is some overlap between the percent saturation ranges found in these two disorders.

3.4 Ferritin Quantitation

Purpose. The serum ferritin level is a measure of the patient's total body iron stores.

Principle, Specimen, and Procedure. See Test 2.3.

Interpretation. The serum ferritin level is characteristically normal to increased in patients with ACD, reflecting their abundant storage iron. The serum ferritin level in patients with iron deficiency anemia is generally markedly decreased.

Notes and Precautions. Because ferritin is an acute-phase reactant, it may be elevated spuriously in patients with acute inflammatory processes. Despite this problem, serum ferritin levels are still of value in patients with possible ACD because they can help distinguish these patients from those with iron deficiency anemia. If results of serum ferritin assays are correlated with erythrocyte sedimentation rate, the distinction between ACD and iron deficiency anemia is enhanced.

Ancillary Tests

The free erythrocyte protoporphyrin level is elevated in ACD because the iron available for hemoglobin synthesis is decreased. Testing for this level, however, is not generally done in the initial evaluation of patients for this disorder.

Course and Treatment

Treatment of the underlying disease is of paramount importance in the care of patients with ACD. Eradication of the underlying disorder results in improvement of the anemia. ACD is often mild and usually does not require specific treatment. Therapies that have been tried and have been generally unsuccessful in these patients include iron and androgen treatment. Transfusion results in temporary improvement but is not recommended unless the patient has symptoms of anemia. Recent evidence suggests that some of these patients will respond to recombinant human erythropoietin.

Anemia With Chronic Renal Disease. The anemia that often occurs in patients with chronic renal disease shares some similarities to ACD. The anemia in these patients is generally normocytic and normochromic, and its severity roughly parallels the severity of the underlying renal disease. As in ACD, multiple factors contribute to the development of anemia in patients with renal disease. Some important pathophysiologic differences exist between these two disorders, however. The primary pathophysiologic mechanism for anemia in these patients is decreased erythropoiesis secondary to either decreased or nonfunctional erythropoietin. In these patients, the bone marrow usually shows erythroid hypoplasia. Azotemia also exacerbates the anemia, because it directly suppresses the bone marrow and because it causes decreased RBC survival. Other manifestations of the anemia associated with chronic renal disease include burr cells in the blood, decreased serum iron level, and decreased transferrin level. Sustained secretion of interleukin-l may be responsible for these iron and transferrin abnormalities. Several additional factors can contribute to a patient's anemia. These patients may have chronic blood loss because of both platelet and vessel defects secondary to the underlying renal disease. Patients undergoing chronic hemodialysis can readily become folate deficient. Finally, patients with renal disease are prone to fluid overload, which can further decrease the hematocrit value.

The treatment of the underlying renal disease is of primary importance in these patients. In addition, the development of recombinant human erythropoietin has resulted in amelioration of the anemia in many patients with chronic renal failure.

Anemia With Chronic Endocrine Disease. Anemia is common in patients with chronic endocrine diseases such as diabetes mellitus and hypothyroidism. The anemia in diabetic patients is characteristically multifactorial. In addition to ACD, diabetic patients may develop enteropathy that leads to poor absorption of iron, vitamin B_{12}, and folate. Likewise, diabetic patients may suffer from chronic blood loss and chronic renal insufficiency. The relative contribution of all of these abnormalities to an anemia varies from patient to patient and varies over time in the same patient.

Likewise, patients with chronic hypothyroidism are also frequently anemic. The various possible factors contributing to an anemia in these hypothyroid patients include decreased oxygen requirements, pernicious anemia, iron deficiency secondary to menorrhagia, and impaired iron absorption. Treatment of the underlying endocrine disorder is of primary importance in the care of these patients. The anemia generally does not require treatment.

Anemia Associated With Liver Diseases. The most common liver disease linked to anemia is alcoholism, and anemia is a very common finding in patients with either acute or chronic alcoholism. Although this anemia is generally mild to moderate, it can periodically become more severe corresponding to the patient's alcohol ingestion and the severity of the patient's liver disease. Although ACD may occur in patients with alcoholism, the anemia in these patients frequently has multiple causes, including direct toxic effects of alcohol, various nutritional deficiencies, RBC survival defects, abnormal iron metabolism, or all of these. The predominant mechanism causing anemia may vary with time. The pathogenesis and morphologic features of the various causes of anemia in patients with alcoholism are shown in Table 3-5.

Alcohol, especially when ingested in large amounts, has a direct toxic effect on hematopoietic elements, resulting in decreased bone marrow cellularity and vacuolization of erythroid precursors. Nutritional deficiencies often found in patients with chronic alcoholism include folate and iron deficiency. Folate deficiency is particularly common in these patients because of decreased ingestion, impairment of folate absorption by alcohol, and antagonism of folate by alcohol. Although typical morphologic features of megaloblastic anemia may be identified in the blood and bone marrow of patients with alcoholism, these changes are often masked by concurrent RBC abnormalities from iron deficiency, hemolysis, or both. Iron stores may be decreased in patients with chronic alcoholism because of decreased ingestion and chronic gastrointestinal blood loss. Hypochromasia is generally present, but the microcytosis of iron deficiency may be masked by the macrocytosis caused by liver disease, folate deficiency, or both. Decreased RBC survival is seen frequently in alcoholic patients with significant hepatic disease. The target cells, spherocytes, spur cells, and microspherocytes that may be identified in the peripheral blood of patients with chronic alcoholism are secondary to extracorpuscular RBC defects caused by congestive splenomegaly, lipoprotein abnormalities in the blood, and severe hypophosphatemia. In addition to iron deficiency, patients with chronic alco-

Table 3-5   Pathogenesis and Morphologic Features of Anemia in Patients With Alcoholism

Mechanism	Morphologic Features	Etiology/Cause
Chronic disease	Normocytic/ normochromic anemia	See earlier discussion
Toxic suppression	Hypocellular bone marrow with vacuolated erythroid precursors	Alcohol toxic to hematopoietic elements
Folate deficiency*	Megaloblastic anemia with oval macrocytes and hypersegmented neutrophils	Decreased ingestion, impaired absorption, and antagonistic action of alcohol vs folate
	Macrocytosis may be masked by concurrent iron deficiency	
Iron deficiency†	Hypochromia present but microcytosis often masked by concurrent macrocytosis from hepatic disease	Decreased ingestion of iron and chronic blood loss via gastrointestinal tract
Decreased red blood cell survival	Target cells, spherocytes, sometimes spur cells and microspherocytes	Extracorpuscular red blood cell defects due to:
		Congestive splenomegaly and portal hypertension
		Lipoprotein abnormalities causing target and spur shapes
		Severe hypophosphatemia
Abnormal iron metabolism	Ring sideroblasts in bone marrow	Complex etiology, not completely known
		Caused in part by decreased functional pyridoxine and inhibition of enzymes involved in hemoglobin synthesis
Hemodilution	None	Portal hypertension associated with fluid overload leading to dilutional anemia

*See Chapter 5 for more details.
†See Chapter 2 for more details.

holism frequently have abnormal iron metabolism that is manifested by ring sideroblasts in the bone marrow. Although the etiology of this phenomenon is not completely understood, the ring sideroblasts are caused in part by decreased functional pyridoxine and decreased activity of the enzymes involved in hemoglobin synthesis. Finally, portal hypertension is often associated with an increase in plasma volume that leads to dilutional anemia.

It is beyond the scope of this chapter to detail the clinical findings and laboratory features of patients with acute and chronic alcoholism. Details of the laboratory evaluation of patients (alcoholic or otherwise) with iron deficiency and folate deficiency can be found in Chapters 2 and 5, respectively. Except for patients with pronounced spur cell formation, marked nutritional deficiency, or gastrointestinal tract bleeding, the anemia associated with chronic alcoholism is generally mild to moderate and does not require treatment. Management of the portal hypertension and congestive splenomegaly is important in ameliorating the RBC survival defects.

Other liver diseases, including postnecrotic cirrhosis, biliary cirrhosis, acute hepatitis, and occasional cases of hemochromatosis, may also be associated with RBC abnormalities and anemia. If severe liver failure results, pronounced acanthocytosis with reduced RBC survival may be evident. Wilson's disease is also linked to hemolytic anemia.

Anemia With AIDS. Cytopenias are common peripheral blood abnormalities in patients with AIDS, and the severity of these cytopenias is roughly correlated with disease status. Consequently, those patients with the most severe cytopenias tend to have advanced disease. As with the other disorders presented in this chapter, the anemia in patients with AIDS is multifactorial, although ACD often predominates (Table 3-6).

In addition, evidence suggests that human immunodeficiency virus (HIV)–1 may invade bone marrow progenitor cells, resulting in multilineage suppression of hematopoiesis. Likewise, immune aberrations characteristic of this disease may result in defective regulation of hematopoiesis. Bone marrow infiltration by secondary tumors may result in impaired hematopoiesis. Bone marrow suppression may also be the consequence of either various sec-

Table 3-6   Causes of Anemia in Patients With AIDS

Anemia of chronic disease
Bone marrow suppression by virus (human immunodeficiency virus–1)
Ineffective regulation of hematopoiesis (T-cell/monocyte defects)
Secondary infections and neoplasms
Various drug treatments
Immune mechanisms (autoantibody production)
Sustained parvovirus infection resulting in prolonged red cell aplasia
Iron deficiency, other nutritional deficiencies
Chronic alcoholism or hepatitis

ondary infections or drug treatments required for secondary infections and/or neoplasms. Autoimmune mechanisms may also be operative in creating blood cytopenias, although the association between Coombs' positivity and hemolytic anemia in patients with AIDS is not clear-cut. The anemia in patients with AIDS is frequently exacerbated by zidovudine therapy, which is also linked to marked macrocytosis.

Various nutritional deficiencies can also develop in AIDS patients secondary to gastrointestinal blood loss, poor intake, or drugs that act as folate antagonists. The secondary infections that patients with AIDS can acquire include parvovirus, which invades erythroid progenitor cells and causes profound red cell aplasia (see Chapter 4). Because patients with AIDS are often unable to mount an immune response to parvovirus, the red cell aplasia is often sustained. Gamma globulin therapy is generally required to ameliorate this secondary viral infection.

References

Brynes RK, Esplin J. Hematologic manifestations of HIV-1 infection. In: Bick RL, Bennett JM, Brynes RK, et al, eds. *Hematology Clinical and Laboratory Practice.* Volume 1. St. Louis: CV Mosby Co, 1993:619-636.

Cash JM, Sears DA. The anemia of chronic disease: Spectrum of associated diseases in a series of unselected hospitalized patients. *Am J Med.* 1989;87:638-644.

Colman N, Herbert V. Hematologic complications of alcoholism: Overview. *Semin Hematol.* 1980;17:164-176.

Dutcher JP. Hematologic abnormalities in patients with nonhematologic malignancies. *Hematol Oncol Clin North A.* 1987;1:281-299.

Eschbach JW, Egrie JC, Downing MR, et al. Correction of the anemia of end-stage renal disease with recombinant human erythropoietin. *N Engl J Med.* 1987;316:73-78.

Foucar K. Anemias. In: *Bone Marrow Pathology.* Chicago, Ill: ASCP Press, 1995: 59-74.

Foucar K. Bone marrow manifestations of systemic infections. In: *Bone Marrow Pathology.* Chicago, Ill: ASCP Press, 1995:497-516.

Girard DE, Kumar KL, McAfee JH. Hematologic effects of acute and chronic alcohol abuse. *Hematol Oncol Clin North Am.* 1987;1:321-334.

Keeling DM, Isenberg DA. Haematological manifestations of systemic lupus erythematosus. *Blood Rev.* 1993;7:199-207.

Le J, Vilcek J. Tumor necrosis factor and interleukin-l: Cytokines with multiple overlapping biological activities. *Lab Invest.* 1987;56:234-248.

Lee GR. The anemia of chronic disease. *Semin Hematol.* 1983;20:61-80.

Means RT, Krantz SB. Progress in understanding pathogenesis of anemia of chronic disease. *Blood.* 1992;80:1639-1647.

Orwoll ES, Orwoll RL. Hematologic abnormalities in patients with endocrine and metabolic disorders. *Hematol Oncol Clin North Am.* 1987;1:261-279.

Paganini EP. Overview of anemia associated with chronic renal disease: Primary and secondary mechanisms. *Semin Nephrol.* 1989;9(Suppl 1):3-8.

4

Aplastic, Hypoplastic, and Miscellaneous Types of Anemia

For clarity, this chapter is organized into three divisions: "Aplastic and Hypoplastic Anemias," "Bone Marrow Replacement Disorders," and "Congenital Dyserythropoietic Anemias."

Aplastic and Hypoplastic Anemias

Both constitutional and acquired disorders of red blood cell (RBC) production have been well-delineated (Table 4-1). These production defects can involve exclusively the erythroid lineage (ie, pure red cell aplasia), or production of all hematopoietic cells may be affected (ie, aplastic anemia). The constitutional (hereditary) types of aplastic anemia include Fanconi's anemia, dyskeratosis congenita, and occasional cases of Shwachman-Diamond syndrome, while Diamond-Blackfan anemia is the only well-established constitutional pure red cell aplasia (Table 4-1). In general, these constitutional disorders are associated with abnormalities in other organ systems, including skeletal and mucocutaneous defects, as well as mental retardation. In addition to the obvious loss of one or more bone marrow lineages, defects in erythrocytes are characteristic of both Diamond-Blackfan and Fanconi's anemia. These RBC defects

Table 4-1 Constitutional and Acquired Aplastic/Hypoplastic Anemias

Type	Clinical Features
Constitutional aplastic anemia	
Fanconi's	Autosomal recessive disease with associated bone, skin, and renal abnormalities
Fetal Hb ↑	Mental retardation
Dyskeratosis congenita	X-linked recessive disorder with skin, nail, and mucosal abnormalities
	Mental retardation
Shwachman-Diamond syndrome	Autosomal recessive; some patients have associated bone abnormalities
Constitutional red cell aplasia	
Diamond-Blackfan anemia	Onset of anemia at birth or early infancy
Fetal Hb ↑	Several genetic types
	Short stature, hypertelorism, retardation
Acquired aplastic anemia	Onset at any age
	Most cases idiopathic
	Other cases linked to infections, toxins, drugs, radiation, immune disorders
Acquired red cell aplasia	
Transient erythroblastopenia of childhood	Patient usually over 1 year old
fetal Hb not increased	
Parvovirus-induced red cell aplasia	Any age, predominates in children
	Patient typically has underlying constitutional anemia
Acquired sustained red cell aplasia	Adolescence through adulthood
	Both idiopathic and secondary types

Table 4-1 *Continued*

Blood	Bone Marrow
Thrombocytopenia is typically initial abnormality	Initially hypercellular
Pancytopenia develops by midchildhood	Eventual aplasia
Decreased reticulocytes	Late development of myelodysplasia or acute myeloid leukemia
Gradual development of pancytopenia	Initially hypercellular
	Eventual aplasia in one half of patients
Decreased reticulocytes	
Neutropenia predominates	Initial abnormalities are granulocytic
One fourth of cases progress to pancytopenia	Eventual aplasia in one fourth of patients
Decreased reticulocytes	
Macrocytic anemia with decreased reticulocytes	Only rare erythroblasts evident
	Other lineages unremarkable
	Increased hematogones
Pancytopenia	Panhypoplasia
Normal morphology	Variable lymphoid infiltrates
Decreased reticulocytes	
Normocytic, normochromic anemia	Only rare erythroblasts evident
	Other lineages unremarkable
Decreased reticulocytes	Variable lymphocytosis
Variable RBC morphology depending on underlying chronic anemia	Only rare erythroblasts evident; these cells contain intranuclear inclusions
	Other lineages usually unremarkable
Decreased reticulocytes	
Normocytic, normochromic anemia	Only rare erythroblasts evident
	Other lineages unremarkable
Decreased reticulocytes	

include increased fetal hemoglobin, expression of i antigen on the surface membrane, and abnormalities of cytoplasmic enzyme levels. Because these disorders are hereditary, disease manifestation occurs in infancy or early childhood. Both pure red cell aplasia and aplastic anemia can also be acquired (Table 4-1). Acquired pure red cell aplasia can be classified into three general types: transient erythroblastopenia of childhood, parvovirus-induced red cell aplasia, and acquired (sustained) pure red cell aplasia. Transient erythroblastopenia of childhood is a self-limited disorder that is likely linked to an antecedent viral infection. Although controversial, many investigators believe the viral infection is different from the parvovirus-induced red cell aplasia. Spontaneous recovery occurs, and these children are otherwise entirely normal.

The parvovirus-induced red cell aplasias more typically occur in children and, occasionally, in adults who have underlying constitutional RBC disorders such as thalassemia, hereditary spherocytosis, or sickle cell anemia. Because of shortened RBC survival times, baseline production of erythrocytes greatly exceeds normal levels in these patients with constitutional anemias. Consequently, the hemoglobin and hematocrit levels plummet when RBC production is halted by parvovirus invasion of erythroid progenitor cells. Viral inclusions within the rare residual erythroblasts can generally be identified, but this diagnosis should be confirmed by serologic studies (Image 4-1). Once the patient mounts an immune response to the parvovirus, this infection is eliminated and erythropoiesis returns. There are also rare reports of parvovirus-induced multilineage aplasia.

In addition to these acquired transient red cell aplasias, both primary and secondary types of acquired (sustained) pure red cell aplasia have been well-described (Table 4-2). Disorders linked to acquired pure red cell aplasia include thymoma, hematopoietic and nonhematopoietic neoplasms, drug treatments (notably diphenylhydantoin), and immune defects.

The causes of acquired aplastic anemia are listed in Table 4-3 and include drug and toxin exposures, various viral infections, immune aberrations, and radiation. In these patients all hematopoietic lineages are either absent or severely attenuated (Image 4-2).

Pathophysiology. For erythropoiesis to occur, the necessary components include adequate stem cells that are capable of

Table 4-2   Types of Acquired Sustained Pure Red Cell Aplasia

Type	Associated Disorders/Conditions
Primary	Idiopathic
Secondary	Thymoma
	Drug treatment
	Hematopoietic neoplasms
	Carcinomas
	Viral infections
	Immune disorders

renewal and differentiation, erythropoietin and other growth factors, appropriate immunoregulation of hematopoiesis, and adequate microenvironment. Deficiencies or defects of all of these components have been suggested in the pathophysiology of the diverse spectrum of congenital and acquired production disorders of erythrocytes.

The congenital hypoplastic anemias may represent stem cell disorders, while acquired anemias such as transient erythroblastopenia of childhood are probably caused by a self-limited, infection-induced, immunoregulatory abnormality. An immunoregulatory abnormality is also the likely cause of many other types of acquired pure red cell aplasia.

The most extensive pathophysiologic studies have been performed on patients with acquired aplastic anemia. Defects described in these patients include deficient or suppressed stem cells, humoral and cellular immunoregulatory defects, and microenvironmental abnormalities. Increased circulating suppressor T cells, which may be responsible for suppressed hematopoiesis, have been identified in some patients with aplastic anemia. In addition, several viral infections have been linked to aplastic anemia, notably hepatitis and Epstein-Barr viruses. One theory regarding viral-induced aplasia states that stem cells are directly suppressed or damaged by these infectious agents. Another theory suggests that these viruses initiate an immune response that suppresses hematopoiesis. Finally, many drug treatments and some toxic exposures have been associated with acquired aplastic anemia caused by either a dose-related or idiosyncratic host response to the drug or toxin.

Table 4-3 Causes of Acquired Aplastic Anemia

Drugs
    Chloramphenicol
    Phenylbutazone
    Anticonvulsants
    Sulfonamides
    Gold
Toxins
    Benzene
    Insecticides
    Solvents
Infections
    Hepatitis
    Epstein-Barr virus
    Influenza
Other conditions/exposures
    Pregnancy
    Radiation exposure
    Immune disorders

Clinical Findings.   Depending on its severity, patients with hypoplastic or aplastic anemia can present with weakness, fatigue, or tachycardia. If pancytopenia is present, additional findings can include petechiae and purpura secondary to thrombocytopenia, and fever and infection secondary to neutropenia. As described earlier, some congenital types of hypoplastic anemias have associated phenotypic abnormalities, including bony defects, mental retardation, and skin and nail abnormalities (Table 4-1). Other clinical features such as hepatosplenomegaly and lymphadenopathy are not evident in patients with uncomplicated hypoplastic or aplastic anemias.

Approach to Diagnosis.   The diagnosis of hypoplastic anemia requires an approach that both identifies the specific type of disorder and excludes other diseases such as bone marrow neoplasms, which can also be manifested by blood cytopenias. This approach to diagnosis generally follows these steps:

1.   Determine the types and severity of the blood cytopenias.

2. Assess the patient for hepatosplenomegaly and lymphadenopathy on physical examination.

3. Evaluate infants and young children for other manifestations of the hereditary hypoplastic disorders, including physical and radiographic defects (Table 4-1).

4. Carefully investigate for evidence of toxin or drug exposure, infectious diseases such as hepatitis or infectious mononucleosis, and recent blood loss.

5. Document bone marrow hypocellularity and rule out an infiltrative or fibrotic process.

6. Use clinical history and other clinical evidence of chronic hemolytic anemia to assess for a possible aplastic crisis of an underlying RBC disorder, such as hereditary spherocytosis or sickle cell anemia.

7. Evaluate adults with pure red cell aplasia for thymoma, other tumors, drug exposure, or infection (Tables 4-1 and 4-2).

Hematologic Findings.   In some types of hypoplastic anemia, only erythropoiesis is reduced; in others, all bone marrow cell lines are affected. Therefore, the hematologic manifestations of these cases can range from isolated anemia to pancytopenia.

Blood Cell Measurements.   Patients with hypoplastic anemias generally have a moderate to severe normochromic anemia that may be normocytic or macrocytic. An elevated mean corpuscular volume (MCV) is characteristic of Diamond-Blackfan anemia and may also be present in some cases of acquired aplastic anemia. Erythrocytes generally show little anisopoikilocytosis, as evidenced by a normal red cell distribution width (RDW). The corrected reticulocyte count is reduced. In patients with either acquired or constitutional aplastic anemia, thrombocytopenia and neutropenia are also present.

Peripheral Blood Smear Morphology.   In the various hypoplastic disorders, erythrocytes, neutrophils, and platelets are generally morphologically unremarkable, except in the cases of parvovirus-induced red cell aplasia that occur in patients with underlying constitutional anemias.

Bone Marrow Examination. Patients with Diamond-Blackfan anemia, transient erythroblastopenia of childhood, and acquired pure red cell aplasia show a marked decrease in erythroid precursors in the bone marrow with essentially normal granulopoiesis and megakaryopoiesis. Erythroid precursors may be totally absent, or only the earliest red cell precursors may be identified. Parvovirus inclusions may be evident in rare erythroblasts in patients with this type of acquired red cell aplasia (Image 4-1). In all types of hypoplastic or aplastic anemias a lymphocytosis with many hematogones may be present, especially in anemias affecting young children. Early in their disease course, patients with Fanconi's anemia may have a hypercellular bone marrow with megaloblastic changes, followed by gradual aplasia. In acquired aplastic anemia and advanced Fanconi's anemia, however, all three cell lines are usually markedly reduced (Image 4-2). There are no specific morphologic abnormalities of the rare residual hematopoietic elements in these patients.

Other Laboratory Tests

4.1 Fetal Hemoglobin Quantitation

Purpose.   Fetal hemoglobin levels in erythrocytes can be used to distinguish between transient erythroblastopenia of childhood and constitutional disorders, such as Diamond-Blackfan and Fanconi's anemias.

Principle, Specimen, Procedure, Notes, and Precautions See Test 10.6.

Interpretation.   Fetal hemoglobin level is characteristically increased in Diamond-Blackfan and Fanconi's anemias, while it is normal in patients with transient erythroblastopenia of childhood. Fetal hemoglobin level may be increased in some cases of acquired aplastic anemia. Usually, only a small population of erythrocytes contains substantial amounts of fetal hemoglobin, and the remainder of erythrocytes contain none.

Ancillary Tests.   Other tests that can be used selectively to distinguish among the various types of aplastic and hypoplastic anemias include the red cell i antigen test and cytogenetic studies. Although not available in most laboratories, red cell i antigen can be detected in patients with Diamond-Blackfan and Fanconi's anemia; i antigen is not present on erythrocytes in patients with transient erythroblastopenia of childhood.

Cytogenetic studies generally reveal chromosomal defects in bone marrow cells of patients with Fanconi's anemia, including increased chromosomal breakage, translocation, sister chromatid exchange, and increased sensitivity to mitomycin C and other agents. Karyotypic abnormalities are not usually found in the other types of hypoplastic and aplastic anemias.

Family studies may be helpful in identifying inheritance patterns associated with constitutional disorders, while serologic studies can be used to document acute parvovirus infection.

Since erythropoietin level is generally increased in all aplastic and hypoplastic anemias, it is not a useful test in distinguishing between these disorders.

Course and Treatment.   The clinical course of hypoplastic and aplastic anemias is diverse. Some patients, such as children with transient erythroblastopenia of childhood, have brief, self-limited episodes of red cell aplasia that require no treatment. Likewise, spontaneous recovery generally occurs in immunocompetent patients with acute parvovirus-induced red cell aplasia.

Children and most adults with either constitutional disorders or acquired aplastic anemia generally require treatment that may include immune modulation, cytokine therapy, androgens, transfusion, or bone marrow transplantation. Any antecedent drug treatment that the patient is receiving should be discontinued, if possible. Suspected toxins should be removed from the patient's environment. In general, blood product transfusions should be reserved for life-threatening situations. Because these transfusions can have a negative effect on the outcome of bone marrow transplantation, they should be used very judiciously in patients likely to require a bone marrow transplant.

The bone marrow of patients with pure red cell aplasia often responds to corticosteroid therapy. If this fails, however, other effective treatments include plasmapheresis, thymectomy (for patients with thymoma-associated acquired red cell aplasia), alkylating agents, azathioprine, cyclosporine, antithymocyte globulin, and danazol therapies. Human recombinant erythropoietin may also be utilized to stimulate erythropoiesis. A careful search for underlying causes of acquired (sustained) pure red cell aplasia should be undertaken.

The clinical course of patients with acquired aplastic anemia depends on the severity of the pancytopenia, the patient's age, and the patient's response to treatment. These patients must be monitored carefully for evidence of infection or bleeding. Various drugs that have been utilized successfully to treat some patients with acquired aplastic anemia include corticosteroids, androgens, lithium carbonate, cyclophosphamide, and human recombinant colony-stimulating factors. Bone marrow transplantation is recommended for those young patients with severe acquired aplastic anemia who have an HLA-matched donor.

There is an increased incidence of acute leukemia in patients who recover from any type of bone marrow hypoplastic disorder. Long-term survivors may also develop myelodysplasia or paroxysmal nocturnal hemoglobinuria–like defects.

Bone Marrow Replacement Disorders

Patients with bone marrow replacement disorders suffer from a failure of hematopoiesis because the medullary portion of the bone marrow has been replaced by fibrosis, neoplastic cells, or nonneoplastic cells (Table 4-4). Even if the neoplastic cells are of hematopoietic origin, they are incapable of producing normal peripheral blood elements. Therefore, patients with bone marrow replacement disorders generally present with cytopenias, ranging from isolated anemia to pancytopenia.

Pathophysiology. Despite the bone marrow's ability to compensate, hematopoiesis will fail once a significant portion of

Table 4-4 Causes of Bone Marrow Failure Secondary to Replacement

---

Neoplastic disorders replacing bone marrow parenchyma
    Acute and chronic leukemias
    Malignant lymphoma (Hodgkin's disease and non-Hodgkin's lymphoma)
    Multiple myeloma
    Metastatic carcinoma and sarcoma
Disorders/therapy causing bone marrow fibrosis
    Agnogenic myeloid metaplasia
    Metabolic bone disorders/endocrine abnormalities
    Following chemotherapy/toxin exposure
Miscellaneous disorders replacing bone marrow parenchyma
    Storage diseases
    Other histiocytic disorders
    Angioimmunoblastic lymphadenopathy
    Mast cell disease

---

the bone marrow medullary space is replaced by tumor or fibrous tissue. This failure of normal hematopoiesis is the primary cause of cytopenias in patients with bone marrow replacement disorders. As described in Chapter 3, however, patients with neoplasms can develop other types of anemia. For example, these patients can suffer from chronic blood loss, anemia of chronic disease, bone marrow suppression by chemotherapy, hypersplenism, and even immune-mediated hemolysis (see Table 3-4).

Clinical Findings. The clinical findings in patients with bone marrow replacement disorders are as diverse as the types of disorders themselves. Most patients with significant bone marrow replacement develop symptoms of cytopenia, most notably malaise and fatigue secondary to anemia. Manifestations of leukopenia and thrombocytopenia, such as infection or bleeding, may also be present. Patients with acute and chronic leukemias, malignant lymphomas, storage diseases, and agnogenic myeloid metaplasia often have significant splenomegaly, which can cause left upper quadrant pain and early satiety. Lymphadenopathy is also present in some of these patients.

Hematologic Findings. Although most patients with bone marrow replacement disorders have cytopenias, some of these patients also have specific morphologic abnormalities that suggest a certain type of bone marrow replacement disorder.

Blood Cell Measurements. A normocytic, normochromic anemia is the most common cytopenia in patients with bone marrow replacement disorders. Although these erythrocytes generally show little anisopoikilocytosis, as manifested by a normal red cell distribution width, some patients, such as those with agnogenic myeloid metaplasia, exhibit marked anisopoikilocytosis. The reticulocyte count is often reduced in these patients, while the white blood cell and platelet counts are highly variable. Patients with leukemias or agnogenic myeloid metaplasia tend to have elevated white blood cell counts. Thrombocytopenia is generally present in patients with bone marrow replacement disorders.

Peripheral Blood Smear Morphology. Most bone marrow replacement disorders have no specific morphologic abnormalities of RBCs, white blood cells, or platelets. Patients with certain hematopoietic replacement disorders, however, such as agnogenic myeloid metaplasia, have pronounced anisopoikilocytosis with teardrop forms, a leukoerythroblastic blood picture, variable basophilia, and large platelets. A leukoerythroblastic blood picture may also be seen in patients with bone marrow involvement by other neoplasms. If the hypoproliferative anemia is complicated by an RBC survival defect, additional morphologic abnormalities will be present. Leukemic or lymphoma cells may be identified in the peripheral blood in patients with this type of replacement disorder.

Bone Marrow Examination. There is a wide spectrum of bone marrow morphologic abnormalities in patients with bone marrow replacement disorders. In some patients, the bone marrow parenchyma is packed with infiltrating tumor cells, while in others it is replaced by collagen. In histiocytic disorders, such as storage diseases, the bone marrow may be replaced by distinctive large, benign-appearing macrophages.

Other Laboratory Tests.   Because this group of disorders is so diverse, there are few individual laboratory tests that can distinguish types of replacement disorders. Many tests can be utilized on a selective basis, however, to help establish the diagnosis of specific bone marrow replacement disorders (see Chapters 28-37).

Course and Treatment.   Fibrotic and benign histiocytic bone marrow replacement disorders tend to exhibit gradually progressive bone marrow infiltration, while neoplasms generally progress more rapidly. The treatment and disease course vary for each type of replacement disorder.

Congenital Dyserythropoietic Anemias

The congenital dyserythropoietic anemias (CDAs) are rare disorders initially described in 1951 and characterized by profound blood and bone marrow RBC morphologic abnormalities and ineffective erythropoiesis. Other features common to this group of disorders include a low corrected reticulocyte count, a mildly elevated indirect bilirubin level, and an elevated lactate dehydrogenase level. In some patients with CDA, an autosomal recessive pattern of inheritance has been determined. Patients with CDA generally have a mild to moderate anemia, with markedly dyspoietic erythrocytes.

At least three types of CDA have been described based on specific morphologic features within the bone marrow. In type I, the erythroid elements within the bone marrow show megaloblastic changes with internuclear chromatin bridges. Type II CDA is characterized by binuclearity and multinuclearity of erythroid precursors. In type III CDA, the multinuclearity is pronounced with up to 12 nuclei present in some erythroid precursors. In all types of CDA, mature erythrocytes are often macrocytic.

The bone marrow in patients with CDA shows erythroid hyperplasia, with asynchrony of nuclear-cytoplasmic maturation. Nuclear abnormalities include variations in size and structure as well as shape abnormalities described above for the CDA subtypes. In addition, mitotic abnormalities, such as lobulation, budding, fragmentation, and karyorrhexis, have also been described. Cytoplasmic abnormalities include vacuolization, basophilic stippling, and excess iron within erythroid precursors.

The pathogenesis of CDA is uncertain, but theories include some primary defect in mitosis or a nuclear or cell membrane defect. Because this type of anemia is mild, these patients are frequently asymptomatic and do not require treatment.

References

Björkholm M. Aplastic anaemia: pathologenetic mechanisms and treatment with special reference to immunomodulation. *J Intern Med.* 1992;231:575-582.

Dessypris EN. The biology of pure red cell aplasia. *Semin Hematol.* 1991;28:275-284.

Foucar K. Aplastic anemia. In: *Bone Marrow Pathology.* Chicago, Ill: ASCP Press; 1995:75-85.

Foucar K. Erythroblastopenic bone marrow disorders. In: *Bone Marrow Pathology.* Chicago, Ill: ASCP Press; 1995:87-94.

Gordon-Smith EC, Rutherford TR. Fanconi anemia: constitutional aplastic anemia. *Semin Hematol.* 1991;28:104-112.

Harris JW. Parvovirus B19 for the hematologist. *Am J Hematol.* 1992;39:119-130.

Liu JM, Buchwald M, Walsh CE, et al. Fanconi anemia and novel strategies for therapy. *Blood.* 1994;84:3995-4007.

Marmont AM. Therapy for pure red cell aplasia. *Semin Hematol.* 1991;28:285-297.

Nissen-Druey C. Pathophysiology of aplastic anemia. *Blood Rev.* 1990;4:97-102.

Rosenfeld SJ, Young NS. Viruses and bone marrow failure. *Blood Rev.* 1991;5:71-77.

Ware RE, Kinney TR. Transient erythroblastopenia in the first year of life. *Am J Hematol.* 1991;37:156-158.

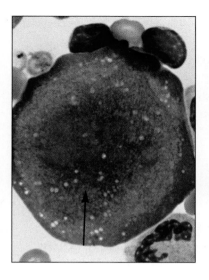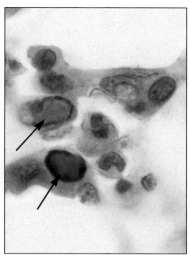

Image 4-1 This composite illustrates intranuclear parvovirus inclusions (↑) within erythroid precursors on bone marrow aspirate smears (left) and biopsy sections (right). (Courtesy of Drs. P. Ward and C. Sever.) (Wright's; H&E)

Image 4-2 The contrast between the bone marrow cellularity of aplastic anemia (left) and normal adult bone marrow (right) is striking on these two bone marrow biopsy sections. (H&E)

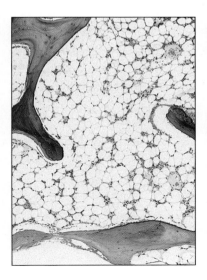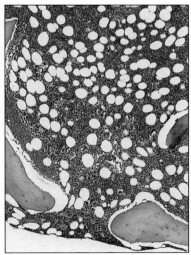

Figure 4-1. ...

5

Megaloblastic Anemias

Megaloblastic anemia occurs when the coenzyme forms of folate and vitamin B_{12} necessary for normal DNA synthesis are deficient. The resultant defective DNA synthesis impairs the ability of all proliferating cells to synthesize enough DNA per unit time to allow for mitosis; as a consequence, there are increased numbers of cells in the DNA synthesis phase of the cell cycle. Since RNA synthesis is not dependent on these coenzymes, an asynchrony between nuclear and cytoplasmic maturation occurs, resulting both in "giantism" of all proliferating cells and in cell nuclei that appear less mature than the cytoplasm. While impaired proliferation of hematopoietic elements is the major clinical manifestation of vitamin B_{12} and folate deficiency, other disorders, such as malabsorption caused by defective production of intestinal epithelial cells, can also develop.

Characteristics of vitamin B_{12} and folate, including dietary sources, recommended daily requirements, normal blood levels, and amounts of stored vitamins, are shown in Table 5-1. Vitamin B_{12} circulates in the peripheral blood bound to various binder proteins. Except in infants, total body stores of vitamin B_{12} are abundant and are sufficient to adequately supply the host for 2 to 5 years. Folate is very heat labile and is destroyed readily in the cooking process. Small

Table 5-1   Characteristics of Vitamin B_{12} and Folate

	Vitamin B_{12}	Folate
Origin	Synthesized exclusively by bacteria	Synthesized by plants and microorganisms
Dietary source	Meat, fish, dairy products (heat stabile)	Vegetables (especially green leafy) and fruits (heat labile)
Parent compound	Cyanocobalamin	Pteroglutamic acid
Recommended daily requirements (μg)		
Infants	0.3	60
Children	0.5-1.0	100
Adults	1-2	200
Pregnant women	2.5-3.0	400
Lactating women	2.5-3.0	300
Normal blood levels	150-1,000 pg/mL	>3.7 ng/mL (red blood cell: 130-640 ng/mL)
Normal total stores* (major storage site)	3,000-5,000 mg (liver)	20-70 mg (liver)
Storage duration on deficient diet	2-5 years	3-5 months

*Total stores are much smaller in infants.

amounts of folate derivatives circulate largely unbound in the blood; greater concentrations of these derivatives are present intracellularly. Except in infants, total body stores of folate are moderate and are sufficient to maintain normal cellular proliferation for approximately 3 to 5 months. Because of the relatively short duration that folate stores will meet host needs, the incidence of folate deficiency is substantially greater than that of vitamin B_{12} deficiency.

Pathophysiology

The physiology and biochemistry of vitamin B_{12} and folate are detailed in Tables 5-2 and 5-3. In patients with vitamin B_{12} deficiency, both the megaloblastic anemia and the neurologic complications appear to be secondary to the defective formation of methionine (Table 5-3). The rate-limiting step in DNA synthesis that requires folate is the conversion of deoxyuridine monophosphate to deoxythymidine monophosphate in pyrimidine synthesis.

Table 5-2 Physiology of Vitamin B_{12} and Folate

	Vitamin B_{12}	Folate
Compounds in food	Several cobalamin forms	Several polyglutamate forms
Physiology of absorption	Vitamin B_{12} released from food by gastric acid, gastric enzymes, and small bowel enzymes → free vitamin B_{12} bound to R-binders primarily; some also binds to IF → pancreatic enzymes degrade R-binder–B_{12} complexes → released B_{12} is then bound to IF	Polyglutamate deconjugated by conjugase enzymes in bile and small bowel lumen
Site of absorption	Vitamin B_{12}–IF complex adheres to receptors on brush border of ileum (pH and calcium-dependent process)	Deconjugated folate absorbed in jejunum
Physiology of circulation	30% of vitamin B_{12} binds to TCII, which delivers it to liver, bone marrow, and other sites 70% of vitamin B_{12} binds to TCI, TCIII, and R-binders, which deliver it exclusively to liver	Folate circulates unbound in blood as 5-methyl THF
Entry into cells	TCII-B_{12} attaches to specific membrane receptors Vitamin B_{12} transferred across plasma membrane (TCII degraded in this process)	Vitamin B_{12} necessary for folate (THF form) to pass across plasma membranes and be retained in cell
Function	Two active forms, methylcobalamin and 5-deoxyadenosyl cobalamin, which facilitate formation of methionine and succinate, respectively	THF essential for all one-carbon transfer reactions in mammalian cells THF required for both purine and pyrimidine synthesis
Excretion	Bile, urine	Urine, sweat, saliva, feces

Abbreviations: IF = intrinsic factor; TC = transcobalamin; R-binder = found in every tissue in body, named for rapid mobility on electrophoresis; THF = tetrahydrofolate.

Table 5-3 Biochemistry of Vitamin B_{12} and Folate Activity

	Vitamin B_{12}	Folate
Biologically active form(s)	Coenzyme B_{12} (5-deoxyadenosyl cobalamin) and methylcobalamin	5-methyl THF
Reactions requiring vitamin B_{12} and/or folate cofactors	I. Homocysteine $\xrightarrow{\text{methylcobalamin}}$ Methionine 5-methyl THF $\nearrow$ $\searrow$ THF Failure in this pathway results in megaloblastosis; reaction also important in central nervous system methylation, and for incorporation of folate into cells II. Methylmalonate $\xrightarrow{\text{Coenzyme } B_{12}}$ Succinate Failure of this reaction not involved in neurologic disease or megaloblastosis	I. Required for both purine and pyrimidine synthesis II. Rate limiting step in DNA synthesis (pyrimidine synthesis) dUMP $\longrightarrow$ dTMP THF $\nearrow$ $\searrow$ DHF III. Folate also essential in amino acid synthesis

Abbreviations: THF = tetrahydrofolate; dUMP = deoxyuridine monophosphate; dTMP = deoxythymidine monophosphate; DHF = dihydrofolate.

Table 5-4 Probable Sequence in Development of Vitamin B_{12} Deficiency

Time Interval After Onset of Intake Failure	Pathologic Abnormality
1-2 years	Vitamin B_{12} level in serum decreased
	Early blood and bone marrow abnormalities, including hypersegmentation and macrocytosis
	Early myelin damage to nerves
2-3 years	Vitamin B_{12} level markedly decreased
	Vitamin B_{12} binders 10% saturated
	Florid megaloblastosis in blood and bone marrow
	Decreased RBC folate, normal to increased serum folate
	Severe damage to myelin

Table 5-5 Sequence in Development of Folate Deficiency

Time Interval After Onset of Intake Failure	Pathologic Abnormality
	3 weeks Decreased serum folate
5-7 weeks	Hypersegmentation of neutrophils in bone marrow and blood
10 weeks	Mild megaloblastic changes in bone marrow
17-18 weeks	Macro-ovalocytes, decreased RBC folate
19-20 weeks	Florid megaloblastosis with anemia

The sequence of events in the development of vitamin B_{12} and folate deficiency is listed in Tables 5-4 and 5-5, respectively. Although folate stores are depleted much more rapidly than vitamin B_{12} stores, the sequence of events in the development of blood and bone marrow abnormalities as deficiency evolves is similar for both vitamins. Hypersegmentation of neutrophils appears early in the development of megaloblastic anemia, while actual anemia is a late event associated with florid megaloblastic morphologic changes. Damage to myelin in peripheral nerves occurs progressively throughout the evolution of vitamin B_{12} deficiency.

Table 5-6   Mechanisms of Vitamin B_{12} Deficiency

	Example	Condition/Disorder
Inadequate intake	Dietary deficiency	Strict vegetarianism
Increased requirement	Growth, development	Pregnancy, lactation
Defective absorption	Decreased IF	Pernicious anemia, congenital IF deficiency
	Decreased pancreatic enzymes	Pancreatitis
	Lack of calcium or abnormal pH	Zollinger-Ellison syndrome
	Defective ileal mucosa	Sprue, regional enteritis, surgical reaction
	Parasitic or bacterial overgrowth	Tapeworm, blind loop
	Drug interference with absorption	Alcoholism, colchicine treatment, PAS treatment
Defective transport	Decreased TCII	Congenital deficiency of TCII
Disorders of metabolism	Suppression or inhibition of metabolic enzymes	Nitrous oxide administration, enzyme deficiencies

Abbreviations: IF = intrinsic factor; TC = transcobalamin; PAS = para-amino salicylic acid.

There are five basic mechanisms leading to vitamin B_{12} deficiency, including inadequate intake, increased requirement, defective absorption, defective transport, and disorders of B_{12} metabolism (Table 5-6). By far, the most common mechanism for vitamin B_{12} deficiency is defective absorption. For vitamin B_{12} absorption to occur, there must be normal amounts of intrinsic factor, sufficient pancreatic enzymes to degrade the vitamin B_{12}-R-binder complexes, appropriate calcium and hydrogen ion concentrations to facilitate the transfer of vitamin B_{12} across plasma membranes, an intact ileal mucosal surface, and lack of competing parasites or bacteria for the ingested vitamin B_{12}. Although abnormalities in any of these components can result in defective absorption, the one most commonly encountered in clinical practice is decreased intrinsic factor in patients with pernicious anemia. Intrinsic factor is secreted by gastric parietal cells stimulated by gastrin and histamine. The antibodies directed against intrinsic factor commonly detected in patients with pernicious anemia may be the cause of the decreased intrinsic factor. Other disorders associated with defective absorption are listed in Table 5-6.

Although vitamin B_{12} deficiency may occur secondary to a lack in dietary intake, a stringent diet deficient in all meat, egg, and milk products must be followed. Because vitamin B_{12} stores are so abundant, the increased requirement for this vitamin during pregnancy and lactation is rarely associated with megaloblastic anemia. Vitamin B_{12} deficiency secondary to transport or metabolic defects is extremely rare.

The major causes of folate deficiency include dietary deficiency and increased requirement, although defective absorption and disorders of metabolism have occasionally been responsible for folate deficiency (Table 5-7). Dietary deficiency of folate is common in chronic alcoholics, drug addicts, and patients of low socioeconomic class who consume inadequate diets. Excessive cooking destroys folate. Increased folate is required by infants, pregnant and lactating women, and patients with malignancies or chronic hemolytic anemias. Premature infants have very low folate stores and are highly susceptible to folate deficiency. Disorders and drug treatment associated with defective absorption of folate and abnormal folate metabolism are listed in Table 5-7.

Clinical Findings

Patients with megaloblastic anemia characteristically present with moderate to severe fatigue and malaise of several months' duration. Their skin may be lemon-yellow because of the combined effects of a moderately increased bilirubin level and the marked pallor of the underlying anemia. Because the defective DNA synthesis affects all proliferating cells, these patients have atrophy of the mucosal surfaces of the tongue, gastrointestinal tract, and vagina. This can cause pain in the mouth and vagina and can lead to a secondary malabsorption in the gastrointestinal tract.

Although the neurologic manifestations of pernicious anemia have been well described, patients with folate deficiency can also develop neuropsychiatric disorders that include irritability, forgetfulness, and sleepiness. Occasionally, patients with folate deficiency will manifest peripheral neuropathy similar to that described in patients

Table 5-7 Mechanisms of Folate Deficiency

	Example	Condition/Disorder
Inadequate intake	Dietary deficiency	Alcoholism, drug addiction, poverty
	Inactivation of folate	Overcooking of food
Increased requirement	Growth, development	Pregnancy, lactation, infancy
	States of increased cell turnover	Chronic hemolytic anemias, malignancies
Defective absorption	Defective jejunal mucosa	Sprue, amyloidosis, lymphoma, surgical resection
	Drug-induced malabsorption	Anticonvulsant, antituberculous, oral contraceptive drug therapy, alcoholism
Disorders of metabolism	Suppression or inhibition of metabolic enzymes	Methotrexate, pyrimethamine treatment, alcoholism
		Congenital disorders of folate metabolism

with vitamin B_{12} deficiency. In pernicious anemia, this peripheral neuropathy is secondary to defective myelin synthesis and is insidious in onset, beginning first in peripheral nerves and gradually progressing to involve the posterior and lateral columns of the spinal cord. The clinical manifestations of peripheral nerve involvement include paresthesias, such as numbness and tingling in the hands and feet; decreased vibration sense; and decreased position sense. With progression to spinal cord involvement, the patient may experience ataxia and eventually symmetrical paralysis. If the megaloblastic anemia is untreated, the patient may eventually develop cerebral involvement, which has been called "megaloblastic madness" and is manifested by mental changes, paranoia, and depression.

Approach to Diagnosis

The approach to the diagnosis of megaloblastic anemia includes:

1. Establishing the presence of a macrocytic anemia
2. Distinguishing between the various causes of macrocytic anemia

3. Determining if the patient is vitamin B_{12} or folate deficient

4. Identifying and treating the underlying disease responsible for the megaloblastic anemia

In addition to megaloblastic anemia, peripheral blood macrocytosis may be seen in patients with alcoholism, liver disease, reticulocytosis, myelodysplastic disorders, and chemotherapeutic effect. Clinical history and a review of the blood smear help exclude these alternate diagnoses. The clinical history should also include questions regarding family history (some very rare types of megaloblastic anemia are secondary to hereditary disorders), drug ingestion, intestinal function, and prior surgical procedures. Evidence of peripheral neuropathy and other neurologic manifestations of vitamin B_{12} or folate deficiency should be assessed by physical examination. Once the diagnosis of megaloblastic anemia has been established, the specific vitamin deficiency causing this anemia must be determined via laboratory tests discussed below. Finally, the cause of the vitamin deficiency must be identified and treated appropriately.

Hematologic Findings

The hematologic findings can be virtually diagnostic in patients with full-blown megaloblastic anemia in whom characteristic abnormalities of erythrocytes and neutrophils can be identified readily. In patients suffering from concurrent iron deficiency anemia, however, the hematologic findings are less predictable. Likewise, the blood of some patients with severe vitamin B_{12} deficiency will fail to exhibit substantial erythrocyte or neutrophil abnormalities.

Blood Cell Measurements. A patient with megaloblastic anemia typically has a moderate to severe normochromic macrocytic anemia with mean corpuscular volumes (MCVs) ranging from 100 to 150 μm^3 (100-150 fL), while the mean corpuscular hemoglobin concentration (MCHC) is normal. Although MCVs at the lower end of this spectrum can be seen in a variety of disorders, a patient with an MCV exceeding 120 μm^3 (120 fL) is very likely to have megaloblastic anemia. Some patients with vitamin B_{12} or folate deficiency will have a normal MCV because these patients also have iron deficiency, inflammatory disorders, or renal failure. The red cell distribution width (RDW) is characteristically markedly elevated in megaloblastic anemia because of extreme anisopoikilocytosis. Circulating macrocytes are often disrupted, producing very small red blood cells. The reticulocyte count is very low; in severe cases, the neutrophil and platelet counts are decreased.

Peripheral Blood Smear Morphology. The peripheral blood smear characteristically contains numerous oval macrocytes as well as schistocytes of various sizes, broken erythrocytes, and even spherocytes (Image 5-1). Red blood cell (RBC) fragmentation occurs because of the increased fragility of these large erythrocytes, which probably are damaged during their passage through the spleen. Basophilic stippling and Howell-Jolly bodies have also been described in RBCs. When the hematocrit value drops below 20% (0.20), nucleated RBCs may be found in the blood. Hypersegmentation of mature neutrophils is a characteristic feature that appears very early in the development of megaloblastic anemia and is a reflection of the nuclear maturation defect. Hypersegmentation can be manifested by cells with six or more nuclear lobes or by an elevation in the mean neutrophil lobe count.

Bone Marrow Examination. The bone marrow in patients with megaloblastic anemia is characteristically hypercellular with erythroid and granulocytic hyperplasia. Mitotic activity is abundant, but there is significant intramedullary cell death secondary to the nuclear maturation defect. The proliferating erythroid and myeloid cell lines show megaloblastic changes. In the erythroid elements, the major morphologic manifestation is nuclear-cytoplasmic asynchrony, in which the nuclei are large with finely dispersed chromatin, while the cytoplasm is more mature with hemoglobinization. The dominant myeloid abnormality is giantism of bands and metamyelocytes and nuclear hypersegmentation of mature granulocytes (Image 5-1). Large megakaryocytes have also been described.

Masking of erythroid megaloblastosis can occur because of concomitant iron deficiency, such as may be seen in pregnant women, patients with various malabsorption disorders, patients with chronic alcoholism, and approximately one third of patients with pernicious anemia. In these patients, the peripheral blood and bone marrow erythroid picture may be intermediate between that described in iron deficiency and in megaloblastic anemia, although the megaloblastic changes in the granulocytic cell line persist.

Other Laboratory Tests

The primary laboratory tests utilized in the diagnosis of megaloblastic anemias include measurements of serum vitamin B_{12}, serum folate, and RBC folate. Some features of these and other ancillary laboratory tests are shown in Table 5-8.

5.1 Serum Vitamin B_{12} Quantitation

Purpose. The level of vitamin B_{12} in the blood is a useful measure of the patient's vitamin B_{12} stores.

Principle. Most laboratories currently utilize a competitive protein-binding assay for this determination. In this assay, the patient's vitamin B_{12} competes with radiolabeled vitamin B_{12} for a fixed number of binding sites. The amount of radiolabeled vitamin B_{12} that is bound is inversely proportional to the patient's vitamin B_{12} level. Many current methodologies accommodate the simultaneous measurement of serum/plasma vitamin B_{12} and folate. (Note: Nonradioactive chemiluminescence techniques are also available.)

Specimen. Either serum or plasma (EDTA) is suitable for this test. Specimen must be separated and frozen if the test cannot be performed within 3 or 4 hours of collection.

Procedure. In this assay, the patient's serum or plasma is mixed with a constant amount of radiolabeled vitamin B_{12}, and boiled

Table 5-8 Laboratory Tests for Diagnosis of Megaloblastic Anemia

Test*	Specimen	Procedure
Vitamin B$_{12}$*	Serum/plasma	Competitive protein-binding assay using radiolabeled B$_{12}$ and purified IF†
Folate*	Serum/plasma	Competitive protein-binding assay using radiolabeled folate and folate-binding proteins†
RBC folate*	Lysed RBCs	Same assay as for folate except that lysed RBCs used†
LDH	Serum/heparinized plasma	LDH catalyzes oxidation of lactate to pyruvate with reduction of NAD to NADH Absorbance of NADH measured
Iron, IBC	Serum/heparinized plasma	See Chapter 2
IF antibodies	Serum	Competitive protein-binding assay
Parietal cell antibodies	Serum	Immunofluorescent test using sections of rat stomach and appropriate control tissues
Indirect bilirubin	Serum	See Chapter 6
Gastrin	Serum	Competitive protein-binding assay

Abbreviations: IF = intrinsic factor; PA = pernicious anemia; IBC = iron-binding capacity; LDH = lactate dehydrogenase; NAD = nicotinamide adenine dinucleotide; NADH = reduced nicotinamide adenine dinucleotide.

*Tests should be performed in all cases of suspected megaloblastic anemia; other tests are helpful in selected clinical settings.

†Nonradioactive chemiluminescence techniques also available.

Table 5-8 *Continued*

Interpretation	Notes and Precautions
Decreased in PA and other anemias secondary to vitamin B_{12} deficiency; may see moderate decrease in patient with severe folate deficiency	Test should use purified IF as binding protein, otherwise may get false normal results
Decreased in anemias due to folate deficiency; normal or increased in PA	False normal results in some patients with concurrent severe iron deficiency Levels fluctuate with diet Falsely elevated level with hemolyzed specimen
Since RBCs are metabolically inactive, RBC folate level reflects patient folate status at time these cells formed; level is decreased in folate and vitamin B_{12} deficiency	Because vitamin B_{12} is required for folate to enter cell, level is decreased in both B_{12} and folate deficiency
LDH is markedly elevated in megaloblastic anemia due to intramedullary destruction of cells	Hemolysis falsely elevates results
Serum iron, storage iron, and IBC all increased in megaloblastic anemias due to decreased iron utilization in erythropoiesis	See Chapter 2
Present in 50% of cases of PA	Very specific for PA but present in only about 50% of cases
Fluorescence of parietal cells in stomach sections (with negative controls) indicates that patient has parietal cell antibodies	Sensitive for PA (positive in 90% of cases) but also found in other disorders
Mildly increased in megaloblastic anemia due to hemolysis of some abnormal RBCs	See Chapter 6
Markedly increased in PA	

to inactivate endogenous binding proteins and to convert all of the vitamin B_{12} to cyanocobalamin. Following cooling, immobilized affinity-purified porcine intrinsic factor is added. This intrinsic factor is covalently coupled to polymer beads. During incubation the endogenous and labeled vitamin B_{12} proteins compete for the limited number of binding sites. The tubes are then centrifuged, decanted, and counted in a gamma counter to evaluate the radioactivity within the pellet. Standard curves are prepared using precalibrated standards.

Interpretation. Decreased vitamin B_{12} levels are seen in patients with pernicious anemia and any other type of megaloblastic anemia caused by vitamin B_{12} deficiency.

Notes and Precautions. The assay must utilize purified intrinsic factor to avoid falsely elevated results secondary to the binding of inactive cobalamin analogues to other binding proteins. In patients with pernicious anemia and coexisting disease, such as iron deficiency, liver disease, hemoglobinopathy, or myeloproliferative disorders, the vitamin B_{12} level may be normal or increased. Falsely low levels may be seen in patients with folate deficiency, pregnant women, women taking oral contraceptives, and patients with transcobalamin deficiency.

5.2 Serum Folate Quantitation

Purpose. Assays of serum folate, in conjunction with RBC folate, are useful in determining the status of the patient's folate stores.

Principle. Serum folate is currently measured using a competitive protein-binding assay analogous to that used for vitamin B_{12}. Using current methodologies, these two assays can be performed simultaneously. The amount of labeled folate that binds to folate-binding proteins is inversely proportional to the amount of the patient's folate. (Note: Nonradioactive chemiluminescence techniques are also available.)

Specimen. Either serum or plasma (EDTA) can be used for this test. The specimen must be separated and frozen if the test cannot be performed within 3 or 4 hours of collection.

Procedure. A constant amount of radiolabeled folate and folate-binding proteins is added to the patient sample. Following boiling to reduce folate, the mixture is cooled and immobilized. Folate binding proteins (coupled to polymer beads) are added. During incubation, the endogenous and labeled folate compete for binding sites on the folate-binding proteins. Following centrifugation, the supernatant is discarded and the radioactivity within the pellet is assessed on a gamma counter. Standard curves are prepared using precalibrated standards.

Interpretation. Decreased serum folate levels are detected in patients with megaloblastic anemia secondary to folate deficiency, while normal or increased levels of serum folate are found in patients with pernicious anemia.

Notes and Precautions. Because serum folate shows significant fluctuation with diet, a patient can have a normal serum folate level and actually be folate deficient. Folate deficiency can also be masked by a concurrent, more severe iron deficiency in which the serum and RBC folate levels may be within normal limits despite the fact that the patient is folate deficient. The reason for this phenomenon is unknown. Hemolyzed samples will give markedly elevated serum folate levels because of the large amounts of folate normally present in erythrocytes. Patients receiving methotrexate or leucovorin treatment will have falsely elevated folate levels secondary to the binding of these drugs to the folate-binding proteins used in the competitive protein-binding assay.

5.3 Red Blood Cell Folate Quantitation

Purpose. RBC folate determination is a more stable measurement of the status of the patient's folate stores than is serum folate. Since RBCs are metabolically inactive, the RBC folate levels reflect the patient's folate status at the time these cells were produced.

Principle.   RBC folate is measured by a competitive protein-binding assay analogous to that utilized for measuring serum folate.

Specimen.   Whole blood is collected in EDTA, which can be frozen or processed immediately. RBCs are lysed with ascorbic acid.

Procedure.   The procedure for the quantitation of RBC folate is the same as that used for serum folate (see Test 5.2).

Interpretation.   Because vitamin B_{12} cofactor is necessary for folate to enter and be retained within RBCs, decreased RBC folate is found in patients with either folate or vitamin B_{12} deficiency. Table 5-9 compares the serum vitamin B_{12}, serum folate, and RBC folate levels in patients with vitamin B_{12} deficiency, folate deficiency, or both.

Ancillary Tests

Several additional laboratory tests, including measurements of serum lactate dehydrogenase, bilirubin, serum and storage iron, intrinsic factor antibody, parietal cell antibody, gastrin, and Schilling and deoxyuridine suppression tests can be useful in evaluating patients with megaloblastic anemia. The expected values for these tests, along with the reason they are abnormal in megaloblastic anemia, are detailed in Table 5-8.

Parietal Cell and Intrinsic Factor Antibodies.   Most patients with pernicious anemia have parietal cell and intrinsic factor antibodies. Although parietal cell antibodies are more sensitive for pernicious anemia, they are also seen fairly frequently in patients with chronic gastritis. Antibodies to intrinsic factor are more specific for pernicious anemia but they are found only in about half of these patients.

Gastrin Test.   Gastrin stimulates parietal cells to secrete intrinsic factor and hydrochloric acid, and serum gastrin levels are typically markedly elevated in patients with pernicious anemia.

Table 5-9 Serum Vitamin B_{12}, Serum Folate, and RBC Folate Levels in Megaloblastic Anemia

Disorder	Serum Vitamin B_{12}	Serum Folate*	RBC Folate
Vitamin B_{12} deficiency	Decreased	Normal or increased	Decreased
Folate deficiency	Normal or decreased	Decreased	Decreased
Deficiency of both vitamin B_{12} and folate	Decreased	Decreased	Decreased

*Fluctuates with changes in dietary folate.

Recent evidence suggests that some parietal cell antibodies may be directed against the gastrin receptor on these cells, which explains the failure of parietal cells to respond to gastrin. The achlorhydria in gastric juices is secondary to the failure of the production of hydrochloric acid by parietal cells.

Schilling Test.   Although the three-part Schilling test is not used consistently today in the initial diagnosis of megaloblastic anemia, it may help to determine the etiology of a megaloblastic anemia in patients with ambiguous results on other tests. The first part of this test measures only the patient's ability to absorb vitamin B_{12}. Intrinsic factor and vitamin B_{12} are given to the patient in the second part of the Schilling test; the third part utilizes antibiotics to destroy bacteria and is designed to detect patients with bacterial overgrowth disorders. The patient ingests radiolabeled vitamin B_{12}, followed by an injection of a loading dose of unlabeled vitamin B_{12}. A 24-hour urine sample is collected and the amount of radioactivity in this sample is measured. In patients with pernicious anemia, the urinary excretion of labeled vitamin B_{12} will be normal only when intrinsic factor is given.

Several problems are common in performing the Schilling test. First, the collection of a 24-hour urine sample is cumbersome, and often an incomplete sample is submitted for evaluation. The patient must have normal renal function and normal intestinal mucosa for the test to be valid. In addition, some patients who cannot absorb dietary vitamin B_{12} can absorb the crystalline vitamin B_{12} that is used, giving a falsely normal result.

Deoxyuridine Suppression Test. A recently developed test of intranuclear vitamin B_{12} and folate levels, referred to as the deoxyuridine suppression test, is based on studies of thymidine synthesis. This test of cultured blood or bone marrow cells is designed to distinguish between the primary and salvage pathways utilized in thymidine synthesis. It assesses both vitamin B_{12} and folate levels, because cofactors of both of these vitamins are required in the primary metabolic pathway of thymidine synthesis. The salvage pathway is favored, however, when a deficiency of either folate or vitamin B_{12} exists. It is possible to test which one of these pathways is operating in the nucleus of the cell, because the salvage pathway can utilize a radioactive deoxyuridine substrate while the primary pathway cannot. If nucleated blood cells are deficient in either vitamin B_{12} or folate, the salvage pathway will be favored, resulting in increased incorporation of radioactive label into the cell's nucleus. With the addition of the deficient vitamin, the metabolic pathway reverts back to the primary synthetic pathway, and the radioactivity within the nucleus decreases. The nuclei of long-lived cells, such as lymphocytes, can be studied to determine the patient's vitamin B_{12} or folate status at the time these cells were last mitotically active. This information can be useful in selected cases when other test results fail to confirm a vitamin B_{12} or folate deficiency. Recent vitamin or folate therapy will not "mask" this test result, because long-lived cells can be studied.

Course and Treatment

Correction of the vitamin deficiency by either parenteral injections of vitamin B_{12} or oral doses of folate results in prompt improvement of the patient's hematologic abnormalities, with normalization of the hemogram within 4 to 8 weeks. Occasionally, patients with folate deficiency will need parenteral therapy until the gastrointestinal tract epithelium has regenerated. Patients with megaloblastic anemia should be evaluated carefully to determine the underlying cause of the vitamin deficiency.

Because the slow development of the anemia has allowed for some compensation, patients with megaloblastic anemia usually do not require transfusion; however, rare patients may present with cardiovascular decompensation requiring immediate treatment. Transfusion in this clinical situation must be considered very carefully because of possible further cardiac decompensation and death secondary to volume overload. Plasmapheresis with RBC infusions may prevent volume overload. Another cardiac complication that occurs in small numbers of patients receiving treatment for megaloblastic anemia is cardiac arrhythmia, which may result in sudden death. The postulated mechanism for this catastrophic complication is the precipitous decrease in potassium level that occurs following vitamin B_{12} therapy. Patients with megaloblastic anemia undergoing therapy may also develop thrombotic complications because of changes in platelet activity associated with restoration of normal vitamin B_{12} or folate levels in platelets.

Following vitamin therapy, there is a rapid and marked decline in the lactate dehydrogenase and plasma iron levels as well as a normalization of the serum bilirubin level. The megaloblastic changes in bone marrow erythroid precursors revert to normal within several days of treatment, followed by reversal of the megaloblastic changes within myeloid precursors a few days later. Reticulocytes can be identified in the peripheral blood within 3 to 5 days after treatment is begun, and they generally peak within 7 to 10 days. The height of the reticulocyte count is inversely proportional to the degree of anemia. Within 1 to 2 months, all peripheral blood parameters will have returned to normal.

In patients with pernicious anemia, the neurologic manifestations of this disorder generally improve substantially with vitamin B_{12} therapy, although they may not resolve entirely. There should be no progression of these neurologic defects, however, while the patient continues to receive parenteral vitamin B_{12} therapy. In patients with pernicious anemia, large doses of folate can reduce the hematologic abnormalities, but the neurologic disease will progress.

Prognosis is good for patients with megaloblastic anemia, provided the vitamin deficiency is adequately treated and the underlying disorder that led to the vitamin deficiency is identified and managed appropriately.

References

Beck WS. Diagnosis of megaloblastic anemia. *Annu Rev Med.* 1991;42:311-322.

Chanarin I, Deacon R, Lumb M, Perry J. Cobalamin and folate: recent developments. *J Clin Pathol.* 1992;45:277-283.

Fairbanks VF. Tests for pernicious anemia: the 'Schilling test.' *Mayo Clin Proc.* 1983;58:541-544.

Herbert V. Biology of disease: megaloblastic anemias. *Lab Invest.* 1985;52:3-19.

Herbert V. Making sense of laboratory tests of folate status: folate requirements to sustain normality. *Am J Hematol.* 1987;26:199-207.

Lindenbaum J. Status of laboratory testing in the diagnosis of megaloblastic anemia. *Blood.* 1983;61:624-627.

Peterson L, McKenna RW. Laboratory evaluation of megaloblastic anemia. In: Bick RL, Bennett JM, Brynes RK, et al, eds. *Hematology Clinical and Laboratory Practice, I.* St Louis, Mo: CV Mosby Co; 1993:459-469.

Scates S, Glaspy J. The macrocytic anemias. *Lab Med.* 1990;21:736-741.

Stebbins R, Scott J, Herbert V. Drug-induced megaloblastic anemias. *Semin Hematol.* 1973;10:235-251.

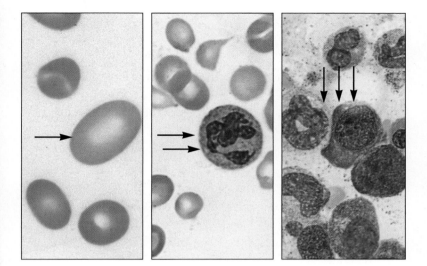

Image 5-1   This composite of blood and bone marrow aspirate smears illustrates the oval macrocytes (↑) , hypersegmentation of neutrophils (↑↑), and florid megaloblastic erythroid and granulocytic elements (↑↑↑) in a patient with megaloblastic anemia. (Wright's)

PART
II

Hemolytic Anemias

6

Accelerated Erythrocyte Turnover

Hemolysis is characterized by premature removal of circulating red blood cells and increased bone marrow production of replacement cells without an overt source of blood loss. This pattern of accelerated erythrocyte turnover is associated with a wide variety of hereditary and acquired hemolytic diseases (Table 6-1) that will be discussed in succeeding chapters.

Pathophysiology

In general, the life span of the red blood cell comprises three components: the bone marrow production phase, the circulating phase, and final removal of senescent or damaged cells. Establishment of a diagnosis of hemolysis requires evaluation of the various phases of the erythrocyte life cycle to demonstrate accelerated red blood cell turnover. Although the actual mechanisms for each phase are not known, their sequence and time course have been determined, allowing normal ranges to be established.

Red blood cells arise from a bone marrow stem cell, requiring approximately 6 days to differentiate from erythroblast to marrow reticulocyte. The daily production of red blood cells is estimated at

Table 6-1   Diseases Associated With Accelerated Erythrocyte Turnover

Inherent Defect in Hemolysis	Result
Hereditary disorders	
Membrane defects	Hereditary spherocytosis, hereditary elliptocytosis
Enzyme defects	G6PD deficiency, pyruvate kinase deficiency, glutathione pathway deficiency, other deficiencies of the pentose pathway
Hemoglobin defects	Amino acid substitutions: hemoglobin S, hemoglobin C, etc; Decreased production: thalassemias
Acquired or extrinsic disorders	
Infection	Bacterial: *Clostridium perfringens* Protozoal: malaria Viral: *Mycoplasma,* infectious mononucleosis
Physiochemical	Burns, benzene derivatives
Mechanical	Heart valve prosthesis (aortic), ulcerative colitis, hemolytic-uremic syndrome, TTP, DIC
Drugs	Interaction with G6PD deficiency, immune complexes
Antibody	Alloantibody: incompatible transfusion, fetal-maternal incompatibility Autoantibody: idiopathic, secondary to malignant lymphomas, collagen vascular diseases, viral infections, secondary to drugs
Membrane defects	Paroxysmal nocturnal hemoglobinuria

Abbreviations: G6PD = glucose-6-phosphate dehydrogenase; TTP = thrombotic thrombocytopenic purpura; DIC = disseminated intravascular coagulation.

3×10^9 cells per kilogram of body weight, which normally equals the rate of red blood cell destruction (1% per day). Marrow reticulocytes expel their nuclei before passing through marrow sinusoids into the peripheral blood as circulating reticulocytes, subsequently shedding the reticular network over 1 to 2 days in the circulation to become mature erythrocytes. Mature red blood cells circulate for about 120 days and are finally removed from circulation by activity of the reticuloendothelial system in the spleen, liver, and bone marrow.

A variety of processes may accelerate red blood cell destruction (Table 6-1). These include inherited or acquired abnormalities in red blood cell shape or size, abnormal membrane characteristics, immune or other physiochemical processes that damage red blood cells, and increased destruction by the spleen and other components of the reticuloendothelial system. The spleen removes marginally damaged red blood cells, the liver removes more severely damaged red blood cells, and intravascular hemolysis occurs with the most severe cell damage.

Red blood cell destruction releases heme, globin, and iron. Heme is broken down into biliverdin, reduced to bilirubin by biliverdin reductase in the reticuloendothelial system, conjugated to soluble monoglucuronides and diglucuronides in the liver, and excreted in the feces as urobilin, urobilinogen, and stercobilinogen. Minimal amounts of the soluble urobilinogen are reabsorbed from the portal circulation and excreted in the urine. Iron released from heme is taken up by the reticuloendothelial cells and is recycled for bone marrow synthesis of new red blood cells, or is stored in the reticuloendothelial cells as ferritin or hemosiderin. The globin peptide chains are degraded to component amino acids that return to the metabolic pool. Enzymes, such as lactate dehydrogenase (LDH), which are normally present within red blood cells, are also released with hemolysis. Accelerated red blood cell turnover results in accumulation of all breakdown products, many of which can be measured with relative ease.

When intravascular hemolysis occurs, free hemoglobin is released into the plasma where it is bound by the $alpha_2$-globulin, haptoglobin. The haptoglobin-hemoglobin complex is then metabolized directly by the reticuloendothelial system. If the binding capacity of haptoglobin is exceeded, free hemoglobin may be seen in the plasma or urine, resulting in hemoglobinemia and hemoglobinuria. Free hemoglobin may also be bound by transferrin and albumin. Oxidation of the ferrous ion of the albumin-heme complexes produces the brown pigment, methemalbumin.

Clinical Findings

A detailed and complete history including drug ingestion, transfusions, medical conditions, operations (such as insertion of heart valves), or a family history of hemolysis or jaundice is extremely important in determining a cause of accelerated red blood cell turnover. This historical information will narrow the large differential diagnosis of hemolysis, facilitating workup and laboratory testing for the patient. Clinical findings depend on the rate of hemolysis and the ability of the bone marrow to compensate for red blood cell destruction by increased red blood cell production. If the bone marrow is able to respond to hemolysis so that the hematocrit remains normal or near normal, the patient is said to have a well-compensated hemolytic anemia and symptoms may be minimal. However, in severe hemolysis when the bone marrow is unable to match the loss of red blood cells, rapid onset of severe anemia may occur. The most common symptoms of anemia are pallor and fatigue. Fever, chills, and headache may be associated with more acute hemolytic episodes. As larger numbers of red blood cells are broken down, there is increased evidence of hemoglobin catabolism. As normal metabolic pathways are overwhelmed, hemoglobinemia or hemoglobinuria results. With long-standing hemolysis, pigment gallstones may be formed.

Splenomegaly is variable. Chronic hemolysis may not be associated with splenomegaly, whereas acute hemolysis with increased reticuloendothelial activity may be associated with mild to moderate splenic enlargement. Hepatomegaly is less common but is usually associated with long-standing hemolysis, reticuloendothelial hyperplasia, and iron deposition. Lymphadenopathy is not characteristic of hemolytic anemia unless there is an underlying lymphoproliferative disorder. Bone pain, secondary to bone marrow erythroid hyperplasia, may be present with long-standing hemolysis.

Approach to Diagnosis

As previously emphasized, a good history and subsequent physical examination of the patient are essential in determining a cause of accelerated red blood cell turnover. The historical and physical information may then direct laboratory testing in an efficient and cost-effective manner (Table 6-2).

If accelerated red blood cell turnover is suspected, the rate of red blood cell turnover can be determined by evaluation of bone marrow production, calculation of circulating red blood cell sur-

Table 6-2   Laboratory Evaluation of Red Blood Cell
Production and Breakdown*

Phase of Life Cycle	Laboratory Tests or Findings
Bone marrow production	**Reticulocyte count**, bone marrow cellularity, ^{59}Fe uptake
Red blood cell circulation	**Hemoglobin/hematocrit**, ^{51}Cr red blood cell survival studies
Red blood cell sequestration	^{51}Cr red blood cell sequestration
Red blood cell breakdown	**Haptoglobin, bilirubin,** hemoglobinemia, methemalbumin, bone marrow iron, **lactate dehydrogenase**
Excretion	**Hemosiderinuria, hemoglobinuria**

*Boldface indicates most useful tests.

vival, and measurement of breakdown products of cell destruction. The following approach provides laboratory information allowing a diagnosis of accelerated red blood cell turnover to be made:

1. Peripheral blood smear morphology and red blood cell indices characterize the anemia. An elevated reticulocyte count indicates accelerated release of new red blood cells to the peripheral blood, and occasionally nucleated red blood cells may be seen.

2. Bone marrow aspiration, including stains for iron, is useful in documenting accelerated marrow erythroid production and breakdown. When the cause of a normochromic anemia is clearly hemolysis (eg, in hemoglobinopathies), bone marrow aspiration may be unnecessary.

3. Hemoglobin breakdown products in the plasma and urine can be measured. Since levels of these compounds increase with rapid destruction of red blood cells, they may provide a means whereby red blood cell destruction can be monitored. Tests for these products and their relative usefulness are summarized in Table 6-3. In episodes of acute hemolysis, bilirubin (total and fractionated), and plasma or urine hemoglobin are most commonly measured. In less acute or chronic compensated hemolysis, urine hemosiderin may be a more sensitive indicator of long-term occult red blood cell degradation.

Table 6-3   Urine and Serum Pigments in Accelerated
Erythrocyte Turnover

Pigment	Normal Range	Comments
Bilirubin, serum	0.5-2.0 mg/dL (8-34 μmol/L)	Limited significance; jaundice seen >3.0 mg/dL (52 μmol/L); fractionation may not be diagnostic in jaundiced patients.
Indirect bilirubin, serum	<0.5 mg/dL (8 μmol/L)	Increased early in hemolysis; physiologic elevation in hereditary conjugation disorders (Crigler-Najjar syndrome, Gilbert's disease)
Hemoglobin, plasma	≤10 mg/dL (1.6 μmol/L)	Significant above 50 mg/dL (8 μmol/L), cherry-red plasma >150 mg/dL (24 μmol/L), binds to haptoglobin, transferrin, or albumin
Hemoglobin, urine	None present	Appears after haptoglobin saturation, hematuria must be excluded, myoglobinuria gives false-positive result on dipstick test
Methemalbumin, serum	None present	Qualitative determination by haptoglobin electrophoresis or spectrophotometric measurement

Determination of bilirubin in compensated hemolytic anemia is of limited usefulness. Tests for urobilin and fecal and urine urobilinogen are unsatisfactory and unnecessary.

4. Serum haptoglobin is a useful test in the absence of overt intravascular hemolysis. Haptoglobin is consumed by the binding of free hemoglobin released from hemolyzed cells.

5. LDH is released into the plasma as red blood cells are rapidly destroyed. LDH_1 is an isoenzyme found predominantly in red blood cells and myocardium. Isoenzyme determinations are useful if the source of total LDH elevation is clearly derived from red blood cells.

6. Radioisotope tracer studies are usually not necessary and are rarely used unless other laboratory tests fail to document accelerated red blood cell turnover in the face of strong clin-

ical suspicion. Radioisotope studies are usually limited to chromium 51 (^{51}Cr)–labeled red blood cell studies, which estimate survival of circulating red blood cells and site of cell sequestration and destruction, and to kinetic studies with iron 59 (^{59}Fe), which is incorporated into precursor erythrocytes and evaluates rate of production, site of production, rate of red blood cell release, and site of sequestration. ^{51}Cr red blood cell survival studies require 3 weeks, but abbreviated tests of 1 hour are also performed. Ferrokinetics using ^{59}Fe are not commonly available, but can be combined with ^{51}Cr sequestration studies to determine sites of production (bone marrow or extramedullary), and are helpful if splenectomy is being considered. Since ^{59}Fe has a longer half-life than ^{51}Cr, ^{59}Fe studies should follow chromium studies.

7. Ancillary screening tests, as summarized in Table 6-4, are used to document the cause of accelerated erythrocyte turnover once its presence has been established. These tests are discussed at greater length in subsequent chapters.

Hematologic Findings

Accelerated red blood cell destruction or loss stimulates increased bone marrow production. This results in premature release of bone marrow reticulocytes that appear on Wright's-stained peripheral smears as polychromatophilic macrocytes. Nucleated red blood cells may also be seen in prolonged or severe hemolytic anemia. With increased cellular destruction and a competent bone marrow, the reticulocyte count is persistently elevated. Reticulocytosis varies with severity and duration of hemolysis. Bone marrow production may increase fourfold to sixfold, permitting reticulocyte counts as high as 60% to 70%. Chronic hemolysis may deplete bone marrow levels of folic acid, decreasing the ability of the bone marrow to mount a reticulocytosis adequate for the degree of anemia. In acute blood loss, the reticulocytosis is of brief duration and usually less than 5%.

The spleen may be enlarged as a result of increased phagocytosis. In some cases, particularly hereditary hemolytic anemias, the liver is also enlarged. Depending on the rate of red blood cell

Table 6-4 Common Screening Tests for Causes of Accelerated Erythrocyte Turnover

Inherent Cause of Hemolysis	Test
Hereditary	
Membrane defects	Red blood cell morphologic studies, osmotic fragility
Enzyme defects	G6PD screening, pyruvate kinase screening
Hemoglobin defects	Hemoglobin electrophoresis, Heinz body test, hemoglobin A_2 and hemoglobin F quantitation
Acquired or extrinsic	
Infection	Red blood cell morphologic studies, malarial smears, cultures
Physiochemical—burns	Red blood cell morphologic studies—spherocytes
Mechanical—intravascular fibrin, prosthetic valves	Red blood cell morphologic studies—schistocytes
Drugs—interaction with enzyme defect	G6PD screening
Drug-induced antibody	Antibody screening with drug-treated cells
Alloantibody or autoantibody	DAT, serum antibody screening, cold agglutinin titer, Donath-Landsteiner test
Membrane defects—PNH	Acid hemolysis test; sucrose lysis test

Abbreviations: G6PD = glucose-6-phosphate dehydrogenase; DAT = direct antiglobulin test; PNH = paroxysmal nocturnal hemoglobinuria.

destruction and the ability of the liver to conjugate and excrete the degradation products, variable degrees of jaundice may be present.

Blood Cell Measurements.   Anemia can be mild (hemoglobin, 11.5 g/dL [115 g/L]) to severe (hemoglobin, 2 g/dL [20 g/L]). Mean corpuscular volume (MCV) is 80 to 110 μm^3 (80-110 fL) as reticulocytes may produce a mild macrocytosis. An MCV greater than 115 μm^3 (115 fL) suggests macrocytic anemia or, rarely, secondary folate depletion. A MCV less than 70 μm^3 (70 fL) in a normochromic anemia suggests hemolysis is due to hemoglobinopathy or paroxysmal nocturnal hemoglobinuria (PNH).

Peripheral Blood Smear Morphology.   Morphologic characteristics generally include polychromatophilia, macrocytes, and nucleated red blood cells in severe cases. The specific appearance of red blood cells is variable, depending on the etiology of red blood cell turnover, and may include:

1. Spherocytes—hereditary spherocytosis, autoimmune hemolytic anemia, ABO fetal-maternal incompatibility, burns.
2. Target cells—hemoglobinopathies, jaundice, postsplenectomy.
3. Cell fragments—hemolytic-uremic syndrome, thrombotic thrombocytopenic purpura (TTP), disseminated intravascular coagulation (DIC), prosthetic valves.

Bone Marrow Examination. The bone marrow is hypercellular with marked normoblastic erythroid hyperplasia. Dyssynchronous nuclear and cytoplasmic maturation may create megaloblastoid cells without giant metamyelocytes or other stigmata of vitamin deficiency. If folic acid or vitamin B_{12} are relatively depleted by prolonged rapid turnover, a true megaloblastic cell population may appear. Bone marrow exhaustion with resultant aplasia can eventually result. Special staining of particle smears with ferroferricyanide (Prussian blue) shows increased reticuloendothelial iron. Sideroblastic iron is often increased and may form ring sideroblasts when ineffective erythropoiesis is present. Absence of stainable iron in hemolysis suggests PNH. In hemolysis, if normoblasts contain stainable iron granules, they are often larger than usual and cover the nucleus.

Other Laboratory Tests

6.1 Serum Bilirubin, Total and Fractionated

Purpose. Increases in indirect bilirubin in the clinical setting of jaundice support the diagnosis of hemolysis.

Principle. Hyperbilirubinemia indicates increased red blood cell destruction, failure of liver conjugation, or block of excretory pathways. In hemolysis, an increased bilirubin load is presented to the liver faster than conjugation can proceed so that non–water soluble (indirect) fraction of bilirubin is increased. In liver failure or obstructive jaundice, conjugation results in direct hyperbilirubinemia.

Specimen.   Serum specimens are stable for days when refrigerated.

Procedure.   Bilirubin levels are measured with an internationally standardized test, generally using the Evelyn-Malloy method or a modification. Bilirubin is coupled with a diazo dye, and the color is quantitated spectrophotometrically at 450 nm at 1 minute. The quick-reacting fraction is considered to be direct (or conjugated) bilirubin. The total bilirubin is measured after the addition of alcohol, and the indirect fraction is calculated by subtracting the amount of direct bilirubin from the total.

Interpretation.   Normal ranges for total bilirubin are 0 to 1.5 mg/dL (0-25.65 µmol/L), and for indirect bilirubin, less than 0.3 mg/dL (5.13 µmol/L). Levels of total bilirubin above 42.75 µmol/L (2.5 mg/dL) are usually associated with clinical jaundice. Bilirubin levels depend on the ability of the liver to compensate for increased levels of heme breakdown products. Initially, more than half the bilirubin will be in the indirect or unconjugated fraction. If liver function is adequate, after several days the hepatic rate of glucuronide conjugation increases so that direct and indirect fractions are nearly equal, and bilirubin fractionation is no longer diagnostic.

In well-compensated hemolytic anemia, levels of total bilirubin may be less than 3 mg/dL (51.3 µmol/L) and no clinical jaundice is seen. Thus, bilirubin levels should not be used to exclude the diagnosis of accelerated red blood cell turnover.

In hemolytic disease of the newborn, the lipid-soluble, indirect-fraction bilirubin is deposited in the striate nucleus of the brain, producing kernicterus. In the newborn, a shift in conjugation from indirect to direct bilirubin usually occurs at 7 to 10 days as liver function matures.

Notes and Precautions.   Misleading elevations of indirect bilirubin can be seen in hereditary disorders of conjugation

(Crigler-Najjar syndrome, Gilbert's disease) and secondary to steroids found in breast milk that interfere with conjugation of bilirubin (breast milk jaundice).

6.2 Plasma Hemoglobin Quantitation

Purpose. Increased plasma hemoglobin indicates intravascular hemolysis. Qualitative assessment is usually sufficient for detecting acute intravascular hemolysis. Quantitation is useful in sera where other pigments (eg, bilirubin) make interpretation of plasma color uncertain.

Principle. Massive red blood cell injury results in intravascular hemolysis, which is seen macroscopically as cherry-red plasma. Free hemoglobin can be quantitated with a modified benzidine reaction that measures oxidation of benzidine by hydrogen peroxide.

Specimen. Five milliliters of blood is collected in heparin or ethylenediaminetetraacetic acid (EDTA). A clot is not a desirable specimen because mechanical hemolysis of red blood cells during clot formation does not allow for the most accurate measurement. Blood must be drawn atraumatically, and plasma should be separated within 1 to 2 hours.

Procedure. A modified benzidine (see "Notes and Precautions") reaction oxidizes a colorless benzidine dye to violet-blue in the presence of hemoglobin and hydrogen peroxide. The color is measured spectrophotometrically at 515 nm or with a photoelectric colorimeter. Quantitation often requires a reference laboratory.

Interpretation. The normal level of plasma hemoglobin is less than 10 mg/dL (1.6 μmol/L). At low levels, test variability is great, and thus the test is only reliable above 50 mg/dL (8 μmol/L), which is the threshold for visual estimation. Free hemoglobin levels less than 30 mg/dL (4.8 μmol/L) are technically inaccurate, and may be seen with difficult venipuncture, mechanical destruction of red blood cells by Vacutainer tubes, or during clotting of the specimen. Hemoglobinemia above 150 mg/dL (24 μmol/L) results in hemoglobinuria. At levels above 200 mg/dL (32 μmol/L), the plasma becomes clear cherry red.

Notes and Precautions. Benzidine may not be available as a result of federal regulations limiting potentially carcinogenic agents in the environment. Ortholidine (*o*-tolidine) may be substituted.

Spectrophotometric results may be falsely high if the serum contains peroxidases or other oxidants that increase the development of color in the benzidine reaction.

6.3   Serum Haptoglobin Quantitation

Purpose. Absence of haptoglobin indicates hemolysis, liver failure, or, rarely, a hereditary variant.

Principle. Haptoglobin is an alpha$_2$-globulin produced in the liver that binds free hemoglobin on a molecule-for-molecule basis. The haptoglobin-hemoglobin complex is metabolized in the reticuloendothelial system, maintaining serum hemoglobin levels below renal thresholds. During intravascular hemolysis, haptoglobin is completely saturated. The excess hemoglobin is then bound by other serum proteins (hemopexin, transferrin, and albumin) before spilling into the urine as hemoglobinuria. Absence of haptoglobin implies saturation and degradation due to hemolysis, or, alternatively, failure of production due to liver failure. Rare abnormal haptoglobins (such as Hp°) are genetic variants that do not bind hemoglobin but are of little clinical significance.

Specimen. Fresh serum is obtained atraumatically. To avoid extraneous hemolysis, serum should not be allowed to remain on red blood cells. Testing specimens with macroscopic hemoglobinemia is superfluous.

Procedure.   The haptoglobin molecule has separate sites for antibody and for hemoglobin binding. Haptoglobin is quantitated with turbidimetric methods using a nephelometer. Antihaptoglobin is added to the patient's serum forming immune complexes with serum haptoglobin (1:1). These immune complexes will scatter light proportionate to their concentration. Most larger hospitals have nephelometers.

Interpretation.   The normal range for haptoglobin is 40 to 180 mg/dL (0.4-1.8 g/L). Less than 25 mg/dL (0.25 g/L) of haptoglobin is consistent with hemolysis. Haptoglobin is an acute-phase reactant, increasing three to four times in inflammation, infection, or tissue necrosis (eg, pneumonia or myocardial infarction). Such increases may mask increased binding of hemoglobin in hemolysis. Haptoglobin levels greater than 200 mg/dL (2.0 g/L) are consistent with inflammation and not helpful in the diagnosis of hemolysis.

Molecular sites for hemoglobin binding are not the same as those for antibody binding by antihaptoglobin. With radial immunodiffusion, false elevations of haptoglobin may appear, since saturated haptoglobin-hemoglobin complexes are also measured if not removed by the reticuloendothelial system.

Haptoglobin is decreased or absent in liver failure, after recent massive transfusion due to removal of senescent transfused red blood cells, and in some abnormally functioning haptoglobin molecules (eg, Hp°).

6.4   Direct Antiglobulin Test (DAT)—Direct Coombs' Test

Purpose.   Detection of globulin adsorbed to the patient's red blood cells suggests immune mechanisms may be an underlying cause of hemolysis.

Principle.   Rabbit antihuman globulin reagent will agglutinate human red blood cells that are coated with human globulin. Broad-spectrum reagents agglutinate cells coated with IgG,

IgM, and/or complement. Monospecific serums agglutinate only red blood cells coated with the specific globulin (ie, IgG, IgM, or complement) to which the reagent is directed.

Specimen. Use of the red blood cells from EDTA specimens prevents nonspecific absorption of complement in specimens. Specimens must be maintained at 37°C until cells and serum have been separated.

Procedure. The patient's red blood cells are saline washed and centrifuged with antiglobulin reagent. Agglutination is graded from 0 to 4+. The adsorbed globulin must be eluted and tested for activity against red blood cells before it is classified as an antibody.

Interpretation. Weakly positive results (+/-) are not usually clinically significant and eluates are generally not successful. Strongly positive tests (2 to 4+) due to antibody may not correlate with the degree of hemolysis. Common causes of positive DAT tests that are not associated with hemolysis include multiple myeloma and cephalosporin therapy. A negative DAT result does not exclude hemolysis if red blood cell destruction has been massive and complete, as in incompatible transfusions.

Notes and Precautions. Refrigeration of blood specimens containing cold agglutinins may cause false-positive results or exaggerates positive results by the cold absorption of the agglutinin and complement.

6.5 Other Serum Pigments

Principle. For the most part, measurement of methemalbumin is not necessary for documentation of hemolysis; however, it may be useful in specialized cases. The presence of methemalbumin indicates chronic or continuing hemolysis, and may be used as a marker of hemolysis, particularly when it is induced by overconsumption of oxidizing agents. Free hemoglobin dissociates into α β dimers and binds to plasma proteins, including haptoglobin, transferrin, and albumin. The ferrous iron of hemoglobin bound to albumin will oxidize to ferric iron, forming methemalbumin, which gives a distinctive rusty appearance to serum. Free hemoglobin in the presence of chloride ion produces hematin, which is bound by the protein hemopexin. Tests for methemalbumin are available in reference laboratories. Methemalbumin is not present in a healthy patient and clears within 4 or 5 days of the cessation of hemolysis. Tests for hemopexin are not generally available. Hemopexin has a normal range of 80 to 100 mg/dL (0.8-1.0 g/L). Levels less than 40 mg/dL (0.4 g/L) indicate hemolysis.

Ancillary Tests

Urine Hemoglobin and Hemosiderin. Hemoglobinuria indicates concurrent or recent hemoglobinemia above the renal excretion threshold of 150 mg/dL (1.5 g/L). It usually appears as cloudy, smoky, dark-red, or cola-colored urine. It may be qualitatively detected by peroxidase reaction of *o*-tolidine or benzidine, which produces a blue color. In the absence of detectable hemoglobin, urine hemosiderin indicates ongoing hemolysis. Even in occult hemolysis, heme is deposited in renal epithelial cells and oxidized to hemosiderin.

In a healthy patient, no urinary hemoglobin or hemosiderin is detectable. Urinary sediments that contain significant numbers of red blood cells usually produce some free hemoglobin in hypotonic or alkaline urines. False-positive results may be seen with hematuria or myoglobinuria, and electrophoresis may be required to identify the process. Hemosiderin granules must be intracellular to have significance.

Total Lactic Dehydrogenase (LDH). LDH increases with either normal or pathologic cell destruction as cytoplasmic glycolytic enzymes, including LDH, are released to the plasma.

Total LDH is usually measured with spectrophotometric kinetic analysis of the reduced form of nicotinamide-adenine dinucleotide (NADH) production. Serum LDH catalyzes the reaction:

$$\text{Lactate} + \text{NAD} \rightarrow \text{Pyruvate} + \text{NADH}$$

NADH absorbs light at 340 nm, so LDH activity can be detected spectrophotometrically by increasing absorbance.

Laboratory Test Selection

Documentation of accelerated red blood cell turnover may usually be made on the basis of peripheral blood smear morphology, red blood cell indices, reticulocyte count, possible bone marrow examination, serum haptoglobin levels, and demonstration of elevation of hemoglobin breakdown products such as serum bilirubin, plasma or urine hemoglobin, or urine hemosiderin. Other tests, such as radioisotopic studies, are rarely required.

Evaluation of accelerated red blood cell turnover may make use of a myriad of different laboratory tests dependent on the etiology of the process. By obtaining a good clinical history and physical examination, test selection can be streamlined and directed to document the cause of hemolysis in a cost-efficient and logical manner. Thus, patients with a family history of hemolysis could undergo workup for heritable disorders of the red blood cell membrane or hemoglobin synthesis, whereas these tests may not be chosen in an elderly patient with acute onset of hemolysis, no family history, and recent onset of generalized lymphadenopathy and splenomegaly.

References

Erslev AJ. Erythrokinetics. In: Williams WJ, Beutler E, Erslev AJ, et al, eds. *Hematology*. 4th ed. New York, NY: McGraw-Hill International Book Co; 1990:414-422.

LaCelle PL. Destruction of erythrocytes. In: Williams WJ, Beutler E, Erslev AJ, et al, eds. *Hematology*. 4th ed. New York, NY: McGraw-Hill International Book Co; 1990:398-406.

Mayer K, Freeman JE. Techniques for measuring red cell, platelet, and WBC survival. *CRC Crit Rev Clin Lab Sci*. 1986;23:201-217.

7

Hereditary Erythrocyte Membrane Defects

Hereditary abnormalities in red blood cell shape include hereditary spherocytosis and hereditary elliptocytosis (ovalocytosis). These are usually secondary to inheritance of abnormal integral proteins underlying the red blood cell membrane that function to maintain cellular shape, membrane stability, or cellular flexibility. Abnormalities in these proteins may lead to increased hemolysis, as in hereditary spherocytosis, or may have little effect on red blood cell life span, as in most cases of hereditary elliptocytosis.

Pathophysiology

The red blood cell membrane is composed of a lipid bilayer with associated proteins overlying and linked to a protein network, called the membrane cytoskeleton. This structural configuration allows the red blood cell to have enough flexibility to squeeze through capillaries without fragmentation, yet regain a stable biconcave shape in larger vessels without loss of cellular integrity. The membrane skeleton is formed by interactions of a number of proteins, including spectrin, actin, ankyrin, and a protein termed band 4.1.

Hereditary spherocytosis is the most common type of hereditary hemolytic anemia among individuals of Northern European origin, but it occurs in all races throughout the world. It is seen in about 1 of 5,000 individuals in the United States. The inheritance is autosomal dominant. Therefore, it is to be expected that one of the patient's parents will be affected and that each of the patient's children will have a 50% chance of inheriting the disorder. In this disease, a primary defect in membrane stability is caused by a quantitative decrease in the amount of spectrin, or more rarely by formation of an abnormal spectrin that does not interact with other proteins within the red blood cell skeleton. This causes a progressive loss of the red blood cell membrane within the circulation, leading to the formation of spherocytes. Spherocytes are less flexible than normal red blood cells, leading to retention within the spleen with further loss of cellular membrane and premature cellular destruction.

Hereditary elliptocytosis is a heterogeneous group of disorders characterized by the finding of elliptocytes in the peripheral blood smear. These represent red blood cells that have failed to regain their normal biconcave shape following passage through the microcirculation. A wide variety of red blood cell membrane skeletal defects have been associated with hereditary elliptocytosis, including dysfunctional spectrin molecules, decreased spectrin content, and band 4.1 defects or deficiency. Unlike patients with hereditary spherocytosis, 90% of patients with hereditary elliptocytosis will not experience clinically significant hemolysis. Hereditary elliptocytosis is also usually inherited as an autosomal dominant trait.

Clinical Findings

The chronic hemolytic state in hereditary spherocytosis varies widely in severity, ranging from an asymptomatic compensated hemolysis to a moderately severe chronic anemia. The age at which the diagnosis is made is usually reflective of the severity of the hemolytic process, with the more severe forms of the disease being diagnosed early in childhood. Clinical manifestations are usually first noted in children or adolescents. Typical complaints include mild jaundice and nonspecific manifestations of anemia, such as weakness. Because of an increased bilirubin turnover, patients with this condition have a high incidence of pigment gallstones. Usually, patients can maintain normal hemoglobin levels due to increased red blood cell production by the bone marrow. However, infection or other stress may lead to acute anemic episodes due to increased splenic activity (hemolytic crisis) or decreased bone marrow production (aplastic crisis). The most consistently positive physical finding is splenomegaly, which may be marked. A variable degree of jaundice and scleral icterus is frequently seen. The most consistent and therapeutically important feature of hereditary spherocytosis is the clinical cure by splenectomy of hemolytic anemia. Red blood cell life span after this procedure is restored to normal or near normal.

Hereditary elliptocytosis may present either as a primary cosmetic disorder with little or no hemolysis, or much more rarely, with a moderately severe hemolytic anemia. Patients with the usual form of hereditary elliptocytosis will have no anemia or splenomegaly. The hemolytic forms of the disease, composing about 10% of cases, may have splenomegaly and often show spherocytes and fragmented red blood cells, in addition to elliptocytes, on the peripheral blood smear.

Approach to Diagnosis

A diagnosis of hereditary spherocytosis should be suspected in patients with chronic hemolytic anemia, especially when spherocytes are seen on the peripheral blood smear. Because of the autosomal dominant inheritance of the disorder, family studies are an important part of the diagnostic evaluation. Sometimes examination of the blood of family members reveals spherocytosis, even when there is no history of anemia, jaundice, or gallstones. This reflects the very mild expression of hereditary spherocytosis in some affected individuals. Rarely, the disorder can arise as a new mutation, without a positive family history.

Splenectomy will abolish the hemolysis in hereditary spherocytosis. If significant hemolysis persists after splenectomy in a patient presumed to have hereditary spherocytosis, the presumptive diagnosis is incorrect. Evaluation of a patient presumed to have hereditary spherocytosis includes the following:

1. Hematologic evaluation, with attention to red blood cell morphologic characteristics, the mean corpuscular hemoglobin concentration (MCHC), and the reticulocyte count.
2. An osmotic fragility test (see Test 7.1) to confirm the presence of spherocytosis.
3. A direct antiglobulin test (see Test 6.4) to rule out autoimmune hemolytic anemia as a cause for spherocytosis.
4. If the diagnosis is in doubt, estimation of red blood cell glycolytic or hexose monophosphate shunt enzyme activities (see Chapters 8 and 9) may be useful.

Elliptocytes are readily identified on the stained blood film (Image 7-1). Because this generally represents a benign anomaly, hereditary elliptocytosis should only be considered the cause of anemia when evidence for hemolysis, such as an elevated reticulocyte count, is found.

Hematologic Findings

Blood Cell Measurements.   Hemoglobin levels in patients with hereditary spherocytosis and hemolytic elliptocytosis frequently range between 9 and 12 g/dL (90-120 g/L), and the mean corpuscular volume (MCV) is usually in the normal range but may be elevated in the presence of prominent reticulocytosis. The MCHC characteristically is elevated to levels as high as 37 g/dL (370 g/L) (normal, 26-34 g/dL [260-340 g/L]) due to membrane loss without loss of cellular hemoglobin. The reticulocyte count usually ranges between 5% and 15% (0.05-0.15). The degree of reticulocytosis is characteristically greater than that in other hemolytic anemias with similar hemoglobin levels.

Peripheral Blood Smear Morphology.   The central morphologic finding in hereditary spherocytosis is the presence of spherocytes on the peripheral blood film. Spherocytes appear as densely staining red blood cells that are slightly smaller than normal with decreased or absent central pallor (Image 7-2). The increased intensity of staining is caused, in part, by increased cellular thickness due to the spherical shape and the increased MCHC. In mild forms of the disease, spherocytes may not be present in large numbers, and the appearance of red blood cells may vary greatly in different parts of the blood smear. Improper technique in preparing the smear may result in the appearance of artifactual spherocytes to an inexperienced observer. Prominent macrocytosis and polychromasia may be present in association with very high reticulocyte counts.

Elliptocytosis is diagnosed when most or all of the cells on the smear have an oval shape with a long diameter that is two or more times the short diameter (Image 7-1).

Bone Marrow Examination. The bone marrow characteristically shows normoblastic erythroid hyperplasia when significant hemolysis occurs. During aplastic crises, erythroid precursors are diminished and evidence of viral infection may be seen.

Other Laboratory Tests

7.1 Osmotic Fragility Test

Purpose. The osmotic fragility test indirectly measures the presence of spherocytes.

Principle. The osmotic fragility test measures the ability of the red blood cell to swell, a property that reflects the cellular surface-to-volume ratio. In a hypotonic medium, red blood cells take up water until the osmotic pressure inside the cell is reduced to that outside the cell. The red blood cell membrane normally has enough redundancy so that the volume of the cell can increase to about 1.8 times the resting volume before reaching the critical hemolytic volume where further entry of water produces lysis. A cell that is spherocytic in the resting state has less membrane redundancy than a normal biconcave cell so that less water can enter before cellular rupture occurs.

Table 7-1 Normal Values for Osmotic Fragility Tests

NaCl (%)	Lysis (%)	
	Fresh	Incubated
0.20	97-100	95-100
0.30	97-100	85-100
0.35	90-99	75-100
0.40	50-90	65-100
0.45	5-45	55-95
0.50	0-5	40-85
0.55	0	15-70
0.60	0	0-40
0.65	0	0-10
0.70	0	0-5
0.75	0	0

Specimen. Blood freshly drawn into heparin or ethylenedi-aminetetraacetic acid (EDTA) is used.

Procedure. The osmotic fragility test is performed by adding small volumes of blood to a series of tubes containing buffered salt solutions with an osmolarity equivalent to that of a 0.2% to 0.9% NaCl solution. A control tube contains distilled water. After standing at room temperature for 1 hour, the tubes are centrifuged, and the percentage of hemolyzed cells is estimated by measuring the amount of hemoglobin released into the supernatant solution by absorbance at 540 nm. The tests should be carried out on freshly drawn blood and, and if necessary, on blood that has been incubated at 37°C for 24 hours. Incubated osmotic fragility tests are more sensitive at detecting low levels of hemolysis. This may be useful when hereditary spherocytosis is suspected clinically, but the levels of hemolysis seen with fresh blood are within normal ranges. However, the increase in sensitivity for detection of osmotic fragility is offset by a loss of specificity in the incubated test.

Interpretation. The normal range of values for the osmotic fragility test is presented in Table 7-1 and Figure 7-1. Increased osmotic fragility is an essential diagnostic feature of hereditary

Figure 7-1 Osmotic fragility of normal red blood cells and those from a patient with hereditary spherocytosis. Normal ranges are shown in the shaded areas for fresh red blood cells (A and C) and for red blood cells incubated at 37°C for 24 hours (B and D). The hemolysis curve for normal red blood cells is shown in A and C. The hemolysis curve for a patient with hereditary spherocytosis is shown in B and D.

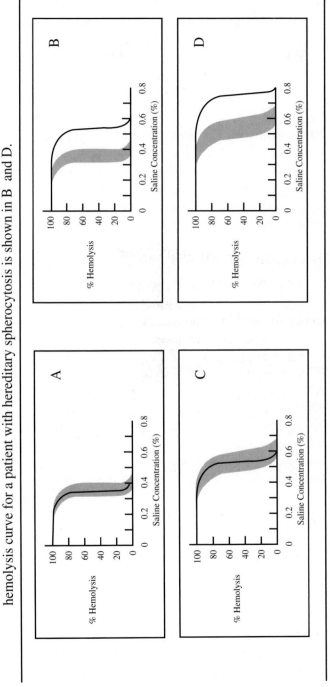

spherocytosis. It is not uncommon, however, in mild forms of the disease to find a minimal increase in osmotic fragility on freshly drawn blood. Incubated osmotic fragility tests are almost always abnormal in such cases. Decreases in hemolysis are seen in thalassemia, iron deficiency, and other conditions where there is an increase in the surface area-to-volume ratio for the red blood cell (eg, in some forms of liver disease).

Notes and Precautions. Because an increased osmotic fragility merely reflects the presence of spherocytes, this finding does not distinguish hereditary spherocytosis from autoimmune hemolytic disease with spherocytosis, in which the osmotic fragility of red blood cells is also increased, although to a lesser degree. Reporting osmotic fragility as percent saline concentrations for beginning and completion of hemolysis is an inadequate representation of test results. Osmotic fragility is best appreciated when reported graphically (Figure 7-1).

Course and Treatment

Both hereditary spherocytosis and elliptocytosis are essentially benign disorders. Complications that may occur include the development of cholelithiasis and cholecystitis, and the occurrence of aplastic or hemolytic crises, particularly after infections. Splenectomy will prolong red blood cell survival in hereditary spherocytosis and hemolytic forms of elliptocytosis. However, this may not be required if the bone marrow can compensate for the anemia by increasing red blood cell production.

References

Davies KA, Lux SE. Hereditary disorders of the red cell membrane. *Trends Genet.* 1989;5:222-227.

Godal HC, Gjonnes G, Ruyter R. Does preincubation of the red blood cells contribute to the capability of the osmotic fragility test to detect very mild forms of hereditary spherocytosis? *Scand J Haematol.* 1982;29:89-93.

Palek J. Hereditary elliptocytosis and related disorders. In: Williams WJ, Beutler E, Erslev A, et al, eds. *Hematology.* 4th ed. New York, NY: McGraw-Hill International Book Co; 1990:569-581.

Palek J. Hereditary spherocytosis. In: Williams WJ, Beutler E, Erslev A, et al, eds. *Hematology.* 4th ed. New York, NY: McGraw-Hill International Book Co; 1990:582-590.

Palek J, Sahr KE. Mutations of the red cell membrane proteins: from clinical evaluation to detection of the underlying genetic defect. *Blood.* 1992;80:308-330.

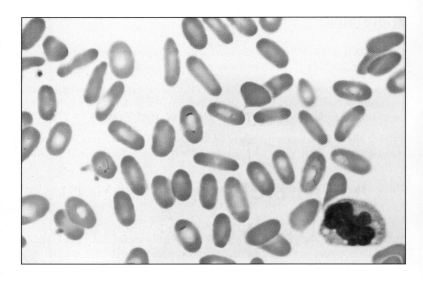

Image 7-1 Elliptocytes.

Image 7-2 Spherocytes. (↑)

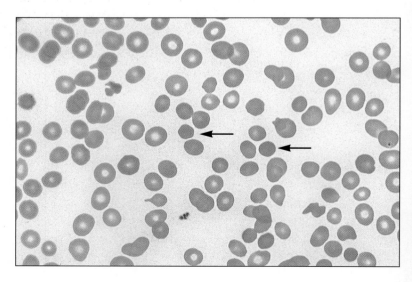

8

Hereditary Erythrocyte Disorders Due to Deficiencies of the Glycolytic Pathway

Mature red blood cells have the capacity for a limited number of enzymatic reactions. Thus, the majority of the cell's energy requirements are met by metabolism of glucose to lactate via the glycolytic or Embden-Meyerhof pathway. Hereditary deficiencies of many glycolytic enzymes have been documented, and several of these deficiencies cause a hereditary nonspherocytic hemolytic anemia. Most of these enzymatic deficiencies are rare, with less than 100 cases in the literature. Pyruvate kinase deficiency is seen slightly more frequently, with more than 300 cases in the literature.

Pathophysiology

Glucose is the main metabolic substrate of red blood cells. Because the mature erythrocyte does not contain mitochondria, it must depend entirely on anaerobic glycolysis to produce energy in the form of adenosine triphosphate (ATP) and reduced nicotinamide-adenine dinucleotide (NADH), an essential coenzyme for the reduction of methemoglobin. About 90% of glucose metabolism occurs by way of the main glycolytic pathway (Embden-Meyerhof pathway), in which glucose is metabolized to lactate in a series of enzymatic reactions (Figure 8-1). There is a net generation of 2 mol of ATP for each mole of glucose that is metabolized. ATP functions in initiating further glycolysis, allowing active cationic transport across the cellular membrane and membrane protein phosphorylation. 2,3-Diphosphoglycerate (2,3-DPG), which alters the hemoglobin oxygen affinity and regulates oxygen delivery to tissues, is an intermediate in this pathway.

About 10% of glucose is metabolized via the hexose monophosphate shunt (HMP shunt), bypassing the early steps of the main glycolytic pathway and generating reduced nicotinamide-adenine dinucleotide phosphate (NADPH). NADPH is required for reduction of glutathione, which is essential for the protection of hemoglobin and red blood cell enzymes from oxidative damage (see Chapter 9).

Hereditary nonspherocytic hemolytic anemia (HNSHA) is characterized by hemolytic anemia, first observed during infancy or childhood, lacking significant numbers of spherocytes and exhibiting normal osmotic fragility. HNSHA is known to be due to a heterogeneous group of disorders, including glycolytic pathway deficiencies (Table 8-1), the most important of which is pyruvate kinase deficiency. Other observed causes of HNSHA include the unstable hemoglobins and disorders of the enzymes of the HMP shunt and glutathione metabolism (Table 8-2).

Clinical Findings

Most cases of HNSHA manifest in childhood or infancy with chronic hemolysis, often associated with splenomegaly. In contrast to deficiencies of the HMP shunt pathway, there is no association with drug ingestion. Patients with triosephosphate isomerase deficiency, phosphoglycerate kinase (PGK) deficiency, or glutathione synthetase deficiency may also have neurologic manifestations associated with their disease.

Most deficiencies of the glycolytic pathway are extremely rare. Pyruvate kinase deficiency, although infrequently seen, is the most prevalent deficiency, accounting for about 90% of cases of HNSHA associated with glycolytic pathway deficiencies. Pyruvate kinase deficiency is inherited as an autosomal recessive trait, similar to most other deficiencies of the glycolytic pathway. Thus, a

Figure 8-1 The glycolytic pathway (Embden-Meyerhof pathway). The enzymes in which a deficiency may lead to a hereditary nonspherocytic hemolytic anemia are underlined.

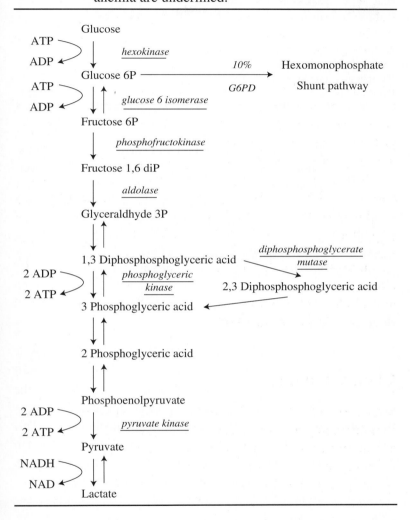

patient must be heterozygous for the trait to be expressed. An exception to autosomal recessive inheritance is PGK deficiency, which is inherited as a sex-linked disorder.

Pyruvate kinase or other glycolytic pathway deficiencies are usually first detected in infancy or later in childhood because of

Table 8-1 Glycolytic Pathway Deficiencies That Cause Hemolytic Anemia

Hexokinase
Glucose-phosphate isomerase
Phosphofructokinase
Aldolase
Triosephosphate isomerase
Diphosphoglycerate mutase
Phosphoglycerate kinase
Pyruvate kinase

anemia, jaundice, development of pigment gallstones, and slight to moderate splenomegaly due to red blood cell retention. The severity of the anemia and other clinical manifestations is widely variable. Severely affected individuals are often jaundiced and anemic at birth, requiring repeated transfusions. Aplastic crises may occur. Less affected individuals may have mild to moderate hemolysis that may or may not require transfusions. Often hemolysis is worsened by infection or other stress.

Approach to Diagnosis

In the autosomal recessive forms of HNSHA, the family history is usually negative unless siblings are affected. Biochemical studies of family members, however, will reveal the hereditary nature of the disorder. A child or infant presenting with a chronic hemolytic anemia must first be evaluated for possible nonheritable causes. This usually involves a direct antiglobulin test (Coombs' test; Test 6.4) to rule out an autoimmune hemolytic process and a sucrose hemolysis test (Test 11.1) to rule out paroxysmal nocturnal hemoglobinuria.

If the anemia is thought to be a hereditary process, it is usually next classified as either a nonspherocytic or spherocytic process. This is usually accomplished by evaluation of the peripheral blood smear for spherocytes. An osmotic fragility test (Test 7.1) will also help rule out hereditary spherocytosis. If the anemia is thought to be a hereditary nonspherocytic hemolytic anemia, hemoglobin electrophoresis to rule out the hemoglobinopathies (Test 10.1) and an isopropanol stability test (Test 10.7) to identify unstable hemo-

Table 8-2   Defects Associated With Hereditary Nonspherocytic Hemolytic Anemia

Enzymatic deficiencies
Glycolytic pathway: most common
Hexose monophosphate shunt pathway: rare variants
Glutathione metabolism: rare
Unstable hemoglobins

globins may be performed. Finally, screening tests for specific enzymatic deficiencies such as glucose-6-phosphate dehydrogenase (G6PD) deficiency (Tests 9.1 and 9.2) and for pyruvate kinase deficiency (Test 8.1) may be performed, followed by appropriate quantitative red blood cell enzyme assays to determine the specific nature of the enzymatic defect.

Hematologic Findings

There are varying degrees of anemia, with hemoglobin levels ranging from 5 to 12 g/dL (50-120 g/L). Reticulocytosis proportional to the severity of the anemia is present (up to 25%) but may be increased to over 50% after splenectomy. Mean corpuscular volume (MCV) may be moderately increased when reticulocytosis is present. In most cases the morphologic characteristics of the red blood cell are unremarkable. Cells are normocytic, normochromic, or, when in association with reticulocytosis, macrocytic with polychromatophilia. Rare spiculated and densely staining red blood cells may be present. Heinz bodies and spherocytes are notably absent. Basophilic stippling of red blood cells is prominent in pyrimidine-5'-nucleotidase deficiency.

Other Laboratory Tests

8.1 Fluorescent Screening Test for Pyruvate Kinase Deficiency

Purpose.   NADH fluorescence detection acts as a screening test useful for the detection of red blood cell enzyme deficiencies.

In practice, it is often enough to know whether the activity of the enzyme in question is markedly deficient. Slight deviations from normal are not likely to be of clinical importance.

Principle. Reduced pyridine nucleotides fluoresce when illuminated with long-wave ultraviolet light, while no such fluorescence occurs with oxidized pyridine nucleotides, providing an indicator of enzymatic activity. Screening procedures are available for pyruvate kinase, glucose-phosphate isomerase, NADH diaphorase triosephosphate isomerase, and G6PD (see Chapter 9). Pyruvate kinase screening is the most commonly used test for a glycolytic pathway deficiency.

Pyruvate kinase catalyzes the phosphorylation of adenosine diphosphate (ADP) to adenosine triphosphate (ATP) by phospho(enol)pyruvate (PEP). This reaction is coupled with the NADH-dependent conversion of pyruvate to lactate:

$$PEP + ADP \xrightarrow{\text{pyruvate kinase}} Pyruvate + ATP$$

$$Pyruvate + NADH + H^+ \xrightarrow{\text{lactate dehydrogenase}} Lactate + NAD^+$$

Thus, there should be a time-dependent loss of ultraviolet fluorescence as NADH is oxidized to NAD, when normal levels of pyruvate kinase activity are present.

Specimen. Whole blood collected in heparin or ethylenediaminetetraacetic acid (EDTA) is suitable for several days at 4°C and for about 1 day at room temperature.

Procedure. The blood sample is centrifuged, the plasma and buffy coat are aspirated. The red blood cell suspension is lysed by a buffered hypotonic screening mixture. The screening mixture provides PEP, ADP, NADH, and $MgCl_2$. It is spotted on filter paper immediately after mixing and every 15 minutes thereafter. After the spots are thoroughly dry, the paper is examined under illumination with long-wave ultraviolet light. The patient's sample is compared with that of a healthy control subject.

Interpretation. The first spot should fluoresce brightly. With the normal sample, fluorescence disappears after 15 minutes of incubation. In contrast, in pyruvate kinase–deficient samples, fluorescence fails to disappear even after 45 or 60 minutes of incubation.

Notes and Precautions. False-negative results may be observed if the patient has received a transfusion recently, so that large numbers of transfused cells containing normal levels of pyruvate kinase are still circulating.

8.2   Red Blood Cell Enzyme Assays

Purpose. Quantitative red blood cell enzyme assays give definitive confirmation of the results of screening tests and allow detection of heterozygotes for possible genetic counseling.

Principle. Most of the quantitative assays of red blood cell enzyme activity use spectrophotometric techniques that depend on the absorption of light of the reduced pyridine nucleotide, NADPH, or NADH at 340 nm spectrophotometrically. Reduction results in the formation of NADPH or NADH, with an increase in optical density, and oxidation results in the formation of NADP or NAD with a decrease in optical density.

Specimen. Blood is collected in EDTA, heparin, or acid-citrate dextrose. Most red blood cell enzymes are stable for several days at 4°C under these conditions. The blood should not be allowed to freeze, since washed red blood cells are used for the enzyme assays and the stability of red blood cell enzymes is usually less in hemolysates than that in intact red blood cells.

Procedure. The procedure for each enzyme measurement is different. See the references for specific methods.

Interpretation. Interpretation differs for each enzyme. In general, only very severe enzyme deficiencies cause hemolytic anemia. Even relatively severe deficiencies of enzymes, such as lactate dehydrogenase, glutathione peroxidase, and inosine triphosphatase, are without known clinical effect.

Notes and Precautions.   Quantitative enzyme assays are best carried out in specialized reference laboratories.

Ancillary Tests

Osmotic fragility testing (Test 7.1) may serve as a useful screening test for identifying hereditary spherocytosis and autoimmune hemolytic anemia with spherocytosis, whereas no increase in osmotic fragility is seen in HNSHA.

The isopropanol stability test (Test 10.7) is used to screen for the unstable hemoglobins.

Course and Treatment

The course of nonspherocytic hemolytic anemia is extremely variable. Severe pyruvate kinase deficiency may require splenectomy early in life. Response to splenectomy is variable. Other patients have a mild, benign course. Genetic counseling and prenatal diagnosis is possible for most of the defects.

References

Beutler E. Red cell enzyme defects. *Hematol Pathol.* 1990;4:103-114.

Beutler E. *Red Cell Metabolism: A Manual of Biochemical Methods.* 3d ed. New York, NY: Grune & Stratton; 1984.

Valentine WN, Tanaka KR, Paglia DE. Hemolytic anemias and erythrocyte enzymopathies. *Ann Intern Med.* 1985;103:245-257.

9

Hereditary Disorders of the Hexose Monophosphate Shunt Pathway: Glucose-6-Phosphate Dehydrogenase Deficiency

Red blood cells lack mitochondria, causing the cell to be dependent on the hexose monophosphate (HMP) oxidative shunt pathway for reduction of nicotinamide-adenine dinucleotide phosphate (NADP) to NADPH. NADPH is an essential reducing agent in circulating red blood cells, allowing for detoxification of oxidated metabolic intermediates and maintenance of the red blood cell membrane. Glucose-6-phosphate dehydrogenase (G6PD) catalyzes the first step of the pathway. Deficiency of this enzyme is the most prevalent inborn metabolic disorder of red blood cells, affecting over 100 million people worldwide, and is an important cause of hemolytic anemia.

Pathophysiology

The HMP shunt pathway functions to produce NADPH by a series of enzymatic reactions (Figure 9-1). In turn, NADPH is utilized as a cofactor for glutathione reductase (GR) to regenerate oxidized glutathione (GSSG) into a reduced state. Normally, red blood cells make use of reduced glutathione (GSH) to detoxify low levels of oxygen radicals that form spontaneously or as a result of drug administration, and reduce oxidized sulfhydryl groups of hemoglo-

Figure 9-1   Hexose monophosphate shunt pathway.

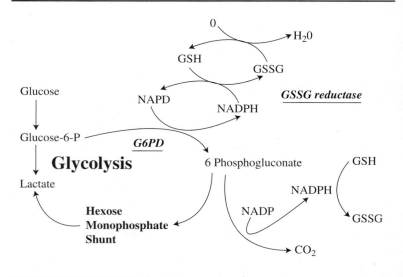

bin, membrane proteins, or enzymes. G6PD-deficient red blood cells are unable to maintain glutathione in its reduced state, impairing the ability of the red blood cell to deal with toxic insults or oxidative stress. This leads to integral membrane damage and the accumulation of oxidized cellular products in the form of Heinz bodies. This will ultimately lead to premature red blood cell lysis in the spleen and hemolytic anemia.

G6PD deficiency results from the inheritance of an abnormal G6PD enzyme. A large number of abnormalities of this gene may give rise to disease (Table 9-1). Normally, the A and B isotypes of G6PD, distinguished by electrophoretic mobility, are seen. The B isoform is the most common type of enzyme found in all population groups. The G6PD A isoform, found in about 20% of black men in the United States, migrates more rapidly on electrophoresis than the normal B enzyme, has similar enzymatic activity to the B isoform, and is not associated with disease. About 11% of US black men have a G6PD variant, G6PD A⁻, that has the same electrophoretic mobility as G6PD A but is unstable, resulting in enzyme loss leading to deficiency as the red blood cell ages. Thus, older circulating red blood cells from individuals with this variant

Table 9-1   Common G6PD Variants

G6PD Variant	Association with Hemolysis	Affected Population
G6PD A	No: normal variant	Blacks
G6PD B	No: normal variant	All
G6PD A⁻	Yes: moderate	Blacks
G6PD^MED	Yes: severe	Whites
G6PD^CANTON	Yes	Asians

Abbreviation: G6PD = glucose-6-phosphate dehydrogenase.

may contain only 5% to 15% of the normal amount of enzymatic activity. G6PD A⁻ is the most common clinically significant type of abnormal G6PD among the US black population. Other G6PD variants predominate in other racial groups, including G6PD Mediterranean (G6PD^MED), found frequently in Sicilians, Greeks, Sephardic Jews, and Arabs. Several other variants, such as G6PD^CANTON or G6PD^MAHIDOL, are common in Asian populations. The population distribution of G6PD deficiency reflects its probable origins in tropical and subtropical areas.

The G6PD gene is carried on the X chromosome, leading to a sex-linked inheritance pattern. Thus, the effect is fully expressed in affected men, who carry only one X chromosome, and inheritance is maternal. In women, only one of the two X chromosomes in each cell is active. Consequently, women who are heterozygous for G6PD deficiency have two populations of red blood cells: deficient and normal cells. The ratio of deficient to normal cells may vary greatly as a result of the variability that is intrinsic to the X-chromosome inactivation process. Some women who are heterozygous for the disease appear to be entirely healthy, whereas others are fully affected.

Deficiencies of other enzymes in the HMP shunt and glutathione metabolism are comparatively rare (Table 9-2). Hereditary GSH deficiency of the red blood cell results from a deficiency of either of the two enzymes of GSH synthesis: gamma-glutamyl cysteine synthetase or GSH synthetase. In some cases, the clinical manifestation of these deficiencies is similar to that of G6PD deficiency; others present with a chronic hemolytic anemia. Dietary deficiencies of flavin-adenine dinucleotide (FAD), which is a

Table 9-2   Enzyme Deficiencies of Hexose Monophosphate Shunt Pathway Clearly Associated With Hemolytic Anemia

Enzyme Deficiency	Occurrence With Hemolytic Anemia
G6PD	Common
Gamma-glutamyl cysteine synthetase	Rare
GSH synthetase	Rare
Glutathione reductase (total deficiency only)	Rare

Abbreviations: G6PD = glucose-6-phosphate dehydrogenase, GSH = reduced glutathione.

cofactor for GSSG reductase, may cause a decrease in enzymatic activity that mimics GSSG reductase deficiency, but may be remedied by dietary manipulation. Actual GSSG reductase deficiency is rare. Other HMP shunt pathway deficiencies are rarely or never associated with hemolytic anemia.

Clinical Findings

G6PD deficiency usually manifests as an episode of acute intravascular hemolysis following ingestion of an oxidant drug or infection in an otherwise apparently healthy person. Hemolysis begins acutely in the case of infection or within 1 to 3 days after administration of an oxidative type drug (Table 9-3), leading to plasma hemoglobinemia (pink to brown plasma), hemoglobinuria (dark or black urine), and jaundice. In severe cases, abdominal or back pain may occur.

In the G6PD A$^-$ deficiency, the hemolytic anemia is self-limited because the young red blood cells produced in response to hemolysis have nearly normal G6PD levels and are relatively resistant to hemolysis, whereas in other types of G6PD deficiency, such as G6PD^{MED}, there may be severe hemolysis, which requires transfusion therapy.

Other stresses that may precipitate acute hemolytic anemia in people who are severely G6PD deficient are the neonatal state and exposure to fava beans. Rare cases presenting as hereditary nonspherocytic hemolytic anemia are also associated with G6PD deficiency (Table 9-4).

Table 9-3   Drugs Commonly Associated With Hemolysis in Glucose-6-Phosphate Dehydrogenase

Antimalarial agents
 Primaquine
 Quinacrine
Sulfonamides
 Sulfanilamide
 Salicylazosulfapyridine
 Sulfacetamide
Other antibacterial agents
 Nitrofurantoin
 Nitrofurazone
 Para-aminosalicylic acid
 Nalidixic acid
Analgesics
 Acetanilid
Sulfones
 Diaminodiphenyl sulfone
 Thiazolsulfone
Miscellaneous agents
 Dimercaprol
 Naphthalene (mothballs)
 Methylene blue
 Trinitrotoluene (TNT)

Approach to Diagnosis

The occurrence of episodic hemolysis raises the suspicion that a patient may be suffering from hereditary deficiency of one of the enzymes of the HMP.

Patients with the most common type of G6PD deficiency present with acute hemolytic anemia. In such cases, a careful history regarding ingestion of drugs is important. Other causes of episodic anemia include paroxysmal nocturnal hemoglobinuria (see Chapter 11), parasitic infections such as malaria, and the presence of some of the unstable hemoglobins (see Chapter 10). When the hemolytic nature of the episodes is less apparent, and particularly in cases associated with infection, differential diagnosis includes an aregenerative crisis that may occur in any of the severe hereditary anemias. The rare variants that present as hereditary nonspherocytic hemolyt-

Table 9-4 Clinical Features of G6PD Variants

Clinical Feature	G6PDA⁻	G6PD^MED	G6PD^CANTON
Drug-induced hemolysis	Common	Common	Common
Infection-induced hemolysis	Common	Common	Common
Favism	Not seen	Common	Not usually seen
Neonatal icterus	Rare	Observed	Observed
Hereditary nonspherocytic hemolytic anemia	Not seen	Seen on occasion	Not seen
Degree of hemolysis	Moderate	Severe	Moderate
Chronic hemolysis	Not seen	Not seen	Not seen

Abbreviation: G6PD = glucose-6-phosphate dehydrogenase.

ic anemia are discussed in Chapter 8. In neonatal icterus, fetal-maternal Rh or ABO incompatibility must be ruled out.

Hematologic Findings

The severity of the anemia is extremely variable. The hemoglobin concentration in the blood may be near normal or as low as 5 g/dL (50 g/L). Examination of the peripheral blood smear usually does not show a distinctive red blood cell appearance. Heinz bodies (particles of denatured hemoglobin and membrane proteins) adhere to the membrane and may be seen initially on supravitally stained preparations prepared for the enumeration of reticulocytes or with crystal violet. They are not seen on Wright's- or Giemsa-stained smears. As hemolysis progresses, Heinz bodies disappear, presumably due to splenic removal of the Heinz body particles or entire red blood cells. Bite cells and/or some spherocytes may be seen. At the beginning of the hemolytic episode, the reticulocyte count may be normal, but if the hemolytic episode has been under-way for several days, the reticulocyte count is usually elevated appropriate to the degree of anemia. Slight macrocytosis may be seen if reticulocytes are present; otherwise, red blood cell indices are normocytic and normochromic. The white blood cell count may be low, normal, or elevated because of granulocytosis.

Other Laboratory Tests

9.1 Fluorescent Screening Test for G6PD Activity

Purpose. The fluorescent screening test that detects formation of NADPH, which fluoresces under ultraviolet (UV) light, is highly reliable for the detection of both severe and mild types of G6PD deficiency in men who do not have an active episode of hemolysis.

Principle. Whole blood or blood hemolysates contain the enzymes of the HMP oxidate shunt pathway. In the presence of NADP, G6PD is oxidized to form 6-phosphogluconate and NADPH. Since phosphogluconate dehydrogenase (6-PGD) is present in virtually all hemolysates, further reduction of NADP occurs in the following reaction:

$$6\text{-phosphogluconate} + NADP^+ \xrightarrow{\text{6-GPD}} \text{Ribulose-5-P} + NADPH + H^+$$

When mildly G6PD-deficient hemolysates are incubated with G6PD and NADP, a small amount of NADPH is formed. In the presence of oxidized glutathione (GSSG), provided in the screening mixture, NADPH is reoxidized in the glutathione reductase reaction to NADP.

Thus, the screening test measures, in effect, the difference between approximately twice the G6PD activity (which forms NADPH) and the glutathione reductase activity (which consumes NADPH).

Specimen. Blood collected in heparin ethylenediaminetetraacetic acid (EDTA) or acid citrate dextrose (ACD) solution is satisfactory. Blood that is several weeks old, and even spots of blood collected on filter paper and dried, may be used.

Procedure.   Whole blood is added to a buffered screening solution containing saponin, G6PD, NADP$^+$, and GSSG. After incubation for 5 to 10 minutes at room temperature, the mixture is spotted on filter paper, allowed to dry, and observed for NADPH fluorescence under long-wave UV light.

In patients with the A$^-$ variant of G6PD who have had a recent episode of hemolysis, the test may be modified by centrifuging the blood sample in a microhematocrit tube and using the bottom 10% of the red blood cell column (representing the reticulocyte-poor, enzyme-deficient cell fraction) for the test.

Interpretation.   Normal samples show a bright fluorescence and deficient samples show little or no fluorescence. No false-positive or false-negative test results are observed. In severe G6PD^{MED} or similar type deficiency in which even very young cells have very low levels of G6PD, a screening test suffices for diagnosis, even in the presence of a severe hemolytic reaction. In patients with the A$^-$ variant of G6PD with ongoing or acute hemolysis, however, the remaining young cells and reticulocytes have normal or near-normal G6PD activity, and most of the enzyme-deficient cells have been removed from the circulation. Diagnosis of G6PD deficiency under these circumstances can be accomplished either by repeating the screening test in 2 or 3 weeks or by modifying the screening test to minimize reticulocyte populations, as previously noted. Recent blood transfusions may also invalidate the results.

Notes and Precautions.   Because G6PD is sex-linked, women who are heterozygous for G6PD deficiency have two red blood cell populations where some of the red blood cells are grossly deficient and others are normal. Although the deficient cells are susceptible to hemolysis, the enzymatic activity, as measured on hemolysates, may be normal, intermediate, or low. The extent of deficiency seen is a function of the proportion of normal and deficient cells in that particular heterozygote. Special methods for the detection of individual cell G6PD activity may be used to help detect heterozygosity.

9.2 Quantitative G6PD Assay

Purpose. In men who are not experiencing hemolysis, the G6PD fluorescent screening test is generally adequate for diagnosis, but quantitative enzyme assays may be useful in the detection of patients who have had an episode of hemolysis and in women with heterozygous disease. The rate of increase of optical density that occurs with the formation of NADPH from NADP in blood hemolysates is measured at 340 nm in a spectrophotometer.

Specimen. Blood collected in EDTA or ACD solution is satisfactory. The G6PD activity is stable for several weeks at 4°C and for several days at room temperature. The blood should not be allowed to freeze, since enzymatic activity is rapidly lost when red blood cells are lysed.

Procedure. The final assay mixture contains 100-mmol/L TRIS with 0.5-mmol/L EDTA buffer (pH 8.0); 10-mmol/L $MgCl_2$; 0.2-mmol/L NADP; and 0.6-mmol/L G6P. The reaction is started by the addition of the G6P, with water being substituted for G6P in the blank cuvette.

Interpretation. Quantitative assay for G6PD activity may reveal the presence of G6PD deficiency in a person who has had a recent episode of hemolysis. Since G6PD is normally an age-dependent enzyme, activity should be increased in a patient with reticulocytosis. Normal or slightly lower than normal G6PD activity in such a patient implies that G6PD deficiency is present. Enzyme activity in women with heterozygous disease may be below the normal range.

Notes and Precautions. The usual assay for G6PD measures the activity of both G6PD and 6-phosphogluconic dehydrogenase, because the product of the G6PD reaction, 6-phosphogluconolactone, is converted rapidly to the substrate for the 6-phosphogluconate dehydrogenase reaction. In practice, this causes no difficulty. Note the precaution in the diagnosis of heterozygosity discussed under Test 9.1 above.

9.3   Glutathione Reductase Assay

Purpose.   The purpose is to determine whether severe glutathione reductase deficiency, a very rare cause of drug-induced hemolytic anemia, is present, and to assess the adequacy of riboflavin nutrition.

Principle.   Glutathione reductase catalyzes the reduction of oxidized glutathione (GSSG) to reduced glutathione (GSH) by NADPH, which is oxidized to NAD in the process. Flavine adenine dinucleotide (FAD) serves as a cofactor for glutathione reductase. The addition of FAD to the system provides information regarding the extent to which the glutathione reductase apoenzyme is saturated with FAD in the red blood cell. This, in turn, reflects riboflavin levels, since riboflavin is a precursor of FAD.

Specimen.   Blood should be collected in EDTA, heparin, or ACD. It can be stored for up to 3 weeks at 4°C or up to 5 days at 22°C.

Procedure.   The following reaction mixture is used: 100-mmol/L TRIS with 0.5-mmol/L EDTA buffer (pH 8.0); 3.3-mmol/L GSSG; and 0.1-mmol/L NADH with or without 1-µmol/L FAD. The rate of increase in optical density at 340 nm is read against a blank from which GSSG has been omitted.

Interpretation.   Severe enzyme deficiency (<5% of normal) may be a cause of drug-induced hemolytic anemia or favism. Stimulation of glutathione reductase activity by riboflavin by more than 50% indicates suboptimal riboflavin intake.

Notes and Precautions.   Modest glutathione reductase deficiency occurs commonly as a result of inadequate riboflavin intake and probably as a result of genetic polymorphisms. It should not be considered a cause of hemolytic anemia.

9.4   Reduced Glutathione (GSH) Determination

Purpose.   Determination of red blood cell GSH levels is useful in the examination of the red blood cells of patients with anemia (see Interpretation).

Principle.   The dithiol compound, dithio-bis-nitrobenzoic acid (DTNB), is reduced by GSH to form a yellow anion, the optical density of which is measured readily at 412 nm.

Specimen.   Whole blood collected in heparin, EDTA, or ACD preservative may be used. GSH levels remain unaltered for 3 weeks in ACD solution or for 1 week in EDTA or heparin solutions at 4°C. At room temperature, the assay should be carried out within a few hours.

Procedure.   In this procedure, 0.2 mL of whole blood is added to 2.0 mL of distilled water. After removal of 0.2 mL of the lysate for hemoglobin determination, 3 mL of a metaphosphoric acid EDTA–sodium chloride precipitating solution is added, and the mixture is filtered. Then, 2 mL of the filtrate is added to 8 mL of 0.3 mol/L Na_2HPO_4 solution, 1 mL of DTNB reagent is added, and the optical density is read at 412 nm.

Interpretation.   The normal red blood cell glutathione concentration is 4.5 to 8.7 µmol/g of hemoglobin. A severe deficiency of glutathione results from a genetic defect in one of the two enzymes of glutathione synthesis: gamma-glutamylcysteine synthetase or glutathione synthetase. Modest reductions of GSH levels and marked instability to challenge by oxidative agents is found in G6PD-deficient red blood cells. Elevated levels of red blood cell glutathione are found in patients with myeloproliferative disorders and in those with pyrimidine-5'-nucleotidase deficiency.

Notes and Precautions. Virtually all of the protein-free DTNB reducing activity in red blood cells is due to glutathione. DTNB is reduced readily by other sulfhydryl compounds, such as cysteine, and thus the degree of specificity will vary from tissue to tissue.

Ancillary Tests

In patients with severe glutathione deficiency, it is desirable to measure the activities of gamma-glutamyl cysteine synthetase and glutathione synthetase. Assay of these enzymes is a relatively difficult radiometric procedure that is best performed by specialized laboratories. Precise identification of the G6PD variants requires electrophoresis, kinetic studies, and other biochemical techniques.

Course and Treatment

Infants with G6PD deficiency and neonatal icterus may require exchange transfusions. Patients with G6PD deficiency should avoid the ingestion of fava beans and the oxidative type drugs. Splenectomy is not usually useful in G6PD deficiency associated with nonspherocytic hemolytic anemia.

References

Beutler E. Glucose-6-phosphate dehydrogenase deficiency. In: Stanbury JB, Wyngaarden JB, Fredrickson DS, et al, eds. *The Metabolic Basis of Inherited Disease*. New York, NY: McGraw-Hill International Book Co; 1983:1629.

Beutler E. *Red Cell Metabolism: A Manual of Biochemical Methods*. 3d ed. New York, NY: Grune & Stratton Inc; 1984.

Chanarin I. *Laboratory Hematology: An Account of Laboratory Techniques*. New York, NY: Churchill Livingstone Inc; 1989.

10

Disorders of Hemoglobin Synthesis

Hemoglobin is a tetrameric protein composed of four globin polypeptides and four heme groups. Abnormalities in hemoglobin synthesis are either qualitative (formation of an abnormal hemoglobin molecule at a normal or near-normal rate) or quantitative with a resultant decrease in the amount of hemoglobin synthesized, as in the thalassemias.

Pathophysiology

The normal adult red blood cell contains predominantly hemoglobin (Hb) A, which is composed of two alpha (α) and two beta (β) globin chains ($\alpha_2\beta_2$). Two other minor adult hemoglobins are HbA_2 (where the beta chain is replaced by a delta [δ] chain), and HbF (where the beta chain is replaced by a gamma [γ] chain). Hemoglobin A_2 is depicted as $\alpha_2\delta_2$ and HbF as a $\alpha_2\gamma_2$ (Table 10-1). At birth, HbF is the predominant type of hemoglobin, but within the first year of life, it is largely replaced by HbA to reflect the adult proportions of approximately 97% HbA, 2% HbA_2, and 1% HbF. HbA_{1c} is a minor hemoglobin that is formed by posttranslational

Table 10-1   Hemoglobin Types Found in a Healthy Adult

Hemoglobin Type	Globin Chains	% Total Hemoglobin
HbA	$\alpha_2\beta_2$	>95
HbA$_2$	$\alpha_2\delta_2$	≤3.5
HbF	$\alpha_2\gamma_2$	≤1

addition of glucose to the N terminal of the HbA beta chains. HbA$_{1c}$ is found in increased amounts in patients with diabetes mellitus.

Each globin chain (alpha, beta, gamma, and delta) has its own autosomal genetic locus. Qualitative alterations in these globin chains arise via genetic mutations of one of the globin chains, usually causing substitution of a single amino acid. The abnormal hemoglobin chains that are formed may or may not alter the functional characteristics of the hemoglobin. If the hemoglobin structural abnormality gives rise to clinical manifestations, the patient is said to have a hemoglobinopathy. The most common hemoglobinopathies are beta chain mutations and include HbS, HbC, and HbE (Table 10-2). These variants may appear as either heterozygous or homozygous defects.

Hemoglobin variants were initially differentiated primarily by their electrophoretic mobility and were assigned letter names (ie, HbC, HbE). Later, when additional hemoglobin variants were discovered with the same mobility, the new variant was distinguished by following the letter previously ascribed to that mobility with the place of discovery of the new variant. Finally, if the exact amino acid structure of a hemoglobin variant was determined, a simple designation was adopted that characterized the amino acid substitution by a superscript to the involved globin chain (ie, for HbS, $\alpha_2\beta_2^{\text{6-glutamic acid}\rightarrow\text{valine}}$).

When an abnormal hemoglobin is synthesized, the clinical manifestations are often determined by the amount of variant present. This is highly influenced by whether the abnormal hemoglobin is inherited as a heterozygote or homozygote. Homozygous inheritance is associated with more severe manifestations. Sickle cell anemia or sickle cell disease refers to the homozygote for HbS, and the sickle cell trait is the heterozygous state. The word "disease" is used for a homozygote with other hemoglobin variants (eg, homozygous HbC disease or HbCC), whereas "trait" refers to the

Table 10-2   Amino Acid Substitutions in the Beta Chains of Common Hemoglobin Variants

Hemoglobin	Position	Amino Acid Substitution
HbS	6	Glutamic acid → valine
HbC	6	Glutamic acid → lysine
HbE	26	Glutamic acid → lysine

heterozygotes (eg, HbC trait or HbAC). The word "disease" is also applied to the HbS heterozygous state when significant clinical findings are associated with the combination (eg, sickle cell-HbC disease). When letter designations are used for the hemoglobins in the heterozygous hemoglobinopathies, the first letter refers to the preponderant hemoglobin found in the red blood cell. Thus, HbAS indicates that the concentration of HbA exceeds that of HbS in the red blood cell of that particular heterozygous variant.

Mutations that decrease or prevent the synthesis of one of the globin chains cause quantitative decreases in structurally normal hemoglobin production. This gives rise to the thalassemia syndromes. The thalassemias are classified according to the chain affected, the most common being alpha-thalassemia and beta-thalassemia. The alpha-thalassemias are most commonly caused by the deletion of one or more of the four alpha globin genes. The beta-thalassemic disorders are usually due to genetic mutations that affect RNA synthesis, processing, or stability; the mutations cause decreased levels of normal protein to be formed. Beta-thalassemias are classified as either minor (heterozygous) or major (homozygous). Heterozygous beta-thalassemia minor is a common disorder. Combined disorders involving the structural variants and the thalassemias are also seen, the most common of which is sickle beta-thalassemia disease.

Clinical Findings

Hemoglobin Disorders Caused by Abnormal Globin Chains. Mutations involving the globin protein genes are usually amino acid substitutions. These may produce pronounced changes in the functional properties of hemoglobin, including solubility and oxygen affinity (Table 10-3).

Table 10-3   Functional Classification of Abnormal Hemoglobins

Type of Abnormality	Functional Effect	Clinical Disorder	Examples
Qualitative Disorders			
Solubility	Aggregation of hemoglobin	Hemolytic anemia	Hemoglobin S, hemoglobin C
Oxidative susceptibility	Oxidative denaturation	Hemolytic anemia	Unstable hemoglobin
Increased oxygen affinity	Decreased oxygen to tissues	Erythrocytosis	Unstable hemoglobin
Decreased oxygen affinity	Premature oxygen release	Cyanosis/anemia	Unstable hemoglobin
Abnormal heme reduction	Inability to carry oxygen	Cyanosis	Methemoglobin
Quantitative Disorders			
Alpha chains	Decreased alpha chains	Range from mild anemia to hydrops fetalis	Alpha-thalassemia
Beta chains	Decreased beta chains	Mild to severe hemolytic anemia	Beta-thalassemia
Beta and delta chains	Decreased beta and delta chains	Thalassemia-like syndrome	Delta-beta-thalassemia
Combined Disorders			
Abnormal hemoglobin and thalassemia	Decreased chain production with altered solubility	Often milder than homozygous structural disorder	Hemoglobin S thalassemia

The most common clinically significant hemoglobinopathy causing changes in hemoglobin solubility is HbS. The heterozygous sickle cell trait is generally considered to be an entirely benign disorder, although hematuria may occur on rare occasions. The homozygous disorder, sickle cell anemia, is a disease characterized by moderately severe hemolysis and painful crises resulting from occlusion of blood vessels by the red blood cells, which assume a sickled shape due to abnormal hemoglobin polymerization. When the gene for HbS is inherited with the gene for certain other abnormal hemoglobins, particularly for HbC (causing HbSC disease) or beta-thalassemia (S-thalassemia), sickle cell diseases that are very similar to sickle cell anemia result. Within the population of black Americans, the HbS gene has a frequency of approximately 9%; the HbC gene, 3%; and the beta-thalassemia gene, 1%. Thus, these mixed disorders are collectively relatively common, affecting approximately 1 in 260 black Americans.

Two other hemoglobins that affect solubility may be seen relatively frequently in the heterozygous state: HbD, which is seen in blacks, and HbE, which is a common mutation in Asian populations. Both of these result in a mild hemolytic anemia, even in the homozygous state. In HbE disease, the anemia is hypochromic and associated with splenomegaly. Hypochromia is also found uniformly in the HbE trait.

The remaining hemoglobinopathies are much less common. Those caused by formation of unstable hemoglobins are usually inherited as autosomal dominant disorders and are characteristically associated with chronic hemolysis. The anemia is often hypochromic. Some unstable hemoglobins are associated with increased oxygen affinity, leading to erythrocytosis and reticulocytosis greater than that usually observed for the degree of anemia seen. Other very rarely seen hemoglobins have decreased oxygen affinity and produce anemia with cyanosis.

A mutant hemoglobin that is unable to maintain heme iron in the reduced state and to bind oxygen, designated as HbM, results in hereditary methemoglobinemia. Methemoglobin is brownish, and patients who inherit this type of hemoglobin have a cyanotic appearance. HbM is inherited as an autosomal dominant disorder.

Thalassemias. The thalassemic syndromes arise from an impairment in the synthesis of the globin chains, leading to a quantitative decrease in the amount of hemoglobin within the cell. Thalassemias are divided into two main categories—alpha-thalassemia and beta-thalassemia—on the basis of which globin chain is affected.

Alpha-thalassemia is a common disorder in many parts of the world. Severe forms of alpha-thalassemia are found in Southeast Asia, but milder disease forms are prevalent among persons of African ancestry. Because of gene duplication of the alpha globin chain genetic locus, most persons have four alpha chain genes with two on each chromosome. Alpha-thalassemia usually results from the deletion of one or more of these genes. The severity of disease is directly correlated with the number of genes deleted. The spectrum of alpha-thalassemic syndromes ranges from deletion of one gene, which causes no clinical disease, to deletion of all four genes, which is incompatible with life.

The most serious clinical consequences result from absence of activity of all four alpha-chain genes, which is a frequent cause of stillbirth in Southeast Asia. The fetal red blood cell hemoglobin is entirely composed of gamma-chain tetramers, designated as hemoglobin Bart's. Since hemoglobin Bart's binds oxygen avidly, it is unable to transport and release oxygen to the fetal tissues. This results in fetal death from hydrops fetalis manifested by severe intrauterine hypoxia, edema, pallor, and hepatosplenomegaly. If one functional alpha-chain gene is present, a less severe disorder occurs, termed HbH disease. At birth, both fetal hemoglobin and hemoglobin Bart's are present in this disorder. In later infancy into adulthood as beta-globin synthesis replaces fetal hemoglobin synthesis, excess unpaired beta chains form beta tetramers designated HbH, which can be detected by hemoglobin electrophoresis, and gives rise to a moderately severe, chronic hemolytic anemia. If two normal alpha-chain genes are present, a mild microcytic anemia designated as alpha-thalassemia minor or alpha-thalassemia trait is observed. In alpha-thalassemia minor, no abnormalities are found on hemoglobin electrophoresis, and the diagnosis is often one of exclusion of other causes of anemia. The presence of three normal alpha chains does not result in a clinically detectable abnormality. The characteristics of the alpha-thalassemias are summarized in Table 10-4.

Beta-thalassemia is common among persons of Mediterranean descent. Beta-thalassemia may arise from gene deletion, or more commonly from point mutations leading to impaired or absent beta-chain synthesis. Mutations leading to complete suppression of beta-chain synthesis are designated as $\beta°$ variants. Other mutations where diminished synthesis of normal beta chains occurs are designated as $\beta+$ variants and may result in milder clinical syndromes than the $\beta°$ variants.

As with the alpha-thalassemias, the degree of disease severity is dependent on the number of abnormal genes inherited. When

Table 10-4   Alpha-Thalassemias

Phenotype	α Globin Output (%)	No. of Functional α Chain Genes and Genotype	Hematologic Findings
Normal	100	4: αα/αα	Normal
Silent carrier	75	3: –α/αα	Normal
α-Thalassemia trait	50	2: –α/–α or --/αα	Mild hypochromic anemia
HbH disease	25	1: –α/--	Hemolytic anemia
Hydrops fetalis	0	0: --/--	Stillborn, severe anemia

Abbreviation: — = deleted or absent α chain; -- = both genes on the locus deleted.

only one beta-thalassemic gene has been inherited (heterozygote), one has a benign, hypochromic microcytic anemia designated beta-thalassemia minor. This anemia is characterized by microcytosis, with a mean corpuscular volume (MCV) of 60 to 70 μm^3 (60-70 fL), a hemoglobin of 10 to 13 g/dL (100-130 g/L), and an elevated or normal red blood cell count. Hemoglobin electrophoresis will usually show increased amounts of HbA_2 due to excess unpaired alpha chains combining with delta chains. Slightly elevated levels of HbF are also present in about 30% of patients with beta-thalassemia minor. Often, patients with beta-thalassemia minor are mistakenly diagnosed as having iron deficiency, because they have a hypochromic microcytic anemia (see Chapter 2).

When two beta-thalassemic genes have been inherited (homozygote), a very serious disorder beginning in infancy and early childhood, called beta-thalassemia major, results. It is characterized by massive hepatosplenomegaly, extreme erythroid hyperplasia in the bone marrow leading to bony deformities, severe hemolytic anemia, and failure to grow or thrive. Hemoglobin electrophoresis shows prominent elevation of the HbF level (ranging from 30%-100%). At the lower end of the spectrum of HbF values, the fetal hemoglobin is distributed heterogeneously among the red blood cell population. This allows beta-thalassemia major to be distinguished from the benign condition designated as hereditary persistence of fetal hemoglobin (HPFH), in which a homogeneous distribution is seen.

Another form of thalassemia, called delta-thalassemia, is associated with suppression of both delta and beta chains synthesis. These disorders are clinically similar to the beta-thalassemias. Patients with heterozygous disease present with thalassemia minor, often with prominent elevation of the HbF level. The patients with homozygous disease, however, present with a clinically milder disease than that usually seen in beta-thalassemia major. The Lepore syndromes, which are often classified in this category, are caused by a mutant hemoglobin, Hb Lepore. This hemoglobin results from a crossover mutation leading to a hybrid globin chain consisting partly of delta chains and partly of beta chains. Hemoglobin Lepore can be detected with electrophoresis.

Approach to Diagnosis

Clinical evaluation and family studies play a particularly important role in evaluating laboratory data in these disorders. Many of the tests can be readily performed. Evaluation of the hemoglobin disorders proceeds with the following:

1. Hematologic evaluation, with attention to red blood cell morphology and indices. Supravital stains may be used to detect inclusion bodies (such as HbH).

2. Hemoglobin electrophoresis for the detection of globin-chain variants with altered electrophoretic mobility and measurement of HbA_2 levels. HbA_2 may also be determined chromatographically.

3. If a hemoglobin with an S-like mobility is encountered, tests of hemoglobin solubility as a means of distinguishing HbS from the electrophoretically similar HbD and less frequent variants may be used. Solubility tests and the sickle test will also screen for sickle cell trait.

4. Alkali denaturation test or the acid elution test (method of Kleihauer and Betke) for fetal hemoglobin evaluation.

5. The isopropanol stability test for detecting unstable hemoglobins.

The following tests may be performed in specialized laboratories:

6. When indicated, spectrophotometric determinations for methemoglobinemia seen with HbMs and measurement of oxyhemoglobin dissociation or $P_{50}O_2$ for detecting hemoglobins with altered oxygen affinity.

7. Globin-chain synthetic studies when thalassemia is suspected but cannot be confirmed by simpler methods, and Southern blotting of alpha-globin genes when additional genetic data are needed.

8. Detailed structural analysis of globin chains using "fingerprinting" of tryptic digests by means of electrophoresis, chromatography, and amino acid sequencing.

Hematologic Findings

The most severe anemia and most striking morphologic changes are seen in the homozygous disorders. Findings in the heterozygous states may be normal or may show minimal hematologic abnormalities. Hematologic abnormalities may be classified into (1) those associated with chronic hemolysis, (2) changes characteristic of a particular disorder, (3) findings seen after splenectomy or (in the case of sickle cell disease) findings related to splenic atrophy, and (4) changes seen with aplastic crises, which may accompany infections.

Blood Cell Measurements. Anemia may be severe, with hemoglobin levels of 5 to 9 g/dL (50-90 g/L) in sickle cell anemia and 2.5 to 6.5 g/dL (25-65 g/L) in thalassemia major. Findings in heterozygotes may be normal, as in sickle cell trait, or they may show mild anemia, as in beta-thalassemia minor. Often the thalassemia syndromes are characterized by decreased hemoglobin levels with normal to slightly increased red blood cell counts and microcytosis out of proportion to the anemia (60-70 μm^3 [60-75 fL]).

Peripheral Blood Smear Morphology. A wide variety of characteristic red blood cell changes are associated with the various disorders of hemoglobin synthesis and are summarized in Table 10-5. Images 10-1 through 10-3 demonstrate the characteristic morphology seen in beta-thalassemia minor, HbC disease, and sickle cell disease. Image 10-4 shows the characteristic appearance of Heinz bodies.

Bone Marrow Examination. Erythroid hyperplasia is proportional to the severity of the hemolysis. A prominent increase in iron deposition is often seen.

Other Laboratory Tests

10.1 Hemoglobin Electrophoresis

Purpose. Hemoglobin electrophoresis is the principal procedure used to separate, detect, and identify abnormal hemoglobins.

Principle. Electrophoresis is the differential movement of charged protein molecules in an electric field. In a basic solution (pH >8) hemoglobins have a negative charge and migrate toward the positive pole or anode. The relative speeds with which different hemoglobins migrate toward the anode are proportional to their net negative charges. Because HbS contains valine in place of the glutamic acid of HbA, it has a smaller negative charge and a slower anodal mobility than HbA in an alkaline medium. At an acid pH, hemoglobins are positively charged, and their relative mobilities in relation to the anode are the reverse of that seen in an alkaline medium.

Specimen. Anticoagulated whole blood or washed red blood cells are used.

Procedure. Electrophoresis on cellulose acetate at a pH 8.4 to 8.8 is the method of choice for initial electrophoretic testing in the general clinical laboratory (Figure 10-1). Patient and control red blood cells are hemolyzed and subjected to elec-

Table 10-5   Red Blood Cell Appearance in Disorders of Hemoglobin Synthesis

Disorder	Morphologic Findings
HbS	Sickle cells
HbC	Target cells, HbC crystals after splenectomy
HbE	Microcytosis, hypochromia, target cells
Unstable Hb	Red blood cell inclusions with supravital dyes
Thalassemia	Microcytosis, target cells, basophilic stippling
Changes due to splenectomy or splenic atrophy	Basophilic stippling, Howell-Jolly bodies, target cells, Pappenheimer bodies, poikilocytosis
Changes associated with hemolysis	Polychromatophilia, fine basophilic stippling, macrocytosis

trophoresis for 15 to 30 minutes. Hemoglobins A, A_2, F, S, and C are most often included as controls. Upon completion of electrophoresis, the membrane is stained and the hemoglobins are identified by their relative positions. The hemoglobins can then be quantitated by elution and spectrophotometric assay or by densitometry scanning. Electrophoresis in citrate agar at pH 6.2 can be used to complement conventional cellulose acetate electrophoresis (see Interpretation; Figure 10-1). The procedure is basically the same as that described for cellulose acetate but requires electrophoresis for 45 to 90 minutes.

Interpretation.   The electrophoretic patterns of some hemoglobin variants on cellulose acetate are shown in Figure 10-2. At an alkaline pH, slow-moving hemoglobins include C, E, A_2, and O; intermediate hemoglobins include D, G, S, and Lepore; hemoglobins A and F are the most anodal. Among the fast-moving hemoglobins are H, I, and Bart's. When a prominent band is found in the HbS region on cellulose acetate electrophoresis at pH 8.6, its identity can be confirmed with electrophoresis on citrate agar at pH 6.2. This will separate HbS from HbD and HbG. Citrate agar also differentiates HbC from HbS, O, E, and A_2 and provides sharp separation of hemoglobins F and A.

Figure 10-1 Comparison of hemoglobin electrophoretic patterns on cellulose acetate and citrate agars.[*]

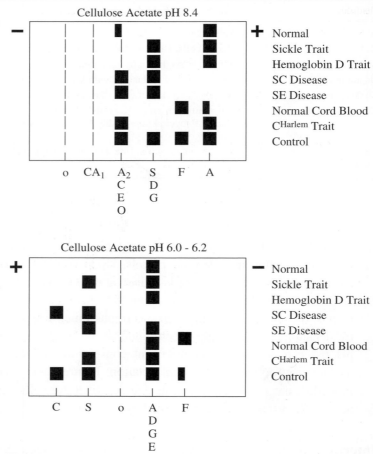

Abbreviation: o = origin.
*Modified with permission from Schmidt RM, Brosious BS: *Basic Laboratory Methods of Hemoglobinopathy Detection.* Publication No. [CDC] 77-8266. Atlanta, DHEW, 1976.

Notes and Precautions. The main limitation of hemoglobin electrophoresis is its inability to detect amino acid substitutions that do not affect charge. Such variants are seen among the unstable hemoglobins and with hemoglobins associated with altered oxygen affinity. Furthermore, as noted previously, different amino acid substitutions may lead to identical changes in electrophoretic mobility.

Figure 10-2 Electrophoretic mobilities of hemoglobins on cellulose acetate (TRIS/EDTA/borate buffer), pH 8.4.*

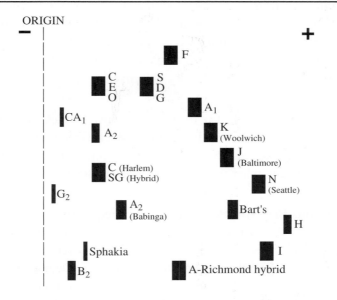

*Modified with permission from Schmidt RM, Brosious BS: *Basic Laboratory Methods of Hemoflobinopathy Detection.* Publication No. [CDC] 77-8266. Atlanta, DHEW, 1976.

10.2 Sickle Cell Test

Purpose. In most cases of sickle cell anemia or the heterozygous sickle disorders (HbSC disease or the S-thalassemias), a few sickled red blood cells are readily seen on the routinely prepared blood smears. In sickle cell trait and in some sickle cell disorders with a lesser propensity for sickling, manipulation is required to induce in vitro sickling.

Principle. When red blood cells containing HbS are deoxygenated, they sickle. Deoxygenation can be accomplished by mixing a drop of blood with a reducing agent on a slide.

Specimen. Venous or capillary blood is used.

Procedure.   The sickle cell test is performed by mixing the amount of blood that adheres to the end of an applicator stick with a drop of freshly prepared 2% sodium metabisulfite solution and covering the suspension with a cover slip. When sickle hemoglobin is present in the red blood cells, they begin to deform within 10 minutes, assuming crescent and holly leaf shapes. The preparation is observed on the microscope within 30 minutes with the high dry objective.

Interpretation.   The test results are positive for sickle cell traits and for all sickle cell disorders in which HbS is present in a concentration of 25% or greater. Sickling has also been described in other relatively rare variants, such as HbC[Harlem].

Notes and Precautions.   The most frequently encountered technical problem resulting in a false-negative test result is outdated metabisulfite reagent that has lost its reducing power. With HbS disorders, test results may not become positive until the infant is 1 or 2 months of age because of the relatively high percentage of HbF in the red blood cells in infancy.

10.3   Solubility Test for HbS

Purpose.   Solubility tests have been used most widely to screen for sickle cell trait, for genetic counseling, and as a means of differentiating HbS from HbD, which are identical on electrophoresis at an alkaline pH.

Principle.   The solubility test is based on the relative insolubility of reduced HbS compared with other hemoglobin variants and HbA in a high-phosphate buffer solution.

Specimen.   Whole blood is used.

Procedure.   A solution of 1.24-mol/L KH_2PO_4 containing saponin to lyse the red blood cells and sodium hydrosulfite (dithionite) to reduce the hemoglobin is used. Blood is added, and the solution is observed for turbidity by the ability to read ruled black lines held behind the test tubes. (Commercial kits are also available.)

Interpretation.   Positive test results are indicated by a turbid suspension through which the ruled lines behind the test tube cannot be seen. Test results are positive for sickle cell trait and sickle cell disorders with rare exceptions (eg, HbC^{Harlem}). Results are negative with all other hemoglobins. The differentiation of sickle cell trait from sickle cell disease may not always be clear since it is based on a quantitative difference in turbidity.

Notes and Precautions.   In the presence of severe anemia, the blood sample usually used may not contain sufficient HbS to yield a turbid solution. With a hemoglobin level less than 7 g/dL (70 g/L), the sample size should be doubled. False-positive results may be seen with lipemic plasma. The solubility test is inadequate as a means of screening for genetic counseling because it fails to detect the important carriers of HbC and beta thalassemia. In general, hemoglobin electrophoresis is needed for a diagnosis of sickle cell anemia, and the sickle cell test and solubility test for HbS are useful only as screening tests.

10.4   Alkali Denaturation Test for Fetal Hemoglobin

Purpose.   Measurement of fetal hemoglobin helps in diagnosis and differentiation of the thalassemias, double heterozygotes with combined thalassemia and a structural hemoglobin variant, as well as in the diagnosis of HPFH. Because the mobility of HbF is close to that of HbA on routine electrophoresis, measurement of HbF based on electrophoretic techniques has not been reliable.

Principle.   HbF is relatively more resistant to denaturation by a strong alkali than other hemoglobins.

Specimen.   Anticoagulated whole blood is used.

Procedure.   Fresh alkali (1.2 N NaOH) is added to a hemolysate. After 1 minute, denatured hemoglobin is precipitated by the addition of ammonium sulfate. The filtrate contains HbF, which is quantitated spectrophotometrically at 415 nm.

Interpretation.   The normal value for HbF is less than 2% (Table 10-6). Patients with beta-thalassemia minor may have elevated HbF levels of 2% to 5%. Those with the less common delta-beta-thalassemia minor may show much higher levels. Patients with homozygous beta-thalassemia show levels of HbF ranging from 30% to 100%. Levels in patients with HPFH range from 15% to 100%. Elevated hemoglobin levels from 2% to 5% have been reported in a large variety of hematologic conditions, including aplastic anemia, pernicious anemia, hereditary spherocytosis, myelofibrosis, leukemia, and metastatic disease with bone marrow involvement.

Notes and Precautions.   The alkali denaturation test is very sensitive at low levels of HbF. At levels greater than 10%, however, the method underestimates HbF, and accurate measurement requires special chromatographic techniques.

10.5   Quantitation of HbA_2 With Chromatography

Purpose.   Levels of HbA_2 are elevated in beta-thalassemia minor. Quantitation of HbA_2 with routine electrophoresis on cellulose acetate has not been uniformly reliable.

Principle.   The most accurate and rapid procedure generally available for measuring HbA_2 is chromatography using an anion exchange column to separate HbA_2 from HbA.

Specimen.   Anticoagulated whole blood is used.

Table 10-6   Hemoglobin Analysis in Beta-Thalassemic Disorders

Classification	Hemoglobin A $\alpha_2\beta_2$	Hemoglobin A$_2$ $\alpha_2\delta_2$	Hemoglobin F $\alpha_2\gamma_2$
Normal	Normal (97%)	Normal (1.5%-3.5%)	Normal (<1%)
Heterozygotes (thalassemia minor)			
Beta-thalassemia	Decreased (>90%)	Increased (3.5%-8%)	Normal or slightly elevated (<5%)
Homozygotes			
Beta$^+$ -thalassemia	Present, decreased	Variably increased	Increased (<100%)
Beta^0 -thalassemia	Absent	Mildly increased (1.5%-4%)	Increased (nearly 100%)
Delta-beta thalassemia	Absent	Absent	Increased (100%)

Beta$^+$ refers to reduced production of beta chains; beta^0, absence of beta chain production.

Procedure.   HbA$_2$ is separated from HbA by use of a column consisting of diethylaminoethyl (DEAE)-cellulose as the ion exchange resin. The resin is equilibrated with a TRIS(hydroxymethyl)-aminomethane phosphate buffer, and the hemoglobin solution is applied. The more strongly charged HbA adheres to the ion exchange resin. HbA$_2$ passes through and is quantitated spectrophotometrically at 415 nm. (Commercial kits with disposable columns are available.)

Interpretation.   The normal range of values for HbA$_2$ is 1.5% to 3.5% (see Table 10-6). In heterozygous beta-thalassemia, the range is 3.5% to 8%.

Notes and Precautions.   A number of hemoglobin variants are eluted from the column under the usual test conditions. These include hemoglobins C, E, O, D, and, to a lesser extent, S. When a value greater than 8% is found, the presence of such a variant is likely. HbA$_2$ may be separated and quantitated in the presence of HbS by eluting the two hemoglobins separately, using buffers with different pH for elution. HbA$_2$ levels may not be elevated in the presence of coexisting iron deficiency.

10.6 Acid Elution Test for Fetal Hemoglobin in Red Blood Cells

Purpose. The acid elution test is used to differentiate HPFH from other states associated with high fetal hemoglobin levels.

Principle. When hemoglobin is precipitated inside the red blood cell and fixed with alcohol, the precipitated HbA and most variants can be solubilized in a buffered solution of citric acid and will be eluted from the cell. HbF remains precipitated inside the cell.

Specimen. Whole blood is used.

Procedure. A blood smear is prepared in the usual manner and fixed in 80% ethanol. It is then treated with a citric acid-phosphate buffer (pH 3.3), which elutes HbA from the red blood cells. The blood film is then stained with eosin, which stains any residual precipitate.

Interpretation. Smears from normal blood show little, if any, staining and appear as ghosts. A heterogeneous distribution of fetal hemoglobin is seen in newborn infants, with fetal-maternal transfusion, and in the thalassemias, with elevated HbF levels. HPFH is the only condition in which HbF is evenly distributed among nearly all of the red blood cells.

Notes and Precautions. The intensity of the staining often differs markedly from one part of the blood film to another, and considerable experience may be required for interpretation.

10.7 Isopropanol Stability Test

Purpose. The isopropanol stability test is used to detect unstable hemoglobins.

Principle. Unstable hemoglobins have reduced stability when compared to normal hemoglobins.

Specimen. Whole blood is used.

Procedure. A hemolysate is added to buffered isopropanol and incubated at 37°C. The preparation is observed for precipitation at 5-minute intervals over 30 minutes.

Interpretation. Unstable hemoglobins generally show turbidity within 5 to 10 minutes, while normal hemoglobins should remain clear for 30 minutes. False-positive test results may be obtained with sickle hemoglobin, fetal hemoglobin, and methemoglobin.

10.8   Test for HbH Inclusion Bodies

Purpose. HbH is an unstable hemoglobin that may be difficult to detect on routine electrophoresis. This test allows detection of HbH and may suggest the presence of other unstable hemoglobins.

Principle. Incubation of whole blood with brilliant cresyl blue causes oxidation and precipitation of HbH, resulting in diffuse stippling.

Specimen. Fresh whole blood is used.

Procedure. Three to four drops of whole blood are incubated with 0.5 mL of a 1% solution of brilliant cresyl blue in citrate-saline solution. Blood films are made at 10 minutes, 1 hour, and 4 hours.

Interpretation. Positive cells show a diffusely clumped pattern of staining throughout the cell, resembling a golf ball, with the reticulum staining light blue (Image 10-5). In HbH disease, 50% or more of the cells on the 1-hour slide may be positive. Results with other unstable hemoglobins are variable, with a longer period of incubation usually required for precipitation and fewer cells staining. The 10-minute slide is a control that shows the number of reticulocytes.

Ancillary Tests

Heinz Bodies.   Heinz bodies are particles of denatured hemoglobins that are attached to the cell membrane (Image 10-4) and are demonstrated with a variety of supravital dyes, such as crystal violet or brilliant cresyl blue. Heinz bodies are found in association with unstable hemoglobin disorders in patients who have undergone splenectomy. They may also be seen during acute drug-induced hemolysis. Incubation of blood with acetylphenylhydrazine or other reagents that cause hemoglobin oxidative damage results in the formation of Heinz bodies in vitro. The pattern of Heinz body formation when such incubation has been carried out under carefully controlled conditions differs in patients with unstable hemoglobins or oxidative hemolysis and normal cells.

Crystal Cells of HbC Disease.   Crystal cells of HbC disease (Image 10.2) are present in as many as 10% of the circulating cells in patients with this disorder who have undergone splenectomy, but these tetrahedral crystals are rare when a functional spleen is present. Crystal cells may be produced in vitro by hypertonic dehydration of red blood cells in a 3% NaCl buffer for 4 to 12 hours.

Course and Treatment

The course and treatment of these hemoglobin synthesis disorders varies greatly depending on which mutation is present. Sickling disorders are characterized by disturbances in the microcirculation since sickle cells are rigid and do not pass through capillaries readily, leading to microinfarction or vaso-occlusion. This may lead to pain or chronic, relentless organ damage. In contrast, the clinical manifestations of HbC disease are minor, being related almost entirely to the moderate anemia that may be present. The thalassemic syndromes also have a wide range of symptoms and clinical severity. The traits are often associated with mild anemia.

In beta-thal-assemia major, transfusions are required to maintain life. This often leads to iron overload, with attendant cardiac damage, requiring lifelong chelation therapy. Patients with hemoglobin H disease should avoid oxidant type drugs, which could precipitate a hemolytic episode. Splenectomy may help to ameliorate the anemia in these patients.

References

Beutler E. The sickle cell diseases and related disorders. In: William WJ, Beutler E, Erslev AJ, et al, eds. *Hematology.* 4th ed. New York, NY: McGraw International Book Co; 1990:613-643.

Bunn HF, Forget BG. *Hemoglobin: Molecular, Genetic, and Clinical Aspects.* Philadelphia, Pa: WB Saunders Co; 1987.

Chanarin I, Waters DAW. Hemoglobin analysis. In: Chanarin I, ed. *Laboratory Hematology.* New York, NY: Churchill Livingstone Inc; 1989:33-54.

Kazazian HH Jr, Boehm CD. Molecular basis and prenatal diagnosis of β-thalassemia. *Blood.* 1988;72:1107-1116.

Stamatoyannopoulos G, Nienhuis AW, Leder P, Majerus PW, eds. *The Molecular Basis of Blood Diseases.* Philadelphia, Pa: WB Saunders Co; 1987.

Weatherall DJ. The thalassemias. In: William WJ, Beutler E, Erslev AJ, et al, eds. *Hematology.* 4th ed. New York, NY: McGraw International Book Co; 1990: 510-539.

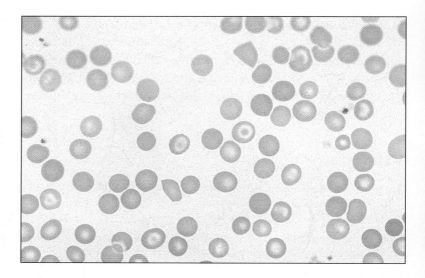

Image 10-1 Beta-thalassemia minor. Microcytosis and a moderate number of target cells are present.

Image 10-2 Hemoglobin C disease. Many target cells and a hemoglobin C crystal cell (↑) are present.

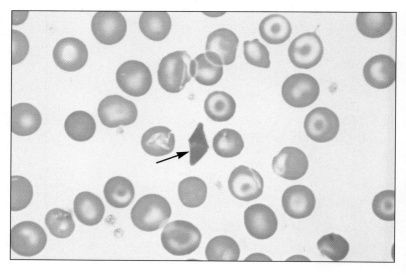

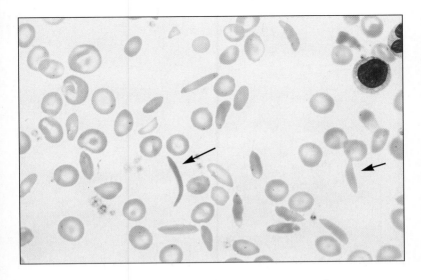

Image 10-3 Sickle cell anemia. Several sickled cells (↑) are seen in addition to target cells and marked anisocytosis.

Image 10-4 Heinz bodies. Supravital staining demonstrates Heinz bodies as coarse, dark dots within the red blood cell.

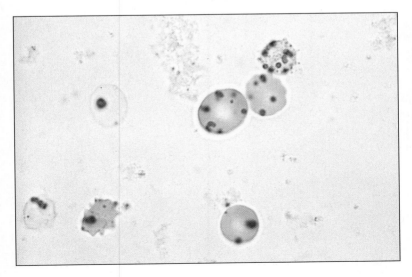

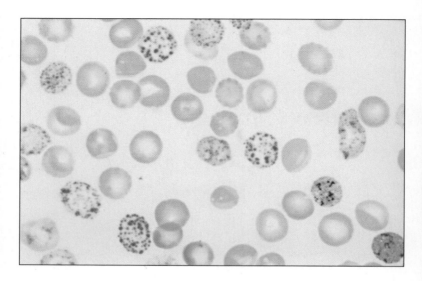

Image 10-5 Hemoglobin H disease. Brilliant cresyl blue staining shows a diffusely clumped staining pattern demonstrating the presence of denatured unstable hemoglobin.

11

Paroxysmal Nocturnal Hemoglobinuria

Paroxysmal nocturnal hemoglobinuria (PNH) is a rare chronic hemolytic disorder in which characteristic episodic hemolysis occurs. Hemolysis is due to acquired deficiencies of red blood cell membrane proteins that predispose the cell to complement-mediated lysis.

Pathophysiology

PNH is an acquired red blood cell membrane disorder, probably arising secondary to a somatic mutation in a pluripotential hematopoietic stem cell. Thus, while white blood cells and platelets are also abnormal, the red blood cell abnormalities usually predominate clinically. This mutation may occur in the setting of bone marrow injury associated with aplastic anemia or bone marrow hypoplasia.

Patients with PNH are deficient in membrane glycoproteins that regulate complement activity including CD59 (membrane inhibitor of lysis), decay accelerating factor (DAF), and homologous restriction factor (HRF), which normally inhibit complement activation. These deficiencies have recently been shown to be due to decreased production of a glycosylphosphatidylinositol anchor which links these proteins to the cell membrane. This leads to enhanced formation of the complement membrane lytic complex on the cell surface. Although red blood cells appear most susceptible to complement-mediated lysis, all hematopoietic cells are similarly affected, which may lead to leukopenia and/or thrombocytopenia in some patients. Hemolysis is sometimes increased at night due to a slight fall in plasma pH that facilitates complement activation.

Clinical Findings

PNH usually begins as insidious onset of anemia. The classically described pattern of episodic hemolysis—increased at night, which causes dark urine after awakening—is often not seen. More often, hemolysis occurs in an irregular fashion, apparently precipitated by events such as infections, operations, and transfusions. Hemoglobinuria or dark urine may be absent. Chronic urinary iron loss, or hemosiderinuria, is a constant feature and may cause the development of iron deficiency anemia.

Abnormal platelet function in these patients is frequently associated with venous thrombosis, which is a major cause of death. Thrombotic events may cause severe episodes of abdominal or back pain or severe, refractory headaches. Thrombophlebitis may occur in the legs or arms and may lead to thromboembolism. Occasionally, patients may experience bleeding due to poor platelet function. Patients are often leukopenic at some stage of the disease, leading to increased susceptibility to infections. In addition, white blood cells show a decrease in leukocyte alkaline phosphatase (LAP) activity.

Approach to Diagnosis

Depending on the predominant features of the presenting illness, PNH may need to be differentiated from other causes of chronic hemolytic anemia, pancytopenia, iron deficiency, or hemoglobinuria. Laboratory evaluation of this disorder is done by the following:

1. Hematologic evaluation with complete blood cell count, peripheral blood morphology, and bone marrow examination.

2. The sucrose hemolysis and urine hemosiderin tests are used as screening tests for PNH.

3. The acid hemolysis test (Ham's test) is a definitive diagnostic test for PNH.

Hematologic Findings

Blood Cell Measurements. The degree of anemia varies widely, with hemoglobin levels ranging from less than 6 g/dL (60 g/L) to normal. The mean corpuscular volume (MCV) may be somewhat increased (with prominent reticulocytosis), or decreased due to iron deficiency anemia. Often, the observed reticulocytosis is low for the degree of anemia. This discrepancy can be attributed to the bone marrow stem cell defect.

Peripheral Blood Smear Morphology. No characteristic morphologic changes are seen. Macrocytosis and polychromatophilia may accompany prominent reticulocytosis. Iron deficiency may result in microcytosis and hypochromia. Spherocytes are absent. Moderate leukopenia and variable thrombocytopenia may be seen.

Bone Marrow Examination. Normoblastic erythroid hyperplasia is the most frequent finding, with adequate numbers of megakaryocytes and myeloid elements. Bone marrow cellularity may be decreased or aplastic in some patients. Stainable storage iron is usually absent, even when clinical iron deficiency is not present.

Other Laboratory Tests

11.1 Sucrose Hemolysis Test

Purpose. The sucrose hemolysis test is the most commonly used screening test for PNH.

Principle. An isotonic sucrose solution of low ionic strength aggregates serum globulins onto the red blood cell surface.

This promotes the binding and activation of complement on the red blood cell membrane. When a small amount of serum (as a source of complement) is added, PNH cells are lysed, whereas normal cells are not.

Specimen. Whole defibrinated blood is used.

Procedure. A small amount of fresh, normal, type-compatible serum is added to a buffered 10% sucrose solution. Washed red blood cells from the patient are added, and the suspension is incubated for 60 minutes at room temperature.

Interpretation. Lysis of greater than 5% of the red blood cells, as detected by release of hemoglobin, which imparts a red color to the supernatant that is detectable by the eye, is compatible with the diagnosis of PNH. Very mild hemolysis, usually amounting to less than 5% of the red blood cells, may be found in the megaloblastic anemias and in autoimmune hemolytic disease. A definitive diagnosis requires performance of the acid hemolysis test (Test 11.2).

Notes and Precautions. It was originally suggested that the sucrose hemolysis test could be carried out using unbuffered sucrose solutions, which may lead to false-negative results. Ethylenediaminetetraacetic acid (EDTA), used in blood collection, will block complement activation and invalidate the test results.

11.2   Acid Hemolysis Test

Purpose. The acid hemolysis test is required to make a definitive diagnosis of PNH.

Principle. Complement fixes to red blood cells at a slightly acidic pH. Cells from patients with PNH will lyse under these conditions, whereas normal red blood cells are resistant to lysis.

Specimen. Whole defibrinated blood is used.

Procedure. The acid hemolysis test is carried out using type-compatible blood from a healthy control subject and blood from a patient with suspected PNH. Red blood cells from the patient or control subjects are suspended in each of the following four serum preparations from both the patient and control subject:

1. Unaltered serum.
2. Serum with a pH adjusted to 6.8 as measured with a pH meter.
3. Serum at pH 6.8 that has been heat inactivated to 56°C for 3 minutes.
4. Heated serum to which guinea pig complement has been added.

Interpretation. A definitive diagnosis of PNH depends on demonstration of all of the following characteristics of in vitro hemolysis:

1. It occurs with patient cells but not with control cells.
2. It is enhanced by slightly acidifying the serum used.
3. It is abolished by heat inactivating the serum at 56°C.
4. Hemolytic activity is not restored to the heated serum by the addition of guinea pig complement.

Some hemolysis may be present in the unaltered serum, but this is generally less than that observed in acidified serum. No hemolysis of control cells should occur in any of the tubes.

Notes and Precautions. Erroneous test results can be obtained by either overacidification or underacidification of serum. In the test as originally described, the pH of the serum was not verified with a pH meter because such instruments were not available. Careful adjustment of the pH of the serum to 6.8 ± 0.1 is necessary if reliable results are to be obtained.

11.3 Test for Urine Hemosiderin

Purpose. Urine hemosiderin is nearly always present in PNH and may provide a valuable screening test.

Principle. Even in the absence of discernible hemoglobinuria, chronic low-grade intravascular hemolysis associated with PNH is sufficient to lead to depletion of serum haptoglobin. This results in the presence of hemoglobin in the plasma, which is reabsorbed by the renal tubules. As the renal tubules become heavily laden with iron, it is excreted in the urine as hemosiderin granules, which are demonstrable with the Prussian-blue stain.

Specimen. A random urine specimen.

Procedure. The presence of hemosiderin in the urine is demonstrated by adding a drop of a mixture of equal parts of 4% hydrochloric acid and 4% potassium ferrocyanide to the sediment of a centrifuged urine specimen. The mixture is incubated at room temperature for 10 minutes, with frequent agitation.

Interpretation. Hemosiderin appears as blue particles. While considerable emphasis has been placed on the intracellular location of hemosiderin in urine, cells containing hemosiderin may have disintegrated in the urine, and free hemosiderin may be the predominant form. Healthy patients' urine does not contain hemosiderin.

Ancillary Tests

Quantitative testing of complement sensitivity may give more precise information regarding the size of the complement-sensitive population; however, it is too complex for routine clinical use. Red blood cell acetylcholinesterase activity and leukocyte alkaline phosphatase activity are diminished in PNH. Flow cytometric techniques for quantification of cell surface decay accelerating factor (CD55) and CD59 levels are being developed.

Course and Treatment

The course may be fulminating or chronic. Occasionally, acute myelogenous leukemia or a myelodysplastic syndrome may supervene. Thrombotic complications, particularly the Budd-Chiari syndrome, may be rapidly fatal. Treatments that have been used include symptomatic blood product transfusions, androgenic steroids to stimulate hematopoiesis, corticosteroids, thrombolytic or anticoagulant agents, and bone marrow transplantation. The latter may be curative.

References

Nicholson-Weller A, Spicer DB, Austen KF. Deficiency of the complement regulatory protein, 'decay-accelerating factor,' on membranes of granulocytes, monocytes, and platelets in paroxysmal nocturnal hemoglobinuria. *N Engl J Med.* 1985;312:1091-1097.

Rosse WF. Paroxysmal nocturnal hemoglobinuria and decay accelerating factor. *Ann Rev Med.* 1990;41:431-436.

Rotoli B, Luzzatto L. Paroxysmal nocturnal hemoglobinuria. *Semin Hematol.* 1989;26:201-207.

Ware RE, Rosse WF, Howard TA. Mutations within the Piga gene in patients with paroxysmal nocturnal hemoglobinuria. *Blood.* 1994;83:2418-2422.

Zalman LS, Wood LM, Frank MM, et al. Deficiency of the homologous restriction factor in paroxysmal nocturnal hemoglobinuria. *J Exp Med.* 1987; 165:572-577.

12

Extrinsic Hemolytic Anemia: General Concepts and Transfusion Reactions

In addition to the intrinsic (inherited) hemolytic anemias and paroxysmal nocturnal hemoglobinuria (PNH), there are a varied group of hemolytic anemias caused by extrinsic factors such as circulating antibodies, chemical, physical, or infectious agents (Table 12-1). In general, antibody-mediated hemolysis is the most common of this group seen clinically. Antibodies can be produced in response to foreign red blood cell antigens (alloantibody), to self-antigens (autoantibody), or to drugs bound to the red blood cell membrane. In this chapter, some of the general features of extrinsic hemolytic anemias will be covered, as well as alloantibody reactions following incompatible transfusion. Subsequent chapters will examine the other primary types of extrinsic hemolytic anemia.

Pathophysiology

Red blood cells contain a large number of cell surface proteins and glycoproteins that are immunogenic, thereby providing the basis for modern day blood banking (Table 12-2). Exposure to a foreign red blood cell surface protein will act as an antigenic stimulus, causing production of either IgG or IgM antibodies (Table 12-3). IgM is a

Table 12-1 Hemolytic Anemia Caused by Extrinsic Factors

Category	Specific Agent
Infectious	Protozoal: malaria
	Bacterial: cholera
	Viral
Physicochemical	Burns
	Chemicals: dose-related toxins (benzenes)
	Drugs: enzyme deficiencies
Antibody-induced	Alloantibody: incomplete transfusion, fetomaternal incompatibility
	Autoantibody: warm-type autoantibodies, cold-type autoantibodies
	Drug-induced antibody: toxic immune complexes (quinidine, quinine); haptens (penicillin); alpha-methyldopa type

Table 12-2 Common Blood Antigens Associated With Clinically Significant Alloantibodies

ABO group antigens
Lewis antigens
Ie antigens
Rh antigens including D/d, C/c, E/e
Kidd group antigens
Duffy group antigens
Kell group antigens

large molecule (molecular weight, 900,000 d) with 10 antigen-binding sites allowing linking together of several cells or agglutination. IgM tends to bind more readily to cells at temperatures below body temperature, hence its association with cold-type immunohemolytic anemia. Complement is activated by IgM binding to the red blood cell surface, and complement-mediated intravascular hemolysis will occur. Clinically important IgM antibodies include the naturally occurring antibodies against red blood cell proteins that allow recognition of foreign blood types, as well as the cold agglutinins that develop following infections or as autoimmune phenomena. In con-

Table 12-3   Properties of Immunoglobulins Acting in Immune Hemolysis by Alloantibodies

Property	IgM	IgG
Size	900,000 d	160,000 d
Antigen binding sites	10	2
Agglutination	Yes	No
Optimal binding temperature	<37°C	37°C
Common antibodies	Blood group antigens	Antigens from previous transfusion or pregnancy
Mechanism of hemolysis	Complement-mediated lysis	Reticuloendothelial cell removal of Ig-coated cells
Type of transfusion reaction	Acute	Delayed

trast, IgG is a much smaller molecule (molecular weight, 160,000 d) with only two antigen-binding sites. Thus, IgG tends to coat red blood cells but does not cause agglutination. Clinically important IgG antibodies causing hemolysis include alloantibodies from previous pregnancy or fetomaternal hemorrhage that cross the placenta and cause hemolytic disease of the newborn, autoimmune or drug-induced hemolytic reactions, and those found in association with lymphoproliferative or chronic inflammatory disorders. However, most of the IgG-mediated hemolytic anemias are idiopathic in cause. Hemolysis is due to removal of the antibody-coated cells by the spleen or cells of the reticuloendothelial system. Large amounts of antibody coating the cells may lead to complement fixation on the cell surface, which will increase the rate of cellular destruction by splenic or liver macrophages, but will not result in complement-mediated lysis.

Physicochemical injury to red blood cells by thermal burn or some chemical agents results in partial loss of red blood cell membrane and spherocytosis, leading to accelerated splenic removal. Full-thickness burns (third-degree) cause damage to red blood cells in the underlying microcirculation. As soon as the damaged cells are removed, the hemolysis stops. Infectious agents (eg, malaria, babesiosis) may disrupt the red blood cell since they proliferate within it, or produce enzymes, such as neuraminidase, that damage the membrane (eg, cholera).

Clinical Findings

Destruction of red blood cells produces anemia, malaise, fatigue, pallor, and weakness. Jaundice is seen with rapid red blood cell destruction, but may be absent in chronic hemolysis. IgM cold active antibodies may lead to vaso-occlusion peripherally in fingers and toes where cooling occurs. Hemolysis ranges from mild to severe. Splenomegaly is uncommon. In contrast, IgG antibodies may result in an acute severe anemia or in a chronic unremitting process. Splenomegaly is common and hepatomegaly may be seen. Lymphadenopathy is rare unless hemolysis is associated with a malignant lymphoma.

Both IgG and IgM alloantibodies act in transfusion reactions. Transfusion reactions may vary from intravascular hemolysis to unexplained shortened red blood cell survival. Acute hemolytic transfusion reactions are usually due to IgM antibodies that recognize transfused red blood cell incompatibility, causing intravascular hemolysis of donor cells. In most cases, this is due to misidentification of blood samples, since crossmatching should help identify most antibodies that would give rise to significant hemolysis. Associated symptoms include fever, chills, facial flushing, hypotension, nausea, vomiting, hemoglobinemia, and hemoglobinuria with subsequent renal shutdown. Delayed hemolytic reactions occur 3 to 14 days after transfusion in patients who have previously been exposed to a blood group antigen via prior transfusion, but do not have detectable antibody at the time of crossmatch. This leads to a secondary, IgG-mediated immune response with attendant hemolysis by the reticuloendothelial system and spleen.

Approach to Diagnosis

A complete history with careful attention to transfusions, drugs, infections, travel, and chronic inflammatory or lymphoproliferative diseases is essential when evaluating an acquired hemolytic process. Infectious diseases, such as bacterial sepsis, causing hemolysis are generally prostrating, and clinical findings separate them from immune hemolysis. Careful examination of the peripheral blood smear and an appropriate travel history helps to establish the diagnosis of malaria or other intraerythrocytic parasites.

Antibody-mediated hemolysis, in particular transfusion reactions, may occur as an acute process or as a delayed process, occurring 3 to 14 days after a transfusion. Historical information, such as sources of exposure to red blood cell products, how recently exposure occurred, and any symptoms associated with the exposure help to guide evaluation of the process. Usually acute transfusion reactions occur due to errors in identification. Delayed type hemolytic reactions occur in patients who have been previously sensitized to red blood cell antigens by pregnancy or previous transfusion, but have antibody levels too low to detect with pretransfusion screens. The transfusion is usually uneventful, but 3 to 14 days later, IgG antibodies are readily detectable and hemolysis occurs. Workup of suspected antibody-mediated or transfusion reaction hemolysis should include the following:

1. Serum antibody screening, which should include several serologic techniques and temperature variations to detect both IgG and IgM antibodies.

2. Pretransfusion or posttransfusion antibody identification combined with appropriate antigen typings of the patient's red blood cells.

3. Direct antiglobulin test (see Test 6.4) if transfusions have been given in the previous 3 to 6 weeks, or if autoimmune hemolysis is suspected.

4 Tests to evaluate acute hemolysis, such as plasma/urine hemoglobin, serum haptoglobin, and serum bilirubin. If intravascular hemolysis has occurred, tests to monitor renal function are also performed.

Hematologic Findings

Often, hematologic tests for transfusion reactions are unrevealing unless transfusions are currently being given. An abrupt fall in hemoglobin up to 14 days after transfusion, a failure to maintain hemoglobin levels after transfusion, or the appearance of jaundice suggest incompatible transfusion. Prolonged administration of incompatible blood can result in splenomegaly and lead to the mistaken diagnosis of autoimmune hemolytic anemia. Intravascular hemolysis may result from ABO incompatible transfusion and with a variety of other antibodies including anti-Kell, anti-Duffy (anti-Fy^a), anti-Kidd (anti-Jk^a or anti-Jk^b), anti-E, anti-C, and anti-S.

Blood Cell Measurements.   Variable anemia is present. One unit of packed red blood cells should increase the hemoglobin (1.5 g/dL [15 g/L]) or the hematocrit (3% [0.03]) in an adult of average size. Acute hemolysis may be associated with leukocytosis and a left shift.

In thermal burns or ABO incompatible transfusions with marked microspherocytosis, the mean corpuscular volume (MCV) may be decreased as low as 60 to 70 µm^3 (60-70 fL).

Peripheral Blood Smear Morphology.   Usually, peripheral smear findings are nonspecific. Transfusions that are ABO incompatible and IgG-mediated hemolysis are associated with microspherocytes. Thermal burns are also associated with transient microspherocytosis lasting 24 to 48 hours. Disseminated intravascular coagulation can be associated with red blood cell fragmentation.

Bone Marrow Examination.   Bone marrow examination is usually not helpful. Prolonged transfusions result in an increase in bone marrow iron. Prolonged hemolysis may also lead to a compensatory erythroid hyperplasia.

Other Laboratory Tests

12.1   Serum Antibody Screening

Purpose.   Serum antibody screening depicts the presence of preformed red blood cell antibodies.

Principle.   Antibody to red blood cell antigens agglutinates or hemolyzes screening cells with the antigen, when the medium of the reaction and the temperature of reaction is appropriate. These tests are widely available, although the reliability of interpretation is variable.

Specimen.   Ten milliliters of serum is obtained fresh to conserve complement, since some antibodies are complement-dependent. If blood must be mailed to a reference laboratory, the serum should be separated from the cells to prevent spurious hemolysis, and both red blood cells and serum must be sent for testing. If serum cannot be tested within 48 hours, it should be stored frozen to conserve complement.

Procedure.   The patient's serum is screened with commercially supplied red blood cells that have most of the 18 major antigen groups represented. Screening cells and serum are incubated at room temperature to detect IgM antibodies, and at 37°C followed by the antiglobulin reaction (indirect Coombs' test) to detect IgG antibodies. IgA antibodies are rarely detected in blood group serology. If antibody is strongly suspected, but not detected, laboratories in larger hospitals or reference laboratories automatically perform tests at 4°C or may use enzyme-treated red blood cells or low ionic strength saline solution (LISS) as the test medium.

Interpretation.   Any degree of hemolysis or agglutination at any stage of the testing is considered positive and graded from 0 to 4+. The antibody must then be identified to assess transfusion hazard and future availability of blood. Results of antibody screening may be negative despite previous reactions to transfusion or incompatible pregnancies, since antibodies may fade completely with time or are of such low titer that they are detectable only with enzyme-treated red blood cells or with cells homozygous for the antigen. Suspicious histories should be reported to the laboratory so that technologists can expand their testing beyond the routine screening procedures. Antigen-incompatible transfusions have diminished red blood cell survival or may have abrupt hemolysis. Antibody is found in 2% to 3% of the previously transfused population, 2% to 3% of those previously pregnant, and less than 1% of all others, for a combined incidence of 5% to 6%.

12.2 Antibody Identification

Purpose. Antibody identification assesses current hazard to transfusion, predicts reliability of crossmatch procedures, evaluates availability of blood (particularly under emergency circumstances), and depicts multiple antibodies.

Principle. The availability and completeness of identification procedures vary in hospital laboratories, and may be best handled by a reference laboratory when specimens with positive results on screening are identified. Depending on distance and complexity of the problem, results may require 1 to 5 days.

Specimen. Serum separated from the clot and a sample of the patient's red blood cells, either from the clot or from a separate anticoagulated (ethylenediaminetetraacetic acid [EDTA]) tube, are used as specimens. If serum cannot be tested within 48 hours, it should be stored frozen to conserve complement.

Procedure. Serum is tested with commercially available panels of nine or ten red blood cell samples for which all antigens are known. Serum is also tested with the patient's own cells and usually with samples of cord blood as well. Serum and cell samples are incubated at room temperature and at 37°C followed by the antiglobulin reaction. The presence of agglutination or hemolysis is noted and graded. Variability in strength of agglutination, temperature of reaction, or medium of reaction may indicate the presence of more than one antibody. Once antibody specificity is known, the patient's red blood cells are typed for the appropriate antigen.

Interpretation. Alloantibody agglutinates specific cells of the panel, but not the patient's own. The pattern of reactive cell samples is compared with the protocol sheet to determine specificity. The patient's own cells should be negative for the particular antigen, and if they are not, the antibody specificity is not confirmed and must be reevaluated.

IgG antibodies are detected at 37°C by indirect antiglobulin, by enzymatic, or by LISS techniques. They usually follow previous transfusion or incompatible pregnancy. Four antibodies: anti-Kell, anti-Fy^a, anti-Jk^a, or anti-Jk^b, are particularly dangerous since they cause intravascular hemolysis and/or disseminated intravascular coagulation (DIC). The Kidd antibodies may not be found during antibody screening, but rapidly increase their titer with incompatible transfusions and may cause intravascular hemolysis beginning as long as 10 days after transfusion when the stimulated antibody titer reaches a critical level. The members of the Rh system (anti-D, -C, -E, -e) follow an immunizing stimulus and destroy cells more slowly by splenic sequestration. Rarely anti-E or anti-C has caused abrupt intravascular hemolysis. IgM antibodies bind complement. Although they may follow incompatible transfusion, they more often appear spontaneously and, therefore, unpredictably. They include anti-Lewis^a and anti-Lewis^b, anti-P1, and anti-M. Many researchers believe that alloantibodies reactive at or below room temperature are not clinically significant. However, if the antibody reacts by the antiglobulin phase, the potential for transfusion reactions exists.

Once identified, antibodies must be permanently recorded, since they may fade with time only to reappear with incompatible transfusions, or are so weak that truly incompatible units appear compatible. The most lethal IgM antibodies are anti-A and anti-B, involved in major blood group incompatibility. Such incompatibility is almost always caused by errors in patient identification. These antibodies are not detectable by antibody identification techniques, because all the test red blood cells are group O.

12.3   Direct Antiglobulin (or Coombs') Test (DAT)

Purpose.   The DAT detects globulin coating of circulating red blood cells, presumably by antibody. It does not distinguish alloantibody from autoantibody. After transfusion, in the absence of autoantibody, the coated red blood cells are donor cells, as confirmed by testing red blood cell antigens.

Principle, Specimen, Procedure.   See Test 6.4.

Interpretation.   Positive results may vary from +/– to 4+, depending on the cause. In autoimmune hemolytic anemia, the DAT tends to be high, whereas in transfusion reactions the DAT is usually 1+ or weaker. The donor cells are a minor population in the patient's circulation, giving a characteristic "mixed-field" appearance. Positive test results may be extremely transient. After massive intravascular hemolysis, the DAT may be negative since all the coated cells are lysed. The antibody specificity of the eluate does not match the patient's red blood cell antigens, although in patients transfused with many units or in those with a DAT of 4+, the antigens may be difficult to determine. Retesting after 4 to 5 days while withholding further transfusions may clarify the picture.

12.4   Serum Haptoglobin

Purpose.   Absence of haptoglobin indicates hemolysis, liver failure, or, rarely, an hereditary variant.

Principle, Specimen, Procedure.   See Test 6.3.

Interpretation.   The normal range of haptoglobin is 40 to 180 mg/dL (0.4-1.8 g/L). Levels less than 25 mg/dL (0.25 g/L) are consistent with hemolysis. Haptoglobin levels may be transiently decreased after massive transfusion as a result of destruction of senescent red blood cells without hemolysis.

12.5   Plasma Hemoglobin

Principle.   IgM antibodies to red blood cell antigens activate the classic complement pathway, resulting in intravascular hemolysis. IgG antibodies of very high titer may also result in intravascular cell destruction.

Purpose, Procedure, Specimen, and Interpretation. See Test 6.2.

12.6 Urine Hemoglobin

Purpose. Free plasma hemoglobin at levels above 150 mg/dL (1.5 g/L) appears in the urine. The test for urine hemoglobin confirms intravascular hemolysis, particularly when venous specimens have been technically difficult to obtain or when obtaining them has been delayed.

Principle. Plasma proteins, haptoglobin, transferrin, and albumin bind free hemoglobin in normal metabolism. When the renal threshold is exceeded, free hemoglobin is detected in the urine. After incompatible transfusion, this is usually a transient occurrence, ending when the incompatible red blood cells have been lysed. With other forms of immune-mediated hemolysis, this may become chronic.

Specimen. Random urine is collected within 2 to 3 hours of the clinical episode.

Procedure. Urine is tested with a dipstick.

Interpretation. Normally, no hemoglobin is present in the urine. Significant reactions are 1+ or greater (scale, 0 to 3+). The urine sediment should be examined for red blood cells (hematuria) not seen with hemolysis but accompanying bladder or prostate surgery and catheters, which may give rise to a false-positive test result. If red blood cell destruction has been occurring slowly over several days, urine hemosiderin may be present without overt hemoglobinuria.

Course and Treatment

Intravascular hemolysis caused by inadvertent ABO incompatibility activates complement and the coagulation cascade to produce disseminated intravascular coagulation. Hypotension, renal failure, and death may follow. The severity of the reaction is dose-related so that treatment requires early recognition to stop the transfusion. Patient hydration must be maintained to avoid renal failure. Osmotic diuresis with 20% mannitol may aid in clearance of plasma hemoglobin. Delayed transfusion reactions produce significant morbidity but less certain mortality. Jaundice and post-transfusion anemia resolve if compatible blood is given. Further transfusion should not be considered until the antibody has been identified and antigen-negative units have been provided.

Hemodialysis may be necessary if renal failure has occurred, and 30% of patients will never regain renal function. In delayed or mild hemolytic transfusion reactions, transfusion with compatible blood and time results in resolution of symptoms and an appropriate posttransfusion hemoglobin level. Treatment of catastrophic infectious disease with hemolysis involves prompt and massive treatment of the underlying organism with appropriate intravenous antibiotic therapy. Malaria is treated with chloroquine, primaquine, or other antimalarial agents, usually with recovery if treated promptly.

References

Issitt PD. *Applied Blood Group Serology.* 3d ed. Miami, Fla: Montgomery Scientific Publications; 1985:99-111.

Kelton JG. Platelet and red cell clearance. *Transfusion Med Rev.* 1987;1:75-84.

Mollison PL. The clinical significance of red cell alloantibodies (and autoantibodies) in blood transfusion. In: Polesky H, Walker R, eds. *Safety in Transfusion Practices.* Skokie, Ill: College of American Pathologists; 1982: 131-150.

Vyas GN. Symposium on transfusion-associated infections and immune response. *Transfusion Med Rev.* 1988;2:193-224.

13

Extrinsic Hemolytic Anemia: Fetomaternal Incompatibility

In fetomaternal incompatibility, or hemolytic disease of the newborn (HDN), the fetus receives antibody passively across the placenta from the mother, who has been exposed to foreign antigens through a previous transfusion or has received small transplacental infusions of red blood cells during the current or a past pregnancy. Many of the characteristics of HDN are similar to those seen in incompatible transfusions.

Pathophysiology

HDN develops due to the transfer of specific red blood cell antibodies across the placenta from the mother to the fetus, which has different red blood cell antigens by virtue of the paternal genetic contribution. Only IgG is capable of crossing the placenta, and the degree of hemolysis is dependent on the amount of antibody as well as the binding avidity of the IgG subtype. Evidence suggests that clinical hemolysis correlates with subtype IgG_3, whereas IgG_1 is not associated with hemolysis. Antibody-coated red blood cells are sequestered in the spleen and liver and destroyed, causing neonatal hepatosplenomegaly.

Maternal sensitization to fetal red blood cell antigens is primarily due to fetomaternal hemorrhage during pregnancy, or more commonly at the time of delivery when the largest blood exchange may occur. The two major types of fetomaternal incompatibility are ABO group incompatibility and Rh incompatibility (Table 13-1).

ABO group incompatibility is very common but usually not clinically severe. The condition is produced by a mother of blood group O with a fetus that is either blood group A or B. It may occur during any pregnancy, even the first, since it is postulated that secreted A or B substance, not just red blood cells, may cross the placenta to induce maternal production of anti-A or anti-B IgG in addition to the IgM anti-A and anti-B normally present. This IgG antibody then recrosses the placenta, attaching to the fetal red blood cells. Antibody avidity is usually poor, so hemolytic disease is slow to appear, usually 3 to 4 days after delivery.

Rh_0 (anti-D) incompatibility appears in pregnancies subsequent to the first as a result of fetomaternal hemorrhage of Rh-positive blood during delivery, thereby sensitizing a Rh-negative mother to produce antibodies. This is much less commonly seen with the current use of prophylactic anti-Rh immune globulin. Given at each abortion or delivery to Rh-negative women, it prevents immune recognition of D antigen by the mother. In 1% of mothers, sensitization may occur in the first pregnancy, but clinical disease in the infant is rare. Occasionally, other antibodies (anti-c, anti-E, and anti-Kell) are involved in fetomaternal incompatibility. The mechanism is the same as that for anti-D, but these antibodies are less efficient at causing neonatal hemolysis and jaundice.

Clinical Findings

Serologic evidence may exist for HDN without clinical evidence of hemolysis, particularly in ABO group incompatibility. Destruction of red blood cells is primarily caused by reticuloendothelial sequestration of IgG-sensitized red blood cells so that the fetal liver and spleen are enlarged and jaundice is present in the neonatal period. In severe Rh-mediated hemolysis, red blood cell destruction occurs in utero. This leads to severe anemia with high output congestive heart failure and anasarca (hydrops fetalis). Jaundice is not seen until after birth, when placental transport of bilirubin is lost

Table 13-1 Characteristics of Hemolytic Disease of the Newborn

Findings	ABO	Rh_0
Clinical		
Pregnancy associated with disease	Any, including the first	After the first pregnancy
Clinical severity	Unpredictable	More severe with each antigen-positive pregnancy
Prenatal evaluation	None needed	Anti-Rh_0 titer, amniocentesis
Onset of jaundice	3-4 wk after delivery	Intrauterine or immediately after delivery
Treatment*	None; phototherapy or rare exchange therapy	None; early delivery, phototherapy, exchange transfusion, or intrauterine transfusion
Laboratory		
Direct Coombs' test	+/− to 1+	2+ to 4+
Fetal blood group	A or B	Rh_0 positive
Antibody	Anti-A or anti-B	Anti-Rh_0 (anti-D)
Maternal blood group	O	Rh_0 negative
Maternal antibody screening	Negative	Positive
Peripheral blood (newborn)	Microspherocytes	Not diagnostic

*Treatment options are listed by increasing severity of hemolysis.

and the neonatal liver assumes bilirubin metabolism. The immature infant liver is initially unable to conjugate bilirubin rapidly enough, leading to high levels of indirect bilirubin and jaundice. The indirect bilirubin is also deposited in the lenticulostriate nucleus of the brain (kernicterus), which may cause mental retardation, motor spasticity, and death.

Approach to Diagnosis

The type of fetomaternal incompatibility producing HDN may be suggested by maternal transfusion and gestational histories. The following tests may be helpful in establishing a diagnosis:

1. Maternal blood group and antibody screening.

2. Newborn blood group.

3. Direct antiglobulin test (DAT) (see Tests 6.4 and 13.3) of newborn cells and eluate of positive red blood cells.

4. Examination of a peripheral blood smear from the infant or cord blood for microspherocytes.

5. If serologic evidence is present for HDN, serial serum bilirubin tests are ordered.

6. The father's blood is tested with the mother's if serologic evidence of HDN is not present, yet the newborn is experiencing hemolysis for undetermined causes and the DAT result is positive. This testing is expected to exclude unusual incompatibilities between paternal antigens (reflected in the child) and maternal antibodies.

7. Although neutralization studies can be performed to classify the maternal antibody as IgG or IgM, knowledge of which helps to estimate likelihood of placental passage, they are rarely necessary or clinically helpful.

Prenatal studies may anticipate clinical disease in the newborn and may direct prenatal or postnatal management. These include titration of anti-D in the maternal serum and amniocentesis to determine levels of intrauterine hemolysis.

Hematologic Findings

There may be a wide spectrum of anemia present, ranging from none to severe. Persistent extramedullary hematopoiesis in an attempt to compensate for hemolysis results in increased circulating nucleated red blood cells (erythroblastosis fetalis). HDN caused by ABO and less common red blood cell antibodies is usually mild. Rh-mediated HDN is progressively severe with each pregnancy, reflected in the severity of fetal anemia.

Blood Cell Measurements. Levels of hemoglobin in mild anemia are 14 to 16 g/dL (140-160 g/L). In moderate anemia, the levels are 10 to 14 g/dL (100-140 g/L); and in severe anemia, they are 8 to 10 g/dL (80-100 g/L). The white blood cell count is 10 to 20 x $10^3/\mu L$ (10-20 x $10^9/L$), and the reticulocyte count is often greater than 10% (0.10).

Peripheral Blood Smear Morphology. The peripheral blood smear shows polychromasia, correlating with the increased reticulocyte count, and nucleated red blood cells greater than 10 per 100 white blood cells (erythroblastosis). Microspherocytes usually indicate ABO hemolytic disease, but usually are not prominent. Thrombocytopenia and leukocytosis are common.

Other Laboratory Tests

13.1 Determination of Blood Group

Purpose.   Testing of the blood group of both the mother and the newborn determines if the mother is negative for antigen and the infant is positive.

Principle.   Maternal red blood cell antigens and newborn antigens are determined for ABO and Rh_0. Tests can be performed for further antigens if indicated.

Specimen.   Red blood cells from clots or anticoagulated specimens are washed well with saline before testing. Specimens are stable for at least 7 days. Cord red blood cells and plasma can be used if the red blood cells are washed well to remove contaminants. Infant heel-stick specimens can also be used.

Procedure.   Standard typing procedures are direct agglutination of red blood cells by anti-A, anti-B, and anti-D antibodies. All Rh(D)-negative cells are tested for D^u, the partial or gene-suppressed D^u antigen.

Interpretation.   In ABO hemolytic disease, the mother's blood is group O (ie, negative for A or B antigens) and the infant's blood is group A or B. In Rh hemolytic disease, the mother is Rh negative and the infant is Rh positive. Where the serologic possibility of both ABO and Rh disease is possible, ie, an O-negative mother with an A- or B-positive child, hemolytic disease is more likely caused by ABO incompatibility, since the group incompatibility has usually lysed Rh-incompatible cells throughout the pregnancy. Mothers who are Rh-positive are not excluded from having infants with hemolytic disease, since they may be negative for minor antigens in the complex (such as C or E) and their offspring positive.

13.2   Maternal Antibody Screening and Identification

Purpose.   A positive antibody screening may indicate anti-Rh_0 type of hemolytic disease rather than ABO type, where screenings are negative.

Principle.   Maternal serum is screened for antibody, usually early in pregnancy and sporadically thereafter to detect IgG or IgM antibodies. The antibody is then identified to assess fetal risk and, if necessary, the father's red blood cell antigens are tested as a predictive measure of fetal involvement.

Specimen.   Serum less than 48 hours old, obtained at the first obstetric visit, is used. A specimen should also be obtained in the third trimester, and more frequently if the early specimen shows positive results, or if the obstetric history warrants it.

Procedure.   Serum is incubated with test red blood cells at room temperature in saline suspension to detect IgM antibodies, and by incubation at 37°C followed by antiglobulin reaction to detect IgG antibodies. All antibodies are identified with the same techniques.

Interpretation.   In ABO hemolytic disease, only the expected anti-A and anti-B antibodies are found in the group O mother, so the antibody screen is negative. In all other types of hemolytic disease, the antibody screen is positive. The antibody must be identified to determine its significance to the newborn. Only IgG antibodies cross the placenta, and they must coat the infant's red blood cells to produce symptoms. Common antibodies found in pregnant women are anti-Lewis[a] and anti-Lewis[b]. These antibodies do not produce neonatal disease because they are IgM and cannot cross the placenta, and because all infants are Lewis[a] and Lewis[b] negative. Thus some antibodies are more significant for the mother in a postpartum hemorrhage than for infant HDN.

The current practice of administering Rh immune globulin at 28 weeks' gestation to prevent erythroblastosis results in positive maternal antibody screening due to weak anti-D (titer, <1:4). Unlike antibody produced as a consequence of natural maternal sesitization, these antibodies do not give a "crisp" pattern of identification.

13.3 Direct Antiglobulin (Coombs') Test in the Newborn

Purpose. The DAT detects globulin coating on the newborn's red blood cells.

Principle. Fetal red blood cells are coated with passively transmitted IgG antibody specific for antigen.

Specimen. Red blood cells from either clotted or anticoagulated cord blood can be used. Small capillary specimens from newborn heel-sticks are also adequate. Cord blood samples are stable for at least 1 week and can be tested if clinical findings appear.

Procedure. Broad-spectrum antiglobulin reagent is centrifuged with the newborn's red blood cells that have been washed with saline to free them of all contaminating substances and serum proteins. Agglutination is graded 0 to 4+. For all tests producing positive results, adsorbed globulin is eluted and tested for antibody specificity.

Interpretation. Infant DAT results are +/– to 1+ for ABO hemolytic disease, 2 to 4+ for Rh hemolytic disease, and 2 to 4+ for hemolytic disease caused by other antibodies. The antibody eluted from the neonatal red blood cells should match that found in the maternal serum. Antibody found only in cord plasma, but not on cord red blood cells, is of doubtful significance, suggesting poor avidity and less likely clinical disease. Antibodies such as anti-c, anti-E, and anti-Kell, adsorbed to fetal red blood cells produce a strong DAT but usually minimal jaundice. Improved antiglobulin reagents make false-negative test results less common, and additional saline washing of the cells diminishes false-negative findings resulting from neutralization of the Coombs' reagent. Rarely, elution of an antiglobulin-negative red blood cell yields antibody because of undetectable numbers of molecules concentrated in the elution process.

Positive DAT results on cord specimens without detectable antibody may indicate adsorption of antibody by Wharton's jelly, but the red blood cell control is usually positive. The test should be repeated on blood from a heel-stick or venous sample. If results are still positive, private antibody limited to this family should be considered, and maternal serum or infant's plasma should be tested against paternal red blood cells for agglutination.

13.4   Acid Elution (Kleihauer-Betke) Stain

Purpose. Fetal-maternal hemorrhage of even small numbers of Rh-positive fetal red blood cells may sensitize the Rh-negative mother unless she is adequately immunized postpartum with Rh immune globulin. Doses are standardized to compensate for fetal hemorrhage volume of 15 mL of packed red blood cells or less. The actual volume of hemorrhage can be calculated by staining a maternal peripheral smear for fetal cells. If the volume of fetal hemorrhage exceeds 15 mL, an increased dosage of the Rh immune globulin should be administered. Intrapartum Rh immune globulin is administered at 20 to 28 weeks' gestation, but Kleihauer-stained peripheral smears are usually not useful at this time because the number of potentially positive cells are so minimal.

Principle.   Fetal hemoglobin is resistant to acid elution, whereas adult hemoglobin is not. A maternal peripheral smear is treated with dilute acid buffer for 10 minutes and then stained. The maternal erythrocyte adult hemoglobin is leached into the buffer leaving red blood cell ghosts, whereas the fetal red blood cells remain as dense red erythrocytes.

Specimen.   Very thin peripheral blood smears fixed in 80% alcohol are prepared from maternal blood collected in ethylenediaminetetraacetic acid (EDTA).

Procedure.   Dried smears are placed in McIlvaine's buffer (pH 3.2) for 10 minutes, followed by washing in distilled water. The smear is then stained with erythrosin and counterstained with hematoxylin. Two thousand cells are counted and the percentage of densely staining cells with fetal hemoglobin (presumably fetal in origin) calculated. The percentage can be converted to milliliters by a nomogram, and 300 mg of Rh immune globulin is administered intramuscularly for each 15 mL of packed red blood cells calculated. Control smears should be made from cord blood specimens (positive) mixed 1 in 10 with adult blood (negative), since questionably positive cells are sometimes seen even with the negative control. Test kits are available using the same principle so that even small laboratories may perform the test.

Interpretation.   Normal adult cells have leaked out hemoglobin and appear as ghosts. Fetal cells are densely pink and refractile. The volume of fetal-maternal hemorrhage is calculated as milliliters of whole blood equal to the percentage of fetal cells x 50. Hemorrhage in excess of 15 mL packed cell volume requires a proportionate increase in Rh immune globulin administered. Since variability in the amount of acid hemoglobin elution may occur even within the same laboratory, it is important that appropriate controls of fetal (cord) blood and adult blood be done to aid in proper interpretation. Work is in progress to develop flow cytometric tests to detect fetal cells, utilizing staining for the Rh antigens, allowing for more extensive evaluation and the ability to detect even a small number of fetal cells within a sample.

Notes.   Adult hemoglobinopathies such as persistent fetal hemoglobin may create a misleading picture. If the volume of fetal cells suggests significant blood loss in an otherwise well infant with normal hemoglobin, the possibility of hemoglobinopathy in the mother should be considered.

Ancillary Tests

Ancillary tests include ultrasonography, which can demonstrate fetal hydrops. Ultrasound localization of the placenta is also necessary prior to amniocentesis for measurement of amniotic fluid pigment, probably bilirubin. This is helpful in estimating the rate of red blood cell destruction and expected degree of fetal anemia. The procedure is undertaken when maternal Rh antibody has been identified and has a significant titer (>1:32). Depending on the titer and the obstetric history, the first procedure is performed at 28 weeks' gestation. At least two specimens are needed to verify an increase in optical density and to determine if the differential absorption is increasing, decreasing, or stable. Specimens are obtained every 1 to 2 weeks, or in borderline cases, every few days.

Amniotic fluid (5-10 mL) is withdrawn and immediately shielded from light, which degrades bilirubin and causes falsely decreased results. The specimen is centrifuged to separate vernix, and the supernatant is scanned in the ultraviolet spectrum from 350 to 700 nm. Bilirubin has a peak absorbance at 450 nm, although the curve is not linear. A tangent is constructed to create a straight line, and the difference in optical density from the tangent to the peak at 450 nm is the Δ OD. Absorbance is plotted vs wavelength. An optical density rise at 450 nm is common early in pregnancy, but decreases after 26 weeks if no red blood cell sensitization is present.

Zones have been determined by Liley that correlate with severity of anemia. If the anemia is severe, and fetal lungs are markedly immature, then intrauterine transfusion is considered. If fetal lung maturation is adequate, then early delivery, which permits extrauterine exchange transfusion, is undertaken. Intrauterine transfusion has a success rate of approximately 85% unless hydrops is present, in which case the success rate is less than 25%.

Notes. False elevations in absorbance are seen when hemoglobin or meconium contaminate the specimen, since one of several hemoglobin A optical peaks occurs at 450 nm. Amniocentesis interpretation is based on experience with anti-D antibody. There is no guaranteed extrapolation to other antibodies nor other causes of hemolysis.

Course and Treatment

Maternal serum is monitored during pregnancy to detect Rh sensitization and follow its course. High Rh antibody titers (>1:32) require amniocentesis to monitor the progression and severity of anemia in the fetus. Rapid progression of hemolysis may require intrauterine transfusion or early delivery with exchange transfusion to treat severe anemia and hyperbilirubinemia. Mild jaundice after birth is controlled with phototherapy, which oxidizes bilirubin in the infant's skin. ABO sensitization is only rarely severe after delivery, often in association with anti-B. No treatment before delivery is necessary, which is also true for HDN caused by other less common antibodies.

References

Blanchette VS, Zipursky A. Assessment of anemia in newborn infants. *Clin Perinatol.* 1984;11:489-510.

Bowman JM. The prevention of Rh immunization. *Transfusion Med Rev.* 1988; 2:129-150.

Levine DH, Meyer HPB. Newborn screening for ABO hemolytic disease. *Clin Pediatr.* 1985;24:391-394.

Mollison PL. Some aspects of Rh hemolytic disease and its prevention. In: Garratty G, ed. *Hemolytic Disease of the Newborn.* Arlington, Va: American Association of Blood Banks; 1984:1-32.

Tannirandorin Y, Rodeck CH. Management of immune hemolytic disease in the fetus. *Blood Rev.* 1991;5:1-8.

Urbaniak SJ. Rh(D) haemolytic disease of the newborn: the changing scene. *Br Med J.* 1985;291:4-6.

14

Drug-Related Extrinsic Hemolytic Anemia

Drugs produce hemolytic anemia by two different mechanisms: by inducing immune-mediated red blood cell destruction or by drug-induced oxidation of hemoglobin in patients with intrinsic defects in hemoglobin synthesis or enzymes needed to protect the cell from oxidative injury. The degree of hemolysis can vary from acute intravascular hemolysis to compensated hemolysis with splenic sequestration. In most cases, the hemolytic anemia is reversible when the drug is withdrawn.

Pathophysiology

Drug-Induced Oxidation of Hemoglobin. A number of drugs have been shown to oxidize hemoglobin in red blood cells. Normally, this does not present a difficulty since the hemoglobin is readily returned to the reduced state. However, in patients with an intrinsic deficiency in the pathways necessary to produce reduced glutathione or in patients with an unstable hemoglobin type, oxidation may lead to hemolysis.

Glucose-6-phosphate dehydrogenase (G6PD) deficiency, which is discussed in more detail in Chapter 9, is the most common enzymatic deficiency associated with drug-induced hemolysis. The inter-action of an oxidant drug with a G6PD-deficient red blood cell leads to depletion of glutathione (GSH) and inadequate production of the reduced form of nicotinamide-adenine dinucleotide phosphate (NADPH). The depletion of GSH is followed by uncontrolled oxi-dation of hemoglobin. Hemoglobin degradation products polymer-ize to form Heinz bodies, with resultant membrane damage and reticuloendothelial phagocytosis by the spleen. Young red blood cells with more NADPH are less susceptible to oxidative damage, so that as reticulocytosis increases, the effect of low doses of the oxidative drug tends to be self-limited. Drugs that induce hemolysis in patients with G6PD deficiency are listed in Table 14-1. These drugs do not uniformly cause hemolysis in any person with G6PD deficiency, nor does every drug analogue in a specific category cause hemolysis.

Patients with unstable hemoglobins, which are discussed in further detail in Chapter 10, may also be more susceptible to oxida-tive damage to hemoglobin. An amino acid substitution in either the alpha or beta chain near the attachment of the heme group of hemoglobin renders the molecule more sensitive to oxidative injury and hemoglobin denaturation. This will lead to the forma-tion of Heinz bodies and hemolysis by reticuloendothelial cells.

Drug-Induced Immune Hemolysis. Drugs can cause immune-mediated hemolysis by a variety of mechanisms, includ-ing drug adsorption to the red blood cell membrane as a hapten, formation of toxic immune complexes, or inducing autoantibodies against the red blood cell membrane (Table 14-2). Except for autoantibody-mediated processes, the drug must be present for hemolysis to occur.

Drugs that cause immune hemolysis often have a benzene ring activated by hydroxyl (–OH), amine (–NH), or sulfur (–S) groups. The drug must bind to a protein carrier, serum proteins, or red blood cell membrane to induce antibody production, and the anti-body produced must have sufficient binding capacity to produce hemolysis. Although by these criteria many drugs are potential causes of hemolysis, most clinically significant cases are caused by penicillin or alpha methyldopa.

Table 14-1   Drugs Commonly Associated With Hemolysis in G6PD

Antimalarial agents
    Primaquine
    Quinacrine
Sulfonamides
    Sulfanilamide
    Salicylazosulfapyridine
    Sulfacetamide
Other antibacterial agents
    Nitrofurantoin
    Nitrofurazone
    Para-aminosalicylic acid
    Nalidixic acid
Analgesics
    Acetanilid
Sulfones
    Diaminodiphenyl sulfone
    Thiazolsulfone
Miscellaneous
    Dimercaprol
    Naphthalene (mothballs)
    Methylene blue
    Trinitrotoluene (TNT)

Abbreviation: G6PD = glucose-6-phosphate dehydrogenase.

Drugs such as penicillin and related antibiotics may also act as haptens by adsorbing to the red blood cell membrane or binding to cell membrane proteins, forming a drug-cell complex that is antigenic. The hapten induces IgG antibody to the penicilloyl moiety, common to drugs of this class and cephalosporins. Drug-coated cells are usually destroyed by the reticuloendothelial system, although intravascular hemolysis can occur. Immune hemolysis occurs only when all three components—drug, protein (or red blood cells), and antibody—are present.

Drug-induced toxic immune complexes are formed following antibody production after a drug binds to a plasma protein to form an immunogen. The drug-protein complex combines with the antibody, and the resultant antigen-antibody complex may attach to the red blood cell, causing activation of complement. Although the immune

Table 14-2 Drug-Mediated Immune Hemolysis and Means of Cellular Destruction

Parameter	Drug Absorption, Hapten Formation	Toxic Immune Complexes	Warm-Type Autoantibodies
Associated drugs	Penicillin and penicillin-type drugs	Quinine, quinidine, nonsteroidal anti-inflammatory agents	Alpha methyldopa, procainamide, mefenamic acid
Role of drug	Binds to red blood cell membrane	Forms antigen-antibody complex that binds to red blood cell	Unknown
Antibody formed	To drug	To drug	To red blood cell
Antibody class	IgG	IgM or IgG	IgG
Proteins detected with direct antiglobulin test	IgG, rarely complement	Complement	IgG, rarely complement
Drug needed for hemolysis	Yes	Yes	No
Mechanism of red blood cell destruction	Splenic sequestration of IgG-coated cells	Complement-mediated lysis and splenic clearance of C_3b-coated cells	Splenic sequestration

complex may then fall off the red blood cell, the complement cascade will continue, causing severe membrane damage and intravascular hemolysis. Thus, a small amount of drug may induce extensive hemolysis. Drugs associated with this type of reaction include quinidine, quinine, and nonsteroidal anti-inflammatory drugs.

Finally, some drugs may induce a true warm-type autoimmune hemolytic anemia, which persists after removal of the drug. The drug most often associated with this type of reaction is alpha methyldopa. The mechanism of antibody production by alpha methyldopa is unknown, although drug-induced alterations of the endoplasmic reticulum of plasma cells have been postulated to explain the persistence of antibody production long after the drug has been discontinued. Clinical hemolysis rarely begins after the drug has been withdrawn, but if hemolysis is already present, it may not resolve for several weeks following discontinuation of the drug.

Clinical Findings

Hemolysis caused by drug interaction with G6PD deficiency or unstable hemoglobins may be an abrupt intravascular event with severe anemia, hemoglobinuria, and jaundice. Anemia occurs 1 to 3 days after beginning treatment with the oxidant drug. If the drug is withdrawn and reticulocytosis begins, the hemolysis will appear to stop.

Drug-induced immune hemolysis is usually less clinically severe, although intravascular hemolysis can occur with all categories of drug-related hemolysis. Hepatosplenomegaly and lymphadenopathy are not associated with drug-induced hemolytic anemia.

Approach to Diagnosis

Proper diagnostic evaluation requires an awareness of drugs that are associated with hemolysis and a high index of suspicion in a patient who is currently receiving, or has recently received, such drugs and who has unexplained anemia. Evaluation proceeds with the following:

1. Hematologic findings, which show a normochromic anemia that may be actively hemolytic. Bone marrow aspiration is usually not needed.

2. Test results for Heinz bodies may be positive in patients with G6PD deficiency or unstable hemoglobins.

3. The direct antiglobulin test result is positive in immunohemolytic processes, although it may be of variable degree depending on the mechanism of drug action.

4. Serum antibody screening tests, which are usually negative with standard reagent red blood cells.

5. Special testing of eluates from Coombs' positive red blood cells in parallel with serum against specific drug-treated red blood cells.

Hematologic Findings

The anemia may be severe, or mild to moderate if well compensated by bone marrow activity. The degree of anemia may also vary depending on the drug mechanism of action, dosage, and the type of antibody evoked. A reactive leukocytosis may appear. In G6PD deficiency and unstable hemoglobins, hemolysis begins as Heinz bodies appear. As the hemolysis persists, Heinz bodies are removed in the spleen and tend to disappear.

Blood Cell Measurements. Hemoglobin can be markedly decreased to 3 g/dL (30 g/L) in severe hemolysis. Elevations in mean corpuscular volume (MCV) to 105 to 110 μm^3 (105-110 fL) reflect reticulocytosis. The white blood cell count is often elevated to 10 to 20 x $10^3/\mu L$ (10-20 x $10^9/L$), and a left shift to the myelocyte stage may be seen.

Peripheral Blood Smear Morphology. Nucleated red blood cells and polychromasia are general findings. Spherocytes may be seen with alpha methyldopa–type autoimmune hemolytic anemias. Target cells are present if jaundice occurs. Bite cells may be seen if Heinz bodies have been extracted in the spleen. Heinz bodies are not seen on Wright's-stained smears, but will be seen on reticulocyte preparations.

Bone Marrow Examination. The bone marrow is hypercellular with normoblastic erythroid hyperplasia and increased iron.

Other Laboratory Tests

For specimen collection in immune hemolysis, whole blood is obtained fresh and allowed to clot at 37°C before the serum is separated. Freezing serum samples should be avoided since this frequently disrupts immune complexes. The red blood cells for testing can be obtained from the clot or from a separately collected ethylenediaminetetraacetic acid (EDTA) specimen, which prevents nonspecific adsorption of complement. Specimens for evaluation in G6PD deficiency may be collected in EDTA.

14.1   Direct Antiglobulin (Coombs') Test (DAT)

Purpose.   The DAT must show positive results for drug-induced immune hemolysis to be considered seriously. Absorbed globulin may be IgG, IgM, or complement.

Principle, Specimen, and Procedure.   See Test 6.4.

Interpretation.   No matter what the mechanism of action, all antibody types have in common antibody globulin and/or complement attached to the red blood cell detectable with the DAT. Without a positive result on the DAT, drug-immune hemolytic anemia is unlikely. The DAT in G6PD drug hemolysis is negative. Often the DAT in drug-induced hemolytic anemias is weakly positive, and use of red blood cell eluates may be necessary for antibody detection. The adsorbed globulin, once detected, is eluted and tested in parallel with the patient's serum against drug-treated red blood cells and untreated red blood cells. The effects of neutralization of the eluate with the suspected drug are also studied. Findings for each category of drug-induced immune hemolysis are summarized in Table 14-2.

14.2   Serum Antibody Tests and Tests With Drug-Treated Red Blood Cells

Purpose.   Agglutination of drug-treated cells by patient serum is consistent with drug-immune hemolysis, but it is not as diagnostic as identifying the globulin actually adsorbed to the red blood cell. For alpha methyldopa, reactions are positive with untreated patient red blood cells, defining the antibody as autoantibody.

Principle.   In general, the organic drug binds with a serum protein or the red blood cell membrane to produce an immunogenic complex. Antibody production, strength, and avidity vary with the drug and with the patient, as well as the duration and route of exposure to the drug. Avidity of the drug (drug adsorption type) or complexes of drug and antibody that fix complement (immune complex type) for the red blood cell membrane appear to be the final common pathway to hemolysis. Some drugs, acting by an unknown mechanism, induce production of a true, warm-type autoimmune hemolytic anemia. Ease of demonstration of the drug antibody varies with the mechanism of action.

Procedure. Tests for the following are available in reference laboratories and most sophisticated hospital blood banks:

1. Drug adsorption. Red blood cells pretreated with weak dilutions of penicillin drugs can be stored in the refrigerator for 2 to 3 weeks for future testing. Treated cells are positive with either direct (IgM) or indirect (IgG) antibody testing. Antibody can be titered against drug-treated cells or neutralized by the appropriate drug.

2. Toxic immune complexes. This is done when the DAT shows coating of the cells with complement. The patient's blood is either pretreated with the drug, or drug is added at the time of the test with patient serum and fresh complement. A DAT is performed. Concentrations of drugs and serum samples are varied to achieve optimum antigen-antibody concentration. Drug neutralization is not demonstrable.

3. True warm-type autoimmune hemolytic anemia (AIHA). The DAT shows agglutination of red blood cells without the drug being present, demonstrating that autoantibodies are present. Weak autoantibodies may require enzyme-treated red blood cells to be demonstrated.

Interpretation.

1. Drug adsorption (penicillins). This type of antibody is common and easily demonstrated. Only IgG antibodies produce significant hemolysis. The antibody may react with one or more penicillin congeners, varying for each patient. Cross-reactions with cephalothin-treated cells occur as a result of

similarities in chemical structure. Antibody titers do not correlate well with clinical hemolysis. The DAT is positive (2 to 4+) with anti-IgG reagents. Weakly positive (±) DAT results are not usually associated with clinical hemolysis. The appearance of a positive DAT is dose- and time-related, usually requiring intravenous antibiotic administration of 10 to 20 million units daily for at least 10 days. Patient red blood cell eluates and the serum react only when the drug is present on the red blood cell membrane, and reactivity is neutralized by high levels of the drug or any cross-reacting drugs, such as methicillin, ampicillin, and oxacillin. Serum antibody alone is not diagnostic because much of the population has IgM antibodies from dietary exposure. Atopic reactions (urticaria, asthma, etc) are unrelated and are caused by IgE antibody.

2. Toxic immune complexes (quinine-quinidine). Negative test results do not exclude the diagnosis of hemolysis since many unknown variables exist. However, this is one of the least common causes of hemolytic anemia in general and of drug-associated immune hemolysis in particular. The DAT result is usually positive, generally because of complement. This can, on rare occasions, provoke intravascular hemolysis not seen in other types of drug-immune hemolytic anemia. If hemolysis has occurred, results of the DAT may be negative. Red blood cell eluates, because they usually contain insignificant amounts of antibody globulin, may not react with drug-treated red blood cells.

3. True warm AIHA (alpha methyldopa). This group is very common and, because antibodies may persist after the drug is withdrawn, its presence is unsuspected until blood is crossmatched for transfusion. The positive DAT results vary from weakly positive to 4+. Formation of autoantibodies is common, and they are found in 10% of patients receiving 1 g/d of the drug or more for longer than 3 months. Direct antiglobulin becomes progressively stronger followed by the appearance of serum antibody. Despite the serologic evidence, only 1% of patients taking alpha methyldopa actually experience hemolysis. These patients should be monitored

with a DAT every 3 to 6 months. Withdrawal of the drug reverses the process, with decrease in serum antibody followed by disappearance of positive DAT results. The presence of antibody and its specificity determines risk with transfusion. Without serum antibodies, transfusion risk is negligible. With serum antibody in a patient with active hemolysis, red blood cell survival is decreased, as for any warm hemolytic anemia.

14.3   Red Blood Cell G6PD Assay

Purpose.   A deficiency of G6PD in a patient with acute hemolysis supports a diagnosis of drug-related hemolysis.

Principle, Specimen, Procedure.   See Test 9.2. Screening tests are available using prepared reagents and fluorometry. These may be followed by quantitative assays.

Interpretation.   The normal range is 2.2 to 5.0 IU/g hemoglobin. Young red blood cells have proportionately more G6PD so that marked reticulocytosis may spuriously elevate the level. Low-normal G6PD levels in the presence of reticulocytosis should be viewed with suspicion and the patient retested in 4 to 6 weeks after likely drugs have been withdrawn. Similarly, if transfusions have been given, retesting must wait for 6 to 8 weeks. Hypochromic anemias may appear to have increased G6PD. Screening tests may miss heterozygote G6PD-deficient red blood cells so that quantitative assays may be necessary.

14.4   Heinz Body Test

Purpose.   G6PD deficiency, as well as other rarer enzyme deficiencies or unstable hemoglobin types are associated with increased numbers of Heinz bodies. This finding is supportive of the diagnosis of drug-induced hemolysis.

Principle. The oxidative pathway of glycolytic red blood cell enzymes maintains hemoglobin stability. In G6PD deficiency, as well as deficiencies of glutathione synthetic enzymes, or unstable hemoglobins, oxidation leads to hemoglobin denaturation. The denatured hemoglobin precipitates, forming Heinz bodies. Normal red blood cells can be induced to form Heinz bodies, but G6PD-deficient cells produce three or four Heinz bodies per red blood cell in the presence of oxidant drugs.

Specimen. Fresh whole blood is collected in EDTA.

Procedure. Methyl violet or neutral red is added to a few drops of blood. Wet mount smears are prepared from the mixture after 15 minutes, 30 minutes, or 1 hour of incubation at room temperature. Red blood cells can also be incubated with phenylhydrazine before preparation of the smears to exaggerate the findings in G6PD deficiency.

Interpretation. Heinz bodies are seen as particles located close to the cellular membrane, ranging in size from 1 to 3 μm. Normal cells may produce a single marginal Heinz body. After phenylhydrazine incubation, G6PD-deficient cells may have three to four Heinz bodies in every cell. If abrupt hemolysis has been present, the test result may be negative because of loss of the Heinz body–positive cells.

Course and Treatment

Immune hemolysis due to drugs is usually mild, although rare cases of severe hemolysis have been reported. All suspicious drugs are immediately discontinued until the cause of hemolysis is determined. If severe intravascular hemolysis has occurred, the patient can be supported with transfusion. In all cases except for those cases where a true warm-type autoantibody has been generated, the antibody is dependent on the presence of the drug and transfusion is tolerated as soon as the drug is cleared from the circulation. With warm-type autoantibodies, such as those seen with alpha methyldopa, antibody persists in the absence of drug. If the DAT result is positive but there is no detectable serum antibody, transfused red blood cells survive normally. However, in the rare instance of acute severe warm-type AIHA, transfused cells have a markedly decreased survival. Therefore, the risk of death from anemia must be weighed against hemolytic complications of transfusion.

Drugs chemically similar to the inciting drug cannot be used again in the patient, since the drug-induced antibody persists for life. When alpha methyldopa or procainamide-type drugs incite a warm-type AIHA, it may be difficult to determine if the hemolysis is caused by unrelated autoimmune disease or by the drug. Active hemolysis of the methyldopa type usually resolves with steroid therapy within 1 to 2 weeks. Steroids can then be tapered without relapse, although the positive DAT result may persist for up to 2 years. If clinical hemolysis is not present, the serologic findings should be allowed to reverse without steroid therapy.

Drug-induced hemolysis in G6PD deficiency is often self-limited as reticulocytes with greater concentrations of enzyme are produced. Drug-induced hemolysis may vary from mild to severe, dependent on the subtype of disease and the oxidative stress (see Chapter 9).

References

Beutler E. Glucose-6-phosphate dehydrogenase deficiency. In: William WJ, Beutler E, Ersley AJ, Lichtman MA, eds. *Hematology*. 4th ed. New York, NY: McGraw-Hill Inc; 1990:591-605.

Chanarin I. *Laboratory Hematology*. New York, NY: Churchill Livingstone Inc; 1989:426-429.

Jandl JH. Heinz body hemolytic anemias. In: *Blood: Textbook of Hematology*. Boston, Mass: Little, Brown, and Co; 1987:335-350.

Packman CH, Leddy JP. Drug-related immunologic injury of erythrocytes. In: William WJ, Beutler E, Ersley AJ, Lichtman MA, eds. *Hematology*. 4th ed. New York, NY: McGraw-Hill Inc; 1990:681-687.

Salama A, Mueller-Eckhardt C. On the mechanisms of sensitization and attachment of antibodies to RBC in drug-induced immune hemolytic anemia. *Blood*. 1987;69:1006-1010.

15

Autoimmune Hemolytic Anemia

Autoimmune hemolytic anemia (AIHA) is caused by antibodies against one's own red blood cell antigens. There are two major sub-categories of AIHA, classified by the temperature at which the autoantibody associates best with the red blood cell antigen. Antibodies that are maximally active at 37°C give rise to warm-type AIHA and clinical syndromes that differ from those autoantibodies that are maximally active at 4°C (cold-type AIHA). The clinical and laboratory characteristics of each type of AIHA are summarized in Tables 15-1 and 15-2.

Pathophysiology

It is unknown why autoantibodies against red blood cells are formed, although a derangement in normal immune function is postulated that allows recognition of self antigens as immunogenic. This may occur as a manifestation of an immune or neoplastic disorder, following the ingestion of certain drugs, following infections, or as an idiopathic process. AIHA can appear at any age, including infancy, although it is more frequent in older age groups. In general,

Table 15-1 Clinical Characteristics of Autoimmune Hemolytic Anemias

Clinical Findings	Warm Type	Cold Type
Onset	Abrupt	Insidious
Jaundice	Usually present	Often absent
Splenomegaly	Yes	Absent
Age	All ages	All ages
Sex	Slightly more women	Women predominate
Origin of autoantibody		
Idiopathic	50%-60%	30%-40%
Drug-induced	25%-30%	1%-5%
Lymphoproliferative disorder	10%-15%	15%-20%
Viral or mycoplasma	0%	25%-35%
Other (inflammatory diseases, other malignancies)	5%-10%	5%-10%

red blood cell lysis occurs following cell membrane binding of IgG or IgM autoantibodies and subsequent complement fixation.

Warm-type AIHA is associated with IgG antibodies in about 90% of cases. Warm reactive autoantibodies coat the cell, leading to increased recognition and subsequent binding by macrophages in the spleen. This enhances the macrophage's ability to phagocytize parts of the red blood cell membrane, leading to the formation of spherocytes and shortened red blood cell survival. If the red blood cell is heavily coated with IgG, complement will also bind to the cell membrane. This usually does not lead to complement-mediated cellular lysis, but the presence of C3 on the cell surface leads to markedly enhanced macrophage binding efficiency and cellular destruction in the liver and spleen. In addition, any process that increases the activity of the mononuclear phagocytic system, such as infection, may further increase hemolysis.

Cold-type AIHA is caused primarily by IgM autoantibodies. Because of the 10 antigen binding sites present on each IgM molecule, they tend to agglutinate red blood cells at low temperatures (<16°C) or in the peripheral areas of the circulation. The agglutinated cells are more susceptible to mechanical trauma and possible hemolysis. If the antibody is active at temperatures approaching

Table 15-2 Laboratory Characterization of Autoimmune Hemolytic Anemias

Laboratory Parameter	Warm Type	Cold Type
Usual immunoglobulin type	IgG	IgM
Direct antibody test	2-4+	2-4+
Monospecific sera		
Anti-IgG only	1+	0
Anti-IgG+ anti-C1	1+	0
Anti-C1 only	Rare	1+
Complement activation	Little or none	Yes
Serum complement levels	Normal or decreased	Decreased
Osmotic fragility	Increased	Normal
Peripheral blood findings	Spherocytes, nucleated red blood cells	Red blood cell agglutination

37°C, it will fix and activate the classic complement cascade on the red blood cell surface, leading either to complement-mediated cellular lysis or increased macrophage-mediated hemolysis in the spleen and liver. In some patients, complement activation will proceed to C3d and stop. Since macrophages have no receptors for this complement component, the cell escapes hemolysis. This effect is seen in ^{51}Cr survival studies when an initial episode of abrupt cell destruction is followed by a slower second phase, where cell survival may approach normal.

AIHA may also be divided by pathogenetic mechanism into either primary (idiopathic) or secondary types. The primary type usually develops in older individuals with no evidence of underlying disease, constituting about 30% of AHIA cases. The remaining 70% of cases are secondary to an underlying disease, drug use, or infection (Table 15-3). Warm-type AIHA is most often associated with autoimmune disorders (such as systemic lupus erythematosus) or neoplastic disorders (such as chronic lymphocytic leukemia or non-Hodgkin's lymphomas). In some cases, the hemolytic anemia may precede the associated disease by several years, necessitating persistent, careful screening for these disorders. Warm-type AIHA secondary to drug use is discussed further in Chapter 14.

Table 15-3 Diseases Associated With Autoimmune Hemolytic Anemia

Disease	Antibody Specificity	
	Warm Antibody	Cold Antibody
Malignancy		
Chronic lymphocytic leukemia	Anti-Rh, LW, Wright[b]	Anti-I
Non-Hodgkin's lymphoma	Anti-u, En[a]	Anti-I
Hodgkin's disease	Anti-Rh	Anti-I
Carcinoma (ovary, thymus, gastrointestinal)	Variable	NA
Inflammatory Disease		
SLE, rheumatoid arthritis, ulcerative colitis	Anti-Rh, LW, Wright[b]	Anti-I, anti-i
Infection		
Mycoplasma	NA	Anti-I
Epstein-Barr virus	NA	Anti-i
Clostridium, Escherichia coli	Anti-T	NA
Drugs		
Methyldopa	Anti-Rh	NA
L-dopa	Anti-Rh	NA

Abbreviations: SLE = systemic lupus erythematosus, NA = not applicable.

Clinical Findings

The clinical history often suggests the type of AIHA. Warm-type AIHA is of abrupt onset, with jaundice and splenomegaly. Anemia may be severe. Cold-type AIHA may also present as an acute onset of anemia, particularly following an infection such as mycoplasma pneumonia, infectious mononucleosis, or cytomegalovirus (CMV). The anemia may range from mild to severe, and intravascular hemolysis may occur. Cold-type AIHA may also have an insidious onset with bone marrow compensation for hemolysis, so that symptoms may be minimal until severe anemia develops. Cold AIHA is usually not associated with jaundice or splenomegaly despite marked anemia.

Most people have low, clinically insignificant titers of cold agglutinins (≤1:32) that bind to red blood cells only at temperatures well below those found even in exposed extremities. When increased production of the IgM leads to higher titers ($\geq$1:256), the temperature of cellular agglutination rises to near 37°C, resulting in complement fixation and a positive direct antiglobulin (direct Coombs') test (see Test 6.4). Clinically, cold-type AIHA can be divided into three categories: acute postviral, chronic idiopathic, and cold agglutinin disease (CAD) (Table 15-4). All three clinical manifestations of cold AIHA produce similar antibodies, but clinical features vary with the cold agglutinin titer. Acute postinfectious cold AIHA is usually seen in younger patients and has an acute, often self-limited course following mycoplasma pneumonia, CMV, or Epstein-Barr virus (EBV) infections. In contrast, chronic idiopathic disease and CAD often occur insidiously in older patients. Chronic idiopathic disease is usually seen in elderly women, whereas cold agglutinin disease is usually associated with an underlying lymphoproliferative malignancy (usually large cell non-Hodgkin's lymphoma).

Paroxysmal cold hemoglobinuria (PCH) is closely related clinically to cold AIHA. It is due to acquisition of an IgG antibody called the Donath-Landsteiner hemolysin. This antibody has a characteristic biphasic mode of action, first adsorbing to red blood cells at low temperature, and then causing intravascular hemolysis and hemoglobinuria as the temperature rises to 37°C. It is important to diagnose PCH since it is usually self-limited and treated by keeping the patient warm.

Approach to Diagnosis

A good clinical history of the hemolytic episode and any other accompanying problems (such as recent infection) combined with pertinent clinical findings (such as the presence of splenomegaly) provide important diagnostic clues as to the cause of the AIHA and will facilitate the workup. Evaluation of the hemolysis proceeds with the following:

1. Hematologic analysis showing a normochromic, normocytic anemia that may be hemolytic in nature. Bone marrow examination is usually not required.

Table 15-4 Characteristics of Cold Agglutinin–Associated Disease

Clinical Parameter	Physiologic	After Infection	Chronic Idiopathic	CAD
Age	Any	Young	Older	Older
Onset	Asymptomatic	Acute, 10-14 days	Insidious	Insidious
Splenomegaly	No	Frequent	No	With lymphoma
Titer	≤ 1:32	≥1:64	≥1:256[*]	>1:10,000[*]
Specificity	Anti-I	Anti-I, anti-i	Anti-I, anti-i	Anti-I
DAT results	Negative	+(G,M,C3)	+(C3)	+(C3)
Intravascular hemolysis	No	40%	No	Rare

Abbreviations: CAD = cold agglutinin disease; DAT = direct antiglobulin test.
*Representative range for titer.

2. Results of direct antiglobulin testing (DAT) or other methods of serum antibody detection should be positive and can identify the absorbed globulins, allowing categorization of the process as a warm-type or cold-type AIHA. If the DAT results are negative, immune hemolysis cannot be proved.

3. If a cold-type AIHA is suspected, further testing may include cold agglutinin titers, the Donath-Landsteiner test to exclude PCH, antibody titers for viruses or mycoplasma, or search for an occult lymphoma or lymphoproliferative disorder in elderly patients to further characterize the type of hemolytic disease.

4. If a warm-type AIHA is suspected, further workup to identify an underlying cause, such as autoimmune disorders, malignancy, lymphoma, or other lymphoproliferative disorder, is required. Possible drug-induced causes should be considered, and use of pertinent drugs discontinued.

Hematologic Findings

Blood Cell Measurements.   Anemia may be severe (hemoglobin level, <3 g/dL [30 g/L]) with normochromic, normocytic indices. There is variable reticulocytosis. In acute hemolysis, a nonspecific stress granulocytosis with a left shift may be present. The leukocytosis can reach leukemoid proportions (>50 x 10^3/mm^3 [50 x 10^9/L]).

Peripheral Blood Smear Morphology. Nucleated red blood cells, marked polychromasia, and anisocytosis are usually seen. In warm-type AIHA, microspherocytes are present, resulting from partial ingestion of antibody-coated red blood cell membrane by the mononuclear phagocytic system. Cold-type AIHA may have similar morphologic changes if it is acutely postinfectious, but the more chronic disease states may have few red blood cell morphologic changes. IgM crosslinking of cells may cause red blood cell clumping in the peripheral smear.

Bone Marrow Examination. The marrow is hypercellular, with marked normoblastic erythroid hyperplasia. Marrow iron is usually markedly increased, reflecting the accelerated erythroid turnover. Prolonged severe hemolysis may result in relative deficiencies of folic acid or vitamin B$_{12}$, causing megaloblastic maturation. Occasionally, bone marrow examination may reveal an underlying lymphoproliferative disorder that is causing the hemolytic disease.

Other Laboratory Tests

Complete evaluation of a hemolytic process suspected to be AIHA by the following tests requires 15 to 20 mL of blood that is obtained and maintained at 37°C until clotted. The serum is promptly removed from the cells and frozen to preserve complement. An ethylenediaminetetraacetic acid (EDTA) specimen is also obtained. EDTA blocks nonspecific absorption of complement, which allows a more accurate assessment of results of the DAT.

15.1   Direct Antiglobulin (Coombs') Test

Purpose.   The DAT depicts globulin adsorbed to the patient's red blood cells and identifies the immunoglobulin class.

Principle, Procedure.   See Test 6.4.

Interpretation.   A clinically significant DAT result is positive (1 to 4+) with broad-spectrum reagents. Monospecific reagents identify the adsorbed globulin type. In warm-type AIHA, monospecific reagents for IgG or IgG and complement are positive. Monospecific reagents in cold-type AIHA show only complement since IgM antibody quickly separates from red blood cells collected at 37°C. C3d is believed to be a clinically significant fraction in AIHA, since it indicates prior absorption of C3 to the red blood cell membrane. Very weak complement reactions (+/–) are not significant, but weak anti-IgG reactions may occasionally be clinically significant.

Very rarely, AIHA is present without a positive DAT result, requiring ultrasensitive methods of Coombs' consumption or radioisotopic analysis to detect antibody molecules on the red blood cells. These tests are not generally available and require the services of a reference laboratory.

15.2   Serum Antibody Detection

Purpose.   These tests detect serum antibody that will coat red blood cells under the test conditions, identify its blood group specificity, and characterize the temperature of reactivity.

Principle.   An indirect Coombs' test—or its modifications—depicts serum antibody binding to red blood cells following incubation of test cells with the patient's serum, followed by washing and addition of direct antibody reagents to detect cell-bound complement and/or immunoglobulin. Enzymatic treatment of cells (by ficin, papain, bromelin, or trypsin) may increase the detection of very low levels of antibody. Alternatively, direct agglutination of saline-suspended cells will also depict serum red blood cell antibodies. If screening tests show positive results, the antibody is identified (see Test 12.2).

Procedure. The patient's serum and red blood cell mixtures are tested with the previously mentioned techniques at 37°C and at 4°C. In addition to panels of reagent red blood cells, the patient's own cells are included as well as specimens of cord blood. The presence of agglutination or of hemolysis is significant and is graded 0 to 4+ (see Test 12.1).

Interpretation. Warm autoantibodies agglutinate test cells by indirect antiglobulin tests and enzyme techniques strongly at 37°C with no increase at 4°C. These are usually IgG. Specific antibody is found in 30% of cases and is usually related to the Rh loci (e, C, D, c), although the appearance of narrow specificity may only reflect differences in titers of antibody components. In the remaining cases, the antibody is directed at some primitive precursor of the Rh system or of the Wright system, and all cells are agglutinated except very rare test cells used at reference laboratories such as Rh null cells.

Since antibodies may be present from previous transfusions concurrent with autoantibodies, specificity should be determined. Although transfusions should be avoided, antibody specificity may help in selection of blood that is least incompatible if life-saving transfusion is needed. With steroids, serum antibodies may change specificity or disappear, although the positive DAT result often persists. The presence of serum antibody correlates more with active AIHA.

Cold autoantibodies are IgM and show strong reactivity at 4°C and weaker reactivity at 37°C. Sometimes this differential is more apparent with diluted serum or in alternative tests that use saline suspensions or enzyme-treated cells. The antibodies may be hemolytic in vitro. Specificity is usually anti-I (reactive with all normal adult cells but not with cord red blood cells). Anti-i specificity (stronger reactions with cord red blood cells than adult cells) is seen with the rare AIHA occurring in infectious mononucleosis. Cold autoantibodies should be titered. To determine whether antibodies are autoantibodies, the patient's red blood cell antigens must be tested and typed for the Rh and I systems.

15.3 Red Blood Cell Eluates

Purpose.   The globin fraction is eluted off the red blood cell membrane to determine if the globulin depicted by the DAT is antibody and to determine the blood group specificity of the globulin.

Principle.   Red blood cell antibody-antigen bonds are disrupted by heat or by destroying the red blood cell membrane, thereby releasing bound antibody so that it can be further analyzed.

Procedure.   The test is usually performed by the blood bank or reference laboratory. When the DAT result is positive, heating the red blood cells at $56°C$ or chemically destroying them with cold organic solvents elutes the adsorbed antibody, which can be tested in parallel with the serum.

Interpretation.   In warm-type AIHA, the eluate antibody identity is the same as that seen in the serum. After recent incompatible transfusion in the absence of AIHA, the DAT may yield positive results because of the presence of coated donor cells, but this represents an alloantibody. Antigen typing of red blood cells in such cases often indicates a mixed field of donor red blood cells and patient cells. After incompatible transfusion in the presence of AIHA, specificity of eluate and serum antibody may not be clarified until transfused cells have been cleared, usually after several days. An eluate that does not react with red blood cells suggests nonspecific globulin absorption, such as that in myeloma or recent cephalothin therapy. In cold-type AIHA antibody, material is not elutable and there is no reaction with red blood cells.

15.4 Cold Agglutinin Titer

Purpose.   The presence of increased cold agglutinins usually establishes that the AIHA is of the cold antibody type. Titers may indicate underlying disease and serve as a means to follow disease status.

Principle.   Cold agglutinins usually have anti-I specificity and will agglutinate saline suspensions of adult red blood cells that have the I antigen on the membrane. Rare cold agglutinins with anti-i specificity will not agglutinate adult red blood cells at the same titer but can be titered with cord blood specimens.

Procedure.   The patient's serum is titered by small-volume serial dilutions (4, 8, 16, 32, etc), and incubated for 2 hours at 4°C with a standard suspension of red blood cells from the patient or of a group O donor (to avoid ABO blood group incompatibility). Cell-serum suspensions are evaluated for agglutination, and the titer is established as the highest serum dilution producing detectable agglutination.

Interpretation.   A low titer of cold agglutinins is normally seen. Clinical significance is associated with titers above 1:256 (Table 15-4). With the increase in titer, the temperature of agglutination often rises toward 37°C, and antibody with complement fixes on the patient's red blood cells as demonstrated by a positive DAT result. Physiologic cold agglutinins have titers of 1:32 or less. Titers of 1:64 or more are seen after recent respiratory viral infections. Titers are 1:256 or more in cold AIHA of elderly women. Viral pneumonia is associated with titers of 1:128 to 1:8,000. In chronic cold agglutinin disease, titers are often 1:50,000 or higher. Progress of cold-type AIHA can be followed up by repeating titers weekly in viral pneumonia or idiopathic disease, and monthly in cold agglutinin disease, particularly in diseases associated with a lymphoproliferative process.

15.5   Donath-Landsteiner Test

Purpose.   The Donath-Landsteiner test facilitates diagnosis of paroxysmal cold hemoglobinuria (PCH), allowing it to be distinguished from cold-type AIHA. PCH is usually a self-limited disease that is treated conservatively by keeping the patient warm.

Principle. The Donath-Landsteiner test reproduces in vitro the biphasic reaction that characterizes PCH. The Donath-Landsteiner hemolysin is a complement-dependent IgG antibody that agglutinates cells at 4°C and lyses them at warmer temperatures (usually considered as 37°C). Other hemolysins may react at a single temperature, 4°C or 37°C, but are not biphasic. The Donath-Landsteiner hemolysin will not lyse cells with reverse incubations of 37°C to 4°C.

Procedure. The patient's serum is incubated with test red blood cells at 4°C and then at 37°C, and the serum cell suspension is observed for hemolysis, which is usually marked (3 to 4+). If biphasic hemolysis is present, it is tested against panels of reagent red blood cells to determine blood group specificity, which is often in the P or I system.

Interpretation. A biphasic hemolysin is diagnostic of PCH, which may occasionally clinically mimic cold-type AIHA. If intravascular hemolysis has recently occurred, the DAT results may be negative. PCH often occurs following a viral infection but can also be seen with congenital syphilis so that definitive syphilitic serologic testing should be performed.

15.6   Ham's Test for Acid Hemolysis

Purpose. A Ham's test is performed to exclude paroxysmal nocturnal hemoglobinuria (PNH), which is caused by an acquired clonal defect of the red blood cell membrane rather than an antibody-mediated process. Whenever antibody hemolysis is suspected, PNH should be considered and excluded.

Principle, Specimen, and Procedure.   See Test 11.2.

Interpretation. False-positive hemolysis results are seen if the acidified sera contain a cold agglutinin. True-positive results occur only with human, not guinea pig, complement. The acid hemolysis test can be confirmed with sucrose lysis.

15.7 Serum Complement Measurement

Purpose. A decrease in serum complement is often associated with IgM antibodies and cold-type AIHA. It may be decreased in some warm-type AIHA.

Principle. Sheep red blood cells are lysed in the presence of rabbit anti-sheep antibody if complement from the patient's serum is present. The reaction can be used to quantitate complement.

Specimen. Fresh serum—separated from red blood cells and immediately frozen.

Procedure. Serum complement is measured spectrophotometrically by lysis of 50% of a red blood cell suspension in 1 hour. This is achieved by 50 to 100 U of complement in most laboratories, but normal ranges must be determined for each individual laboratory.

Interpretation. Serum complement is decreased in cold AIHA since the antibodies bind complement. Levels may also be decreased in warm AIHA when complement is fixed to the cell membrane. Lytic complement tests are not easily performed and often require reference laboratories.

15.8 Serum Haptoglobin Quantitation

Purpose. Haptoglobin is decreased or absent in hemolysis or in liver failure. A low serum haptoglobin level indicates that hemolysis may be present if liver function is normal.

Principle, Procedure, and Specimen. See Test 6.3.

Interpretation. Normal values are usually 40 to 80 mg/dL (0.4-1.8 g/L), with active hemolysis values less than 10 mg/dL (0.1 g/L). In cold-type AIHA secondary to viral or mycoplasma pneumonia, haptoglobin may be increased as an acute reactant protein, obscuring expected decreases seen with hemolysis.

15.9   Osmotic Fragility Test

Purpose.   This test detects spherocytes, which are more sensitive to osmotic lysis than normal red blood cells.

Principle, Specimen, and Procedure.   See Test 7.1.

Interpretation.   Hemolysis increases with the presence of spherocytosis, usually seen in warm-type AIHA. Review of the peripheral smear should show spherocytes, and it is usually not necessary to confirm this finding by osmotic fragility testing.

15.10   Antibody Titers for Mycoplasma and Viruses

Purpose.   Testing for mycoplasma and virus antibody titers identifies (often in retrospect) possible infectious agents as the cause of cold-type AIHA.

Principle.   These antibodies require acute- and convalescent-phase sera obtained 7 to 10 days apart to show a rise in titer of antibody for specific organisms.

Procedure.   The tests are usually performed at county or state reference laboratories, which require both specimens to be submitted. The agent suspected should be specified. The most common etiologic agents of interest are *Mycoplasma*, and less frequently EBV or CMV.

Interpretation.   A three-dilution rise in titer is required for the test to aid diagnosis, since previous exposure to these viruses is fairly common. IgM antibody suggests recent infection.

15.11   Antinuclear Antibody Test

Purpose.   Antinuclear antibody by indirect immunofluorescence should be ordered when warm-type AIHA is diagnosed, particularly in young women, to determine if systemic lupus erythematosus (SLE) or other collagen vascular disease is an underlying cause for warm-type AIHA. It should be kept in mind that the hemolysis frequently precedes SLE by months or even years.

Principle.   The patient's serum contains autoantibody to nuclear material. If nuclear material is present, the antibody binds to it and can be depicted with fluorescence.

Procedure.   The patient's serum is incubated with a source of nuclear antigen (tissue culture cells, rat kidney, human granulocytes). The antigen-antibody combination is demonstrated by an antiglobulin reagent tagged with a fluorescent dye. The patient's serum can then be titered.

Interpretation.   Titers above 1:20 in most laboratories are suspicious and titers of 1:80 or greater are considered diagnostic of SLE. Suspicious positive test results may be seen in up to 3% of older individuals. High antinuclear antibody titers in the elderly suggest drug-induced AIHA of the methyldopa type (see Chapter 14). Supplemental tests for anti-DNA or anti-Sm may confirm the diagnosis of SLE.

15.12   Evaluation of Occult Lymphoma

Purpose.   Warm-type AIHA may precede lymphoma by years, but AIHA may be the only recognizable sign in concomitant unsuspected disease.

Physical examination and radiologic evaluation of all lymph node areas, liver, and spleen may help detect an unsuspected lymphoma. A biopsy should be performed when adenopathy or hepatosplenomegaly is found.

Course and Treatment

Warm-type AIHA usually responds in 7 to 10 days to high-dose steroid therapy, which suppresses antibody production and inhibits macrophage adherence. In steroid-resistant cases, immunosuppressive medication or splenectomy to decrease reticuloendothelial activity is usually successful.

There is little therapy available for cold-type AIHA. It does not respond to steroid therapy, immunosuppressive drugs, or splenectomy. Postinfectious AIHA is usually self-limited, but in some severe cases, plasmapheresis may help to decrease antibody levels. In CAD associated with a lymphoproliferative disorder, treatment of the underlying disease often results in improvement of cold agglutinin titers. Chronic idiopathic cold AIHA seen in elderly women waxes and wanes, possibly in relation to infections or other stresses.

PCH is usually treated by keeping the patient warm. It is self-limited, responding to recovery from the underlying infection. Aggressive therapy should therefore be avoided.

Although as many as 30% of patients may show no reaction to transfusion, it should generally be avoided in both warm- and cold-type AIHA to minimize formation of further alloantibodies, which can complicate crossmatching. In addition, transfusion may increase autoantibody titers and avidity for red blood cells, accelerating hemolysis. Red blood cell survival is less than 1 week in warm-type AIHA and may be minutes or hours in cold-type AIHA, making transfusions of limited usefulness unless symptoms of impending stroke or myocardial infarction are present.

References

Issit PD. *Applied Blood Group Serology.* 3rd ed. Miami, Fla: Montgomery Scientific Publications; 1985:72-104, 664-665.

Jandl JH. *Blood: Textbook of Hematology.* Boston, Mass: Little, Brown and Co; 1987:297-318.

Petz LD, Garratty G. Serologic investigation of autoimmune hemolytic anemia. In: *Acquired Immune Hemolytic Anemia.* New York, NY: Churchill Livingstone Inc; 1980:139-184

PART
III

Reactive Disorders of Granulocytes and Monocytes

16 ✓

Neutrophilia

The normal range for absolute neutrophil count shows prominent age variation. For example, a brisk neutrophilia, often exceeding $30 \times 10^3/mm^3$ ($30 \times 10^9/L$), is typical at birth. Shortly after birth, the absolute neutrophil count plummets and lymphocytes predominate by 2 weeks of age. The normal range for absolute neutrophil count in infants is approximately $2.5\text{-}7.0 \times 10^3/mm^3$ ($2.5\text{-}7.0 \times 10^9/L$), while the normal range for children and adults is approximately $1.5\text{-}7.0 \times 10^3/mm^3$ ($1.5\text{-}7.0 \times 10^9/L$). These normal ranges reflect only the circulating pool of neutrophils, while an equal number of neutrophils are attached to the vascular endothelium, the so-called marginated pool.

Neutrophilia is defined as an absolute neutrophil count that exceeds $10 \times 10^3/mm^3$ ($10 \times 10^9/L$) for patients beyond the neonatal period. The causes of reactive neutrophilia are listed in Table 16-1 and include a variety of disorders ranging from infections to metabolic defects. The most common causes of reactive neutrophilia in clinical practice include bacterial infections, therapeutic or endogenous drugs or hormones, and acute tissue necrosis (Images 16-1, 16-2). An absolute neutrophilia is also common in patients with a variety of hematopoietic neoplasms, especially chronic myelopro-

Table 16-1   Reactive Neutrophilias

Infections
    Primarily bacterial
    Less common in viral, mycobacterial, leptospiral, or toxoplasmal infections
Drugs, hormones
    Excess CSF (therapeutic, CSF-producing tumors)
    Epinephrine (therapeutic or endogenous production)
    Corticosteroids (therapeutic or endogenous production)
    Lithium
    Poisons/toxins/venoms
Tissue necrosis
    Acute gout
    Burns
    Trauma
    Infarct
Inflammatory disorders
    Collagen vascular disorders
    Other autoimmune disorders
Miscellaneous
    Stress/severe exercise
    Pregnancy
    Smoking
    Acute hemorrhage/hemolysis
    Postsplenectomy
Metabolic
    Ketoacidosis
    Uremia
    Eclampsia
    Thyrotoxicosis

Abbreviations: CSF = colony-stimulating factor.

liferative disorders. In these patients the neutrophils are part of the neoplastic process. Because chronic myeloproliferative disorders represent clonal stem cell defects, the mature red blood cells, white blood cells (WBCs), and platelets within the peripheral blood are all derived from the neoplastic clone.

Pathophysiology

For granulopoiesis to occur, the bone marrow must contain sufficient stem cells and progenitor cells, an adequate microenvironment for hematopoiesis, and sufficient regulatory factors. Granulopoiesis is an exquisitely regulated system of cell proliferation and maturation. Regulation of granulopoiesis is largely achieved by factors produced within the bone marrow microenvironment. The most well characterized of these regulatory factors is a family of glycoproteins termed "colony-stimulating factors" (CSFs). By binding to an appropriate surface receptor on progenitor cells, these regulatory proteins stimulate production of granulocytes (G-CSF), monocytes (M-CSF), or both (GM-CSF). CSFs also induce a hyperfunctional state in mature neutrophils and monocytes, cells which also express CSF receptors. The hyperfunctional state of these mature cells is linked to morphologic changes such as toxic granulation, Döhle bodies, and prominent cytoplasmic vacuolization. CSFs are produced by a variety of cells within the bone marrow microenvironment, including monocytes-macrophages and T lymphocytes.

Although specific stages of granulocyte maturation have been defined, this process is a biologic continuum characterized by both progressive decrease in nuclear size with eventual segmentation and progressive increase in cytoplasmic granularity. The arbitrarily defined stages of granulopoiesis consist of myeloblasts, promyelocytes, myelocytes, metamyelocytes, band neutrophils, and segmented neutrophils. Myeloblasts, promyelocytes, and myelocytes are capable of mitotic division, while metamyelocytes, band neutrophils, and segmented neutrophils have lost this capability. Primary granules are initially recognized in "late" myeloblasts and promyelocytes. These lysosomal granules contain numerous cytolytic enzymes, the most notable of which is myeloperoxidase. Secondary granules are first apparent at the myelocyte stage of maturation, and these granules eventually outnumber primary granules, giving the cytoplasm a homogeneous pink blush. Like primary granules, these secondary lysosomal granules contain numerous cytolytic enzymes. The most commonly evaluated secondary granule enzyme is leukocyte alkaline phosphatase.

The time required for granulopoiesis is highly variable, ranging from 1 to 3 weeks. Once neutrophils are released into the peripheral blood, they circulate for only a few hours before egressing to tissues. Homeostatic rates of neutrophil production exceed $1\text{-}2 \times 10^9$ neutrophils per kilogram per day.

Baseline granulopoiesis can be stimulated in many infectious and inflammatory conditions. The primary mechanisms for neutrophilia include demargination of the marginated pool, release of the bone marrow maturation-storage compartment, and increased neutrophil production. Demargination of neutrophils is caused by epinephrine release and can occur within minutes. Because the circulating and marginating pools are approximately equal, this mechanism would be predicted to double the absolute neutrophil count. Greater increases in the absolute neutrophil count result from release of the bone marrow maturation storage compartment, a phenomenon induced by corticosteroids, acute infections, and acute inflammation. In addition to a substantial absolute neutrophilia, a left shift with circulating band neutrophils, metamyelocytes, and even myelocytes is a predictable finding in patients in whom mobilization of the bone marrow maturation storage compartment has occurred.

For a neutrophilia to be sustained, increased bone marrow production must occur. This mechanism of neutrophilia is the slowest to occur but results in a substantial sustained neutrophilia. Increased bone marrow neutrophil production is mediated by CSFs, and conditions linked to sustained increased CSF production include chronic infections, chronic inflammation, CSF-producing tumors, and therapy with recombinant human CSF.

Clinical Findings

The clinical findings in patients with reactive neutrophilia are diverse, depending on the underlying disorder. Fever is a hallmark of acute infection, while various other signs and symptoms are linked to the specific site of infection. Patients in whom the neutrophilia is part of a bone marrow neoplasm (ie, patients with chronic myeloproliferative disorders) generally present with symptoms of fatigue and malaise. Fever is not present, unless these patients have developed a secondary infection. Splenomegaly and variable hepatomegaly are common clinical findings in patients with chronic myeloproliferative disorders.

Approach to Diagnosis

The evaluation of a patient with an increase in absolute neutrophil count must include both the distinction between a reactive and neoplastic process and the determination of the likely cause of a reactive neutrophilia. The distinction between a reactive neutrophilia and a chronic myeloproliferative disorder, notably chronic myelogenous leukemia (CML), is based on the assimilation of a variety of clinical, hematologic, and chemical parameters (Tables 16-2, 16-3). In general, pronounced toxic changes, a limited left shift, and lack of basophilia characterize a reactive neutrophilia, while CML is characterized by a strikingly elevated WBC count, lack of toxic changes, left shift including blasts, abnormalities in other lineages, and basophilia.

The following approach to diagnosis should be considered:

1. Assess complete blood count with differential.

2. Evaluate morphology for toxic changes and for evidence of multilineage abnormalities.

3. Conduct appropriate microbacterial studies to evaluate for a possible infection.

4. Integrate blood findings with clinical features and chemical analyses.

5. Measure leukocyte alkaline phosphatase, examine bone marrow, or conduct cytogenetic evaluation *in selected cases* in which a neoplastic disorder cannot be excluded.

Hematologic Findings

Blood Cell Measurements. In a reactive neutrophilia the WBC count rarely exceeds 30 x 10^3/mm^3 (30 x 10^9/L). In exceptional cases, including young children and patients receiving CSF therapy, the WBC count may exceed 50 x 10^3/mm^3 (50 x 10^9/L). A neoplastic disorder should be strongly considered when the WBC count exceeds 100 x 10^3/mm^3 (100 x 10^9/L).

Depending on the underlying disorder, the hemoglobin, hematocrit, and platelet values are highly variable in patients with reactive neutrophilia. For example, if an infectious or inflammatory

Table 16-2   Morphologic Features of Reactive Neutrophilia

Blood	Comments
Leukocytosis	Usually <30 x 10³/mm³ (<30 x 10⁹/L); higher WBC count in young children
	Rarely exceeds 50 x 10³/mm³ (50 x 10⁹/L) except in patients receiving CSF therapy (or with CSF-producing tumor)
Left shift	Bands and metamyelocytes typical; may also see myelocytes
	In septic neonates may see circulating myeloblasts along with other granulocytic elements
Döhle bodies	Retained portion of cytoplasm from more immature state of maturation
Toxic granulation	Etiology controversial; either retained primary granules or altered uptake of stain by secondary granules
Cytoplasmic vacuoles	Prominent neutrophil vacuoles correlate with sepsis
Other lineages	Thrombocytosis common; if DIC develops thrombocytopenia is found
	Eosinophilia or monocytosis may accompany neutrophilia
	Basophilia not present

Abbreviations: CSF = colony-stimulating factor; DIC = disseminated intravascular coagulation.

condition is long-standing, an anemia of chronic disease may have developed (see Chapter 3). In patients with severe infections and secondary disseminated intravascular coagulation, red blood cell fragmentation and thrombocytopenia may be evident. Thrombocytosis, however, accompanies many cases of reactive neutrophilia that are secondary to acute stress.

Peripheral Blood Smear Morphology.   The morphologic features of reactive neutrophilia are listed in Table 16-2. Although highly variable, the WBC count usually does not exceed 30 x 10³/mm³ (30 x 10⁹/L); exceptions do occur, especially in patients receiving CSF therapy. In addition to an increase in mature neutrophils, a left shift including bands and metamyelocytes is typical in patients with a marked reactive neutrophilia. In septic newborns, circulating blasts and promyelocytes may also be evident.

Table 16-3   Comparison of Reactive Neutrophilia to Chronic
Myelogenous Leukemia (CML)

Parameter	Reactive Neutrophilia	CML
WBC	Usually <30 x 10^3/mm^3 (<30 x 10^9/L)	Usually >50 x 10^3/mm^3 (>50 x 10^9/L)
Toxic neutrophils	Present	Usually absent
Left shift	Includes myelocytes	Includes blasts
Basophilia	Absent	Present
Platelet count	Variable, decreased with sepsis	Increased
Platelet morphology	Unremarkable	Abnormal, variable micromegakaryocytes
Nucleated erythroid cells in blood	Absent	Present
Splenomegaly	Absent	Present
Fever	Usually present	Usually absent
Uric acid	Normal	Increased
LAP	Increased	Low
Karyotype	Normal	Philadelphia chromosome

However, circulating blasts are not a typical feature of reactive neutrophilia in adults, except in those receiving recombinant human CSF. Toxic changes within the cytoplasm of reactive neutrophils include Döhle bodies, toxic granulation, and, when sepsis is present, prominent cytoplasmic vacuoles. Some cases of reactive neutrophilia are characterized by nuclear hyposegmentation (pseudo–Pelger-Huët change). The absolute neutrophilia may be accompanied by eosinophilia or monocytosis in a variety of infectious and inflammatory processes. Notably, basophilia is not a feature of a reactive neutrophilia.

In patients with chronic myeloproliferative disorders, toxic changes are not present, the left shift includes blasts, and basophilia is common. Morphologic abnormalities of platelets and red blood cells are common, and both circulating erythroid and megakaryocytic precursors may be evident.

Bone Marrow Examination.   In a straightforward reactive neutrophilia, bone marrow examination is generally not necessary. In patients with a sustained reactive neutrophilia, the predicted bone marrow findings would include a granulocytic hyperplasia. However, bone marrow examination may be warranted for culture or to exclude a possible neoplastic process.

Other Laboratory Tests

16.1   Leukocyte Alkaline Phosphatase (LAP)

Purpose.   The LAP test is useful in differentiating CML from leukemoid reactions (see also Test 34.1).

Principle.   LAP is an enzyme present within the secondary granules of maturing neutrophils from the myelocyte stage onward. Stimulated neutrophils contain increased amounts of LAP. Therefore, the test helps distinguish reactive neutrophilia (increased LAP) from the abnormally maturing clonal granulocytes of CML (decreased LAP).

Procedure.   LAP is usually determined semiquantitatively by specific cytochemical staining of peripheral blood smears. The LAP present in the neutrophils hydrolyzes a substrate that is then coupled to a dye, forming brown-to-black particles in the cytoplasm of these cells at the enzyme sites. The smears are then counterstained, examined microscopically, and 200 segmented or band neutrophils are counted and graded 0 to 4+ by evaluating the number of the cytoplasmic particles. The LAP score is calculated by addition of the number of cells times the grade, as shown in the following example. The range of normal scores is 13 to 130, although there may be slight variation in each laboratory.

No. Cells x Grade	Score
10 x 0	0
30 x 1	30
30 x 2	60
20 x 3	60
10 x 4	40
100 cells	190 = LAP score

Table 16-4   Leukocyte Alkaline Phosphatase Scores

Low score
   CML (very low score)
   Other hematopoietic neoplasms (rare)
   Rare infections
   Rare toxic exposures
High score
   Infections
   Chronic myeloproliferative disorders (not CML)
   Inflammatory processes/some nonhematopoietic neoplasms
   Pregnancy
   Stress
   Oral contraceptives
   Drug treatments (lithium, corticosteroids, estrogen, colony-stimulating
      factor)

Abbreviation: CML = chronic myelogenous leukemia.

Specimen.   Freshly prepared patient and control blood smears
   are obtained from fingerstick capillary blood. Blood smears
   should be dried at least 1 hour before fixation. If not stained
   immediately, fixed slides may be stored overnight in a freezer
   without significant loss of enzyme activity.

Interpretation.   The general LAP scores in reactive conditions,
   pregnancy, and chronic myeloproliferative disorders are listed
   in Table 16-4. The LAP score may be increased in CML
   patients with secondary infections. A rising LAP score also
   characterizes some cases of CML in early blast crisis.

Notes and Precautions.   Improperly stored smears lose enzymatic   activity   and   give   falsely   low   LAP   scores.
   Ethylenediaminetetraacetic   acid   (EDTA)   anticoagulant
   inhibits this reaction.

Ancillary Tests

A variety of other laboratory tests may be used to evaluate selected patients with neutrophilia. For example, serologic tests for col-

lagen vascular disorders, uric acid levels, and gallium scans may be warranted for specific clinical indications. Both routine cytogenetic studies or molecular analyses for BCR/ABL gene rearrangements may be useful in patients with suspected malignancies.

Course and Treatment

The course and treatment of neutrophilia depends on the underlying disease process.

References

Dale DC. Neutrophilia. In: Williams WJ, Beutler E, Erslev AJ, Lichtman MA, eds. *Hematology*. 4th ed. New York, NY: McGraw-Hill; 1990:816-820.

Foucar K. Constitutional and reactive myeloid disorders. In: *Bone Marrow Pathology*. Chicago, Ill: ASCP Press; 1995:99-119.

Kerrigan DP, Castillo A, Foucar K, et al. Peripheral blood morphologic changes after high-dose antineoplastic chemotherapy and recombinant human granulocyte colony-stimulating factor administration. *Am J Clin Pathol*. 1989;92:280-285.

Kitamura H, Kodama F, Odagiri S, et al. Granulocytosis associated with malignant neoplasms: a clinicopathologic study and demonstration of colony-stimulating activity in tumor extracts. *Hum Pathol*. 1989;20:878-885.

Peterson L, Foucar K. Granulocytosis and granulocytopenia. In: Bick RL, ed. *Hematology: Clinical and Laboratory Practice*. St Louis, Mo: CV Mosby Co; 1993:1137-1154.

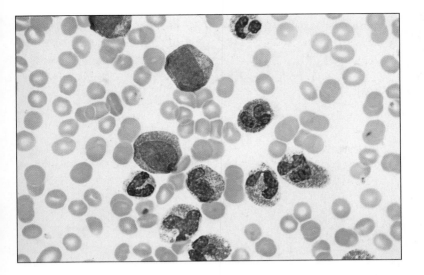

Image 16-1 A striking leukocytosis with pronounced toxic changes and left shift is evident on this blood smear from a patient receiving pharmacologic doses of recombinant human granulocyte–colony-stimulating factor. (Wright's)

Image 16-2 Both toxic neutrophilia and ingested organisms (↑) are present on this blood smear from a patient with ehrlichiosis. (Courtesy of Dr. P. Ward.) (Wright-Giemsa)

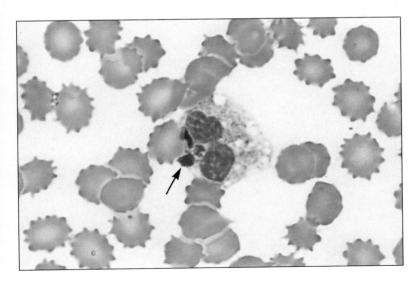

17

✓

Eosinophilia

Eosinophils are normally present in the blood in low numbers, and there are no age variations in normal eosinophil counts. Eosinophilia is defined as an absolute eosinophil count exceeding $0.6 \times 10^3/mm^3$ ($0.6 \times 10^9/L$). Causes of reactive eosinophilia are summarized in Table 17-1. The most common causes are drug treatments, allergies, or parasites. Parasites must invade tissues to produce eosinophilia. Recently identified causes of reactive eosinophilia include eosinophilia-myalgia syndrome secondary to L-tryptophan ingestion; therapy with pharmacologic doses of recombinant human interleukins is also associated with a brisk, reactive eosinophilia.

In addition, various nonhematopoietic neoplasms can be associated with either reactive peripheral blood eosinophilia or eosinophilic infiltrates within the neoplasm itself. Both tumor-associated blood eosinophilia and tumor-associated tissue eosinophilia are linked to factors produced by the tumor cells that induce eosinophil production. Tumor-associated blood eosinophilia is generally associated with more advanced disease and an overall worse prognosis. In these patients, the sustained blood eosinophilia with

Table 17-1 Causes of Reactive Eosinophilia

Allergic and hypersensitivity reactions
Drug allergies
Cytokine therapy (recombinant human interleukins)
Parasitic infections
Cutaneous disorders
Connective tissue diseases/collagen vascular diseases
Neoplasms (carcinoma, lymphoma, Hodgkin's disease, acute lymphoblastic
  leukemia)*
Immunodeficiency disorders
Sarcoidosis

*Increased eosinophil production secondary to cytokines released by neoplastic cells; eosinophils are
  not neoplastic.

subsequent degranulation can result in tissue damage, further compromising the overall debilitated condition of the patient.

Finally, increased blood eosinophils can be a feature of a variety of hematopoietic neoplasms, including chronic myeloproliferative disorders and certain acute myeloid leukemias (Table 17-2). In these patients, the eosinophils are part of the neoplastic clone and often exhibit morphologic abnormalities.

Pathophysiology

Although eosinophils are derived from the same progenitor cells that give rise to other granulocytic elements within the bone marrow, eosinophil production is influenced by interleukin-1, interleukin-3, and interleukin-5 produced in the bone marrow microenvironment. Like other regulatory factors, these interleukins not only stimulate production of eosinophils, but functional activity of mature eosinophils is enhanced, most notably by interleukin-5. Although the distinctive granule used to identify the eosinophil is a secondary granule, the stages of eosinophil maturation are presumed to parallel other granulocytic cells, and include myeloblasts, promyelocytes, eosinophilic myelocytes, eosinophilic metamyelocytes, and mature eosinophils. These mature eosinophils characteristically have bilobed nuclei and contain abundant large, refractile eosinophilic granules.

Table 17-2   Hematopoietic Neoplasms Demonstrating Mature
Blood Eosinophilia

Chronic myeloproliferative disorders
    Chronic myelogenous leukemia
    Chronic eosinophilic leukemia
    Idiopathic hypereosinophilic syndrome
    Other chronic disorders
Acute leukemias
    Acute myelomonocytic leukemia with eosinophilia (variable blood
      eosinophilia)
    Other myeloid leukemias
    Acute lymphoblastic leukemia with eosinophilia*

*Evidence regarding whether the eosinophils are part of a neoplastic clone is controversial.
Eosinophils may be reactive, nonclonal.

Eosinophils are present in low numbers in the peripheral blood, and normal eosinophil function is dependent on migration to solid tissue. Eosinophils demonstrate two main functions: (1) modulation of immediate hypersensitivity reactions and (2) destruction of parasites. Release of eosinophil secondary granules plays a key role in both of these functions. These secondary granules contain major basic protein, peroxidase, arylsulfatase, histamine oxidase, and eosinophil cationic protein. In addition, the surface membranes of eosinophils express Fc receptors for IgE, IgG, and certain complement components.

Clinical Findings

The cause of eosinophilia may be either clinically obvious or obscure. In addition to the clinical features of the diverse disorders that cause eosinophilia, the eosinophilia itself can produce distinctive clinical manifestations. A sustained peripheral blood eosinophilia can result in endothelial and endomyocardial damage from intravascular degranulation of these cells. The potent cytolytic enzymes contained within eosinophil secondary granules damage endothelial cells throughout the body. As a consequence, either thrombosis or endomyocardial fibrosis may result. Although both neoplastic and reactive eosinophils can be associated with this type of tissue damage, it is far more common in patients with neoplastic eosinophilic disorders such as idiopathic hypereosinophilic syndrome, chronic eosinophilic leukemia, or other chronic myeloproliferative disorders with a prominent eosinophilic component. Patients with these chronic myeloproliferative disorders may also exhibit organomegaly, pulmonary infiltrates, and central nervous system disease, in addition to the more common thrombotic and cardiac disorders.

Eosinophilia-myalgia syndrome is a recently identified cause of peripheral blood eosinophilia, linked to L-tryptophan ingestion. These patients, usually women, present with severe myalgia and arthralgia, fatigue, peripheral blood eosinophilia, and, less frequently, respiratory disorders, skin changes, and neuropathy. Eosinophilia-myalgia syndrome has been linked to L-tryptophan produced by a single Japanese manufacturer and is thought to be caused by a toxic contaminant.

Approach to Diagnosis

In any patient with a sustained eosinophilia, it is important to distinguish a reactive process from a chronic myeloproliferative disorder with an eosinophilic component. Once an eosinophilia is determined to be reactive, the underlying cause must be identified.

The following approach to diagnosis should be considered:

1. Perform clinical evaluation and assess history of drug treatments.
2. Evaluate for possible parasitic infection, including history of travel to foreign countries.
3. Perform appropriate laboratory tests for possible parasitic infection if clinically warranted.
4. Perform physical examination for evidence of organomegaly or pulmonary infiltrates.
5. Chest x-ray may be warranted in patients with possible pulmonary infiltrates.
6. Evaluate for neoplasms associated with blood eosinophilia as a consequence of cytokine production by the tumor.

Hematologic Findings

Blood Cell Measurements. Eosinophilia is present when the absolute eosinophil count exceeds $0.6 \times 10^3/mm^3$ ($0.6 \times 10^9/L$). Eosinophils have a diurnal variation, highest in the morning, decreasing in the afternoon.

Blood Morphology. In reactive eosinophilias, the peripheral blood eosinophils are generally morphologically unremarkable, although hypodense or degranulated eosinophils may be noted occasionally (Image 17-1). Recent studies suggest that eosinophils become hypodense when exposed to recombinant human interleukin-3.

In contrast, like neutrophils, neoplastic mature eosinophils may be a component of acute myeloid leukemias, chronic myelogenous leukemias, and other chronic myeloproliferative disorders, including those previously called idiopathic hypereosinophilic syndromes (Table 17-2). The eosinophils in these neoplasms are often atypical, exhibiting both nuclear and cytoplasmic abnormalities (Image 17-2). Hypersegmented, hypogranular, degranulated, or vacuolated eosinophils are especially prominent in the chronic myeloproliferative disorders previously termed "idiopathic hypereosinophilic syndromes."

Bone Marrow Examination. Bone marrow examination is generally not required in patients with clear-cut reactive eosinophilia. However, both bone marrow examination and cytogenetic studies are valuable in those patients with a likely myeloproliferative disorder.

Ancillary Tests

1. If parasitic infection is suspected, both stool examination for ova and parasites and serologic tests for parasites may be warranted.

2. Although nonspecific, the determination of serum IgE levels may be useful in selected situations.

3. Nasal smears or sputum cytology for eosinophils may be use-

ful in selected patients. Nasal eosinophilia is common in allergic rhinitis, while abundant eosinophils in sputum may be evident in patients with Löffler's pneumonia. Charcot-Leyden crystals may be present.

4. A chest radiograph is useful to evaluate for either Löffler's pneumonia or sarcoidosis.

5. Biopsy of the gastrocnemius muscle, diagnostic in most cases of trichinosis, is used only in severely ill patients in whom the diagnosis is in doubt.

6. Serologic tests for collagen vascular disorders may be helpful in some patients.

Course and Treatment

Treatment of reactive eosinophilia depends on the underlying cause. Those eosinophilias that are a manifestation of a chronic myeloproliferative disorder often require therapy to arrest the tissue damage from intravascular eosinophil degranulation.

References

Caulfield JP, Hein A, Rothenberg ME, et al. A morphometric study of normodense and hypodense human eosinophils that are derived *in vivo* and *in vitro*. *Am J Pathol.* 1990;137:27-41.

Enokihara H, Kajitani H, Nagashima S, et al. Interleukin 5 activity in sera from patients with eosinophilia. *Br J Haematol.* 1990;75:458-462.

Kamb ML, Murphy JJ, Jones JL, et al. Eosinophilia-myalgia syndrome in L-tryptophan–exposed patients. *JAMA.* 1992;267:77-82.

Liesveld JL, Abboud CN. State of the art: the hypereosinophilic syndromes. *Blood Rev.* 1991;5:29-37.

Noguchi H, Kephart GM, Colby TV, Gleich GJ. Tissue eosinophilia and eosinophil degranulation in syndromes associated with fibrosis. *Am J Pathol.* 1992;140:521-528.

Rothenberg ME, Owen WF Jr, Silberstein DS, et al. Human eosinophils have prolonged survival, enhanced functional properties, and become hypodense when exposed to human interleukin 3. *J Clin Invest.* 1988;81:1986-1992.

Sanderson CJ. Interleukin-5, eosinophils, and disease. *Blood.* 1992;79:3101-3109.

Stefanini M, Claustro JC, Motos RA, Bendigo LL. Blood and bone marrow eosinophilia in malignant tumors: role and nature of blood and tissue eosinophil colony-stimulating factor(s) in two patients. *Cancer.* 1991;68:543-548.

Varga J, Uitto J, Jimenez SA. The cause and pathogenesis of the eosinophilia-myalgia syndrome. *Ann Intern Med.* 1992;116:140-147.

Weller PF, Bubley GJ. The idiopathic hypereosinophilic syndrome. *Blood.* 1994;83:2759-2779.

Zucker-Franklin D. Eosinophils: morphology, production, biochemistry, and function. In: Williams WJ, Beutler E, Erslev AJ, Lichtman MA, eds. *Hematology.* 4th ed. New York, NY: McGraw-Hill; 1990:835-839.

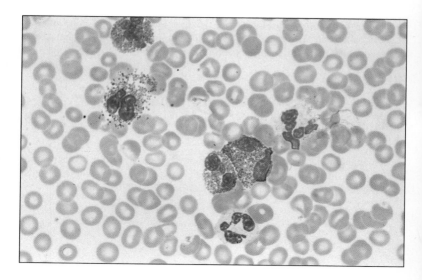

Image 17-1 An increase in relatively normal-appearing eosinophils is present on this blood smear from a female patient who was taking L-tryptophan. (Wright's)

Image 17-2 A striking dysplastic blood eosinophilia characterizes this chronic myeloproliferative disorder termed idiopathic hyper-eosinophilic syndrome. Note prominent degranulation. (Wright's)

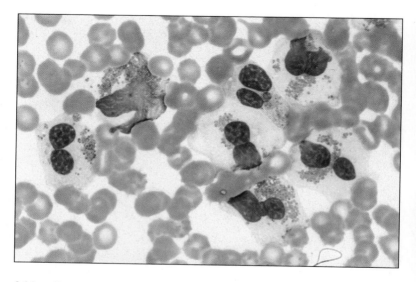

18

Basophilia

Basophils are the least numerous granulated cell within the peripheral blood. These cells generally account for less than 2% of white blood cells, and the absolute basophil count is characteristically less than $0.1 \times 10^3/mm^3$ ($0.1 \times 10^9/L$). There are no established age-related variations in absolute basophil count.

Basophilia is defined as an absolute basophil count that exceeds $0.2 \times 10^3/mm^3$ ($0.2 \times 10^9/L$). The reactive disorders associated with an increase in mature basophils are uncommon, and the absolute basophil counts are generally only moderately increased in these conditions (Table 18-1). These reactive conditions include allergic disorders and hypersensitivity reactions, inflammatory disorders such as ulcerative colitis and rheumatoid arthritis, chronic renal disease, and rare infections including influenza, chicken pox, and smallpox. The absolute basophil count may also be increased following radiation.

In contrast, neoplastic disorders with a mature basophilic component are much more frequently encountered in clinical practice than reactive basophilias. Furthermore, the absolute basophil count is substantially higher in patients with these neoplastic conditions. Chronic myeloproliferative disorders, especially chronic myeloge-

Table 18-1   Causes of Reactive Basophilia

Allergic or hypersensitivity reactions
Inflammatory disorders (collagen vascular disease)
Endocrinopathy
Renal disease
Rare infections
Irradiation
Rare carcinomas

nous leukemia (CML), are the most common malignancies in which an absolute basophilia is present. Even though the percentage of basophils is generally less than 10% of the white blood cells in patients with CML, because of the marked leukocytosis, the absolute basophil count is strikingly elevated. A rising absolute basophil count can precede overt blast crisis in some CML patients. Basophilia is a consistent feature in the blood of patients with CML, while only about one third of patients with other chronic myeloproliferative disorders will demonstrate this finding. In addition, various acute leukemias can also exhibit a basophilic component, but these cells are generally very immature-appearing, requiring special studies for their identification.

Pathophysiology

Although the mechanisms responsible for basophil production have not been completely delineated, regulatory factors currently thought to play a role in basophil production include interleukin (IL)-3, granulocyte-monocyte colony-stimulating factor (GM-CSF), IL-4, and IL-5. Even though the earliest stages of maturation are not distinguishable from other myeloid lineages, the proposed stages of basophil maturation include myeloblast, promyelocyte, basophilic myelocyte, basophilic metamyelocyte, and mature basophil. Basophils are recognized in the peripheral blood and bone marrow by their distinctive secondary granule, which is large, deeply basophilic, and often obscures the segmented nucleus. These secondary granules contain numerous proteins that are essential for basophil function. These proteins include heparin, histamine, eosinophil chemotactic factor, arylsulfatase A, slow-reacting substance of anaphylaxis, as well as many other substances.

Basophils appear to be closely related to tissue mast cells. Despite the differences in immunophenotype and morphology between basophils and mast cells, the granule contents of these two cells are remarkably similar. Likewise, both of these cells function in immediate hypersensitivity reactions via granule release. Basophil degranulation occurs in response to the binding of IgE antibodies to Fc receptors on the cell membrane.

Clinical Findings

The clinical findings in patients with reactive basophilia are quite variable, reflecting the spectrum of disorders associated with this blood abnormality. Some patients with allergic and hypersensitivity reactions may have urticaria, while patients with collagen vascular disorders, endocrinopathy, or renal disease will exhibit very diverse symptomatology and clinical findings.

The clinical features of patients with neoplastic mature basophilia are more distinctive. As described earlier, a striking mature basophilia is typical of CML, and these patients frequently have marked splenomegaly at presentation. These patients may also complain of malaise, fatigue, and left upper quadrant pain. Hepatomegaly is variable, but present in a substantial number of CML patients (see Chapter 34).

Approach to Diagnosis

Reactive basophilias must be distinguished from chronic myeloproliferative disorders with a mature basophilic component. A variety of clinical and hematologic parameters are useful in making this distinction.

The following approach to diagnosis should be considered:

1. Perform a complete blood count with differential.

2. Determine absolute basophil count and assess morphology of basophils.

3. Evaluate other lineages for evidence of a chronic myeloproliferative disorder. For example, in patients with CML, a

marked leukocytosis with left shift to myeloblasts is characteristic. In addition to an absolute basophilia, eosinophilia is also common. Likewise, most CML patients will demonstrate a marked, atypical thrombocytosis.

4. Correlate with clinical features; assess for splenomegaly.
5. Evaluate chemical indicators of increased cell turnover such as uric acid.

Hematologic Findings

Blood Cell Measurements. Basophils are noteworthy when the absolute basophil count exceeds 0.2 x 10^3/mm^3 (0.2 x 10^9/L). Most reactive basophilias are characterized by a modest increase in basophils, while in neoplastic disorders, the absolute basophil count is often strikingly increased. Except for anemia (usually anemia of chronic disease), other peripheral blood abnormalities are not generally present in patients with reactive basophilia.

Blood Morphology. Basophils are morphologically unremarkable in reactive basophilia. In contrast, a variety of morphologic abnormalities may be present in the blood of patients with chronic myeloproliferative disorders (see Chapters 31, 32, 34).

Bone Marrow Examination. Bone marrow examination is not generally required in the evaluation of patients with a reactive basophilia. In contrast, bone marrow examination with cytogenetic studies is often essential in establishing the diagnosis of various chronic myeloproliferative disorders.

Course and Treatment

The clinical course for reactive basophilia is related to the underlying disorder. Likewise, treatment of these patients is determined by the underlying disorder. In general, the increase in basophils within the peripheral blood is not associated with any disease manifestations. The treatment of chronic myeloproliferative disorders, such as CML, is often directed toward lowering the white blood cell count, reducing splenomegaly, and ameliorating other symptoms. In recent years, curative therapy has been attempted in these patients (see Chapter 34).

References

Bodger MP, Newton LA. The purification of human basophils: their immunophenotype and cytochemistry. *Br J Haematol.* 1987;67:281-284.

Denburg JA. Basophil and mast cell lineages *in vitro* and *in vivo. Blood.* 1992; 79:846-860.

Galli SJ, Dvorak AM, Dvork HF. Morphology, biochemistry, and function of basophils and mast cells. In: Williams WJ, Beutler E, Erslev AJ, Lichtman MA, eds. *Hematology.* 4th ed. New York, NY: McGraw-Hill; 1990:840-845.

Lichtman MA. Basophilopenia, basophilia, and mastocytosis. In: Williams WJ, Beutler E, Erslev AJ, Lichtman MA, eds. *Hematology.* 4th ed. New York, NY: McGraw-Hill; 1990:849-855.

Zucker-Franklin D. Basophils. In: Zucker-Franklin D, Greaves MF, Grossi CE, et al, eds. *Atlas of Blood Cells: Function and Pathology.* 2nd ed. Philadelphia, Pa: Lea & Febiger; 1988:287-320.

19

Monocytosis

Although generally present in low numbers, monocytes and related cell types are ubiquitous inhabitants of all organ systems in the body. Monocytes generally comprise only 2% to 9% of white blood cells, with an absolute count of 0.1-$0.9 \times 10^3/mm^3$ (0.1-$0.9 \times 10^9/L$). Slightly higher numbers of monocytes may be identified within the blood of normal infants. However, there are no striking age-related variations in normal absolute monocyte count.

A monocytosis is defined as an absolute monocyte count that exceeds $1.0 \times 10^3/mm^3$ ($1.0 \times 10^9/L$) in adults and $1.2 \times 10^3/mm^3$ ($1.2 \times 10^9/L$) in neonates. Both neoplastic and nonneoplastic disorders are associated with an absolute monocytosis (Tables 19-1, 19-2). The most common cause of a reactive monocytosis is a chronic infection secondary to many agents, including tuberculosis, *Listeria*, syphilis, subacute bacterial endocarditis, and certain protozoal and rickettsial infections. In general, a chronic infection is more likely to exhibit monocytosis than an acute infection. Other causes of reactive monocytosis include nonhematopoietic neoplasms such as Hodgkin's disease and occasional non-Hodgkin's lymphomas. Often recovery from agranulocytosis is preceded by monocytosis; this is common in patients with cyclic neutropenia. A variety of immune-

Table 19-1   Causes of Reactive Monocytosis

Chronic infections, many agents
Hodgkin's disease
Recovery of agranulocytosis
Collagen vascular diseases
Gastrointestinal disorders (immune-mediated)
Non-Hodgkin's lymphomas
Sarcoidosis
Multiple myeloma
Hemolytic anemia
Chronic neutropenia
Rare carcinomas
Splenectomy
Immune thrombocytopenic purpura

mediated disorders are also associated with a mature reactive monocytosis, including collagen vascular diseases and gastrointestinal disorders such as ulcerative colitis and regional enteritis. Other less
common causes of reactive monocytosis include hemolytic anemia,
chronic neutropenia, and postsplenectomy states.

Likewise, patients with hematopoietic neoplasms can exhibit a
peripheral blood monocytosis, but in these disorders the monocytes
are part of the neoplastic clone (Table 19-2). For example, monocytosis is a defining feature of myelodysplastic disorders such as
chronic myelomonocytic leukemia. In addition, both acute
myelomonocytic and acute monocytic leukemias demonstrate a
monocytic component. However, in these acute leukemias the
monocytes demonstrate marked immaturity, while more mature-
appearing circulating monocytes are evident in chronic
myelomonocytic leukemia and chronic myelogenous leukemia.
Other chronic myeloproliferative disorders can sometimes demonstrate an increase in peripheral blood monocytes, and circulating
neoplastic monocytic/histiocytic cells may be occasionally identified in the peripheral blood of patients with malignant histiocytosis.

Pathophysiology

Monocytes are derived from bone marrow myeloid progenitor cells,
and regulatory factors linked to monocyte production include gran-

Table 19-2   Disorders With Circulating Neoplastic Monocytes

Myelodysplasia, especially chronic myelomonocytic leukemia
Acute myelomonocytic leukemia
Acute monocytic leukemia
Chronic myelogenous leukemia
Other chronic myeloproliferative disorders
Malignant histiocytosis

ulocyte-monocyte colony-stimulating factor and monocyte colony-stimulating factor. The proposed stages of monocyte differentiation within the bone marrow include monoblasts, promonocytes, and mature monocytes, although neither monoblasts nor promonocytes are typically identified in normal bone marrow specimens.

Monocytes circulate briefly in the peripheral blood and migrate to tissues where they mature into a variety of cells comprising the monocyte/histiocyte/immune accessory cell system. Members of this diverse cell family exhibit a variety of functions in both cellular and humoral immunity, as well as phagocytic and antimicrobial activities. Monocytes and other cells within this lineage secrete hundreds of proteins that modulate immune function, regulate hematopoiesis, stimulate inflammatory reactions, provide host defense against tumors, and remove either senescent blood cells or infectious organisms by phagocytosis. A partial list of proteins produced by cells within this complex lineage includes complement components, interferons, interleukins, prostaglandins, tumor necrosis factors, and colony-stimulating factors. Like neutrophils, monocytes contain granules within their cytoplasm that play a major role in the cell's function. These granules contain numerous enzymes including lysozyme, acid phosphatase, collagenase, and elastase.

Clinical Findings

The predicted clinical features in patients exhibiting reactive monocytosis are diverse, because of the large variety of disorders linked to this relatively nonspecific peripheral blood finding. The most common cause of reactive monocytosis is chronic infection, and these patients are likely to be febrile with other symptomatology related to the specific type of chronic infection. In patients in whom the monocytosis is a component of a hematopoietic neoplasm, additional blood abnormalities are expected. The clinical features in patients with either myelodysplasia or acute leukemia often include fatigue, fever, malaise, and signs of organ infiltration.

Approach to Diagnosis

Since blood monocytosis occurs frequently in certain hematologic neoplasms, it is imperative that a distinction between a reactive and neoplastic monocytosis be made. In patients with hematologic neoplasms such as chronic myelomonocytic leukemia, acute myelomonocytic and monocytic leukemias, and chronic myelogenous leukemia, the monocytes are an integral part of the neoplastic clone. The determination of the reactive or neoplastic nature of a blood monocytosis often requires the integration of a variety of hematologic, morphologic, and other laboratory and clinical parameters. A general approach to monocytosis includes:

1. A complete blood count with differential
2. Evaluating monocytes for evidence of nuclear immaturity or other atypical features
3. Evaluating other peripheral blood cells for evidence of atypia, dysplasia, or immaturity
4. Correlating clinical and hematologic findings
5. Appropriate cultures to assess for possible chronic infection
6. Bone marrow examination for culture or assessment for hematopoietic neoplasm
7. Cytogenetic evaluation for possible hematopoietic neoplasm

Hematologic Findings

Blood Cell Measurements. In healthy children and adults, the absolute monocyte count is characteristically less than $1.0 \times 10^3/\text{mm}^3$ ($1.0 \times 10^9/\text{L}$). Depending on the cause of the monocytosis, many other peripheral blood abnormalities may be evident. For example, a reactive monocytosis secondary to infection may be accompanied by a neutrophilia (Image 19-1). In these patients, the platelet count is highly variable, and a mild to moderate anemia (most likely anemia of chronic disease) may also be evident. The white blood cell count is also highly variable in patients with a neoplastic monocytosis. However, the white blood cell count is typically elevated, with increased numbers of monocytes and a variable proportion of immature myeloid and monocytic elements. In these patients with hematopoietic neoplasms, the hemoglobin, hematocrit, and platelet count may be markedly reduced.

Peripheral Blood Smear Morphology. Evidence of monocyte immaturity, such as finely dispersed nuclear chromatin, nucleoli, and variable abnormal nuclear configurations, suggests that the monocytes are part of a neoplastic process (Image 19-2). Circulating monoblasts also suggest a neoplastic process. Reactive monocytes characteristically exhibit a relatively mature nuclear chromatin configuration, while the cytoplasm is frequently vacuolated (Image 19-1). Cytoplasmic granulation may also be prominent. In addition to evaluating monocyte morphology, an evaluation of the morphology of other cell types in the peripheral blood can be helpful in distinguishing a benign from a neoplastic monocytosis. If there is prominent dyspoiesis of neutrophils, erythrocytes, or platelets, the patient in all likelihood has a neoplastic hematologic disorder with involvement of many cell lines, including the monocyte lineage. This multilineage dyspoiesis with atypical monocytes is especially prominent in myelodysplastic disorders.

Bone Marrow Examination. Bone marrow examination may be warranted in selective patients with a blood monocytosis. Indications for bone marrow examination in this patient population include culture or evaluation for a possible hematopoietic neoplasm.

Ancillary Tests

1. Blood or bone marrow culture
2. Serologic studies for infectious agents
3. Cytogenetics in cases of possible hematopoietic neoplasm

4. Urine/serum lysozyme levels (highest in monocytic leukemias)

Course and Treatment

The clinical course varies with the underlying disorder, as does the treatment in patients with monocytosis. In general, patients with a neoplastic monocytosis follow an aggressive disease course requiring antileukemic therapy.

References

Douglas SD, Hassan NF. Morphology of monocytes and macrophages. In: Williams WJ, Beutler E, Erslev AJ, Lichtman MA, eds. *Hematology.* 4th ed. New York, NY: McGraw-Hill; 1990:858-868.

Foucar K, Foucar E. The mononuclear phagocyte and immunoregulatory effector (M-PIRE) system: evolving concepts. *Semin Diagn Pathol.* 1990;7:4-18.

Johnston RB Jr. Monocytes and macrophages. *N Engl J Med.* 1988;318:747-752.

Johnston RB, Zucker-Franklin D. The mononuclear phagocyte system: monocytes and macrophages. In: Zucker-Franklin D, Greaves MF, Grossi CE, et al, eds. *Atlas of Blood Cells: Function and Pathology.* 2nd ed. Philadelphia, Pa: Lea & Febiger; 1988:323-357.

Maldonado JE, Hanlon DG. Monocytosis: a current appraisal. *Mayo Clin Proc.* 1965;40:248-259.

Nathan CF. Secretory products of macrophages. *J Clin Invest.* 1987;79:319-326.

Papadimitriou JM, Ashman RB. Macrophages: current views on their differentiation, structure, and function. *Ultrastruct Pathol.* 1989;13:343-372.

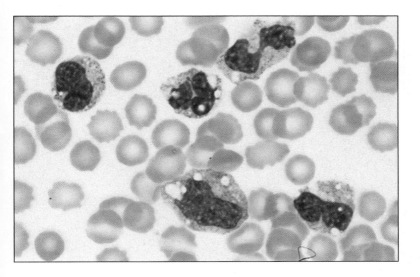

Image 19-1 Prominent cytoplasmic vacuolization of both neutrophils and monocytes is evident on this blood smear from a septic infant. (Wright's)

Image 19-2 On this blood smear from a child with chronic myelomonocytic leukemia, a striking monocytosis with some nuclear immaturity and dyspoiesis is evident. (Wright's)

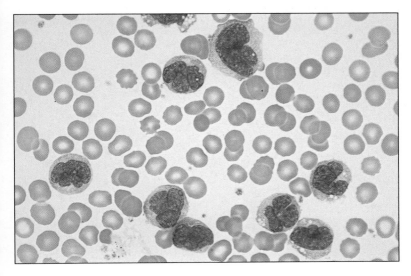

20

Neutropenia

In normal adults, the range for absolute neutrophil count is 1.5-7.0 x 10^3/mm^3 (1.5-7.0 x 10^9/L). Both patient age and race have an impact on the established lower limit of normal range for absolute neutrophil count. For example, in neonates and infants, the lower limit of normal range for absolute neutrophil count is approximately 2.5 x 10^3/mm^3 (2.5 x 10^9/L), while the lower limit of normal for children and adults is 1.5 x 10^3/mm^3 (1.5 x 10^9/L). Approximately one fourth of healthy black children and adults demonstrate an absolute neutrophil count that ranges from 1.0-1.5 x 10^3/mm^3 (1.0-1.5 x 10^9/L). Because these patients demonstrate no evidence of clinically significant neutropenia, this value is presumed to represent a normal race variation.

Consequently, the definition of neutropenia varies by patient age and race. An absolute neutrophil count below 2.5 x 10^3/mm^3 (2.5 x 10^9/L) constitutes neutropenia in infants, while an absolute neutrophil count less than 1.5 x 10^3/mm^3 (1.5 x 10^9/L) is generally used to define neutropenia in other patient groups. Neutropenias are subclassified into mild, moderate, and severe based on the absolute neutrophil count. A mild neutropenia generally ranges from 1.0-1.5 x 10^3/mm^3 (1.0-1.5 x 10^9/L), while moderate neutropenias range from 0.5-1.0 x 10^3/mm^3 (0.5-1.0 x 10^9/L). Patients with severe neutropenia (<0.5 x 10^3/mm³ [<0.5 x 10^9/L]) are at the greatest risk for serious bacterial infection, usually of endogenous origin.

Causes of neutropenia are listed in Table 20-1. Neutropenia can be the result of either a constitutional bone marrow defect or an acquired abnormality, and there are prominent age variations in the most common causes of neutropenia. In addition, an isolated neutropenia must be distinguished from multilineage cytopenias. The primary causes of neutropenia, based on patient age, are listed in Table 20-2. Infection is by far the most common cause of neutropenia in neonates. Neonates may also develop neutropenia from maternal factors such as hypertension, drug treatments given to the mother during late gestation, and maternal antibodies that cross the placenta and attack fetal granulocytes. In addition, a variety of constitutional neutropenic disorders have been well-described, although these disorders are rare and seldom encountered in clinical practice. Of these rare hereditary disorders, the more prevalent are cyclic neutropenia, Kostmann syndrome, and Chédiak-Higashi syndrome (see Chapter 22 for illustration and description). Severe sustained neutropenia characterizes Kostmann syndrome and Chédiak-Higashi syndrome, while patients with cyclic neutropenia exhibit episodic loss of neutrophils followed by a rebound recovery.

Infection is also a common cause of neutropenia in older children. Other causes of neutropenia in infants and children include autoimmune disorders, bone marrow neoplasms, myeloablative therapy, and idiosyncratic drug reactions. In adults, idiosyncratic drug reactions are the most common cause of neutropenia in ambulatory patients. Numerous drug treatments are linked to acquired neutropenia and patients should always be queried regarding medications. Other common causes of neutropenia in adults include infections, bone marrow replacement disorders, myeloablative therapy, megaloblastic anemia, and various autoimmune/immune disorders including acquired white cell aplasia. Splenic pooling of neutrophils can be present in patients with hypersplenism.

Pathophysiology

Normal numbers of circulating neutrophils are maintained by adequate bone marrow proliferation, unimpeded bone marrow matu-

Table 20-1   Causes of Neutropenia

Infections
Idiosyncratic drug reactions
Autoimmune/other immune disorders
Neoplasms replacing bone marrow
Megaloblastic anemia
Constitutional neutropenic disorders
Hypersplenism
Acquired idiopathic neutropenia
Bone marrow ablative therapies

ration and release into blood, and normal survival time in blood. Defects both within and outside the bone marrow may be responsible for neutropenia, and these mechanisms can be broadly classified as proliferation, maturation, survival, and distribution defects (Table 20-3). Often, more than one of these mechanisms is operational in the production of neutropenia. For example, a patient with an infection may develop a neutropenia because of bone marrow suppression by the infectious agent, decreased neutrophil survival, and increased egress of neutrophils from the blood to sites of infection. Likewise, the mechanisms that are operative in patients who develop neutropenia secondary to idiosyncratic drug reactions are also variable. In some of these patients, the drug causes abrupt loss of the granulocyte lineage (ie, proliferation defect), while drug-induced immune-mediated neutrophil destruction is operative in other patients (ie, a survival defect).

Clinical Findings

Because of the variety of underlying causes, patients with neutropenia have diverse clinical manifestations. However, all neutropenic patients must be assessed for possible underlying infections that may be either the cause or the consequence of the neutropenia. Secondary infections in neutropenic patients are often derived from endogenous organisms, and commonly involved sites include skin, oral pharynx, gingiva, gastrointestinal tract, and the anal region. The detection of infection may be challenging in neutropenic patients, because many of the clinical "clues" to a specific site of infection are the conse-

Table 20-2   Age-Related Causes of Neutropenia

Patient Age	Causes of Neutropenia Listed in Order of Frequency
Neonate	Infection
	Maternal hypertension and/or drug treatment
	Maternal antibody production
	Constitutional disorders such as cyclic neutropenia, Kostmann syndrome, and Chédiak-Higashi syndrome
Infant/Child	Infection
	Autoimmune neutropenia
	Neoplasms replacing bone marrow
	Idiosyncratic drug reactions
	Myeloablative therapies
	Constitutional neutropenic disorders (rare)
	Megaloblastic anemia (rare)
	Copper deficiency (rare)
Adult	Idiosyncratic drug reactions
	Infections
	Neoplasms replacing bone marrow
	Myeloablative therapies
	Autoimmune disorders including white cell aplasia
	Aplastic anemia
	Hypersplenism
	Megaloblastic anemia
	Large granular lymphocytosis

quence of the migration of huge numbers of neutrophils to that site. In neutropenic patients, findings such as swelling, induration, erythema, and even infiltrates on chest roentgenogram are less conspicuous.

Approach to Diagnosis

The evaluation of a patient with neutropenia requires the integration of multiple clinical and laboratory parameters. Although the appropriate workup varies with patient age, in general, the evaluation of a neutropenia should include:

1. Detailed history for evidence of recurrent infections, findings suggestive of a constitutional disorder, symptoms of a current infection, and symptoms of an underlying immunologic disorder or occult neoplasm.

2. Investigation for drug therapy, toxin, or alcohol exposure.

Table 20-3 Mechanisms Causing Neutropenia

Mechanism	Comments
Proliferation defect	Failure of granulocytic lineage
	Often only scattered myeloblasts and promyelocytes present
	Occurs in many constitutional neutropenias, many idiosyncratic drug reactions, bone marrow replacement disorders, aplastic anemia, and following myeloablative therapy
Maturation defect	Granulocytic lineage abundant but maturation does not proceed normally and many cells die within the bone marrow
	Occurs in neutropenias associated with megaloblastic anemia and rare constitutional disorders such as myelokathexis
Survival defect	Bone marrow production and release of neutrophils is increased, but cells are rapidly removed from blood
	Occurs in many infections and immune disorders characterized by antineutrophil antibody production
Distribution abnormality	Total body granulocyte pool is normal, but number of circulating neutrophils is reduced
	Occurs in patients with hypersplenism and patients with defective release of bone marrow neutrophils (rare)
	Seldom the primary mechanism responsible for neutropenia

3. Physical examination for possible splenomegaly, evidence of occult infection or neoplasm.

4. Complete blood count with differential; serial complete blood counts may be necessary to document either a cyclic pattern or to document neutrophil recovery in patients with transient neutropenia.

5. Morphologic review of blood smear for evidence of hematopoietic neoplasms, infection-related changes, megaloblastic features, and evaluation of other lineages.

6. Laboratory workup for possible infection, if clinically suspected.

7. In selected patients, laboratory assessment of immune status, tests for collagen vascular disorders, or serologic studies for viral agents.

8. Various radiographic studies in selected individuals, including those patients with suspected constitutional neutropenic disorders.

9. Bone marrow examination. This is generally required in adult patients with new-onset neutropenia. Likewise, bone marrow evaluation is necessary in children with suspected neoplasms, aplasia, and selected infections. However, many children develop transient neutropenia following viral infections. In these children, who are otherwise healthy and who have only isolated neutropenia, a "watch and wait" approach is often taken. A bone marrow examination will not likely be considered in these children unless spontaneous neutrophil recovery is not evident within 1 to 2 months.

Hematologic Findings

Blood Cell Measurements. The neutrophil count is less than $1.5 \times 10^3/mm^3$ ($1.5 \times 10^9/L$). Depending on the cause of the neutropenia, the other hemogram parameters are highly variable.

Peripheral Blood Smear Morphology. Although the total number is decreased, the morphology of granulocytes is normal. In infected patients, toxic changes and left shift may be evident. Monocytosis may be present and is partly compensatory.

Bone Marrow Examination. Bone marrow findings vary with the mechanism responsible for the neutropenia. In patients with proliferation defects, the granulocytic lineage is largely absent. This may be the consequence of some hematopoietic regulatory defect or the bone marrow may be effaced by a neoplasm or fibrosis. In patients with maturation defects, the granulocytic lineage is hyperplastic and morphologic abnormalities are generally prominent. In patients with survival defects, the granulocytic lineage is likewise hyperplastic. However, as a consequence of rapid release of mature forms into the blood, the granulocyte maturation pyramid may be left-shifted in patients with survival defects. If the survival defect is immune-mediated, bone marrow macrophages may contain ingested neutrophils (Image 20-1).

Ancillary Tests

Numerous ancillary tests may be warranted in selected neutropenic patients, including tests for folate and vitamin B_{12} levels, collagen vascular disease, immune status, granulocyte antibody studies, cytogenetics, serologic tests for infectious agents, neutrophil survival studies, and copper levels.

Course and Treatment

The management of a patient with neutropenia includes:

1. Prompt antibiotic therapy for infected patients.
2. Determination and management of the underlying cause of neutropenia.
3. Possible human recombinant colony-stimulating factor therapy to stimulate neutrophil production.

The development of recombinant human colony-stimulating factor has been a major breakthrough in the treatment of neutropenias of diverse etiology, including both constitutional and acquired neutropenic disorders. The most consistent increases in absolute neutrophil count are achieved with granulocyte colony-stimulating factor therapy. In these patients, a brisk neutrophilia with prominent toxic changes results from pharmacologic doses of granulocyte colony-stimulating factor (see Chapter 16).

References

Baley JE, Stork EK, Warkentin PI, Shurin SB. Neonatal neutropenia: clinical manifestations, cause, and outcome. *Am J Dis Child.* 1988;142:1161-1166.

Bux J, Mueller-Eckhardt C. Autoimmune neutropenia. *Semin Hematol.* 1992; 29:45-53.

Dale DC, Hammond WP IV. Cyclic neutropenia: a clinical review. *Blood Rev.* 1988;2:178-185.

Foucar K. Constitutional and reactive myeloid disorders. In: *Bone Marrow Pathology*. Chicago, Ill: ASCP Press; 1995:99-119.

Foucar K, Duncan MH, Smith KJ. Practical approach to the investigation of neutropenia. *Clin Lab Med*. 1993;13:879-894.

Jonsson OG, Buchanan GR. Chronic neutropenia during childhood: a 13-year experience in a single institution. *Am J Dis Child*. 1991;145:232-235.

Julia A, Olona M, Bueno J, et al. Drug-induced agranulocytosis: prognostic factors in a series of 168 episodes. *Br J Haematol*. 1991;79:366-371.

Lyall EGH, Lucas GF, Eden OB. Autoimmune neutropenia of infancy. *J Clin Pathol*. 1992;45:431-434.

Peterson L, Foucar K. Granulocytosis and granulocytopenia. In: Bick RL, Bennett JM, Brynes RK, et al, eds. *Hematology: Clinical and Laboratory Practice*. St Louis, Mo: CV Mosby Co; 1993:1137-1154.

Pisciotta AV. Drug induced agranulocytosis peripheral destruction of polymorphonuclear leukocytes and their marrow precursors. *Blood Rev*. 1990;4:226-237.

Reed WW, Diehl LF. Leukopenia, neutropenia, and reduced hemoglobin levels in healthy American blacks. *Arch Intern Med*. 1991;151:501-505.

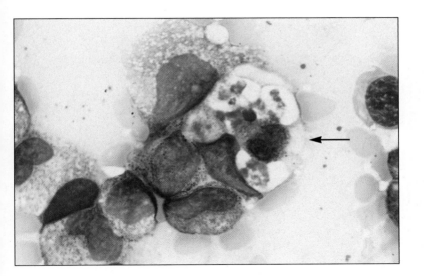

Image 20-1   On this imprint smear of bone marrow from a child with autoimmune neutropenia, a macrophage contains numerous ingested neutrophils (↑). (Wright's)

21

Functional Defects of Granulocytes

In this chapter disorders linked to impaired neutrophil function will be reviewed. Adequate neutrophil function is essential for protection from invading bacteria and fungi. As predicted, patients with significant neutrophil function defects are susceptible to recurrent bacterial and fungal infections. All genetic disorders of neutrophil function are extremely rare and not usually encountered in clinical practice. Acquired neutrophil function defects are much more common but are generally not severe.

Pathophysiology

Neutrophil function is a very complex and highly regulated process that requires normal levels and functional activity of various cytoplasmic components and membrane proteins, as well as an external environment that contains adequate chemotactic factors, complement levels, cytokines, and normal endothelial cell function. A series of interrelated activities are required to accomplish neutrophil destruction of invading bacteria and fungi. Neutrophils must be produced in adequate numbers by the bone marrow and appropriately released into the peripheral blood (see Chapters 16 and 20).

Circulating neutrophils must be able to sense chemotactic factors released in the vicinity of bacterial or fungal invasion. Appropriate ligands on the surface of the neutrophil are necessary to bind these chemotactic factors, which include immunoglobulins, complement components, bacterial metabolites, and denatured neutrophil proteins. These neutrophils must then attach to endothelial cells, egress through the blood vessel wall, and migrate to the specific site of invasion. Adhesion of neutrophils to endothelial cells is accomplished by binding of neutrophil adhesion molecules (integrins such as CD11b/CD18) to ligands on the surface of the endothelial cells. Neutrophils must subsequently recognize, bind, phagocytize, and finally destroy these invading bacteria or fungi.

Both chemotaxis and microbial phagocytosis/destruction require the integrated activity of cytoplasmic cytoskeletal proteins, cytoplasmic granules, and surface membrane constituents of neutrophils. The complement system is essential for many of these neutrophil activities. In addition, cytokines such as the colony-stimulating factors not only induce neutrophil production within the bone marrow, but enhance functional activities of mature neutrophils. Both of these effects of colony-stimulating factors are achieved by binding to a specific surface membrane receptor on either immature or mature cells. Once microorganisms have been engulfed by neutrophils, an oxidative reaction (so called respiratory burst) is often required for their destruction.

Any abnormality in this complex series of neutrophil functional activities can result in an increased susceptibility to bacterial or fungal infections, including infections with low-virulence organisms. These neutrophil functional abnormalities can be either constitutional (genetic) or acquired, and are generally classified as defects in adhesion, mobility, granule formation, and phagocytic/killing activity (Table 21-1). In some disorders, more than one type of defect is evident. Because sophisticated methodologies to investigate neutrophil function are relatively new, multiple types of neutrophil function defects have been only recently categorized. In addition to intrinsic neutrophil abnormalities, disorders in the complement cascade and immunoglobulins are also a cause of neutrophil dysfunction.

All constitutional neutrophil functional defects are exceedingly rare, and hereditary disorders are typically manifested during

Table 21-1   Classification of Constitutional and Acquired
Functional Defects of Neutrophils

General Type of Defect	Constitutional Disorders	Acquired Disorders/Conditions
Adhesion defects	Leukocyte adhesion deficiency	Aging Alcohol-induced drug effects (corticosteroids, epinephrine, aspirin) Diabetes Renal disorders Paraproteinemias Sickle cell anemia
Defects in granule structure/ function	Chédiak-Higashi syndrome Specific granule deficiency	Chronic myeloproliferative disorders Severe burns
Mobility defects	Chédiak-Higashi syndrome Complement disorders Neutrophil actin deficiency Other actin and microtubular defects Specific granule deficiency Hyperimmunoglobulin E syndrome	Autoimmune disorders (collagen vascular disorders) Diabetes Chronic renal failure Infections including HIV-1 Malnutrition Thermal injury After bone marrow transplant Graft-versus-host disease Recombinant interleukin-2 therapy
Phagocytic/ killing defects	Chronic granulomatous disease Complement disorders Myeloperoxidase deficiency Other neutrophil enzyme deficiencies Immunodeficiency disorders with decreased immunoglobulins Thalassemia major	Autoimmune disorders (collagen vascular disorders) Thermal injury Diabetes After bone marrow transplant Graft-versus-host disease Malnutrition HIV-1 infection Sickle cell anemia

Abbreviation: HIV-1 = human immunodeficiency virus–1.

infancy and early childhood. These hereditary neutrophil function disorders are often severe, and, consequently, patients develop numerous recurrent and progressive bacterial and fungal infections, often associated with poor wound healing.

Chédiak-Higashi syndrome was the first recognized constitutional neutrophil function disorder. This autosomal recessive, multisystem disease is the consequence of defects in granule structure and function that affect many cells throughout the body. Because of abnormalities in melanosome structure, these patients often have oculocutaneous albinism. Abnormal granules are apparent within all granulated hematopoietic cells and even within lymphocytes (see Chapter 22). Because of this abnormal cytoplasmic granulation, many cells die within the bone marrow, resulting in peripheral blood neutropenia. Although neutrophil defects are primarily responsible for the increased susceptibility to infection in patients with Chédiak-Higashi syndrome, functional defects of eosinophils, basophils, and monocytes are also present. The abnormal cytoplasmic granulation in Chédiak-Higashi syndrome results in both impaired mobility (ie, defective chemotaxis) and defective degranulation.

Chronic granulomatous disease is another type of constitutional neutrophil function disorder that may be rarely encountered in clinical practice. Most cases of chronic granulomatous disease are X-linked recessive disorders, although both autosomal recessive and autosomal dominant subtypes of chronic granulomatous disease have also been described. The onset of disease is characteristically within the first year of life, and patients with this disease frequently have lymphadenopathy, hepatosplenomegaly, and anemia of chronic disease. Dominant sites of recurrent infection include lung, lymph node, and skin. Older patients often demonstrate restrictive lung disease, while severe gastrointestinal disease is evident in a smaller proportion of these patients. Patients with chronic granulomatous disease demonstrate mutations that result in defective generation of NADPH oxidase leading to a failure to undergo oxidative reactions (failure of so-called respiratory burst). Consequently, ingested organisms are not killed.

In general, acquired disorders of neutrophil function are less severe than constitutional defects and are often transient. The acquired conditions and disorders associated with various neutrophil function defects are listed in Table 21-1.

There are also physiologic age variations in neutrophil function. Normal neonates frequently demonstrate impaired functional activities of neutrophils and monocytes, including defects in bone marrow release, cellular activation, and chemotaxis. This, in part, explains the increased susceptibility of newborns to serious bacterial infections. Likewise, elderly patients may also develop aberrations in neutrophil adhesion, resulting in mild functional impairment.

Clinical Findings

Most constitutional neutrophil functional defects are manifested in infancy or early childhood, while acquired neutrophil functional defects are more prevalent in adults. Depending on the severity of the functional defect, the clinical findings are variable. However, patients with profound neutrophil functional defects characteristically present with severe, recurrent bacterial and, less often, fungal infections that involve skin, oral cavity, sinuses and lung, lymph nodes, and the gastrointestinal tract. Progressive organ damage can be the consequence of these recurrent infections. Bronchiectasis can result from recurrent pneumonias, while fistulas and abscesses may result from recurrent infections along the gastrointestinal tract.

In patients with either adhesion or mobility defects, inadequate numbers of neutrophils reach sites of infection. The lack of pus is a unique feature in these patients, and there may be few localizing clinical signs and symptoms.

Approach to Diagnosis

Although a neutrophil functional defect should be considered in children and adults with severe, recurrent bacterial and fungal infections, in actual practice most patients with recurrent infections do not exhibit a demonstrable neutrophil function defect. However, in that subgroup of patients with a likely defect, the approach should include both the distinction between a constitutional and acquired defect, and an attempt to categorize the nature of the neutrophil function abnormality. In general, the evaluation of these patients should include:

1. Complete blood count with differential.

2. Morphologic evaluation of neutrophils, evaluation of other lineages.

3. Detailed history regarding the frequency, severity, sites of infection, and types of recurrent infections, age of onset, and family history.

4. Physical examination to assess for scars, abscesses, pulmonary infiltrates; careful evaluation of skin, oral cavity, and respiratory tract.

5. Evaluation for other features of constitutional neutrophil function defects.

6. Evaluation for evidence of underlying disorders and drug treatments that are linked to acquired neutrophil function defects in adults.

7. Assessment of immune status, complement component levels, immunoglobulin levels, and CH_{50}.

8. Human immunodeficiency virus–1 testing in appropriate situations.

A variety of specialized tests of neutrophil function should also be considered. However, the sequence of this specialized neutrophil function testing should be determined on an individual case basis. These specialized tests of neutrophil function include:

1. Nitroblue tetrazolium dye test (indirect measurement of respiratory burst activity).

2. Myeloperoxidase stain of neutrophils.

3. Flow cytometric evaluation of expression of CD11/CD18 (adhesion molecules) on neutrophil surface membranes.

4. Assessment of neutrophil mobility, chemotaxis, and adhesion properties.

5. Superoxidase generation (other tests of oxidation).

6. Rebuck skin window to assess if neutrophils migrate to sites of infection (not commonly used today).

7. Electron microscopy to evaluate neutrophil granules.

Hematologic Findings

Blood Cell Measurements. Depending on both the nature of the neutrophil functional defect and whether the patient is actively infected, the blood cell measurements are variable. Patients with ongoing infection will often demonstrate an absolute neutrophilia with toxic changes. Extremely high elevations of the absolute neutrophil count are characteristic of constitutional leukocyte adhesion disorders. In these patients, the absolute neutrophil count may exceed $100 \times 10^3/\text{mm}^3$ ($100 \times 10^9/\text{L}$). In contrast, neutropenia is a frequent finding in Chédiak-Higashi syndrome. Patients with recurrent infections may also develop anemia of chronic disease.

Peripheral Blood Smear Morphology. Except for the massively enlarged granules that characterize Chédiak-Higashi syndrome, other morphologic findings in patients with neutrophil functional defects are not distinctive.

Bone Marrow Examination. Granulocytic hyperplasia is an anticipated finding in patients with neutrophil functional defects who suffer from recurrent infections. In addition, granulomas may be evident, especially in patients with recurrent fungal infections. Indications for bone marrow examination in patients with neutrophil function abnormalities include assessment for infection, unexplained blood to cytopenia, and evaluation for possible secondary hemophagocytic syndrome or lymphoproliferative disorder (notably in patients with Chédiak-Higashi syndrome).

Other Laboratory Tests

21.1   Nitroblue Tetrazolium Dye Test

The nitroblue tetrazolium (NBT) test is used to indirectly detect the production of superoxide by neutrophils.

Principle.   NBT is a soluble, yellow dye that is converted to an insoluble blue-black compound when neutrophils are capable of undergoing oxidative metabolism. This insoluble material precipitates within neutrophil cytoplasm and can be seen by light microscopy. Neutrophils that fail to reduce NBT lack this oxidative capability.

Specimen.   Heparinized blood can be utilized for activated NBT tests.

Procedure.   Stimulated neutrophils are incubated with NBT. This dye is reduced by oxidative enzymes contained within granules in neutrophils and monocytes. Following incubation, blood smears are prepared and stained with Wright's stain. A differential cell count is performed by separating neutrophils into those either containing or lacking the blue-black precipitate. Appropriate controls are utilized.

Interpretation.   Indirect evidence of production of superoxide is present when neutrophils contain the blue-black precipitate. Neutrophils that fail to reduce NBT are evident in patients with chronic granulomatous disease, as well as in other neutrophil enzyme deficiency disorders, some complement deficiency conditions, and agammaglobulinemias. Normal ranges are determined within individual laboratories.

Notes and Precautions.   The NBT test cannot be performed on ethylenediaminetetraacetic acid (EDTA)–anticoagulated specimens. Likewise, heparin forms complexes with NBT that are ingested by neutrophils, making heparin an undesirable anticoagulant for examining spontaneous NBT-reducing activity. However, the incubated NBT-reducing activity utilizing stimulated neutrophils is not affected by heparin anticoagulation.

21.2   Myeloperoxidase Stain

Purpose.   This cytochemical stain is used to evaluate the presence of myeloperoxidase within neutrophil granules.

Principle.   The myeloperoxidase enzyme of granulocyte primary granules reduces substrate dyes in a colorimetric reaction
producing an insoluble compound that precipitates within the
cytoplasm of neutrophils.

Specimen.   Freshly prepared blood smears.

Procedure.   A colorless substrate (usually benzidine dihy-
drochloride) and hydrogen peroxide are layered on the peripheral blood smear. During the incubation, the myeloperoxidase
present within neutrophil primary granules converts hydrogen
peroxide into water and oxygen, which oxidizes the substrate
producing a blue-black precipitate. After counterstaining, cells
are viewed under a light microscope, and the proportion of
positive neutrophils is determined.

Interpretation.   Normal neutrophils demonstrate strong positive granular reactivity throughout the cytoplasm. In patients
with myeloperoxidase deficiency, no staining or only weak
staining may be identified.

Notes and Precautions.   Optimal pH is essential for this enzymatic reaction. Myeloperoxidase is degraded by exposure to
light, and this enzyme stain should generally be performed
within a few hours of obtaining the specimen.

Ancillary Tests

Many tests have been developed that assess different types of
neutrophil functional activities (see "Approach to Diagnosis"
above). The decision to perform these sophisticated tests
should be determined on a case-by-case basis. Likewise, the
sequence of testing strategies in patients with a presumed neutrophil function abnormality should be determined on a case-
by-case basis. Additional specialized tests of neutrophil function include:

1. Adherence of neutrophils to nylon wool fiber or to plastic tissue culture plates.

2. Neutrophil aggregation studies.

3. Ingestion of particles by neutrophils.

4. Measurements of various granule constituents, in addition to myeloperoxidase.

5. Assessment of bacterial killing ability.

Course and Treatment

Patients with severe neutrophil function defects (typically constitutional defects) often succumb to recurrent bacterial or fungal infections, and prompt antibiotic therapy for established or suspected infections is essential. In addition, antibiotic prophylaxis is commonly used. These patients may also develop severe organ failure, most commonly pulmonary failure, as a consequence of tissue destruction from repeated infections. Some response to immune-modulating agents such as human recombinant interferon γ has been achieved in patients with chronic granulomatous disease. Finally, bone marrow transplantation has been attempted in small numbers of patients with constitutional neutrophil function defects.

References

Berkow RL, Howard TH. Laboratory evaluation of qualitative neutrophil disorders. In: Bick RL, Bennett JM, Brynes RK, et al, eds. *Hematology Clinical and Laboratory Practice*. St Louis, Mo: CV Mosby Co; 1993;2:1123-1135.

Curnutte JT. Disorders of phagocyte function. In: Hoffman R, Benz EJ, Shattil SJ, et al, eds. *Hematology Basic Principles and Practice*. New York, NY: Churchill Livingstone; 1991:571-589.

Curnutte JT. Disorders of granulocyte function and granulopoiesis. In: Nathan DG, Oski FA, eds. *Hematology of Infancy and Childhood*. 4th ed. Philadelphia, Pa: WB Saunders Co; 1993;1:904-977.

Granger DN, Kubes P. The microcirculation and inflammation: modulation of leukocyte-endothelial cell adhesion. *J Leuk Biol*. 1994;55:662-675.

Lisiewicz J, Bick RL. Morphology and biochemistry of the myeloid series. In: Bick RL, Bennett JM, Brynes RK, et al, eds. *Hematology Clinical and Laboratory Practice*. St Louis, Mo: CV Mosby Co; 1993;2:1053-1075.

Metcalf JA, Gallin JI, Nauseef WM, Root RK. *Laboratory Manual of Neutrophil Function.* New York, NY: Raven Press; 1986:1-191.

Newburger PE, Malawista SE, Dinauer MC, et al. Chronic granulomatous disease and glutathione peroxidase deficiency, revisited. *Blood.* 1994;84:3861-3869.

Shearer WT, Paul ME, Smith CW, et al. Laboratory assessment of immune deficiency disorders. *Immunol Allergy Clin N Am.* 1994;14:265-299.

Watts RG, Howard TH. Functional disorders of granulocytes and monocytes. In: Bick RL, Bennett JM, Brynes RK, et al, eds. *Hematology Clinical and Laboratory Practice.* St Louis, Mo: CV Mosby Co; 1993;2:1099-1121.

Yang KD, Hill HR. Functional biology of the granulocyte-monocyte series. In: Bick RL, Bennett JM, Brynes RK, et al, eds. *Hematology Clinical and Laboratory Practice.* St Louis, Mo: CV Mosby Co; 1993;2:1077-1092.

22 ✓

Leukocytic Disorders of Abnormal Morphology

Both hereditary and acquired disorders are associated with morphologic abnormalities of neutrophils (Tables 22-1, 22-2). These abnormalities include both nuclear and cytoplasmic aberrations. Nuclear defects include hyposegmentation and hypersegmentation, while cytoplasmic abnormalities include various types of inclusions, hypergranular cytoplasm, and hypogranular cytoplasm.

Although all hereditary disorders with abnormal neutrophils are rare, the more prevalent of these genetic disorders include Pelger-Huët anomaly, May-Hegglin anomaly, Chédiak-Higashi syndrome, and Alder-Reilly anomaly (Table 22-1). Pelger-Huët anomaly is characterized by either bilobed or nonsegmented neutrophil nuclei. The nuclear chromatin of these cells tends to be uniformly dense. The cytoplasm of these neutrophils is unremarkable, and these cells demonstrate no functional abnormalities. The neutrophils in May-Hegglin anomaly contain large blue cytoplasmic inclusions that resemble Döhle bodies. Similar inclusions are also evident in other granulated cells. Additional hematologic abnormalities include thrombocytopenia, enlarged platelets, and variable neutropenia. Many of these patients are asymptomatic. In contrast, patients with Chédiak-Higashi syndrome suffer from frequent pyogenic infections

Table 22-1   Hereditary Granulocyte Disorders of Abnormal
Morphology

Disorder	Granulocyte Feature
Pelger-Huët anomaly	Bilobed or nonsegmented neutrophil nuclei; cytoplasm normal
May-Hegglin anomaly	Large blue cytoplasmic inclusions resembling giant Döhle bodies
Chédiak-Higashi syndrome	Giant cytoplasmic granules
Alder-Reilly anomaly	Intense azurophilic granulation of neutrophil cytoplasm
Myelokathexis	Shape abnormalities, pyknotic nuclei, hypersegmentation

Table 22-1 *Continued*

Other Blood, Bone Marrow Abnormalities	Inheritance	Other Findings
No other lineage abnormalities No functional abnormalities	Autosomal dominant	No associated findings
Thrombocytopenia Enlarged platelets Variable neutropenia Inclusions also in eosinophils, basophils, and monocytes	Autosomal dominant	Many patients are asymptomatic
Neutropenia, thrombocytopenia All granulated cells and even lymphocytes affected Represent fused lysosomes Functional defects of neutrophils Some patients develop infection-associated hemophagocytic syndrome or Epstein-Barr virus–induced lymphoproliferative disorders	Autosomal recessive	Partial oculocutaneous albinism Frequent pyogenic infections
Eosinophils and basophils contain large basophilic granules Vacuolated/abnormally granulated lymphocytes in some cases	Autosomal recessive	Associated with several different types of genetic mucopolysaccharide disorders
Striking bone marrow abnormalities affecting all stages of granulopoiesis Neutropenia; intramedullary death of granulocytes Functional defects of neutrophils and monocytes	Not well characterized	Growth retardation Skeletal abnormalities

Table 22-2   Acquired Neutrophil Disorders with Abnormal Morphology

Morphologic Abnormality	Other Hematologic Findings	Comments
Pseudo–Pelger-Huët change	Dependent on underlying cause	Found in patients with hematologic neoplasms (myelodysplasia, AML, CML)
		Result of drug exposure (colchicine, sulfonamides)
		Linked to mycoplasma infection
		Rare finding after bone marrow transplantation
Hypersegmentation of neutrophils	Varies depending on cause:	Vitamin B_{12} or folate deficiency
	Pancytopenia, macrocytosis in patients with folate or vitamin B_{12} deficiency	Myelodysplasia, acute myeloid leukemia, other myeloid neoplasms
	Cytoplasmic hypogranulation common in myelodysplasia or myeloid leukemias	Steroid therapy, certain chemotherapeutic agents
Hypogranular cytoplasm	Often found in association with nuclear segmentation abnormalities	Myelodysplasia
		Acute myeloid leukemias
		Chronic myeloid neoplasms, often in transformation
Intense cytoplasmic granulation	Marked neutrophilia with left shift	Pharmacologic doses of recombinant human CSF
		Neoplasms producing CSF

Abbreviations: AML = acute myeloid leukemia; CML = chronic myelogenous leukemia; CSF = colony-stimulating factor.

and often die in childhood. Chédiak-Higashi syndrome is characterized by giant cytoplasmic granules that are present within all granulated cells and even lymphocytes within the blood and bone marrow. These giant granules represent fused lysosomes and are linked to many functional defects. Other abnormalities include neutropenia and thrombocytopenia. As a consequence of immunosuppression, patients with Chédiak-Higashi syndrome may develop secondary viral infections that induce either florid hemophagocytic syndromes or lymphoproliferative disorders. Intense azurophilic granulation of neutrophil cytoplasm characterizes the Alder-Reilly anomaly, a finding that is associated with several different types of genetic mucopolysaccharide disorders. Abnormalities of eosinophils, basophils, and lymphocytes are also evident in patients with these genetic mucopolysaccharide disorders.

Acquired morphologic abnormalities of neutrophils are substantially more common than hereditary disorders (Table 22-2). Morphologic abnormalities of both neutrophil nuclei and cytoplasm are common in patients with hematologic neoplasms such as myelodysplasia, acute myeloid leukemias, and chronic myeloid leukemias, especially in transformation. For example, patients with these hematologic malignancies may demonstrate both neutrophil pseudo–Pelger-Huët nuclei in conjunction with hypogranular cytoplasm. Less commonly, nuclear hypersegmentation may be evident in neutrophils from these patients. Other causes of acquired neutrophil hypersegmentation include vitamin B_{12} or folate deficiency, and occasional drug treatments. Acquired Pelger-Huët change is also associated with certain drug exposures, notably colchicine and sulfonamide therapy. This nuclear segmentation defect can also be found in patients with mycoplasma infection and in rare bone marrow transplant recipients. Finally, intense cytoplasmic granulation is an acquired abnormality in patients receiving pharmacologic doses of recombinant human colony-stimulating factor.

Pathophysiology

The pathophysiology of hereditary granulocyte disorders is linked to the underlying genetic defect. The cause of acquired neutrophil abnormalities is not always clear-cut. In patients with vitamin B_{12}

or folate deficiency, the basic defect is an inability to undergo mitosis (see Chapter 5), while the various nuclear and cytoplasmic abnormalities identified in patients with hematologic neoplasms are the consequence of these acquired clonal genetic disorders. The cause of those morphologic abnormalities of neutrophils linked to drug treatments or infection is less clear-cut, but these changes should regress following successful treatment of the infection or cessation of the drug treatment.

Clinical Findings

Associated clinical findings in patients with hereditary neutrophil disorders are listed in Table 22-1. The clinical findings in patients with acquired neutrophil disorders are variable, linked to the specific underlying disorder. Patients with hematologic neoplasms often experience fatigue, malaise, and fever if secondary infection has occurred. Likewise, splenomegaly and hepatomegaly may be evident in some of these patients.

Approach to Diagnosis

When a morphologic abnormality of neutrophils is encountered, it is essential to determine if this is a hereditary or acquired defect. The integration of clinical findings, other hematologic parameters, history, and physical examination generally allow for this distinction. The cause of an acquired neutrophil abnormality must also be determined. Emphasis should be placed on distinguishing neoplastic from nonneoplastic causes of acquired morphologic abnormalities of neutrophils. The evaluation of a patient with neutrophil morphologic abnormalities generally includes:

1. Complete blood count (CBC) with differential.
2. Morphologic review of neutrophils and other lineages.
3. Family history and possible evaluation of other family members.
4. Evaluation for evidence of infection.
5. Evaluation for evidence of bleeding.
6. Assessment for drug treatments linked to morphologic abnormalities.

7. Evaluation for hematopoeitic neoplasm.

8. Evaluation of patients for phenotypic abnormalities that occur in genetic neutrophil disorders.

9. Evaluation for possible secondary neoplasms or infection-associated hemophagocytic syndrome in selected patients.

Hematologic Findings

Blood Cell Measurements. Several of the hereditary and acquired granulocyte disorders with abnormal morphology are associated with cytopenias, most notably neutropenia and/or thrombocytopenia. Anemia may also be evident in patients with recurrent chronic infections and in patients with underlying hematologic malignancies.

Peripheral Blood Smear Morphology. The various morphologic abnormalities of neutrophil nuclei and cytoplasm in patients with either hereditary or acquired granulocyte disorders are delineated in Tables 22-1 and 22-2 (Image 22-1). In addition, enlarged platelets characterize May-Hegglin anomaly, while cytoplasmic abnormalities of other granulated cells or lymphocytes may be encountered in patients with May-Hegglin anomaly, Chédiak-Higashi syndrome, and Alder-Reilly anomaly (see Table 22-1). In patients with acquired neutrophil abnormalities, other blood findings suggestive of myeloid neoplasms may be evident.

Bone Marrow Examination. Bone marrow examination is generally not required in patients with hereditary granulocyte disorders, unless warranted for cultures, assessment for a secondary neoplasm, or possible infection-associated hemophagocytic or lymphoproliferative disorder. In contrast, bone marrow examination may be necessary to determine if an acquired neutrophil disorder is the consequence of a hematologic neoplasm.

Ancillary Tests

Various tests of neutrophil function may be warranted in selected patients with morphologic abnormalities of neutrophils. In addition, assessment of vitamin B_{12} or folate levels is appropriate in selected patients. Cytogenetic studies are also warranted for patients with possible hematologic neoplasms.

Course and Treatment

The clinical course is highly variable in patients with hereditary and acquired morphologic disorders of neutrophils. For example, patients with Pelger-Huët anomaly and most patients with May-Hegglin anomaly are asymptomatic. In contrast, patients with Chédiak-Higashi syndrome experience severe recurrent infections, infection-associated hemophagocytic syndrome, and secondary neoplasms. Likewise, patients with hematologic neoplasms demonstrate a variable disease course, typically requiring multi-agent chemotherapy or possible bone marrow transplant (see Chapters 28, 29, 34).

References

Bassan R, Viero P, Minetti B, et al. Myelokathexis: a rare form of chronic benign granulocytopenia. *Br J Haematol.* 1984;58:115-117.

Brunning RD. Morphologic alterations in nucleated blood and marrow cells in genetic disorders. *Hum Pathol.* 1970;1:99-124.

Davey FR, Erber WN, Gatter KC, Mason DY. Abnormal neutrophils in acute myeloid leukemia and myelodysplastic syndrome. *Hum Pathol.* 1988;19:454-459.

Eichacker P, Lawrence C. Steroid-induced hypersegmentation in neutrophiles. *Am J Hematol.* 1985;18:41-45.

Lindenbaum JL, Nath BJ. Megaloblastic anaemia and neutrophil hypersegmentation. *Br J Haematol.* 1980;44:511-513.

van Hook L, Spivack C, Duncanson FP. Acquired Pelger-Huët anomaly associated with *Mycoplasma pneumoniae* pneumonia. *Am J Clin Pathol.* 1985;84:248-251.

West BC. Chédiak-Higashi syndrome neutrophils are characterized by the absence of both normal azurophilic granules. *Am J Pathol.* 1986;122:177-189.

White JG, Clawson CC. The Chédiak-Higashi syndrome: the nature of the giant neutrophil granules and their interactions with cytoplasm and foreign particulates. *Am J Pathol.* 1980;98:151-196.

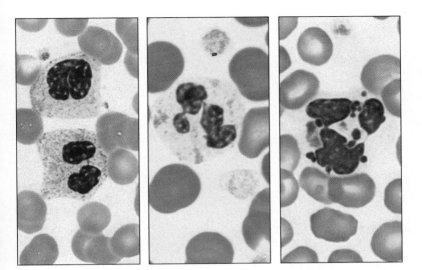

Image 22-1   These blood smears illustrate morphologic abnormalities in Pelger-Huët anomaly (left), May-Hegglin anomaly (center), and Chédiak-Higashi syndrome (right; Courtesy of Dr. P. Ward). (Wright's)

PART
IV

Reactive Disorders of Lymphocytes

23

Reactive Disorders of Lymphocytes

A peripheral blood lymphocytosis in adults is usually defined as any lymphocyte count in excess of $4 \times 10^3/mm^3$ ($4 \times 10^9/L$). Normal lymphocyte counts are considerably higher in infants and children (Table 23-1). Therefore, the age of the patient must be considered when the blood is evaluated for lymphocytosis.

About 60% to 80% of circulating blood lymphocytes are T lymphocytes, 10% to 20% B lymphocytes, and 5% to 10% natural killer (NK) cells. The T-cell population consists of T-helper cells (CD4+) and T-suppressor cells (CD8+), with the former outnumbering the latter approximately two to one.

Pathophysiology

Benign peripheral blood lymphocytoses are polyclonal increases in lymphocytes and usually represent responses to underlying disorders or conditions (Table 23-2). Most benign lymphocytoses are characterized morphologically by reactive-appearing lymphocytes, although mature lymphocytoses also occur.

The most common cause of a reactive lymphocytosis is infectious mononucleosis (IM) caused by primary Epstein-Barr virus

Table 23-1   Age-Related Reference Values for Lymphocyte Count

Age	Absolute Number of Lymphocytes, x 10^3/mm^3 (x 10^9/L)
Birth	2.0-11.0
14 days	2.0-9.0
4 years	2.0-7.0
≥16 years	1.0-4.0

(EBV) infection (see Chapter 24). Even though the EBV infects B cells, the circulating reactive lymphocytes in this disorder are predominantly T cells of the cytotoxic/suppressor phenotype (CD8). This population of cells is expanded in response to the EBV-infected B cells and is the predominant immunologic mechanism for bringing the acute infection under control.

Infections with several other agents, primarily viruses, have also been associated with a lymphocytosis. In some of these disorders, the clinical and peripheral blood picture is similar to that of EBV-IM. These disorders are referred to as IM-like syndromes (Table 23-2). The most common of these is caused by an acute cytomegalovirus (CMV) infection. The pathogenesis of CMV infection is less well understood than EBV-IM, but the peripheral lymphocytosis, like that of EBV-IM, is a T-cell response consisting primarily of T-cytotoxic/suppressor cells.

A transient stress lymphocytosis is occasionally observed in some patients with acute noninfectious medical conditions. The lymphocytosis in this situation represents an expansion of the normal lymphocyte population and is thought to be secondary to epinephrine release. The lymphocytosis resolves quickly, often within a few hours, followed by a neutrophilia.

Acute bacterial infections rarely cause a lymphocytosis. An exception is whooping cough, in which a striking lymphocytosis may be seen. The causative organism, *Bordetella pertussis*, produces a soluble factor that appears to play a role in the accumulation of lymphocytes in the blood by preventing them from homing normally back to lymphoid tissue. Surface marker studies show that these cells are predominantly of T-helper (CD4+) phenotype.

Table 23-2 Causes of Benign Lymphocytosis

Reactive lymphocytosis
   Infectious mononucleosis (EBV)
   Infectious mononucleosis–like syndromes
       Cytomegalovirus
       Toxoplasmosis
       Adenovirus
       Acute HIV infection
       Human herpesvirus-6
   Other viral infections
       Viral hepatitis
       Rubella
       Roseola
       Mumps
       Chickenpox
   Drug reactions
   Transient stress lymphocytosis
Mature lymphocytosis
   Whooping cough
   Infectious lymphocytosis
   Cigarette smoking

Abbreviations: EBV = Epstein-Barr virus; HIV = human immunodeficiency virus.

The pathogenesis of the lymphocytosis reported in rare individuals who smoke cigarettes is unknown, but a polyclonal increase in B cells occurs.

Clinical Findings

The clinical signs and symptoms of patients with a reactive lymphocytosis vary depending on the underlying cause. Most are acute, self-limited infectious diseases.

Infectious Mononucleosis (EBV). This disorder typically occurs in teenagers and young adults and is characterized by fever, sore throat, headache, malaise, nausea, and anorexia. Lymphadenopathy is almost always present, and splenomegaly may also be observed.

Infectious Mononucleosis-like Syndromes. CMV-induced IM-like syndromes usually occur in adults between the ages of 20 and 30 years old. The clinical syndrome may be indistinguishable from EBV-IM, but pharyngitis and lymphadenopathy are typically less severe than in EBV infection. *Toxoplasma gondii* infection is a rare cause of IM-like syndrome; lymphadenopathy without lymphocytosis is more common. Patients undergoing seroconversion to the human immunodeficiency virus (HIV) may present with an IM-like illness. Widespread lymphadenopathy with varying combinations of sore throat, fever, and malaise are often present. Rarely, infection with human herpes virus–6 causes an IM-like syndrome. This virus is also the causative agent of roseola. Infection with adenovirus has been associated with an IM-like syndrome.

Other Causes of a Reactive Lymphocytosis. Occasionally, patients with viral hepatitis present with a reactive lymphocytosis. Patients with rubella, roseola, mumps, and chickenpox may have a reactive lymphocytosis. A reactive lymphocytosis may also be seen in patients with drug reactions. A transient stress lymphocytosis is occasionally observed in patients presenting with trauma, myocardial infarction, status epilepticus, and other acute medical conditions.

Whooping Cough. Whooping cough (pertussis) is usually seen in infants and young children who have not been immunized, and is characterized clinically by severe paroxysmal coughing and prominent lymphocytosis.

Infectious Lymphocytosis. Infectious lymphocytosis is a benign illness of young children presumably of viral origin. The patients are often asymptomatic, but fever, abdominal pain, or diarrhea may be present. Organomegaly does not occur. The symptoms resolve within a few days. The lymphocytosis may persist for several weeks.

Lymphocytosis and Smoking. Persistent polyclonal lymphocytosis has been reported rarely in individuals who smoke cigarettes. Small numbers of binucleate forms of lymphocytes are reported in these patients.

Approach to Diagnosis

Accurate diagnosis of a patient with a benign peripheral blood lymphocytosis requires correlation of the clinical and laboratory findings. The diagnostic approach begins with the following:

1. Clinical history, including age of the patient, symptoms, and physical examination.

2. Complete blood cell count with differential to determine magnitude of lymphocytosis and other cell counts.

3. Morphologic examination of blood smear to evaluate lymphocytes.

4. Additional laboratory tests to determine the cause of the lymphocytosis.

The clinical history, physical findings, and hematologic abnormalities often suggest the most likely diagnosis and determine which additional tests are needed to identify the cause of the lymphocytosis. For example, if a patient has clinical manifestations consistent with IM and a reactive lymphocytosis, the diagnostic tests should include a test for the heterophil antibody (Table 23-3). Since EBV-IM is the most common cause of a reactive lymphocytosis, the test result will likely be positive and a definitive diagnosis will be made. If, however, the heterophil test is negative, acute CMV infection, heterophil-negative EBV-IM, and other conditions associated with a reactive lymphocytosis should be considered. For a more detailed discussion of the diagnostic approach to a patient with IM or IM-like syndrome, see Chapter 24. In other conditions associated with lymphocytosis (see Table 23-2), the clinical findings may be highly suggestive of the underlying disorder, will determine the necessity of additional laboratory testing, or may even establish the diagnosis.

The differential diagnosis of a patient with a reactive lymphocytosis sometimes includes a malignant lymphoproliferative disorder, most notably acute lymphoblastic leukemia (ALL) and chronic lymphocytic leukemia (CLL). Confusion of a reactive lymphocytosis with ALL is most likely to occur when the leukocyte count is unusually high (ie, >30 x 10^3/mm^3 [>30 x 10^9/L]). This problem is

Table 23-3 Selected Tests in the Differential Diagnosis of Benign Lymphocytosis

Disease	Test	Interpretation
Infectious mononucleosis (EBV)	Heterophil test (see Test 24.1)	Positive results in association with characteristic blood smear morphology indicate EBV-IM
	EBV-specific serologic tests (see Test 24.2)	IgM and IgG antibodies to viral capsid antigens indicate acute infection
Cytomegalovirus (CMV)	Culture via shell vial technique or polymerase chain reaction	Positive results indicate acute infection
	Serologic tests via complement fixation, immunofluorescence, and ELISA	CMV-specific IgM indicates recent infection
Toxoplasmosis	Serologic tests via indirect fluorescent antibody test or ELISA	Elevated IgM antitoxoplasma antibody indicates acute infection
Adenovirus	Culture	Positive results in acute infection
Acute HIV infection	Antibody to HIV via Western blot; test for p24 antigen with ELISA	Positive results indicate infection with HIV
Human herpesvirus-6	Test for antibody via immunofluorescence or ELISA	Significant IgM antibody or increases in IgG suggest acute infection
Hepatitis A, B, C	Serologic tests with ELISA or radioimmunoassay	Hepatitis A–specific IgG and IgM are positive in acute infection
		Presence of hepatitis B surface antigen (HBsAg) in absence of antibody indicates acute infection
		Antibody to hepatitis C virus is present in acute infection
Rubella	Culture of virus; test for antibody using hemagglutination inhibition, ELISA, or complement-fixation procedures	Isolation of virus or rise in antibody titer indicates acute infection
Bordetella pertussis	Culture of nasal swab; direct fluorescent antibody staining procedure of clinical specimens or cultures	Identification of bacteria indicates acute infection

Abbreviations: EBV = Epstein-Barr virus; IM = infectious mononucleosis; ELISA = enzyme-linked immunosorbent assay; HIV = human immunodeficiency virus.

compounded when the serologic test results are negative. Familiarity with the morphologic appearance of reactive lymphocytes, however, will aid in this differential diagnostic dilemma. In addition, anemia and thrombocytopenia are almost always present in acute leukemia, but usually absent or mild in benign reactive conditions such as IM. Moreover, the diagnosis of ALL should not be confirmed without a bone marrow aspirate and biopsy and other ancillary studies, including immunophenotypic analysis (see Chapter 30).

A benign reactive lymphocytosis can occasionally be difficult to distinguish from chronic lymphoproliferative disorders such as CLL. This is more of a problem in patients over the age of 40 years because of the relative frequency of CLL in comparison to reactive disorders such as IM in this age group. In addition, when IM does occur in the older patient, the clinical findings may be atypical for IM. The morphologic characteristics of the lymphocytes in CLL may be helpful in this differential diagnosis since, in general, they appear more monotonous than the lymphocytes in a reactive process. In some cases, however, immunophenotypic studies and a bone marrow biopsy may be necessary to differentiate these two disorders (see Chapter 35).

Hematologic Findings

Blood Cell Measurements.   Anemia is usually absent. The platelet count is usually normal, although mild thrombocytopenia not less than $100 \times 10^3/mm^3$ ($100 \times 10^9/L$) may be present. The absolute lymphocyte count in IM and IM-like syndromes usually exceeds $4.0 \times 10^3/mm^3$ ($4.0 \times 10^9/L$) with total leukocyte counts ranging from about 10 to $30 \times 10^3/mm^3$ (10.0-$30.0 \times 10^9/L$). Leukocyte counts above this level are rare. Patients with viral hepatitis, rubella, roseola, mumps, and chickenpox may have an absolute lymphocyte count greater than $4.0 \times 10^3/mm^3$ ($>4.0 \times 10^9/L$), but the degree of elevation is less and the duration of the lymphocytosis more transient than that in IM. In addition, plasma cells are often more prominent. In patients with drug reactions, an eosinophilia and neutrophilia may accompany the lymphocytosis with variability in the leukocyte counts. These patients also frequently exhibit circulating plasma cells. In transient stress lymphocytosis, the lymphocytosis is mild to moderate, averaging about 6.0 to 8.0 x 10^3/mm³ (6.0-8.0 x 10^9/L).

In whooping cough, the peak lymphocyte counts average about 10.0 x 10^3/mm³ (10.0 x 10^9/L); counts above 30.0 x 10^3/mm³ (30.0 x 10^9/L) are not unusual. A neutrophilia may also be present. Leukocyte counts in infectious lymphocytosis range from 35.0 to 100.0 x 10^3/mm³ (35.0-100.0 x 10^9/L). Absolute lymphocyte counts in polyclonal lymphocytosis associated with smoking are usually mildly elevated but may exceed 10.0 x 10^3/mm³ (10.0 x 10^9/L) with total leukocyte counts greater than 15.0 x 10^3/mm³ (15.0 x 10^9/L).

Peripheral Blood Morphology. In most benign lymphocytoses, the lymphocytes appear morphologically reactive (Image 23-1). Other terms used for these cells include atypical, variant, Downey, and transformed. The morphologic features of these cells and the morphologic characteristics of IM are discussed in Chapter 24. The appearance of the lymphocytes in the IM-like syndromes, including acute CMV infection, is indistinguishable from that in IM. The morphologic features of viral hepatitis, rubella, roseola, mumps, and chickenpox are also similar to IM, but the lymphocytosis is often less intense and not as long-lasting, and circulating plasma cells are frequently prominent. Plasma cells are also often prominent in patients with drug reactions and a reactive lymphocytosis; an eosinophilia and neutrophilia may also be present.

The lymphocytes in transient stress lymphocytosis consist of mature or mildly reactive-appearing lymphocytes. Large granular lymphocytes are occasionally prominent in these patients.

Unlike the previous disorders, the lymphocytes in whooping cough appear mature with condensed chromatin patterns and scant cytoplasm; they frequently exhibit cleaved or convoluted nuclei (Image 23-2). The lymphocytes in infectious lymphocytosis appear mature and an eosinophilia may be present in the later stages of the disease. The lymphocytes in lymphocytosis associated with cigarette smoking appear mature, with binucleate forms described.

Bone Marrow Examination. Bone marrow biopsy is usually not indicated in disorders characterized by a benign or reactive lymphocytosis in the blood. It should be done, however, if a malignant process is suspected.

Other Laboratory Tests

23.1 Serologic Tests, Cultures, and Other Methods for Identification of an Acute Infection

Purpose. Serologic tests, cultures, or other techniques may be performed to determine a specific cause of the lymphocytosis.

Principle. After individuals have been exposed to infectious agents, specific antibodies are produced. These can be detected with several types of serologic tests and used to diagnose a current or recent infection. Some organisms can be cultured from blood or tissue samples and are diagnostic of an acute infection. Some agents or specific antigens can be detected with direct and indirect fluorescent antibody tests, radioimmunoassay (RIA), enzyme-linked immunoabsorbent assay (ELISA), and polymerase chain reaction (PCR).

Specimen. Serum is used for the serologic tests. Both acute and convalescent serum are sometimes necessary to interpret the results. Blood or other tissue is used for culture techniques. Serum or tissue is used for antigen tests.

Procedure and Interpretation. See Table 23-3.

Course and Treatment

The clinical course depends on the underlying cause of the lymphocytosis. Many are acute, self-limited disorders, and only symptomatic therapy is indicated. Antiviral therapy (eg, ganciclovir) may be used for some viral infections, such as CMV. Zidovudine is the current antiviral therapy for human immunodeficiency virus infection.

Infection with hepatitis B virus is serious. The disease resolves in 90% of patients, but 1% have a fulminant hepatitis and 9% develop chronic hepatitis. Effective therapy is not available; therefore, prevention is the best approach. Hepatitis B vaccine is effective.

Erythromycin eradicates the causative organism in whooping cough, although it may not alter the clinical course of the disease.

References

Brunell PA. Rubella (German measles). In: Wyngaarden JB, Smith LH, Bennett JC, eds. *Cecil Textbook of Medicine.* 19th ed. Philadelphia, Pa: WB Saunders Co; 1992:1827-1829.

Cohen JI, Corey RC. Cytomegalovirus infection in the normal host. *Medicine.* 1985;64:100-114.

Gordon DS, Jones BM, Browning SW, et al. Persistent polyclonal lymphocytosis of B lymphocytes. *N Engl J Med.* 1982;307:232-236.

Groom DA, Kunkel LA, Brynes RK, et al. Transient stress lymphocytosis during crisis of sickle cell anemia and emergency trauma and medical conditions. *Arch Pathol Lab Med.* 1990;114:570-576.

Horwitz CA, Henle W, Henle G, et al. Heterophil-negative infectious mononucleosis and mononucleosis-like illnesses. *Am J Med.* 1977;63:947-957.

Horwitz CA, Henle W, Henle G, et al. Infectious mononucleosis in patients aged 40 to 72 years: report of 27 cases, including 3 without heterophil-antibody responses. *Medicine.* 1983;62:256-262.

Hutchinson RE, Kuree AS, Davey FR. Lymphocytic surface markers in lymphoid leukemoid reactions. *Clin Lab Med.* 1988;8:237-245.

Johnston RB Jr. Whooping cough (pertussis). In: Wyngaarden JB, Smith LH, Bennett JC, eds. *Cecil Textbook of Medicine.* 19th ed. Philadelphia, Pa: WB Saunders Co; 1992:1674-1676.

Kubic VL, Kubic PT, Brunning RD. The morphologic and immunophenotypic assessment of the lymphocytosis accompanying *Bordetella pertussis* infection. *Am J Clin Pathol.* 1990;95:809-815.

McMonigal K, Horwitz CA, Henle W, et al. Post-perfusion syndrome due to Epstein-Barr virus: report of two cases and review of the literature. *Transfusion.* 1983;23:331-335.

Ockner RK. Acute viral hepatitis. In: Wyngaarden JB, Smith LH, Bennett JC, eds. *Cecil Textbook of Medicine.* 19th ed. Philadelphia, Pa: WB Saunders Co; 1992: 763-770.

Peterson L, Hrisinko MA. Benign lymphocytosis and reactive neutrophilia: laboratory features provide diagnostic clues. *Clin Lab Med.* 1993;13:863-877.

Steeper TA, Horwitz CA, Ablashi DV. The spectrum of clinical and laboratory findings resulting for human herpesvirus-6 (HHV-6) in patients with mononucleosis-like illnesses not resulting from Epstein-Barr virus or cytomegalovirus. *Am J Clin Pathol.* 1990;93:776-783.

Steeper TA, Horwitz CA, Hanson M, et al. Heterophil-negative mononucleosis-like illnesses with atypical lymphocytosis in patients undergoing seroconversions to the human immunodeficiency virus. *Am J Clin Pathol.* 1988;90:169-174.

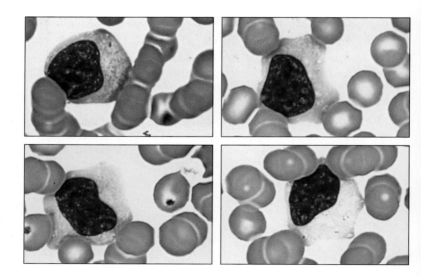

Image 23-1   Reactive lymphocytes from a patient with infectious mononucleosis.

Image 23-2   Blood smear from a child with whooping cough shows lymphocytes with scant cytoplasm, condensed chromatin, and cleaved nuclei.

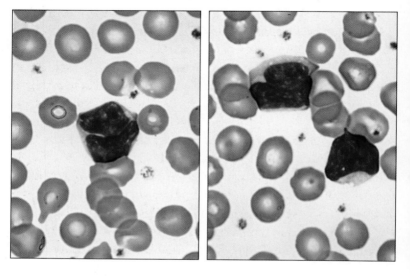

24

Infectious Mononucleosis

Infectious mononucleosis (IM), is an acute, self-limited febrile illness caused by primary infection by the Epstein-Barr virus (EBV).

Pathophysiology

EBV is a ubiquitous virus that infects B lymphocytes. The route of transmission of EBV appears to be by intimate contact with saliva from a previously infected person. EBV-infected lymphocytes from the oropharynx disseminate the virus throughout the reticuloendothelial system, provoking an intense immunologic response. In the early phases of the infection, T lymphocytes become activated and restrain viral replication in B lymphocytes. The lymphocytosis characteristic of this period consists primarily of T lymphocytes with cytotoxic/suppressor phenotype. A humoral response is also present during acute IM and is characterized by non-EBV–specific responses such as the production of heterophil antibody and EBV-specific antibodies including those directed against viral capsid antigen (VCA), early antigen (EA), and Epstein-Barr nuclear antigen (EBNA). The humoral response appears to be important in preventing recurrent infection, but it is the cellular response that is responsible for control of the acute infection. Latent EBV infection persists after resolution of symptoms, but cycles of replication of the virus do not occur in patients with intact immunologic systems.

Clinical Findings

IM typically occurs in teenagers and young adults between the ages of 10 and 25 years. Characteristic symptoms include sore throat, fever, headache, malaise, nausea, and anorexia. Lymphadenopathy, usually cervical, is almost always present. Over 50% of patients have splenomegaly, and mild hepatitis may be present. Acute EBV infections are also common in early childhood, but are often asymptomatic or characterized by clinical symptoms not recognized as IM. IM is rare over age 40 years, since most patients are immune to the virus by that time. When it does occur, the presenting features may be atypical, including prolonged fever, often without pharyngitis and lymphadenopathy.

Approach to Diagnosis

In a patient suspected of having IM, the initial laboratory workup should include the following:

1. Complete blood cell count with leukocyte differential.
2. Morphologic examination of the peripheral blood smear.
3. Test for IM heterophil antibody.

The appearance of increased numbers of reactive lymphocytes in the blood is one of the earliest laboratory signs of IM and is essential for the diagnosis. Minimal morphologic criteria for the diagnosis of IM (Table 24.1) have been established and will be discussed in the section on peripheral blood smear morphology.

The diagnosis of IM is confirmed by detection of heterophil antibodies specific for the disease (see Test 24.1). When serial studies are done, heterophil antibody tests are positive in over 96% of teenagers and young adults with IM.

In the majority of cases, the diagnosis of IM is straightforward.

Table 24-1   Minimal Morphologic Criteria for Diagnosis of
Infectious Mononucleosis

≥50% mononuclear cells (lymphocytes and monocytes) in blood smear
At least 10 reactive lymphocytes per 100 leukocytes
Marked lymphocyte heterogeneity

However, difficulties may arise, especially if the heterophil test is negative. This occurs more often in young children, since heterophil positivity is less frequent, with about 75% positivity at ages 2 to 4 years and less than 25% positivity in children under the age of 2 years. Heterophil-negative EBV-IM is unusual but is occasionally seen in teenagers and young adults. When the heterophil antibody cannot be detected, EBV-specific serologic tests can be used to confirm the diagnosis of EBV-IM. These tests are based on the detection of antibodies produced against specific antigens encoded by the EBV such as VCA, EA, and EBNA (see Test 24.2). There are also several disorders that have clinical and morphologic features indistinguishable from EBV-IM that should be considered in patients who clinically appear to have EBV-IM but in whom the heterophil test is negative. These are discussed in Chapter 23, the most common being acute CMV infection.

A practical diagnostic approach for IM that is useful in most clinical settings is shown in Table 24-2. This approach uses both the blood smear morphologic findings and a commercially available rapid test for heterophil antibody as the initial diagnostic workup. Four diagnostic possibilities exist:

1. If the peripheral blood smear does not exhibit the morphologic features of IM and the results of the rapid test are negative for heterophil antibody, the diagnosis of IM is usually excluded and no further testing for IM is indicated. Other causes for the patient's symptoms should be considered.

2. If the morphologic features of IM are present in the blood smear and the results of the rapid test for heterophil antibody are positive, the diagnosis of IM is confirmed. No further testing is required. Determination of heterophil titer is unnecessary since it does not correlate with clinical course.

Table 24-2   Workup of Patients With Clinically Suspected Infectious Mononucleosis (IM)*

Reactive Lymphocytosis[†]	Rapid Test for Heterophil Antibody	Diagnosis of IM	Further Diagnostic Tests
Absent	Negative	Not confirmed	Not indicated
Present	Positive	Confirmed	Not indicated
Absent	Positive	Inconclusive	Reference tube test or EBV serologic tests
Present	Negative	Suspicious of IM or IM-like illness	Repeat rapid heterophil test in 1-2 weeks, EBV serologic tests, tests for CMV, etc (see text)

Abbreviations: EBV = Epstein-Barr virus; CMV = cytomegalovirus.
*Modified from Horwitz CA. Practical approach to diagnosis of infectious mononucleosis. *Postgrad Med.* 1979;65:179-184.
†Blood smear meets minimal morphologic criteria for IM (see Table 24-1).

3. When the results of the rapid test are positive for the heterophil antibody but the blood smear lacks the morphologic characteristics of IM, the diagnosis of IM is not confirmed. Testing for the heterophil antibody by the reference tube test (see Test 24.1) is useful in these situations. If results with the reference tube test are negative, the results of the rapid test can be presumed to be falsely positive. If the tube test results are positive, another blood smear should be evaluated because occasionally the appearance of reactive lymphocytes lags behind positive serologic findings. Since heterophil antibodies in some individuals may persist for over a year after acute IM, it may also be useful to question the patient about past symptoms of IM. EBV-specific serologic tests can be used in place of the reference tube test in this situation.

4. If the blood smear meets the minimal morphologic criteria for IM and the results of the rapid test for heterophil antibody are negative, the diagnosis of IM should still be suspected. The serologic findings frequently lag behind the

appearance of reactive lymphocytes and retesting may yield a positive result in 1 to 2 weeks. If a negative rapid test result persists, the patient may still have IM, but may not produce the heterophil antibody. In this instance, EBV-specific serologic tests may be necessary to establish the diagnosis. Other disorders that may result in an IM-like syndrome unrelated to EBV such as acute CMV infection should also be considered (see Chapter 23).

Hematologic Findings

Blood Cell Measurements. Hemoglobin and hematocrit levels are usually normal in IM. Mild hemolysis is occasionally seen in persons with IM, but clinically significant anemia is uncommon, occurring only in about 1% to 3% of patients. When anemia is present, it is usually an autoimmune hemolytic anemia caused by red cell autoantibodies. Red cell autoantibodies with anti-i, anti-N, and anti-I specificities have been described in IM.

An absolute lymphocytosis, usually greater than 4.0 x 10^3/mm^3 (4.0 x 10^9/L), is present. The total leukocyte count is increased and ranges from 10 to 30 x 10^3/mm^3 (10.0-30.0 x 10^9/L); counts exceeding this are rare. The leukocytosis begins about 1 week after the onset of symptoms, peaks during the second or third weeks, and persists for 2 to 8 weeks. A mild-to-moderate neutropenia is often present and is most prominent in the third or fourth week of the illness. Rarely, agranulocytosis may complicate IM. Mild thrombocytopenia (100-150 x 10^3/mm^3 [100-150 x 10^9/L]) is present in about one third of patients with IM; severe thrombocytopenia is rare. Both the neutropenia and thrombocytopenia are apparently secondary to an immune mechanism.

Peripheral Blood Smear Morphology. The erythrocytes are usually normochromic and normocytic, but spherocytes and increased polychromasia may be apparent if an autoimmune hemolytic anemia is present.

The most striking morphologic finding in the peripheral blood smear is the presence of increased numbers of reactive lymphocytes. Reactive lymphocytes are benign, activated lymphocytes with a characteristic morphologic appearance. Other terms used to describe these cells include variant, atypical, transformed, or Downey cells. Reactive lymphocytes are present in the blood of healthy individuals, but usually represent less than 10 per 100 leukocytes.

More than 60 years ago, Downey and McKinley examined Wright's-stained blood smears from patients with IM and classified reactive lymphocytes into three groups: Downey I, Downey II, and Downey III—based solely on morphologic features.. This classification can facilitate recognition of the varied appearance of reactive lymphocytes.

The Downey type I cell (Image 24-1) is a small lymphocyte with minimal basophilic cytoplasm, condensed chromatin, and indented or lobulated nuclei. This type of cell is uncommon in IM, but may be prominent in some patients, especially young children. The Downey type II cell (Image 24-2) is the most commonly encountered reactive lymphocyte in IM. It is a large cell with abundant pale blue cytoplasm and coarse, but dispersed chromatin. Nucleoli are absent or indistinct. Peripheral or radiating basophilia of the cytoplasm is often present, and scattered azurophilic granules may be noted. The Downey type III cell (Image 24-3) is a medium-to-large lymphocyte with moderate amounts of basophilic cytoplasm, round-to-oval nuclei with coarsely reticular chromatin patterns, and visible nucleoli. These cells are commonly referred to as immunoblasts. They are present in very low numbers in IM, usually only 1% or 2% of the total lymphocytes, but are almost always present, especially early in the disease. Transitional forms of these three types of reactive lymphocytes occur in IM and contribute to the heterogeneity of the morphologic features of the lymphocytes in this disorder. In addition, circulating plasma cells may be present in small numbers in IM.

Minimal morphologic criteria (Table 24-1) for the diagnosis of IM have been established and include (1) at least 50% mononuclear cells in the blood smear, (2) at least 10 reactive lymphocytes per 100 leukocytes, and (3) marked lymphocyte heterogeneity.

Bone Marrow Examination. A bone marrow biopsy is usually not indicated in infectious mononucleosis.

Other Laboratory Tests

24.1 Tests for Detection of Heterophil Antibody

Purpose. Heterophil antibodies are produced in EBV-IM; they appear within the first 2 weeks of illness and are usually undetectable 3 to 6 months after the acute illness. The diagnosis of IM is confirmed by detection of heterophil antibodies.

Principle. The IM heterophil antibody is of the IgM class and reacts with beef, sheep, and horse erythrocytes; it does not react with guinea pig kidney. This characteristic separates the IM heterophil antibody from cross-reacting, Forssman-type antibodies.

Specimen. Serum inactivated for complement is used for the reference tube test for heterophil antibody. Serum or plasma may be used for rapid slide tests.

Procedure. Two types of tests are available for heterophil antibodies:

1. The original reference tube test (Paul-Bunnell-Davidsohn) is a sheep cell agglutination test. Serial dilutions of the patient's serum are incubated with sheep red blood cells to determine the titer at which the sheep red blood cells agglutinate. Serum aliquots are then absorbed individually with guinea pig kidney or beef cells and retitered against the sheep red blood cells. A markedly reduced agglutination titer following beef red blood cell absorption but not guinea pig kidney absorption indicates a positive test. The sensitivity of this test is improved by substituting horse erythrocytes for sheep erythrocytes.

2. Most clinical laboratories use one of the commercially available rapid tests to depict heterophil antibodies. Several commercial kits are available and most are based on the same principle as the original reference tube test. The Monospot test (Ortho Diagnostics Inc), as an exam-

ple, incorporates preserved horse cell stroma for sensitivity and fine suspensions of guinea pig kidney and beef cells for specificity.

Interpretation. The presence of the heterophil antibodies in conjunction with the characteristic peripheral blood are highly specific for the diagnosis of IM. False-positives occur but are not common. Heterophil antibodies are not present in other conditions associated with a reactive lymphocytosis such as the CMV-mononucleosis-like syndrome. A small percentage of teenagers and young adults with IM will not produce a heterophil antibody even though they have EBV-IM. These cases represent heterophil-negative IM and can be diagnosed with EBV-specific serologic tests (see Test 24-2). As noted earlier, the incidence of heterophil positivity is much lower in infants and young children.

24.2 EBV-Specific Serologic Tests

Purpose. EBV-specific serologic tests can be used to establish the diagnosis of EBV-IM. These tests are especially useful in patients with heterophil-negative EBV-IM.

Principle. EBV-specific serologic tests are based on the detection of antibodies produced against specific antigens encoded by the virus. During the EBV infection, there is sequential appearance and disappearance of different antibodies (Figure 24-1). Almost all patients develop antibodies of both IgG and IgM type to VCA early in the course of the disease. The IgM anti-VCA titers diminish rapidly during convalescence and are usually undetectable at 12 weeks, while the IgG anti-VCA titers persist for life. Antibody to early antigen (anti-EA) appears during the acute phase of the disease and then declines. Antibodies to EBNA do not appear until symptoms have resolved and then persist indefinitely.

Procedure. Assays for EBV-specific antibodies are usually done with indirect immunofluorescence microscopy. Enzyme-

Figure 24-1 Sequential appearance and disappearance of heterophil and Epstein-Barr virus–specific antibodies during acute Epstein-Barr virus infection.*

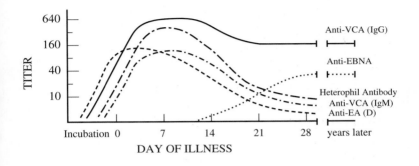

* Used with permission from Stein R, Linder J. Mononuclear leukocytosis and infectious mononucleosis. In: Koepke J, ed. *Laboratory Hematology*. New York, NY: Churchill Livingstone Inc; 1984.

linked immunoassays (ELISA), Western blot analysis, and other immunoassays are also available.

Interpretation.   An acute primary infection is indicated by the following: (1) the presence of IgM anti-VCA, (2) high titers of IgG anti-VCA, (3) detection of anti-EA, and (4) the absence of anti-EBNA. The presence of IgG anti-VCA and anti-EBNA with absence of IgM anti-VCA indicates a remote infection.

Course and Treatment

IM is a self-limited disease, lasting an average of 2 to 3 weeks. Only symptomatic therapy is usually indicated. Steroid therapy is controversial but is occasionally used for the treatment of severe complications related to IM, including severe pharyngitis with obstructing tonsils, autoimmune hemolytic anemia, and other severe cytopenias. Other rare complications include splenic rupture, neurologic complications, myocarditis, and pericarditis. In patients with normal immunity, the syndrome resolves within days or weeks; persistence of symptoms beyond several months is unusual.

References

Cheeseman SH. Infectious mononucleosis. *Semin Hematol.* 1988;25:261-268.

Henle W, Henle GE, Horwitz CA. Epstein-Barr virus specific diagnostic tests in infectious mononucleosis. *Hum Pathol.* 1974;5:551-565.

Horwitz CA, Henle W, Henle GE, et al. Clinical and laboratory evaluation of infants and children with Epstein-Barr virus-induced infectious mononucleosis: report of 32 patients (aged 10-48 months). *Blood.* 1981;57:933-938.

Horwitz CA. Practical approach to diagnosis of infectious mononucleosis. *Postgrad Med.* 1979;65:179-184.

Horwitz CA, Henle W, Henle GE, et al. Heterophil-negative infectious mononucleosis and mononucleosis-like illnesses. Laboratory confirmation of 43 cases. *Am J Med.* 1977;63:947-957.

Horwitz CA, Henle W, Henle GE, et al. Infectious mononucleosis in patients aged 40 to 72 years: report of 27 cases, including 3 without heterophil antibody responses. *Medicine.* 1983;62:256-262.

Peterson L, Hrisinko MA. Benign lymphocytosis and reactive neutrophilia: laboratory features provide diagnostic clues. *Clin Lab Med.* 1993;13:863-877.

Straus SE, Cohen JI, Tosato G, et al. Epstein-Barr virus infections: biology, pathogenesis, and management. *Ann Intern Med.* 1993;118:45-48.

Thorley-Lawson DA. Basic virologic aspects of Epstein-Barr virus infection. *Semin Hematol.* 1988;25:247-260.

Tomkinson BE, Sullivan JL. Infectious mononucleosis and other Epstein-Barr virus-associated infections. In: Hoffman R, Benz EJ, Shattil SJ, Furie B, Cohen HJ, eds. *Hematology—Basic Principles and Practice.* New York, NY: Churchill Livingstone Inc; 1991:627-635.

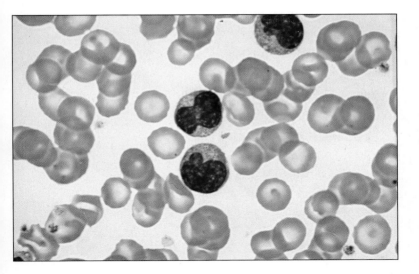

Image 24-1   Reactive lymphocytes classified as Downey type I cells. These cells are rare in infectious mononucleosis but may be prominent in young children.

Image 24-2   Reactive lymphocyte in a blood smear from a patient with infectious mononucleosis. This is a Downey type II reactive lymphocyte.

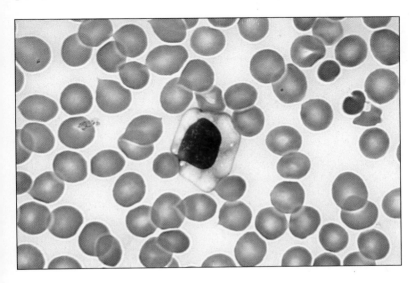

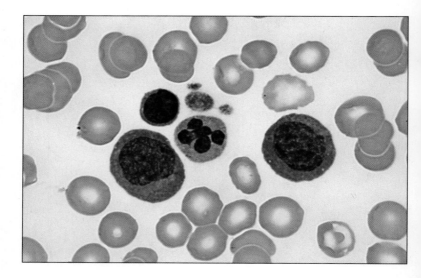

Image 24-3   Two large Downey type III reactive lymphocytes along with a neutrophil and lymphocyte. This type of reactive lymphocyte is commonly referred to as an immunoblast.

25

Lymphocytopenia

Lymphocytopenia in adults is usually defined as a total lymphocyte count less than $1.0 \times 10^3/mm^3$ ($1.0 \times 10^9/L$). In children younger than 16 years, absolute lymphocyte counts are higher, with the lower reference value being about $2.0 \times 10^3/mm^{3}$ [3] ($2.0 \times 10^9/L$). Since T cells are the predominant lymphocytes in the blood, lymphocytopenia is usually associated with disease processes in which these cells are decreased.

Pathophysiology

Lymphocytopenia results from three types of abnormalities: (1) decreased production, (2) increased loss or destruction, and (3) changes in lymphocyte distribution. In some cases, it is not possible to classify the pathogenesis of the lymphocytopenia. Table 25-1 categorizes major causes of lymphocytopenia according to pathogenic mechanism.

Decreased Production. Severe combined immunodeficiency disease (SCID) is a syndrome characterized by profound defects in cellular and humoral immunity caused by a heteroge-

Table 25-1   Causes of Lymphocytopenia

Decreased production
    Severe combined immunodeficiency
    Protein-calorie malnutrition
    Zinc deficiency
Increased destruction
    AIDS
    Radiation therapy
    Neoplastic chemotherapy
    Antilymphocyte globulin
    Systemic lupus erythematosus
    Thoracic duct drainage or rupture
    Loss from intestinal lymphatics
    Wiskott-Aldrich syndrome
Redistribution
    Glucocorticoid therapy
    Anesthesia and surgery
    Tuberculosis
    Influenza
    Sarcoidosis
    Burns
Unknown mechanism
    Hodgkin's disease
    Myasthenia gravis
    Renal insufficiency
    Cancer
    Felty's syndrome
    Acute bacterial infections in the elderly

neous group of genetic abnormalities. The classic example of SCID, Swiss-type agammaglobulinemia, is autosomal recessive and is characterized by severe lymphocytopenia involving both T and B cells. The pathogenesis of this disorder is not completely clear, but it is thought to be secondary to an absence of lymphoid stem cells or a defect in development with depletion of both T and B lymphocytes. Other hematopoietic lineages are spared.

Deficiency of adenosine deaminase, an enzyme involved in the purine salvage pathway, is another cause of SCID. This disorder is inherited as autosomal recessive. The enzyme deficiency results from a mutation of the adenosine deaminase gene and causes accumulation of adenosine metabolites that may be toxic to normal maturation of the cell. These patients have varying degrees of lymphopenia, with T cells usually more deficient than B cells.

Nutritional deficiencies may cause decreased production of lymphocytes. Protein-calorie malnutrition is a common cause of lymphocytopenia worldwide. Deficiency of zinc, an element required in protein synthesis, is also associated with lymphocytopenia with decreased numbers of circulating T-helper cells and increased T-suppressor cells.

Increased Loss or Destruction. Lymphocytopenia is prominent in AIDS and is due to selective loss of the helper/inducer subset of T lymphocytes. The lymphocytopenia in AIDS is probably due to a direct cytopathic effect of human immunodeficiency virus (HIV). Radiotherapy induces a lymphocytopenia through death of lymphocytes by direct exposure. T-helper lymphocytes are more sensitive than T-suppressor cells; the helper/suppressor ratio can be decreased for months after exposure to radiation. Chemotherapeutic agents, especially alkylating agents, can cause profound lymphocytopenia that may persist for years. The administration of antilymphocyte globulin leads to lymphocytopenia by destruction of lymphocytes. The lymphocytopenia in systemic lupus erythematosus is caused by cytotoxic antilymphocyte antibodies that act through complement-mediated cell lysis. Both T and B lymphocytes may be lost from the body because of structural defects (ie, fistulas) or damage to the thoracic duct. Lymphocytes may also be lost through intestinal lymphatics in association with protein-losing enteropathies, severe congestive heart failure, or other primary diseases of the gut or intestinal lymphatics. In Wiskott-Aldrich syndrome, an X-linked immunodeficiency disease, lymphocytopenia is thought to be caused by premature destruction of the lymphocytes secondary to a membrane defect.

Redistribution. Redistribution of lymphocytes appears to be the primary mechanism by which glucocorticoids cause lymphocytopenia. Lymphocytopenia is often associated with anesthesia and surgical stress and is secondary to redistribution, perhaps related to endogenous steroid release. Patients with various inflammatory conditions, including tuberculosis, influenza, and sarcoidosis, may have lymphocytopenia. The cause of the decrease in circulating lymphocytes is not clear, but may be due to relocation of lymphocytes to the sites of inflammation. Lymphocytopenia is associated with burns and may be related to changes in the trafficking patterns of the lymphocytes.

Unknown Pathogenesis. In many conditions associated with lymphocytopenia, the mechanisms responsible are unknown (Table 25-1).

Clinical Findings

The signs and symptoms present in patients with lymphocytopenia are those characteristic of the underlying disease process associated with the lymphocytopenia. Whether the patient exhibits clinical signs of immunodeficiency depends on the pathophysiology of the disease, the duration of the disorder, the lymphocyte subsets affected, and the degree to which cellular or humoral immunity is functionally disturbed. In general, patients with cellular immunodeficiency disorders suffer from recurrent infections with low-grade or opportunistic infectious agents. In congenital disorders, this is often accompanied by growth retardation, wasting, and a short life span. A high incidence of malignancies, especially lymphomas, is also observed in some patient groups.

Severe combined immunodeficiency is the most severe congenital immune deficiency state involving both cellular and humoral immunity. Affected patients suffer from recurrent bacterial, fungal, viral, or protozoan infections starting as early as 3 months of age. Transfusion with nonirradiated blood products may lead to severe graft-vs-host reactions. Persistent pulmonary infection, diarrhea, and wasting dominate the clinical picture. Wiskott-Aldrich syndrome also appears in early childhood with a triad of eczematoid dermatitis, thrombocytopenia with bleeding, and recurrent opportunistic infections. Patients are at high risk for developing malignancies, most commonly lymphomas and leukemias.

Patients with AIDS suffer from repeated life-threatening infections. Opportunistic infections are prominent and include *Pneumocystis carinii* pneumonia, *Mycobacterium avium* complex pneumonia or disseminated disease, cryptosporidiosis diarrhea, oral candidiasis, hepatitis B, and cytomegalovirus and herpes virus infections. Malignancies (Kaposi's sarcoma, lymphoma), autoimmune diseases (thrombocytopenia), and neurologic disorders also occur in patients with AIDS.

Protein-calorie malnutrition resulting in lymphocytopenia is an important underlying factor of infection worldwide.

Approach to Diagnosis

Clinical history—including the age and sex of the patient, family history, history of medication, social and medical history, and physical examination—is needed to determine the subsequent workup. Unless the cause of the lymphocytopenia is clinically apparent or the lymphocytopenia is transient, the approach to the diagnosis should involve a comprehensive assessment of the integrity of the immune system. A thorough workup of patients with immunodeficiency diseases such as the congenital disorders can be complex and in many cases should be performed at referral medical centers with expertise and experience in the diagnosis and treatment of these disorders.

In many cases the workup of patients with lymphocytopenia will include:

1. Complete blood cell count with differential and platelet count. A bone marrow aspirate and biopsy should be performed if the reason for the lymphocytopenia is unclear or to confirm a suspected diagnosis.

2. Quantitative immunoglobulin determination.

3. Immunophenotypic analysis of peripheral blood lymphocytes.

4. Ancillary tests such as skin tests to evaluate cellular immunity.

5. Other tests dependent on the clinical setting to determine the underlying cause. These could include tests for HIV, antinuclear antibodies (systemic lupus erythematosus), lymph node biopsy (sarcoidosis), etc.

6. Cultures in patients suspected of having infection.

Hematologic Findings

Blood Cell Measurements. In adults, the lymphocyte count is less than $1.0 \times 10^3/mm^3$ ($1.0 \times 10^9/L$) in lymphopenia. In children it is less than $2.0 \times 10^3/\text{mm}^3$ $(2.0 \times 10^9/\text{L})$. Granulocytopenia may also be present. The presence or absence of thrombocytopenia depends on the underlying condition. Thrombocytopenia is frequently present in congenital immune deficiency states; it is also common in AIDS. A normochromic, normocytic anemia is present in many of the diseases associated with lymphocytopenia.

Bone Marrow Examination. Findings will depend on the underlying disorder and recent therapeutic approaches. In some congenital immunodeficiency states, lymphocytes may be decreased.

The bone marrow in patients with HIV is usually hypercellular, even in the setting of peripheral cytopenias. Dysplasia is often present in all cell lines. Plasma cells are frequently increased. Lymphohistiocytic aggregates are frequent in bone marrow core biopsy specimens and may be large and atypical. These must be distinguished from lymphomas since lymphomas are increased in AIDS and also frequently involve the bone marrow. Disseminated infections, especially *Mycobacterium avium* complex and histoplasmosis, often involve the bone marrow. The marrow granulomas in association with these agents may be loosely formed or even absent.

Other Laboratory Tests

25.1 Quantitation of Immunoglobulins

Purpose. Immunodeficiency states associated with lymphocytopenia are typically combined with deficient production of immunoglobulins. In AIDS, a polyclonal hypergammaglobulinemia is often present.

Principle. Immunoglobulin production is altered when there is a defect in the B-cell population alone or when a combined defect involving both B and T lymphocytes exists. Defects in antibody production can also result from severe defects in T lymphocyte function, since, in humans, all antigens appear to be T-lymphocyte dependent.

Procedure, Specimen, and Interpretation
See Test 38.5.

25.2 Immunophenotypic Analysis of Peripheral Blood Lymphocytes

Purpose. Lymphocyte markers are used to identify and enumerate lymphocyte subsets. This aids in diagnosing and classifying disorders associated with lymphocytopenia.

Principle. Labeled monoclonal antibodies bind to determinants on T cells, B cells, their subsets, and other hematopoietic cells (Table 25-2). Labeled cells can then be enumerated with flow cytometry.

Specimen. Fresh peripheral blood sample anticoagulated with heparin.

Procedure. Flow cytometry involves a fluid system that delivers the cell sample past an excitation light beam in a single-file stream. The scattered light and any fluorescence emitted from this interaction (from dyes used to stain specific cell molecules) are collected and converted to electrical signals. They can then be analyzed to give quantitative information about specific cell characteristics.

Interpretation. About 60% to 80% of circulating lymphocytes are T cells, 10% to 20% B cells, and 5% to 10% natural killer (NK) cells. The T-cell population consists of T-helper (CD4+) and T-suppressor (CD8+) cells, with the T-helper cells outnumbering the T-suppressor cells two to one.

In Swiss-type SCID and in adenosine deaminase deficiency, both T and B lymphocytes are profoundly depleted or absent. Natural killer cell levels may be normal. In Wiskott-Aldrich syndrome, T cells may be normal at first but diminish with age with frequent inversion in the CD4 to CD8 ratio.

In AIDS, CD4+ cells are depleted. In patients with HIV, there is a strong association between CD4+ lymphocyte levels

Table 25-2   Monoclonal Antibodies Commonly Used for the Characterization of Lymphocytes and Other Hematopoietic Cells

Antigen (CD)	Major Reactivity
1	Cortical thymocytes, Langerhans cells, interdigitating reticulum cells
2	T cells, natural killer (NK) cells
3	T cells
4	Helper/inducer T cells
5	T cells, B-cell subset
7	T-cell subset
8	Cytotoxic/suppressor T cells
10	Lymphoid progenitor cells, germinal center B cells, granulocytes
11c	Monocytes, granulocytes, NK cells
13	Monocytes, granulocytes
14	Monocytes
15	Granulocytes
16	NK cells, granulocytes
19	B cells, except plasma cells
20	B cells, except plasma cells
21	Mature B cells
22	B cells, except plasma cells
23	Activated B cells
24	B cells, granulocytes
25	Activated T and B cells, macrophages
30	Activated T and B cells
33	Monocytes, myeloid progenitor cells
34	Hematopoietic precursor cells
35	Granulocytes, monocytes, B cells, some NK cells, erythrocytes
38	Plasma cells, thymocytes, activated T cells
41	Platelets
43	T cells, granulocytes
45	Leukocyte-restricted
56	NK cells
57	NK cells, T-cell subset
61	Platelets and megakaryocytes
71	Activated T and B cells, macrophages, proliferating cells

and development of opportunistic infections, progression to AIDS, and eventual death. Measurement of the CD4 subset is not only useful in assessing prognosis but is also useful in management decisions and in evaluating response to therapy.

Course and Treatment

The clinical course and treatment of lymphocytopenia depends on the underlying cause. The prognosis of patients with SCID is dismal without therapy. However, bone marrow transplantation has been successful with histocompatible sibling donors. Patients with Wiskott-Aldrich syndrome have progressive loss of T-cell function with increasing infectious complications. Bleeding complications are also prominent. About 10% of patients develop a malignancy, the majority being leukemias and lymphomas. Children with this disorder rarely survive beyond their teens; however, bone marrow transplantation in children with this syndrome has produced encouraging results.

Patients with HIV are currently being treated with zidovudine. Patients with AIDS eventually succumb to infection and/or malignancies associated with AIDS.

References

Bagby GC. Leukopenia. In: Wyngaarden JB, Smith LH, Bennett JC, eds. *Cecil Textbook of Medicine*. 19th ed. Philadelphia, Pa: WB Saunders Co; 1992:907-914.

Buckley RH. Primary immunodeficiency diseases. In: Wyngaarden JB, Smith LH, Bennett JC, eds. *Cecil Textbook of Medicine*. 19th ed. Philadelphia, Pa: WB Saunders Co; 1992:1446-1453.

Geha RS, Rosen FS, Chatila T. Primary immunodeficiency diseases. In: Nathan DG, Oski FA, eds. *Hematology of Infancy and Childhood*. Philadelphia, Pa: WB Saunders Co; 1993:1033-1057.

Hoxie JA. Hematologic manifestations of AIDS. In: Hoffman R, Benz EJ Jr, Shattel SJ, Furie B, Cohen H, eds. *Hematology: Basic Principles and Practice*. New York, NY: Churchill Livingstone Inc; 1991:1759-1780.

Johnson RL. Flow cytometry: from research to clinical laboratory application. *Clin Lab Med*. 1993;13:831-852.

Pirruccello SJ, Johnson DR. Reagents for flow cytometry: monoclonal antibodies and hematopoietic cell. In: Keren DF, Hanson CA, Hurtubise PE, eds. *Flow Cytometry and Clinical Diagnosis.* Chicago, Ill: ASCP Press; 1994:56-91.

Sadler DA, Keren DF. Surface marker assays in immunodeficiency diseases. In: Keren DF, Hanson CA, Hurtubise PE, eds. *Flow Cytometry and Clinical Diagnosis.* Chicago, Ill: ASCP Press; 1994:309-356.

Schoentag RA, Cangiarella J. The nuances of lymphocytopenia. *Clin Lab Med.* 1993;13:923-936.

Toft P, Suendsen P, Tonnesen E, et al. Redistribution of lymphocytes after major surgical stress. *Acta Anaesthesiol Scand.* 1993;37:245-249.

Weinberg KI, Parkman R. Congenital immunodeficiency states. In: Williams WJ, Beutler E, Erslev AJ, Lichtman MA, eds. *Hematology.* 4th ed. New York, NY: McGraw-Hill Publishing Co; 1990:967-972.

PART
V

Reactive Disorders of
Lymph Nodes

26

Reactive Disorders of Lymph Nodes

The term lymphadenopathy refers to an enlarged lymph node or group of nodes. It is a common physical finding that requires an explanation as to its cause. Lymphadenopathy is often a transient response to localized infection, and in these patients the pathologic condition should be sought in the area drained by the node. In other patients, the lymphadenopathy may be due to metastatic malignancy or response to a systemic disease. Lymphadenopathies caused by neoplastic proliferation of lymphoid cells are known as malignant lymphomas and will be discussed in Chapters 36 and 37.

Pathophysiology

Enlargement of lymph nodes is caused by proliferation of lymphoid cells and the associated cells of the mononuclear phagocytic system. In addition there is frequently a variable degree of vascular proliferation. The intensity and pattern of reaction depends on the nature and duration of the antigenic stimulus, and on the age and immune status of the patient.

As noted in Table 26-1, a large variety of disorders may be associated with lymphadenopathy. These disorders may be divided

Table 26-1   Causes of Lymphadenopathy

Infections
  Viral
    Infectious mononucleosis,* cytomegalovirus,* HIV,† postvaccinal
      lymphadenitis‡
  Bacterial
    Staphylococcus, Streptococcus*; *Mycobacterium tuberculosis,** cat
      scratch disease,‡ syphilis,* chancroid‡
  Protozoal
    Toxoplasmosis*
  Fungal
    Cryptococcus,* histoplasmosis,* coccidioplasmosis*
  Chlamydial
    Lymphogranuloma venereum‡
Autoimmune
  Rheumatoid arthritis,* systemic lupus erythematosus,* Sjögren's
    syndrome‡
Iatrogenic
  Drug hypersensitivity (phenytoin, carbamazepine),* serum sickness,*
    silicone‡
Malignant
  Hodgkin's disease,* non-Hodgkin's lymphoma,* acute and chronic
    leukemias,* metastatic cancer*
Other disorders
  Castleman's disease,* Kikuchi-Fujimoto lymphadenitis,‡ sarcoidosis,*
    dermatopathic lymphadenopathy,‡ histiocytosis X,* sinus histiocytosis
    with massive lymphadenopathy,* Kimura's disease,‡ angioimmunoblastic
    lymphadenopathy,* abnormal immune response*

*Localized or generalized lymphadenopathy.
†Generalized lymphadenopathy.
‡Localized lymphadenopathy.

into five categories: infections, autoimmune, iatrogenic, malignant, and others. In approximately 40% to 60% of patients who undergo lymph node biopsy, no specific diagnosis can be reached. Of the specific benign lymphadenopathies, the most common causes encountered are infectious mononucleosis, toxoplasmosis, tuberculosis, and human immunodeficiency virus (HIV) infection.

Clinical Findings

The cause of the lymphadenopathy is frequently not apparent from the changes observed under the microscope in a lymph node biopsy specimen alone. The patient's clinical history, physical examination, and the results of other investigations are usually essential for an accurate diagnosis. Certain benign lymphadenopathies, such as Kikuchi's lymphadenitis, are much more common in women than in men (4:1), while malignant lymphadenopathies are more common in men. Infectious mononucleosis is rarely seen in patients older than 35 years of age. Sexual behavior, drugs, previous surgery/biopsy, vaccination, occupation, exposure to pets, and duration of lymphadenopathy are important aspects of the clinical history (Table 26-2).

Fever and weight loss are common symptoms in many benign and malignant lymphoproliferative disorders. A sore throat is frequently present in infectious mononucleosis. The presence of toothache, earache, or other lesions in the region drained by the enlarged lymph nodes may explain the cause of lymphadenopathy in some patients.

Once a significant lymph node enlargement has been detected, a careful physical examination must be done in search of other sites of lymphadenopathy, and the presence or absence of splenomegaly should be noted. With inguinal lymphadenopathy, a genital and perineal examination is imperative. In inflammatory disorders, the lymph nodes are frequently tender, while in malignant lymphomas they are usually firm, rubbery, and usually painless. A rock-like, hard lymph node usually indicates metastatic tumor. A careful ear, nose, and throat examination is indicated in patients with cervical lymphadenopathy in search of a possible source of infection or a primary tumor.

Approach to Diagnosis

Following a clinical history and physical examination, the workup of a patient with lymphadenopathy should proceed in the following fashion:

1. Complete blood cell count, including evaluation of the peripheral blood smear.
2. Erythrocyte sedimentation rate (ESR).
3. Throat culture and culture for gonorrhea (if clinically indicated).

Table 26-2   Useful Clinical Information in the Evaluation of Lymphadenopathy

Clinical Parameter	Description
History	Sex, age, duration of lymphadenopathy, symptoms, sexual behavior, drug history, pets, occupation
Physical examination	Location of lymphadenopathy; size, tenderness, and texture of lymph node; presence or absence of splenomegaly; ear-nose-throat examination or genital-pelvic examination (depending on site of lymphadenopathy)

4. Chest roentgenogram and computed tomography (CT) when needed.

5. Serologic tests for infectious disorders and autoimmune disorders.

6. Blood chemistry tests including transaminase levels, serum calcium, and angiotensin-converting enzyme levels (test for sarcoidosis).

7. Lymph node fine needle aspiration.

8. Lymph node biopsy for histologic examination and culture.

9. Tuberculin skin test.

10. Bone marrow aspirate and biopsy examination.

Hematologic Findings

The hematologic findings in reactive lymphadenopathies are quite variable depending on the cause. The examination of the peripheral blood smear may be particularly helpful.

Blood Cell Measurements.   When anemia is present it is usually mild, normochromic, and normocytic. The leukocyte count is usually elevated. The platelet count may be normal, decreased, or increased depending on the cause of the lymphadenopathy.

Peripheral Blood Smear Morphology.   The red blood cells are usually normochromic, normocytic, or sometimes macrocytic as seen in patients with acquired immunodeficiency syndrome

(AIDS). In pyogenic infections or in the early stages of viral infections such as infectious mononucleosis, neutrophilic leukocytosis is often present. The presence of many reactive (atypical) or transformed lymphocytes together with the characteristic clinical setting suggest infectious mononucleosis. Such lymphocytosis is also frequently found in cytomegalovirus infection and toxoplasmosis.

Bone Marrow Examination. Examination of the bone marrow aspirate is rarely helpful. The bone marrow biopsy specimen may show granulomas in patients with tuberculosis, sarcoidosis, or disseminated fungal disease. Special stains for organisms and cultures may occasionally be helpful in the diagnosis.

Erythrocyte Sedimentation Rate (ESR). Although the ESR is a nonspecific test, persistently elevated levels would indicate that the patient needs further investigation.

Other Laboratory Tests

26.1 Serologic Tests for Infectious Agents

Purpose. A variety of infectious diseases and autoimmune disorders associated with lymphadenopathy may be detected with immunoassays.

Principle. The presence of specific and nonspecific antibodies produced by various organisms is detected by methods such as complement fixation and enzyme immunoassay (enzyme-linked immunosorbent assay) methods.

Specimen. Serum is used as a specimen. Specimens from the acute and convalescent phases are needed to detect rises in titer in complement fixation tests.

Procedure. A variety of methods can be used. The indirect immunofluorescent technique is performed by incubation of serum dilutions with organisms fixed to glass slides. Specific antibody adheres to the organism. In complement fixation tests, specific antibody attaches to antigen (organism) with complement binding.

Enzyme-linked immunosorbent assay (ELISA) methods are extremely sensitive and are used for detecting antibodies to a variety of bacteria, viruses, and parasites. In this technique, an enzyme, such as alkaline phosphatase, is conjugated to an antispecies immunoglobulin, such as antihuman IgG or IgM. An antigen specific of the infectious agent is used to coat a polystyrene well. Dilutions of the unknown serum are added and allowed to react. Excess serum is removed by washing. To detect the antibody specific to the infectious agent, the enzyme-linked antihuman immunoglobulin is then added and allowed to bind. Unbound immunoglobulin is removed by washing. Then the appropriate substrate for the enzyme is added to measure the enzyme activity of the bound antihuman immunoglobulin.

Other tests include Western blot (for HIV infection) and polymerase chain reaction (PCR) technology.

Interpretation. Infectious mononucleosis, cytomegalovirus lymphadenitis, HIV lymphadenitis, toxoplasmosis, histoplasmosis, lymphogranuloma venereum, cat scratch disease, syphilis, and autoimmune disorders such as rheumatoid arthritis, systemic lupus erythematosus, and Sjögren's syndrome are disorders for which serologic tests are available. A variety of techniques are used, including immunofluorescence, complement fixation, latex fixation, and more recently ELISA. When interpreting the results, it should be noted that even when the same basic procedure is used, the results from different laboratories may vary; reference values are frequently changing due to modification in techniques and reagents. It is therefore important to be familiar with the particular method used and the reference values given by the laboratory.

In children and young adults with lymphadenopathy, the detection of heterophile antibodies (Monospot test) may be very helpful in the diagnosis of infectious mononucleosis. It is important to note that this test may be negative in approximately 50% of patients in the first 2 weeks of illness. Tests for Epstein-Barr virus (EBV) and/or cytomegalovirus (CMV) may also be useful. Other serologic tests which may be helpful include ELISA for HIV, toxoplasmosis, and cat scratch disease.

26.2   Lymph Node Biopsy

Purpose.   Lymph node biopsy is the final step in the investigation of a patient with lymphadenopathy. It is done to provide a histopathologic diagnosis and, if indicated, sterile tissue should be submitted for culture.

Principle.   Biopsy should be performed when a significantly enlarged lymph node persists and/or increases in size and other tests have failed to provide a diagnosis. A lymph node biopsy should not be performed if a viral infection, such as infectious mononucleosis, is suspected because histopathologic features often resemble malignant lymphoma.

Specimen.   Lymph node biopsy. If several enlarged lymph nodes are present, an attempt should be made to remove the largest node.

Procedure.   Histologic interpretation of lymph node biopsy specimens is often difficult, and special care is required in the handling of the specimen. The major reason for difficulty in the interpretation is still technical in nature and results from improper handling of the biopsy specimen. It is extremely important that the complete lymph node be submitted intact to the pathology laboratory. There a portion of fresh tissue should be frozen for possible immunologic or molecular studies. If clinically indicated, sterile culture should be performed. A portion of the tissue should then be fixed in formalin and another portion should be fixed in B5. For a more detailed discussion in the handling of a lymph node specimen, see Chapter 36.

Interpretation.   Optimal interpretation of a lymph node biopsy specimen often requires collaboration of an experienced surgeon, a hematopathologist, and a hematologist/oncologist. Reactive lymphoproliferative disorders may be difficult to differentiate from malignant disorders, both in lymph nodes and extranodal sites. Detailed clinical information, excellent histologic sections and sometimes immunologic studies are important to attain a correct diagnosis.

The most helpful approach to the histologic diagnosis is the pattern approach, ie, the low-magnification appearance of the lymph node. Table 26-3 presents the most common patterns seen and the disorders associated with a particular pattern of cellular infiltrate. Once the general pattern is determined at low power, a higher-power examination will determine the cellular components present. Table 26-4 outlines features that may be useful in differentiating benign from malignant disease. For a detailed histopathologic description of the various disorders listed in Table 26-3, see textbooks on lymph node pathology. Images 26-1 to 26-6 illustrate the characteristic morphologic features observed in several benign lymph node disorders.

Notes and Precautions.   As previously noted, a number of benign disorders may both clinically and histopathologically closely resemble a malignant lymphoproliferative disorder. Therefore, a hematopathologist should be consulted if the primary pathologist reviewing the tissue does not have experience in examining lymph nodes. In addition, if adequate specimen is available, a fresh tissue specimen should be frozen for possible future phenotypic and genotypic studies. Immunoperoxidase studies, in situ hybridization studies, and gene rearrangement studies can be extremely helpful in the final diagnosis in difficult cases. These studies are described in more detail in Chapter 36.

Fine needle aspiration (FNA) of lymph nodes, when performed by a cytopathologist with experience in the interpretation of lymph node cytologic findings, can in selected cases be helpful. The diagnosis of metastatic carcinoma to lymph nodes for example can usually be facilitated by FNA, obviating surgical biopsy.

Table 26-3   Patterns Observed in Reactive Lymphadenopathies

Follicular pattern
    Nonspecific hyperplasia
    Rheumatoid arthritis
    AIDS
    Castleman's disease
    Toxoplasmosis
    Syphilis
Macronodular pattern
    Progressive transformation of germinal centers
Interfollicular pattern
    Viral lymphadenitis (infectious mononucleosis, cytomegalovirus)
    Dermatopathic lymphadenitis
    Postvaccinal lymphadenitis
Mixed pattern (follicular and interfollicular)
    Viral lymphadenitis (infectious mononucleosis, cytomegalovirus)
    Toxoplasmosis
    Kimura's disease
    Lymphogranuloma venereum
Sinusoidal pattern
    Nonspecific histiocytosis
    Sinus histiocytosis with massive lymphadenopathy
    Langerhans cell histiocytosis (histiocytosis X)
    Whipple's disease
    Monocytoid B-cell hyperplasia
    Lymphangiogram effect
Diffuse pattern
    Infectious mononucleosis
    Angioimmunoblastic lymphadenopathy
    Abnormal immune response
    Drug reactions
Necrotizing pattern
    Cat-scratch disease
    Kikuchi-Fujimoto lymphadenitis
    Infarction
Granulomatous pattern
    Sarcoidosis
    Tuberculosis
    Fungal disease
    Leprosy

Table 26-4 General Features Differentiating Benign From Malignant Disease in Lymph Node

Feature	Benign	Malignant
Architecture	Distorted	Often effaced
Sinuses	Open or focally compressed	Often obliterated
Normal cell components	Hyperplastic	Often obliterated
Cell type	Mixture, often transformed cells	Atypical, often monomorphic cells
Immunophenotype	Polyclonal	Usually monoclonal

Ancillary Tests

Chest Roentgenogram. A chest roentgenogram, although normal in most cases, is usually indicated because it may show enlarged mediastinal lymph nodes, which may indicate malignant lymphoma, tuberculosis, sarcoidosis, histoplasmosis, or metastatic malignancy. In addition, primary lung parenchymal lesions may be detected.

Serum Chemistry. Elevated serum calcium levels and angiotensin-converting enzyme may suggest a diagnosis of sarcoidosis. Elevated transaminase levels are frequently seen in infectious mononucleosis.

Tuberculin Skin Test. A positive tuberculin skin test may be helpful in differentiating tuberculosis from sarcoidosis.

Course and Treatment

As expected, the clinical course and treatment of lymphadenopathy is dependent on the cause.

References

Fessas PH, Pangalis GA. Non-malignant lymphadenopathies: reactive non-specific and reactive specific. In: Pangalis GA, Pollack A, eds. *Benign and Malignant Adenopathies: Clinical and Laboratory Diagnosis.* London, England: Hardword Academic Publishers; 1993:19-29.

Ioachim HL. *Lymph Node Biopsy.* 2d ed. Philadelphia, Pa: JB Lippincott Co; 1994.

Jaffe ES. *Surgical Pathology of Lymph Nodes and Related Organs.* Philadelphia, Pa: WB Saunders Co; 1985.

Lukes RJ, Collins RD. Tumors of the hematopoietic system. In: *Atlas of Tumor Pathology.* 2d series. Fascicle 28. Washington, DC: Armed Forces Institute of Pathology; 1992.

Pangalis GA, Boussiotis VA, Fessas PH, et al. Clinical approach to patient with lymphadenopathy. In: Pangalis GA, Pollack A, eds. *Benign and Malignant Lymphadenopathies: Clinical and Laboratory Diagnosis.* London, England: Hardword Academic Publishers; 1993:19-29.

Peterson BA, Frizzera G, eds. Benign lymphoproliferative disorders. *Semin Oncol.* 1993;20:553-657.

Said JW. AIDS-related lymphadenopathies. *Semin Diagn Pathol.* 1988;5:365-378.

Swerdlow SH, Sukpanichnant S, Glick AD, Collins RD. Reactive states in lymph nodes resembling lymphomas or progressing to lymphomas: a selective review. *Mod Pathol.* 1993;6:378-391.

Van der Valk P, Meijer CJLM. The histology of reactive lymph nodes. *Am J Surg Pathol.* 1987;11:866-878.

Williamson HA. Lymphadenopathy in a family practice. *J Fam Pract.* 1985;20:449-452.

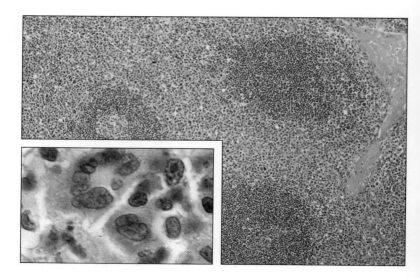

Image 26-1 Low-power view of a lymph node section from a patient with infectious mononucleosis. There is a prominent interfollicular infiltrate of large cells. Inset shows high-power view of atypical large cells, which resemble those seen in non-Hodgkin's anaplastic large cell lymphoma.

Image 26-2 High-power view of a lymph node section from a patient with infectious mononucleosis shows florid immunoblastic cell proliferation. Inset shows an immunoperoxidase study with many immunoblasts showing immunoreactivity with antibody to CD30 (Ki-1). The lesion could be mistaken for non-Hodgkin's large cell lymphoma.

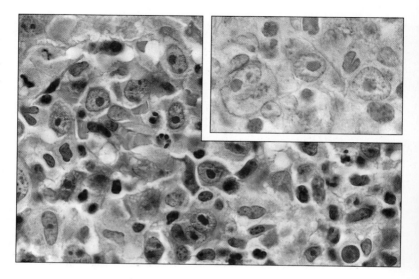

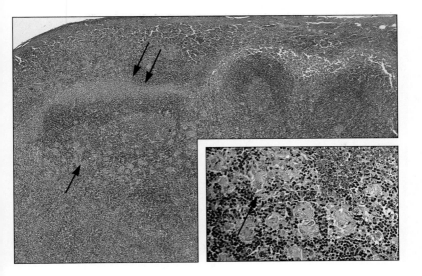

Image 26-3 Low-power view of a lymph node section from a patient with toxoplasmosis. The morphologic features include follicular hyperplasia, epithelioid histiocytes encroaching on germinal centers (↑), and monocytoid B cells within sinusoids (↑↑). Inset shows high-power view of epithelioid histiocytes (↑) in germinal center.

Image 26-4 Low-power view of a lymph node section from a patient with Kikuchi-Fujimoto lymphadenitis. There is follicular hyperplasia and extensive necrosis (↑). Inset shows high-power view of associated large cell infiltrate, which may be mistaken for non-Hodgkin's large cell lymphoma.

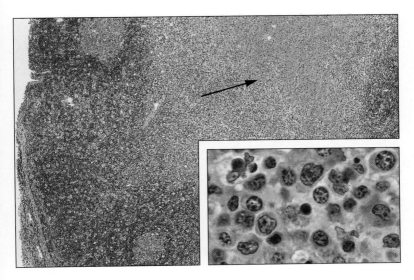

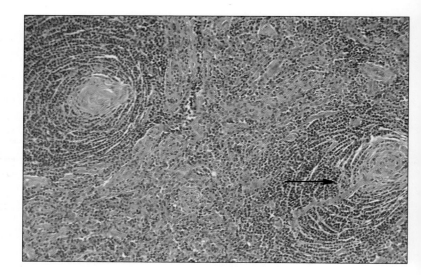

Image 26-5 Section of lymph node from patient with Castleman's disease (giant lymph node hyperplasia). The two follicles present show an onionskin type arrangement of the mantle cells, surrounding atrophic, hyalinized germinal centers. A vascular twig is seen extending into one follicle (↑).

Image 26-6 Low-power view of a lymph node section shows progressive transformation of germinal centers. A large nodule is seen containing predominantly small lymphocytes (↑).

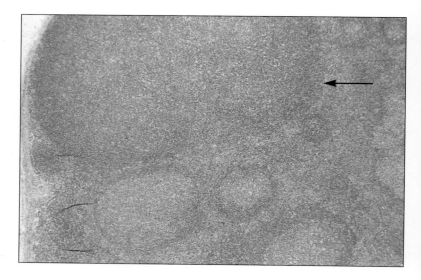

PART VI

Disorders Involving the Spleen

27

Hypersplenism

Hypersplenism is classically defined by the following four criteria: (1) reduction in one or more cellular elements in the peripheral blood, (2) bone marrow hyperplasia in response to the cytopenia, (3) splenomegaly, and (4) correction of the cytopenias by splenectomy.

Pathophysiology

The spleen is a 50- to 250-g encapsulated vascular organ containing both red and white pulp. The red pulp is a system of vascular sinuses supported by the cords of Billroth. The vascular sinuses are lined by endothelial cells on top of a fenestrated basement membrane. The cords of Billroth are lined by reticuloendothelial cells and macrophages. The white pulp is lymphoid tissue composed of perivascular T lymphocytes and lymphoid follicles of B lymphocytes. Blood enters via the arterial circulation into the sinusoidal spaces, and then percolates by the splenic cords, returning through splenic veins to the peripheral circulation. Red blood cells that are senescent or damaged are lysed within the acidotic, hypoxic environment found within the cords of Billroth. Red blood cells that contain particulate inclusions of nuclear debris, siderotic granules, or denatured hemoglobin (Heinz bodies) or have excessive membrane material will have this material removed by partial phagocytosis or "pitting" of the cell by macrophages. The red blood cell is not lysed, but will return to the peripheral circulation. The normally sluggish flow through the 3-μm sinusoidal fenestrations to the splenic cords requires red and white blood cells that are properly deformable if they are to make the transit through the spleen. Abnormal red blood cells, such as spherocytes or target cells, will become trapped in the splenic sinusoids and are more readily destroyed. An increase in splenic size slows the cellular transit time, enhancing cellular removal. In addition, any condition that increases macrophage phagocytic activity will decrease the survival of blood elements.

The white pulp lymphocytes function immunologically to recognize antigens, with subsequent production of antibodies. Antigenic stimulation results in follicular hyperplasia with formation of germinal centers composed of immunologically competent T and B lymphocytes. The follicular proliferation can result in lymphoid hyperplasia, with or without splenomegaly.

The cause of hypersplenism varies with the underlying disease (Table 27-1). In most patients with hypersplenism, splenomegaly of varying degree is present, although hypersplenism can result from an overactive reticuloendothelial system with minimal enlargement of the spleen. Hypersplenism can give rise to anemia, leukopenia, or thrombocytopenia or combinations of these cytopenias. The mechanisms of cell loss include macrophage ingestion of damaged or globulin-coated cells; mechanical blockade by fibrosis or by thickened splenic cords due to abnormal storage products within reticuloendothelial cells (mucopolysaccharides, hemosiderin, etc); and increased transit time following increases in spleen size and/or volume.

Clinical Findings

Almost all patients with hypersplenism have splenomegaly of some degree. Dependent on the mechanism of splenic enlargement, other physical findings may be present. Liver disease may be associated with hepatomegaly early in the disease process, but with advancing

Table 27-1   Mechanisms of Splenic Enlargement and Hypersplenism

Mechanism	Associated Diseases

Functional-reticuloendothelial hyperplasia or hyperfunction	Hemolytic anemias
	  Immune-mediated
	  Hemoglobinopathy
	  Enzyme defects
	  Hereditary spherocytosis
	Infections
	  Infectious mononucleosis
	  Bacterial endocarditis
	  Malaria
	  Miliary tuberculosis
	Collagen vascular disorders
	Rheumatoid arthritis
	  (Felty's syndrome)

Congestion (Banti's syndrome)	Cirrhosis Portal vein thrombosis

Infiltrative diseases	Neoplasms
	  Leukemia, acute and chronic
	  Lymphomas
	Extramedullary hematopoiesis
	  Myelofibrosis
	Metabolic disorders affecting
	  Macrophage function
	    Gaucher's disease
	    Niemann-Pick disease
	    Hemochromatosis

cirrhosis, the liver may decrease in size. Lymphadenopathy may accompany lymphoid neoplasms. Jaundice may be seen in several of the diseases associated with hypersplenism (hereditary spherocytosis, malaria, pernicious anemia, or advanced cirrhosis), but it is not a primary manifestation of hypersplenism.

Approach to Diagnosis

A diagnosis of hypersplenism is based on the clinical history and documentation of peripheral blood cytopenias in the face of an appropriate bone marrow response (the "full marrow, empty blood syndrome"). The approach to diagnosis includes the following:

1. Hematologic findings show a decrease in one or more peripheral blood cell lines associated with normal or increased bone marrow production of that cell lineage.

2. Splenomegaly is usually determined by physical examination and detection of a palpable spleen tip. In the obese patient, it may be confirmed by radioactive scans of spleen and/or liver with technetium 99m.

3. Radioactive studies with chromium 51 determine sites of red blood cell sequestration and are used if the diagnosis of hypersplenism is in doubt or splenectomy is being considered.

4. The underlying disease determines the diagnostic approach so that history of alcohol abuse, present or past infection, hepatitis, or a positive family history (as in the storage diseases) is helpful. Diagnosis of the underlying cause may require ancillary testing such as liver function tests or radiologic imaging in cirrhosis, blood cultures to diagnose subacute bacterial endocarditis (SBE), or heterophile tests for infectious mononucleosis.

Hematologic Findings

The most common findings in hypersplenism are normochromic anemia and mild to moderate thrombocytopenia. Red blood cells are usually sequestered first, followed by platelets, and then white blood cells.

Blood Cell Measurements. Normochromic anemia, with levels of hemoglobin at 9.0 to 11.0 g/dL (90-110 g/L) is usually seen. Mild to moderately severe decreases in platelet count (30-100 x 10^3/mm^3 [30-100 x 10^9/L]) are also common. Leukocytes may be decreased, but show a normal differential count.

Peripheral Blood Smear Morphology. The appearance of the blood smear varies with the underlying causes of hypersplenism. Some common associations include:

1. Spherocytes: hereditary spherocytosis.
2. Target cells: liver disease (congestive splenomegaly).
3. Teardrop and hand mirror red blood cells: myelofibrosis.
4. Leukoerythroblastosis with nucleated red blood cells and immature granulocytes: extramedullary hematopoiesis associated with myelofibrosis (myeloid metaplasia).
5. Atypical lymphocytes: chronic infections or infectious mononucleosis.
6. Circulating lymphoma cells: non-Hodgkin's lymphomas.
7. Blasts: acute leukemia.

Bone Marrow Examination. Bone marrow aspiration shows normal to moderate hypercellularity (80%), with all cell lines increased and maturing normally. Hyperplasia of one or more cell lines may be seen, in an attempt to compensate for peripheral cytopenias.

Other Laboratory Tests

27.1 Chromium 51 Labeling

Purpose. Test uses chromium 51–labeled red blood cells to measure red blood cell survival and splenic uptake of the radioactive label.

Principle Specimen. Chromium 51 is used to label red blood cells or platelets. Wherever red blood cells are trapped or lysed, ^{51}Cr is released and can be detected with external monitoring. Increased splenic sequestration of labeled red blood cells in the absence of antibody-mediated hemolysis implies hypersplenism. Frequent sampling and gamma counting of the peripheral blood determines the half-life of red blood cells, which is decreased in hemolysis and in hypersplenism. Radioactive uptake by the spleen is compared to a baseline (precordium) and to the liver to establish ratios of ^{51}Cr uptake. Splenic size can be estimated with radioscintigraphy using 1 to 2 mCi of ^{99}mTc, a nuclear medicine procedure that requires only 1 or 2 minutes.

Specimen.   Small, equal volume (3-mL) aliquots of heparinized blood should be refrigerated and counted simultaneously to minimize specimen variability. Specimens can be counted as whole blood or as red blood cells, excluding counts leaching into plasma as the result of mechanical hemolysis.

Procedure.   Performed in a nuclear medicine facility, tests with ^{51}Cr–labeled red blood cells require 3 weeks for a complete study. If hemolysis is present, the study may be completed sooner. A sample of the patient's own red blood cells is withdrawn, labeled with 50 μCi ^{51}Cr, and reinjected. Serial 3-mL aliquots of blood are drawn over a period of 21 to 26 days to determine the cell half-life. External counting is done over the precordium, spleen, and liver every 2 days for 3 weeks to determine sites and rate of uptake. Radioactive counts are plotted against time. Ratios of radioactivity between the liver and spleen are calculated for selected points during the 3-week period. Suspensions of donor platelets can be labeled similarly and platelet half-life studied. Leukocyte sequestration studies have not been established and are not commonly available.

Interpretation.   Normal labeled red blood cell half-life is 26 days with a spleen/liver ratio of 1.0. In hypersplenism, the spleen/liver ratio is 1.5 to 2.0, and in hemolysis the spleen/liver ratio is above 3.0.

Normally there is a steady decrease in precordium and peripheral blood radioactivity, with a steady, slow increase in spleen and liver (reticuloendothelial) counts. In splenic enlargement caused by hypersplenism, peripheral blood radioactivity declines in proportion to decreasing counts in the heart and liver. Since splenic blood flow is increased, counts increase rapidly proportionate to its size and remain constant thereafter, reflecting circulating intact red blood cells rather than accumulations seen with red blood cell degradation as in hemolysis. If radiolabeled donor red blood cells rather than autologous red blood cells are used, they must be compatible, since antibody will lead to splenic sequestration and a false interpretation of hypersplenism.

Notes and Precautions. The patient's blood volume must remain constant without blood loss or transfusion during the 21 to 26 days of the test. Use of other gamma-emitting radioisotopes as used in lung, liver, or spleen scans must be avoided during the 3 weeks of the test. If platelet concentrates are labeled, they should be relatively free of erythrocytes, which are preferentially labeled. This test is rarely necessary, since good clinical correlation of cytopenias with splenic enlargement demonstrable with physical examination or computed tomography (CT) scans are usually sufficient to allow a diagnosis of hypersplenism.

Course and Treatment

The course of hypersplenism varies with the underlying disorder. Treatment of infectious diseases with the appropriate antibiotic results in resolution of splenic hyperfunction. In cases associated with hereditary metabolic diseases or hematopoietic diseases, splenic enlargement is usually relentless. Anemia and leukopenia in such disorders may remain moderate, but thrombocytopenia may become severe. When appreciable decreases in peripheral blood cell counts occur, splenectomy may have a dramatic effect in restoring normal cell counts. Splenectomy is most successful when splenomegaly causes mechanical destruction or cellular sequestration, as in hereditary spherocytosis or storage diseases. It is of less predictable benefit in immune-mediated hemolytic anemias, but succeeds in improving cytopenias in 50% of the patients who fail to respond to steroid therapy. In hematologic disorders, splenectomy may be a temporizing treatment, as in chronic leukemias, or be a part of the diagnostic evaluation, as in lymphomas. In myelofibrosis, the advantage of relieving thrombocytopenia by splenectomy must be weighed against losing a major source of extramedullary hematopoiesis. Splenectomy is associated with side effects of decreased immune functioning, particularly with respect to encapsulated microorganisms such as *Pneumococcus*. In the elderly, bedridden patient, splenectomy may cause a temporary increase in circulating platelets, which may be associated with thrombotic events. After splenectomy, the pitting function of the spleen is lost, so that red blood cells with Howell-Jolly bodies or nucleated red blood cells are seen circulating in the peripheral blood.

References

Erslev AJ. Hypersplenism and hyposplenism. In: Williams WJ, Beutler E, Erslev AJ, Lichtman MA, eds. *Hematology.* New York, NY: McGraw-Hill Inc; 1990: 694-699.

Wolf BC, Neiman RS. *Disorders of the Spleen.* Philadelphia, Pa: WB Saunders Co; 1989:20-38.

PART
VII

Acute Leukemias

28

Myelodysplastic Syndromes

Myelodysplastic syndromes (MDS) are bone marrow stem cell disorders that lead to ineffective and disorderly hematopoiesis. They manifest as irreversible quantitative and qualitative defects of hematopoietic cells caused by abnormal division, maturation and production of erythrocytes, granulocytes, monocytes, and platelets. In some cases the clinical and morphologic features are similar to those of acute myeloid leukemia (AML).

Pathophysiology

The mechanisms that contribute to the development of an MDS are poorly understood. It is possible that some are caused by exposure to agents that have adverse effects on hematopoietic stem cells, which leads to the disruption of normal hematopoiesis. The cytotoxic effects of alkylating agents and radiotherapy clearly play an important role in the etiology of secondary (therapy-related) MDS.

Regulatory abnormalities in the production of hematopoietic growth factors may contribute to the etiology of the stem cell defect in MDS. In MDS and AML the absence of growth-inducing bone marrow proteins can uncouple the orderly pattern of growth and differentiation of myeloid hematopoietic cells. Because some growth factors such as interleukin-6 and colony-stimulating factor 1 are produced by bone marrow fibroblasts, defects or alterations in the supportive marrow stromal elements may contribute to the pathogenesis of MDS.

Somatic mutation of *ras* oncogenes occurs frequently in AML and in a small percentage of cases of MDS, most commonly in chronic myelomonocytic leukemia (CMML). The role that mutations of *ras* or other oncogenes play in the development of MDS is not clear, but they may be useful as clonal markers of malignancy.

Numerous and complex cytogenetic abnormalities are associated with MDS. Whether these cytogenetic changes are a cause or a result of MDS is uncertain, however. None of the presently recognized cytogenetic changes appear to be specific for MDS.

Clinical Findings

The median age at which MDS is diagnosed is between 60 and 75 years. Few patients are less than 50; however, people may be affected at any age and rare cases are even reported in children. Males are afflicted slightly more often than females. Signs and symptoms are nonspecific and generally relate to the blood cytopenias. Fatigue, weakness, and malaise are common. Less frequently, patients present with infections or manifestations of hemorrhage. A small percentage of patients have splenomegaly, most commonly those with CMML. Hepatomegaly is rare.

Approach to Diagnosis

A diagnosis of MDS should be considered for any patient over 50 years of age with unexplained blood cytopenias and/or monocytosis. A complete blood count and careful examination of a blood smear and bone marrow aspirate smears and trephine biopsy sections are essential for diagnosis and classification. The type and severity of the changes vary for different classes of MDS. Some patients present with profound dysplastic changes and increased myeloblasts. Others present with only subtle changes, and diagnosis may be delayed for several months or until other causes of the cytopenias have been eliminated.

After a clinical history and physical examination, laboratory diagnosis of MDS should proceed as follows:

1. A complete blood cell count.

2. A blood smear examination for dysplastic changes.

3. Studies to assess vitamin B_{12}, folate, and other potential deficiency states.

4. Bone marrow aspiration and trephine biopsy morphologic examination.

5. Bone marrow cytogenetic studies.

6. Other studies as clinically indicated for serum biochemical parameters and to evaluate for possible toxic exposure (eg, arsenic poisoning and infectious disease). When available, in vitro bone marrow culture studies may be performed as clinically indicated.

Hematologic Findings

The hematologic findings in MDS are highly variable. In some patients, diagnosis is obvious on examination of the blood smear. Other patients require a thorough evaluation to rule out secondary causes of cytopenias and dyshematopoiesis. The features generally used to define an MDS include various combinations of blood cytopenias, ineffective hematopoiesis, dyserythropoiesis, dysgranulopoiesis, dysmegakaryopoiesis, and increased myeloblasts. Ineffective hematopoiesis characterized by blood cytopenias, bone marrow hypercellularity, and increased numbers of hematopoietic precursors is found in the majority of cases and is most often typified by anemia with reticulocytopenia and erythroid hyperplasia in the bone marrow.

Blood Cell Measurements. The complete blood count (CBC) generally reveals a normocytic or mildly macrocytic anemia with a low or normal reticulocyte count. The red cell distribution width (RDW) is often elevated as a result of red cell anisocytosis. Leukocyte counts vary from normal to markedly reduced. In a minority of cases the leukocyte count is elevated, most often due to monocytosis. The platelet count may be reduced or normal; patients rarely present with thrombocytosis.

For the more indolent and prognostically favorable categories of MDS, anemia may be the only significant cytopenia. Patients with the less favorable types of MDS almost always present with pancytopenia or bicytopenia. The cytopenias typically progress with time, but the rate of progression is variable.

Blood Smear Morphology. The spectrum of morphologic changes observed on blood smears are listed in Table 28-1. The description of the various categories of MDS in the section on classification of MDS provides more detail (Images 28-1 to 28-3).

Bone Marrow Examination. In most cases, the bone marrow is hypercellular or normocellular; however, examples of hypocellular MDS may be encountered as well. Iron stores are often increased. Myelofibrosis is occasionally observed, most often in cases of secondary (therapy-related) MDS. The most important findings in the bone marrow are the dysplastic changes and, in some cases, increased myeloblasts (Table 28-1).

Dyserythropoiesis: Dyserythropoiesis is the most common morphologic change. Many cases of refractory anemia and refractory anemia with ringed sideroblasts involve only mild dyserythropoietic changes. In the more severe categories of MDS, profound dyserythropoiesis with bizarre erythroid precursors is often observed (Image 28-4). Ringed sideroblasts may be found in any of the MDS but are most striking in refractory anemia with ringed sideroblasts (RARS) (Image 28-5).

Dysgranulopoiesis: Dysgranulopoiesis varies from absent to severe (Image 28-6). The types of changes are listed in Table 28-1. Abnormally localized immature precursors (ALIP) is the term used to refer to the distribution of granulocytes on bone marrow trephine biopsy sections. The most immature granulocyte precursors are normally located in groups along the bone trabecula. As the granulocytes mature, they extend toward more central areas between bone trabeculae. In some MDS the most immature granulocyte precursors are found in large numbers or in groups remote from the usual location adjacent to the trabecula. Some investigators have

Table 28-1 Hematologic Findings in Myelodysplastic Syndromes

Blood	Bone Marrow
Dyserythropoiesis	
Anemia	Erythroid hyperplasia (occasionally hypoplasia)
Anisopoikilocytosis	Nuclear-cytoplasmic asynchrony
Oval macrocytes	Megaloblastic(oid) chromatin
Hypochromic cells	Karyorrhexis
Dimorphic populations	Multinuclearity
Decreased polychromatophilic cells	Nuclear fragments
Basophilic stippling	Ringed sideroblasts
Nucleated red blood cells	Vacuolated red blood cells
Howell-Jolly bodies	PAS positive erythroblasts
Dysgranulopoiesis	
Neutropenia	Increased myeloblasts and immature granulocytes
Rarely neutrophilia	Abnormally localized immature precursors
Immature granulocytes	Maturation defects
Hypogranularity	Hypogranularity
Nuclear hyposegmentation	Abnormal granules
(pseudo–Pelger-Huët change)	Abnormal nuclei
Occasionally hypersegmentation	
Circulating myeloblasts (<5%)	Myeloperoxidase-deficient neutrophils
	Increased monocytes
	Increased basophils
Dysmegakaryopoiesis	
Thrombocytopenia	Increased or decreased megakaryocytes
Large platelets	Clusters of megakaryocytes
Hypogranular platelets	Micromegakaryocytes
Vacuolated platelets	Large mononuclear forms
Abnormal platelet granules	Odd numbered nuclei
Micromegakaryocytes	Multiple small nuclei

associated ALIP with a poor prognosis and a greater likelihood of transformation to AML.

Dysmegakaryopoiesis: Dysmegakaryopoiesis is found in many of the MDS (Table 28-1). In some cases, dysmegakaryopoiesis may be the primary manifestation (Image 28-7).

Increased Myeloblasts: Increased myeloblasts are found in some MDS. The percentage of bone marrow myeloblasts is one of the defining features of the classification. Myeloblasts should not exceed 5% in the blood or 30% in the bone marrow.

Classification of the Myelodysplastic Syndromes

The classification of the MDS that is most commonly used is the French-American-British (FAB) Cooperative Group Classification, published in 1982. The first five categories listed in Table 28-2 are based on this classification system. In addition to the five FAB classes, many people also use the designation "chronic myelomono-cytic leukemia in transformation" (CMML-T).

A significant number of cases of MDS either do not fulfill all of the FAB criteria for a given group or overlap two or more categories. For these cases the designation "myelodysplastic syndrome, unclassified" is appropriate. Cases of secondary (therapy-related) MDS are often difficult to classify according to FAB criteria and might best be considered a separate category. Table 28-3 compares the categories of MDS.

Refractory Anemia. The major manifestation of refractory anemia (RA) is ineffective erythropoiesis characterized by erythroid hyperplasia, anemia, and reticulocytopenia. The anemia may be normocytic or macrocytic with anisopoikilocytosis; oval macrocytes are common. Some degree of neutropenia or thrombocytopenia may be present. In rare cases, when patients present with neutropenia or thrombocytopenia without anemia, the term "refractory cytopenia" may be descriptively more appropriate. There is little or no evidence of dysplastic changes in the neutrophils or platelets. Myeloblasts are rarely identified in the blood smear.

The bone marrow is hypercellular or normocellular with erythroid hyperplasia or, rarely, hypoplasia. Dyserythropoiesis may be noted but is usually not severe. Ringed sideroblasts are occasionally observed, but they number less than 15% of the erythroblasts. Dysgranulopoiesis and dysmegakaryopoiesis are absent. The bone marrow may contain normal or slightly increased numbers of myeloblasts but never more than 5%.

Table 28-2   Classification of Myelodysplastic Syndromes*

Refractory Anemia (RA)
Refractory Anemia With Ring Sideroblasts (RARS)
Refractory Anemia With Excess Blasts (RAEB)
Refractory Anemia With Excess Blasts in Transformation (RAEB-T)
Chronic Myelomonocytic Leukemia (CMML)
Chronic Myelomonocytic Leukemia in Transformation (CMML-T)
Myelodysplastic Syndrome Unclassified

*Modified from Bennett JM, Catovsky D, Daniel HT, et al. Proposals for the classification of the myelodysplastic syndromes. *Br J Haematol.* 1982;51:189-199.

Table 28-3   Morphologic Features of Myelodysplastic Syndromes*

FAB Category	Blasts	Sideroblasts	Monocytosis	Dyspoiesis
RA	<5%	<15%	–	+
RA-S	<5%	>15%	–	+
RAEB	5%-19%	Variable	–	++
RAEB-T	20%-29%	Variable	+/–	++
CMML	1%-19%	Variable	+	++
CMML-T	20%-29%	Variable	+	++

*Modified from Bennett JM. The classification of myelodysplastic syndrome. In: Schmalzl F, Mufti GJ, eds. *Myelodysplastic Syndromes.* New York, NY: Springer-Verlag NY Inc; 1992:3-10.

Refractory Anemia with Ringed Sideroblasts (RARS).

The clinical and morphologic features of RARS are similar to those for RA. However, in RARS 15% or more of the bone marrow erythroblasts are ringed sideroblasts (Image 28-5). There is commonly a dimorphic anemia with normal erythrocytes and microcytic and/or hypochromic poikilocytes. Coarse basophilic stippling (including Pappenheimer bodies) is observed in some of the erythrocytes. Neutropenia or thrombocytopenia are present in a minority of patients.

The bone marrow is hypercellular or normocellular with erythroid hyperplasia and markedly increased iron stores. The numerous ringed sideroblasts are the most prominent feature. Mild dyserythropoiesis may be observed but dysplastic changes in granulocytes and megakaryocytes are usually not present. Myeloblasts are rarely increased and never exceed 5%.

Refractory Anemia With Excess Blasts (RAEB).   Pancytopenia or bicytopenia are characteristic of RAEB. Dysplastic changes are commonly observed in erythrocytes, granulocytes, and platelets. Nucleated red blood cells and immature granulocytes, including myeloblasts and, occasionally, micromegakaryocytes, may be found in the blood smears; myeloblasts constitute less than 5% of the leukocytes.

The bone marrow is normocellular or hypercellular, and granulocytic and/or erythroid hyperplasia are noted. Myeloblasts are increased to at least 5% but less than 20%. Auer rods are not observed. Dyserythropoiesis is more severe than in RA or RARS. Dysgranulopoiesis is often prominent. Megakaryocytic hyperplasia with dysmegakaryopoiesis and megakaryocytic clusters on biopsy sections may be observed. The features that distinguish RAEB from RA and RARS include the severity of the pancytopenia or bicytopenia, the profound dysplastic changes, and the presence of 5% or more myeloblasts in the bone marrow.

Refractory Anemia With Excess Blasts in Transformation (RAEB-T).   RAEB-T bridges MDS and AML. It is the designation used for cases in which many of the morphologic features suggest a diagnosis of AML but the percentage of bone marrow myeloblasts is less than 30%. The morphologic and clinical features of RAEB-T are similar to those of RAEB, with the addition of one or more of the following three criteria: (1) 5% to 29% myeloblasts in the blood; (2) 20% to 29% myeloblasts in the bone marrow; (3) the presence of Auer rods.

Chronic Myelomonocytic Leukemia (CMML).   T h e morphologic features of CMML are similar to those of RAEB with the addition of monocytosis. The FAB criteria for diagnosis of CMML include more than $1.0 \times 10^3/mm^3$ $(1.0 \times 10^9/L)$ blood monocytes, increased serum and urine lysozyme levels, and a hypercellular bone marrow. Anemia and thrombocytopenia are less common than in RAEB. The total leukocyte count in CMML is variable and may be elevated, which is generally not true of the other MDS; occasionally there is marked leukocytosis. Hepatomegaly and/or splenomegaly are present in one third to one half of patients. The bone marrow myeloblast count is frequently less than 5%, and dysplastic changes in the developing erythrocytes, granulocytes, and megakaryocytes are often less severe than in RAEB and RAEB-T.

CMML is associated with a broad spectrum of clinical and hematologic presentations. The designation CMML appears to encompass both myelodysplastic and chronic myeloproliferative syndromes. Some patients present with the clinical and morphologic features typical of MDS (eg, blood cytopenias, dysplastic hematopoiesis, and increased bone marrow myeloblasts). Others present with marked monocytosis, organomegaly, and minimal or no increase in blasts. There is controversy over whether these should be regarded as MDS or as chronic myeloproliferative syndromes. Some cases that were previously designated Philadelphia chromosome negative chronic myeloid leukemia (CML) have the clinical and morphologic features of CMML.

Chronic Myelomonocytic Leukemia in Transformation (CMML-T). Patients with CMML-T have hematologic manifestations similar to CMML with the addition of one or more of the same three criteria that distinguish RAEB-T from RAEB.

Secondary (Therapy-Related) Myelodysplastic Syndrome. Secondary MDS occurs in patients previously treated with chemo-therapy and/or radiotherapy. Alkylating drugs and the epipodo-phyllotoxins appear to be the agents most commonly implicated. The median onset of secondary MDS is approximately 5 years after initiation of alkylating agents and 2.5 to 3 years after first use of epipodophyllotoxins. In many patients there is evolution to frank AML in a short time. Patients present with unexplained cytopenias. The dysplastic changes in the blood and marrow cells are similar to those in RAEB and are often severe; however, the bone marrow myeloblast percentage is frequently less than 5%. Myelofibrosis, hypocellularity, and ringed sideroblasts are encountered more frequently than in primary MDS.

Myelodysplastic Syndrome, Unclassified. The FAB criteria for diagnosis and classification of the MDS apply to most patients. However, a significant minority of cases fulfill most of the criteria for an MDS but differ from any of the FAB categories in one or more major features. Some of the more common reasons for difficulty in classifying an MDS are listed in Table 28-4. Cases with these features may be designated "MDS, unclassified," or the most closely applicable FAB category may be used with notation of the variant features.

Cases are commonly encountered in which there are severe dysplastic changes in all marrow cell lines and profound pancytopenia but no increase in myeloblasts. The features that distinguish these cases from RA or RARS are the severity of the pancytopenia and the degree of dysgranulopoiesis and dysmegakaryopoiesis. Clinically and morphologically, these cases most closely resemble RAEB; however, they lack excess blasts. This presentation is typical of secondary (therapy-related) MDS but may also be encountered in primary MDS.

MDS, unclassified, may also be the appropriate designation for rare cases in which patients present with neutropenia or thrombocytopenia without anemia. The terms refractory cytopenia, refractory neutropenia, and refractory thrombocytopenia have all been used to describe these cases. A diagnosis of MDS in patients with neutropenia or thrombocytopenia without anemia should be made with caution, and only when there is convincing evidence of dysplasia and other causes have been ruled out.

One FAB criterion for every class of MDS is bone marrow hypercellularity or normocellularity. It is clear, however, that some patients with the morphologic and clinical features of an MDS have a moderately to markedly hypocellular bone marrow. It seems appropriate to give these cases a specific identification by designating them hypocellular MDS.

On rare occasions, patients with features of RAEB or RA also present with leukocytosis or thrombocytosis instead of the expected cytopenias. The presence of leukocytosis has been noted in CMML but is not a feature included in the descriptions of the other FAB categories of MDS. These cases may be designated MDS, unclassified, or they may be placed in the most appropriate FAB category with notation of the unusual finding.

Myelofibrosis is relatively common in cases of secondary MDS and may be encountered in primary MDS. Characterization

Table 28-4 Features That May Cause Difficulty in the Classification of a Myelodysplastic Syndrome

Severe generalized dyshematopoiesis and pancytopenia with no increase in bone marrow blasts
Refractory neutropenia or thrombocytopenia only
Hypocellular bone marrow
Significant leukocytosis or thrombocytosis
Myelofibrosis

of the MDS may be problematic because of the difficulty involved in obtaining a marrow aspirate adequate for morphologic examination and for determining the percentage of myeloblasts. Some of these cases can be subclassified, but in many cases the designation "myelodysplasia with myelofibrosis" is more appropriate.

Myelodysplasia in Children. Myelodysplastic syndromes are primarily diagnosed in older adults and are rarely encountered in pediatric patients. However, the features and course of disease in children are similar to those found in adults. The median survival period is about 1.5 years, and about one third to one half of cases evolve to an acute myeloid leukemia. In reports on childhood MDS in which cases are classified by FAB criteria, the categories of RAEB and RAEB-T seem to be most common. The most common cytogenetic abnormalities are monosomy 7 and trisomy 8.

Isolated monosomy 7 syndrome of childhood often presents with features of an MDS. Recurrent infections and hepatosplenomegaly are common findings and neurofibromatosis has been observed. Patients usually have anemia and leukocytosis; thrombocytopenia is present in about half of the patients. Monocytosis and leukoerythroblastosis are common, as is defective neutrophil function. Dysplastic changes are generally observed, but myeloblasts are uncommon in the blood and only slightly elevated in the bone marrow. The bone marrow is hypercellular, and slight reticulin fibrosis may be present. Monosomy 7 syndrome of childhood is similar in many respects to juvenile chronic myeloid leukemia (JCML). The features that distinguish them are the markedly elevated hemoglobin F levels in JCML and the absence of an isolated monosomy 7. These disorders should be considered pediatric subtypes of MDS. Although both may resemble some cases of CMML in adults, patients with JCML or monosomy 7 syndrome may have a worse prognosis than patients with CMML.

Ancillary Tests

Cytogenetics. Bone marrow clonal chromosome abnormalities are found in approximately 30% to 40% of patients with a primary MDS. Patients with RAEB and RAEB-T have a higher incidence of chromosome abnormalities than patients in the other classes of MDS. In these groups the incidence of cytogenetic changes may be 45% to 60%. In secondary MDS cytogenetic abnormalities are observed in nearly 100% of cases.

Multiple cytogenetic changes have been identified, including deletion, trisomies, monosomies, and complex structural anomalies. The majority of patients show a loss of chromosome material rather than the reciprocal translocations or inversions that are common in patients with acute leukemia. Some of the most common recurring chromosome defects in primary MDS are listed in Table 28-5. The most common defect appears to be 5q⁻ alone or in combination with other chromosome abnormalities. It has been found in association with all classes of MDS. 5q⁻ as a single abnormality is associated with RA, characteristic megakaryocytic abnormalities, thrombocytosis, and a stable clinical course (5q⁻ syndrome).

The recurring chromosome defects found in primary MDS have also been identified in secondary (therapy-related) MDS. Complete or partial loss of chromosomes 5 or 7 is found in a very high percentage of cases of secondary MDS.

In Vitro Bone Marrow Cell Culture Studies. The colony-forming capacity of hematopoietic cells is diminished or absent in the majority of patients with MDS. A leukemic type in vitro growth pattern is often observed and is most commonly encountered in the more severe categories of MDS. In vitro culture of hematopoietic precursors may be valuable in assessing disease progression and prognosis.

Other Ancillary Laboratory Findings. Abnormalities in neutrophil function are reported in about half of the cases of MDS. Aberrant myeloid antigen expression may be identified.

Table 28-5   Cytogenetic Abnormalities in Myelodysplastic
                  Syndromes*

Complete or partial loss of chromosomes 5 or 7
Trisomy 8
Deletion or translocation 11q
Deletion or translocation 12p
Other complex chromosome defects

*Modified from Sandberg AA, Wullich B. Myelodysplastic syndromes: cytogenetic anomalies and
their clinical significance. In: Schmalzl F, Mufti GJ, eds. *Myelodysplastic Syndromes*. New York,
NY: Springer-Verlag NY Inc; 1992:165-177.

Occasionally, neutrophil myeloperoxidase staining is decreased or
absent, and alkaline phosphatase levels may be increased,
decreased, or normal. Red blood cell metabolic abnormalities,
changes in red blood cell membrane antigens, elevated levels of
hemoglobin F, a positive acid hemolysis (Ham) test, and various
platelet function abnormalities have all been reported.

Differential Diagnosis of Myelodysplastic Syndromes

MDS must be distinguished from other myeloproliferative disorders and from a variety of causes of secondary myelodysplasia,
including nutritional deficiency states, infectious processes, drug
effects, and toxic exposures. These conditions are often associated
with one or more blood cytopenias and dysplastic changes that
may be identical to those observed in MDS. A thorough historical
assessment and laboratory evaluation for secondary, potentially
reversible causes of myelodysplasia must always be performed
before a diagnosis is made. Table 28-6 lists conditions that may be
considered in the differential diagnosis of MDS.

Course and Treatment

Many treatment regimens have been tried on patients with MDS.
Most have been ineffective; at best they have resulted in limited
clinical improvement. Protocols involving chemotherapeutic agents
are generally reserved for patients with increased myeloblasts

Table 28-6 Considerations in the Differential Diagnosis of
Myelodysplastic Syndromes (MDS)

Megaloblastosis due to vitamin B_{12} or folate deficiency
Heavy metal intoxication: arsenic, lead, etc
Acute alcohol intoxication
Drug effects: primarily antineoplastic
Congenital dyserythropoietic anemia
Chronic infectious disease
Acquired immune deficiency syndrome
Acute myeloid leukemia (M2, M4, M6)
Any other condition with unexplained cytopenias or myelodysplasia

and/or severe pancytopenia. Conventional antileukemic chemotherapy is generally ineffective. However, some investigators report success in patients less than 50 years old. Patients in this younger age group may be candidates for bone marrow transplantation, which has been curative in some individuals.

Growth factors (colony-stimulating factor) that regulate hematopoiesis by promoting proliferation and differentiation of progenitor cells are currently being investigated as a possible treatment for MDS. Granulocyte-macrophage colony-stimulating factor (GM-CSF), which enhances function of mature granulocytes and monocytes and stimulates proliferation of the hematopoietic progenitor colonies, has been shown to increase neutrophil counts in MDS. However, its effect appears to be temporary.

Prognosis and Prognostic Indicators in MDS. In the majority of cases the course of disease is chronic with gradually worsening blood cytopenias. Survival varies from several years to only a few weeks or months. Death results from evolution to AML or from complications of blood cytopenias due to progressive bone marrow failure. Table 28-7 compares the incidence of evolution to AML and length of survival for the FAB categories of MDS. Secondary MDS has a similar incidence of evolution to AML as RAEB, approximately 30% to 40%.

Features with prognostic significance in primary MDS are shown in Table 28-8. A predominance of good prognostic indicators are found in patients with RA and RARS. Mostly poor indica-

Table 28-7   Survival and Evolution to Acute Myeloid
Leukemia in Patients With Myelodysplastic
Syndromes*

FAB Type (% of Patients)	Leukemic Evolution (%)	Median Survival (Months)	Survival Range (Months)
RA (28)	12	50	18-64
RARS (24)	8	51	14-76+
RAEB (23)	44	11	7-16
RAEB-T (9)	60	5	2.5-11
CMML (16)	14	11	9-60+

*From Third MIC Cooperative Study Group. Recommendations for a morphologic, immunologic, and cytogenetic (MIC) working classification of the primary and therapy related myelodysplastic disorders. *Cancer Genet Cytogenet.* 1988;32:1-9.

Table 28-8   Indicators of Good and Poor Prognoses in
Myelodysplastic Syndromes

Good

Younger age

Normal or moderately reduced neutrophil and platelet counts

Low blast counts in the bone marrow (<20%) and no blasts in the blood

No Auer rods

Ringed sideroblasts present

Normal karyotypes or mixed karyotypes without complex chromosome abnormalities

In vitro bone marrow culture reveals nonleukemic growth pattern

Poor

Advanced age

Severe neutropenia (<0.5 x 10^3/mm³[0.5 x 10^9/L]) or thrombocytopenia (<50 x 10^3/mm³ [50 x 10^9/L])

High blast count in the bone marrow (20%-30%) or blasts in the blood

Auer rods

Absence of ringed sideroblasts

Abnormal localization of immature granulocyte precursors on bone marrow sections

All or mostly abnormal karyotypes or complex marrow chromosome abnormalities

In vitro bone marrow culture reveals leukemic growth pattern

tors are found in patients with RAEB, RAEB-T and CMML, CMML-T, and secondary MDS.

References

Bennett JM. The classification of myelodysplastic syndrome. In: Schmalzl F, Mufti GJ, eds. *Myelodysplastic Syndromes*. New York, NY: Springer-Verlag NY Inc; 1992:3-10.

Bennett JM, Catovsky D, Daniel HT, et al. Proposals for the classification of the myelodysplastic syndromes. *Br J Haematol.* 1982;51:189-199.

Brunning RD, McKenna RW. Tumors of the bone marrow: myelodysplastic syndromes. *Atlas of Tumor Pathology*. 3rd Series. Washington, DC: Armed Forces Institute of Pathology; 1994:143-194.

Foucar K, Langdon RM, Armitage JO, et al. Myelodysplastic syndromes: a clinical and pathologic analysis of 109 cases. *Cancer.* 1985;56:553-561.

Gadner H. Pediatric experiences in myelodysplastic syndromes. In: Schmalzl F, Mufti GJ, eds. *Myelodysplastic Syndromes*. New York, NY: Springer-Verlag NY Inc; 1992:31-37.

Groupe Français de Morphologie Hematologique: French Registry of Acute Leukemia and Myelodysplastic Syndromes. Age distribution and hemogram analysis of the 4496 cases recorded during 1982-1983 and classified according to FAB criteria. *Cancer.* 1987;60:1385-1394.

Guyotat D, Campos L, Thomas X, et al. Myelodysplastic syndromes: a study of surface markers and *in vitro* growth patterns. *Am J Hematol.* 1990;34:26-31.

Janssen JWB, Buschle M, Layton M, et al. Clonal analysis of myelodysplastic syndromes: evidence of multipotent stem cell origin. *Blood.* 1989;73:248-254.

Juneja SK, Imbert M, Jouault H, et al. Haematological features of primary myelodysplastic syndromes (PMDS) at initial presentation: a study of 118 cases. *J Clin Pathol.* 1983;36:1129-1135.

Krsnik I, Srivastava PC, Galton DAG. Chronic myelomonocytic leukemia and atypical chronic myeloid leukemia. In: Schmalzl F, Mufti GJ, eds. *Myelodysplastic Syndromes*. New York, NY: Springer-Verlag NY Inc; 1992:131-139.

Michels SD, McKenna RW, Arthur DC, et al. Therapy-related acute myeloid leukemia and myelodysplastic syndrome: a clinical and morphologic study of 65 cases. *Blood.* 1985;65:1364-1372.

Sandberg AA, Wullich B. Myelodysplastic syndromes: cytogenetic anomalies and their clinical significance. In: Schmalzl F, Mufti GJ, eds. *Myelodysplastic Syndromes*. New York, NY: Springer-Verlag NY Inc; 1992:165-177.

Third MIC Cooperative Study Group. Recommendations for a morphologic, immunologic, and cytogenetic (MIC) working classification of the primary and therapy related myelodysplastic disorders. *Cancer Genet Cytogenet.* 1988; 32:1-9.

Tricot G, Vlietinck R, Boogaerts MA, et al. Prognostic factors in the myelodysplastic syndromes: importance of initial data on peripheral blood counts, bone marrow cytology, trephine biopsy and chromosomal analysis. *Br J Haematol.* 1985;60:19-32.

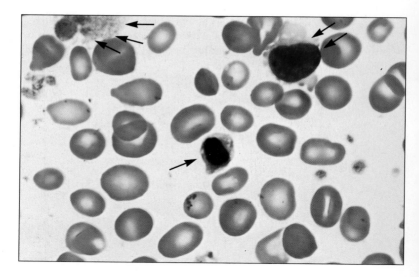

Image 28-1 Blood smear from a patient with a myelodysplastic syndrome. There is red cell anisopoikilocytosis with oval macrocytes. A nucleated red blood cell is illustrated in the center of the field (↑) and a micromegakaryocyte near the top (↑↑). Atypical platelets are at the upper left (↑↑↑).

Image 28-2 Blood smear from a patient with a myelodysplastic syndrome showing a hypogranular pseudo–Pelger-Huët neutrophil (↑) and a lymphocyte.

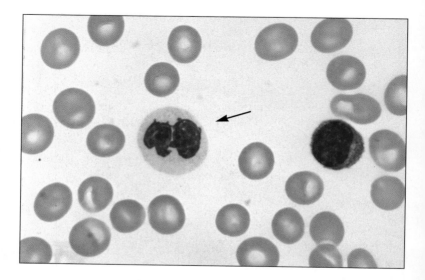

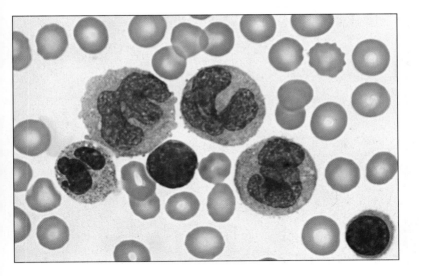

Image 28-3 Blood smear from a patient with CMML. Three atypical monocytes, two small lymphocytes, and a neutrophil are illustrated.

Image 28-4 Bone marrow smear from a patient with a myelodysplastic syndrome. There is dyserythropoiesis with a multinucleate megaloblastoid erythroid precursor (↑).

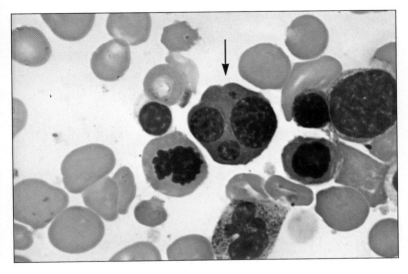

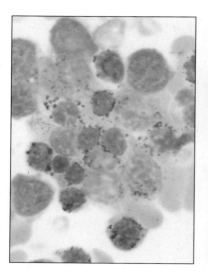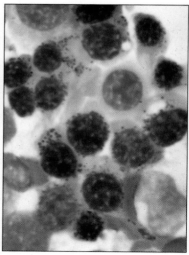

Image 28-5 Iron stains on a bone marrow smear from a patient with refractory anemia with ringed sideroblasts (RARS). Numerous ringed sideroblasts are visible. The smear on the right has a Wright's counter stain.

Image 28-6 A bone marrow aspirate smear from a patient with a myelodysplastic syndrome (CMML) shows markedly dysplastic neutrophils and monocytes.

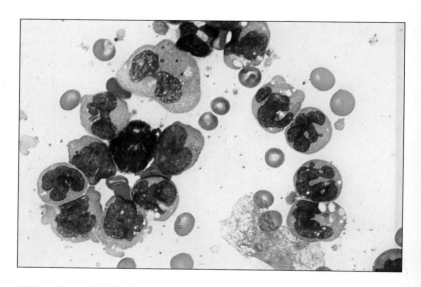

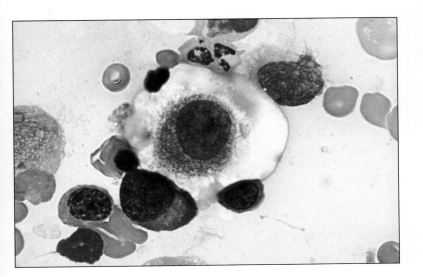

Image 28-7 A bone marrow aspirate smear from a patient with RAEB shows a dysplastic megakaryocyte and dyserythropoiesis. The megakaryocyte is uninucleate, small, and exhibits zoning of the cytoplasm.

29

Acute Myeloid Leukemia

Acute myeloid leukemias (AMLs) are neoplastic proliferations arising in hematopoietic precursor cells. They result in overgrowth of myeloblasts and other immature cells of myeloid lineage. The malignant cells replace the bone marrow, circulate in the blood, and may accumulate in other tissues, including lymph nodes, liver, and spleen. The overall incidence of AML in the United States is about 2.1 per 100,000 population per year. The age-specific incidence rate increases with age through the eighth decade. Eighty to ninety percent of acute leukemias in adults are AMLs.

Pathophysiology

The cause of AML is unknown, but studies suggest that genetic, environmental, and occupational factors may contribute to the etiology in some cases. Persons with Down syndrome, Bloom syndrome, Fanconi's anemia, neurofibromatosis, and several other genetic diseases are at higher risk of developing AML. Exposure to benzene and radiation and treatment with alkylating agents and epipodophyllotoxin drugs increases the risk of AML.

Table 29-1 Clinical Features of Acute Leukemia Related to Pathophysiology

Pathophysiology	Clinical Features
Anemia	Weakness and pallor
Thrombocytopenia (occasionally DIC)	Bleeding or bruising
Granulocytopenia (immunosuppression)	Fever, infections
Leukemic infiltrates	Bone or joint pain, lymphadenopathy, hepatosplenomegaly
Leukemic cells in CSF (leptomeningeal leukemia infiltrates)	Neurologic symptoms (headache, vomiting, visual disturbance, etc)

Abbreviations: DIC = disseminated intravascular coagulation; CSF = cerebrospinal fluid.

AML originates in deranged clones of hematopoietic stem cells. Cell kinetic studies have shown that the rate of maturation of normal marrow cell lines is markedly reduced, leading to overgrowth of the malignant clone. The neoplastic cells replace the normal bone marrow cells, resulting in anemia, neutropenia, thrombocytopenia, and an outpouring of the neoplastic blasts into the peripheral blood. Death results from bone marrow failure, which leads to profound blood cytopenias, severe infections, and bleeding. The variants of AML are thought to represent maturation blocks that affect different stages of stem cell maturation.

Clinical Findings

Onset of symptoms may be insidious or abrupt; fatigue, malaise, pallor, weakness, and fever are the most common. An infection secondary to neutropenia is the initial manifestation in some patients. Hemorrhage in the form of petechiae, ecchymosis, or epistaxis is seen in less than 50% of patients. Bleeding is a particular problem in patients with acute promyelocytic leukemia (M3), which is associated with disseminated intravascular coagulation.

Physical examination may reveal splenomegaly and lymphadenopathy, but both are usually less remarkable than in acute lymphoblastic leukemia (ALL). Sternal tenderness is common, and gingival hyperplasia may be a presenting sign in monocytic leukemias. Occasionally, accumulation of blasts results in the formation of an extramedullary tumor mass or "granulocytic sarcoma." These tumors may form in any part of the body and occasionally precede other manifestations of leukemia by several months. The clinical features and their relationship to pathophysiology are summarized in Table 29-1.

Approach To Diagnosis

The clinical manifestations detailed above are indications of a possible acute leukemia and dictate the series of laboratory tests that should be performed. After a complete history and physical examination, the laboratory evaluation for AML should proceed as follows:

1. A complete blood count.
2. Examination of a blood smear.
3. Bone marrow aspiration and trephine biopsy morphologic examination.
4. Cytochemical studies on blood and bone marrow.
5. Immunophenotyping of leukemic blasts by flow cytometry or immunocytochemistry.
6. Bone marrow cytogenetic studies.
7. Electron microscopy and molecular diagnostic studies in special cases.
8. Radiographic studies for assessment of extramedullary mass disease as clinically indicated.
9. Other laboratory tests as clinically indicated, including coagulation studies, serum biochemistry studies, and febrile evaluation.

Hematologic Findings

The hematologic findings vary among cases. In many patients the diagnosis is obvious from the blood smear examination. In others the changes are more subtle, and careful examination of blood smears and bone marrow by experienced individuals is required to make a diagnosis. Of first importance in the diagnosis is distinguishing AML from a reactive or other nonneoplastic condition. Secondly, AML must be distinguished from ALL because therapy differs significantly. Lastly, the subclassification of AML may provide prognostic or therapeutic insights.

The features that distinguish AML and ALL are listed in Table 29-2. These, combined with the cytochemical and immunophenotypic studies, facilitate correct diagnosis and classification in nearly all cases.

Blood Cell Measurements.   Blood counts are abnormal in almost every case. In most patients there is a reduction in at least two of the major normal cell types and often all three are reduced—ie, the patient has anemia, neutropenia, and thrombocytopenia. The anemia is usually normocytic and normochromic. The leukocyte count is elevated in more than 50% of patients due to the circulating blasts and other immature myeloid cells. Only about 20% of patients have leukocyte counts that exceed 100 x 10^3/mm^3 (100 x 10^9/L).

Blood Smear Morphology.   The decrease in the number of normal blood cells is apparent from examination of the blood smears. Red blood cells are usually normochromic-normocytic, with variable anisocytosis and poikilocytosis, and nucleated red blood cells are often present. Neutropenia and thrombocytopenia are present in most cases. Dysplastic changes in the form of hypogranular and hyposegmented neutrophils and large atypical platelets may be observed. The number of leukemic blasts varies from numerous, with leukocyte counts of more than 100 x 10^3/mm^3 (100 x 10^9/L), to rare or absent. When blasts are sparse on the blood smear the diagnosis of acute leukemia may only be possible with a bone marrow examination.

Bone Marrow Examination.   A bone marrow examination should always be performed when a diagnosis of acute leukemia is considered. Complete clinical information is essential to the individual interpreting the bone marrow slides. Most errors

Table 29-2 Cytologic Features of Blasts in Acute Myeloid and Acute Lymphoblastic Leukemias

Feature	Acute Myeloid Leukemia	Acute Lymphoblastic Leukemia
Blast size	Larger, usually uniform	Variable, small to medium size
Nuclear chromatin	Usually finely dispersed	Coarse to fine
Nucleoli	1 to 4, often prominent	Absent or 1 or 2, often indistinct
Cytoplasm	Moderately abundant, fine granules often present	Usually scant, coarse granules sometimes present (~ 7%)
Auer rods	Present in 60%-70% of cases	Not present
Other cell types	Often dysplastic changes in maturing myeloid cells	Myeloid cells not dysplastic

in the diagnosis and classification of acute leukemia result from incomplete or erroneous clinical information, inadequate specimens, and technically poor blood and marrow preparations. The optimal morphologic evaluation for leukemia includes examination of well-prepared blood and bone marrow smears and trephine biopsy sections.

Bone marrow smears are hypercellular in most cases and consist predominantly of blasts and other immature and abnormal cells. Normal hematopoietic precursors are markedly reduced. There is retarded maturation of myeloid cells and variable dysplastic changes in granulocytic, erythroid, and megakaryocytic precursors. The number of blasts varies, but 30% or more are generally required for a diagnosis of AML. Auer rods may be found in myeloblasts in 60% to 70% of cases.

The morphologic description of the blasts in the various categories of AML is provided below in the following section. The cytologic features that help distinguish AML and ALL on blood and bone marrow smears are shown in Table 29-2. All morphologic criteria should be considered contemporaneously when making an interpretation. Although there are general differences between the two types of leukemia in each of the morphologic parameters, only the presence of unequivocal Auer rods always distinguishes AML from ALL. When the morphologic findings are not distinctive for one of these major categories of acute leukemia, additional diagnostic studies must be performed.

Table 29-3 French-American-British (FAB) Classification of
Acute Myeloid Leukemia

Myeloblastic leukemia minimally differentiated	M0
Myeloblastic leukemia without maturation	M1
Myeloblastic leukemia with maturation	M2
Hypergranular promyelocytic leukemia	M3
Microgranular (hypogranular) M3 variant	
Myelomonocytic leukemia	M4
With marrow eosinophilia (M4e)	
Monocytic leukemia	M5
Poorly differentiated (M5a)	
Differentiated (M5b)	
Erythroleukemia	M6
Megakaryoblastic leukemia	M7

Trephine biopsy sections are usually markedly hypercellular, but occasionally a normocellular or hypocellular marrow is encountered. Normal hematopoietic cells are replaced by a diffuse proliferation of leukemic cells. Scattered individual or clusters of megakaryocytes and other normal bone marrow elements may be observed.

Morphologic Classification of Acute Myeloid Leukemia

The French-American-British (FAB) Cooperative Group classification of the acute leukemias and myelodysplastic syndromes has gained international acceptance and is the one most widely used. This classification system is based primarily on morphology and cytochemistry, but immunophenotyping and other studies help define some of the categories. The FAB classification has provided common terminology for hematologists and hematopathologists and a uniform base of comparison for studies in the literature. The FAB classification of AML is shown in Table 29-3. The case distribution of the FAB categories of AML is given in Table 29-4.

The FAB classification system requires that blasts constitute 30% or more of the bone marrow nucleated cells for a diagnosis of AML. This criterion distinguishes between acute leukemia and a

Table 29-4   The Distribution of FAB Categories of AML

FAB Category	Sultan et al (n = 250)	Stanley et al (n = 358)
M0*	?	?
M1	21%	10%
M2	32%	45%
M3	16%	10%
Hypergranular		(7%)
Microgranular		(3%)
M4	16%	19%
With eosinophilia		(6%)
M5	12%	10%
Poorly differentiated		(6%)
Differentiated		(4%)
M6	3%	6%
M7*	?	?

Abbreviation: AML = acute myeloid leukemia
*Not included in these studies. The incidence of M0 is approximately 3% of AMLs. The incidence of M7 is up to 10% of AML in children.

myelodysplastic syndrome. There are exceptions to this rule that will be addressed in the discussions of the individual categories of AML that follow.

Minimally Differentiated AML (M0).   Criteria for the diagnosis of M0:

- Blasts are agranular and may resemble L2 or, rarely, L1 ALL.
- Less than 3% of blasts are myeloperoxidase or Sudan black B positive.
- Blasts are negative for expression of B and T lymphocyte associated antigens.
- Expression of at least one myeloid antigen, CD13 or CD33.
- Other myeloid markers may be positive (eg, CD14, CD11b)
- Blasts may express myeloperoxidase by immunohistochemical methods or by electron microscopy.

Minimally differentiated AML includes the small number of cases that have a demonstrable myeloid lineage by immunophenotypic or ultrastructural findings but lack definitive cytologic and cyto-chemical criteria (Image 29-1). Two to three percent of cases of AML are M0. There should be no expression of lymphocyte asso-ciated antigens by the leukemic blasts, with the exceptions of ter-minal deoxynucleotidyl transferase (TdT), CD2, CD4, and CD7. Antibodies to these antigens react in some cases of AML. Expression of one of these markers in AML should not be consid-ered evidence of mixed lineage leukemia.

Myeloblastic Leukemia Without Maturation (M1).
Criteria for the diagnosis of M1:

- Sum of myeloblasts must be 90% or more of the nonery-throid cells.
- The remaining cells must be either maturing granulocytes from promyelocytes onwards or monocytes.
- At least 3% of blasts must be myeloperoxidase or Sudan black B positive.

The morphologic spectrum of myeloblasts may vary consider-ably in cases of M1 (Image 29-2). The blast nucleus is general-ly round. The cytoplasm may or may not contain azurophilic granules. Auer rods are found in varying numbers of myeloblasts in approximately 50% of cases. Evidence of maturation to promyelocytes may be minimal or absent. In many cases the myeloblasts appear undifferentiated and the myeloid nature of the leukemia is identified only after the myeloperoxidase stains are examined. When only 3% to 10% of the blasts are myeloper-oxidase reactive, immunophenotyping studies should be per-formed to confirm the diagnosis.

Myeloblastic Leukemia With Maturation (M2).
Criteria for the diagnosis of M2:

- The sum of myeloblasts is from 30% to 89% of the nonery-throid cells.
- Granulocytes from promyelocytes to mature neutrophils con-stitute more than 10% of cells.
- Monocytic precursors are less than 20%.

M2 is characterized by evidence of maturation beyond the myeloblast stage of development (Image 29-3). The maturing neutrophils often show dysplastic changes. Erythroid and megakaryocyte precursors may be dysplastic, and a frank panmyelopathy is observed in some cases. Auer rods are found in about 70% of cases. Because of the obvious maturation in M2, the myeloid nature of the disease is not in question. The finding of myeloperoxidase reactivity in the myeloblasts merely confirms the morphologic diagnosis.

A t(8;21)(q22;q11) bone marrow chromosome rearrangement is found in 20% to 25% of cases of M2. These cases are characterized by large leukemic blasts, prominent Auer rods, and markedly dysplastic changes in developing neutrophils.

Hypergranular Promyelocytic Leukemia (M3).

Criteria for the diagnosis of M3:

- The majority of cells are abnormal promyelocytes with a characteristic pattern of heavy cytoplasmic granulation.
- The nucleus of the leukemic promyelocytes is often reniform.
- Cells containing multiple Auer rods are usually present.
- In microgranular (hypogranular) variant there are smaller and fewer cytoplasmic granules.

M3 has distinctive clinical, morphologic, ultrastructural, and cytogenetic features. The blood leukocyte count is usually reduced at presentation. The leukemic cell population in the bone marrow is composed predominantly of abnormal promyelocytes (Image 29-4). Myeloblasts are a minor component in most cases and rarely reach 30%. In M3 the abnormal promyelocytes are considered comparable to blasts for the diagnosis of acute leukemia. The promyelocytes are characterized by numerous red to purple cytoplasmic granules. The granules are often larger and darker staining than normal, and may be so numerous as to obscure the nuclear borders. Cells containing multiple intertwined Auer rods are found in approximately 90% of cases, and large globular inclusions of Auer-like material may be observed.

A variant form of M3 designated microgranular or hypogranular M3 is characterized by leukemic cells with sparse and/or fine granulation and strikingly irregular nuclear shape (Image 29-5). Their identity as abnormal promyelocytes may be obscured by these features. Cells containing multiple Auer rods are present in the majority of cases but are usually less abundant than in typical hypergranular M3. Unlike typical M3, patients with the microgranular variant generally have a moderately to markedly elevated blood leukocyte count.

A t(15;17)(q22;q12-21) bone marrow chromosome rearrangement is found in nearly 100% of cases of both typical and microgranular M3. The chromosome break points correspond with the promyelocytic leukemia (PML) gene on chromosome 15 and the retinoic acid receptor-α (RARα) gene on 17, which results in a PML-RARα fusion gene.

The most outstanding clinical features associated with both typical and microgranular M3 are the high frequency of disseminated intravascular coagulation (DIC) and the response to treatment with all-trans retinoic acid. In most patients there is severe DIC and hemorrhage prior to or during induction therapy. Hemorrhage is the cause of early death in some patients. When DIC and hemorrhage are adequately controlled patients have an excellent chance for complete remission and prolonged survival. All-trans retinoic acid appears to interact with the PML-RARα fusion gene to induce maturation of the leukemic promyelocytes. Complete but transient clinical remissions are frequently achieved with high doses of retinoic acid therapy.

Myelomonocytic Leukemia (M4).   Criteria for the diagnosis of M4:

- The sum of myeloblasts and monoblasts is 30% or more.
- The sum of myeloblasts and granulocytes is 20% to 80%.
- 20% to 80% of the bone marrow cells are of monocyte lineage, as demonstrated by the nonspecific esterase stain or a serum lysozyme level that exceeds three times normal.
- If fewer than 20% of the marrow cells are monocytes, the diagnosis is still M4 if the blood monocyte count exceeds 5 x 10^3/mm^3 (5 x 10^9/L).

Both granulocytic and monocytic differentiation are observed in varying proportions in the bone marrow (Image 29-6). The major criterion distinguishing M4 from M2 is the proportion of monoblasts, promonocytes, and monocytes, which collectively must equal 20% or more. Monoblasts and early promonocytes cannot always be distinguished from granulocyte precursors in routine marrow smears. For this reason the additional criteria of nonspecific esterase reactivity in 20% or more of the cells or an elevated lysozyme are included. Auer rods are present in the myeloblast component in approximately 60% of cases. The blood leukocyte count is often markedly elevated. Organomegaly, lymphadenopathy, and other tissue infiltration are common.

A variant of M4 with increased and dysplastic bone marrow eosinophils and an abnormality of chromosome 16 is designated M4 with eosinophilia (M4e) (Image 29-7). The major features of this variant are shown below.

Features of M4 With Eosinophilia (M4e)

- Usual criteria for M4
- Increased bone marrow eosinophils
- Dysplastic eosinophils; primarily abundant large, basophilic staining granules
- Abnormalities of chromosome 16, either inv(16)(p13q22) or del(16)(q22)

M4e constitutes approximately 30% of cases of M4. The incidence of extramedullary disease is higher (54%) than for most types of AML; lymphadenopathy and hepatomegaly are particularly common. Granulocytic sarcoma concurrent with or preceding bone marrow involvement is more common than in most other leukemias. There is a high incidence of central nervous system relapse with intracerebral myeloblastomas in addition to leptomeningeal leukemia. This M4 variant has a high complete remission rate (76% to 92%) and a longer median survival time than other types of AML.

Monocytic Leukemia (M5). Criteria for the diagnosis of M5:

- 80% or more of all nonerythroid cells in the bone marrow are monoblasts, promonocytes, or monocytes.
- M5–Poorly differentiated (M5a): 80% or more of the monocytic cells are monoblasts.
- M5-Differentiated (M5b): Less than 80% of all monocytic cells are monoblasts; the remainder are promonocytes and monocytes.

M5-Poorly differentiated is characterized by a predominance of monoblasts that are large and have moderately abundant, variably basophilic cytoplasm, which frequently contains delicate peroxidase negative azurophilic granules (Image 29-8). Auer rods are not observed. The nucleus is round with reticular chromatin and one or more prominent nucleoli. Because the morphology of the blasts is poorly differentiated in routine smears, the diagnosis is often made only with the aid of cytochemical stains. Monoblasts are nonspecific esterase positive and myeloperoxidase negative.

The leukemic cells in M5-differentiated manifest more obvious cytologic evidence of monocytic features. The nuclei have delicate chromatin and a characteristic folded or cerebriform appearance (Image 29-9). The promonocyte cytoplasm is less basophilic than monoblasts are and contains a variable number of azurophilic granules. Auer rods are rarely observed. The promonocytes are usually nonspecific esterase positive; some exhibit weak myeloperoxidase activity. In most cases of M5b, monoblasts constitute less than 30% of the marrow cells. Promonocytes are considered comparable to monoblasts for purposes of distinguishing leukemia from a myelodysplastic syndrome. The combination of monoblasts and promonocytes totals 30% or more.

M5 is associated with the highest incidence of organomegaly, lymphadenopathy, and tissue infiltration of all the categories of AML. The first clinical manifestations of leukemia are often extramedullary tissue infiltrates, particularly in children with M5a.

Erythroleukemia (M6).   Criteria for the diagnosis of M6:

- 50% or more of all nucleated bone marrow cells are erythroblasts.
- 30% or more of the remaining cells (nonerythroid) are myeloblasts.
- Dyserythropoiesis is prominent.

Most patients with M6 present with pancytopenia and erythroblastosis. Some cases evolve from a myelodysplastic syndrome or present as a secondary leukemia in patients with prior alkylating agent chemotherapy. The predominant leukemic cell in the marrow is the erythroblast. Myeloblasts are often less than 30% of the total bone marrow cells but must constitute 30% or more of the nonerythroid cells. There is striking erythroid hyperplasia and dyserythropoiesis characterized by abnormalities of nuclear development, including megaloblastoid changes and karyorrhexis. Gigantoblasts with multiple nuclei are commonly present (Image 29-10). The leukemic erythroblasts may contain cytoplasmic vacuoles that are PAS positive. There is often evidence of dyspoietic megakaryocytes and platelets. Auer rods are present in myeloblasts in about 50% of cases. In rare cases nearly 100% of the bone marrow cells are leukemic erythroblasts; the designation erythremic myelosis has been used for this rare form of acute myeloid leukemia.

Megakaryoblastic Leukemia (M7).   Criteria for the diagnosis of M7:

- 30% or more blasts in the bone marrow.
- Blasts are identified as being of megakaryocyte lineage by expression of megakaryocyte specific antigens and platelet peroxidase reaction on electron microscopy.

In blood and bone marrow smears megakaryoblasts are usually medium to large cells. Nuclear chromatin is dense and homogeneous. Nucleoli are variably prominent. There is scant to moderately abundant cytoplasm, which may be vacuolated. An irregular cytoplasmic border is often noted, and occasionally projections resembling budding platelets are present. Transition forms between poorly differentiated blasts and recognizable micromegakaryocytes are often observed (Image 29-11). In some cases the majority of the leukemic cells consist of small lymphoid-like blasts. A marrow aspirate may be difficult to obtain because of frequent myelofibrosis. Trephine biopsy sections often reveal morphologic evidence of megakaryocytic differentiation that is not appreciated in the marrow aspirate smears.

Although many cases of M7 consist predominantly of poorly differentiated blasts, clues to their identity are often present. These include the presence of circulating micromegakaryocytes, atypical platelets, pseudopod projections on the surface of the blasts or zoning of the cytoplasm, myelofibrosis, and clusters of small megakaryocytes in trephine sections. More precise identification is accomplished with immunophenotyping or electron microscopy and ultracytochemistry.

Acute Basophilic Leukemia. Although the existence of rare cases of acute leukemia with primarily basophil differentiation has been generally recognized, basophilic leukemia is not an FAB category at present (Image 29-12). Recently, reports of cytologically undifferentiated leukemias with ultrastructural evidence of basophil differentiation have appeared. These poorly differentiated, acute basophilic leukemias would most likely be classified as MO without electron microscopic confirmation of basophil lineage. Some cases may be classified as acute lymphoblastic leukemias in the absence of immunophenotyping. The characteristics of acute basophilic leukemia are listed below.

Criteria for the diagnosis of acute basophilic leukemia:

- Differentiated: basophil granules by light microscopy.
- Poorly differentiated: no or minimal basophil granules by light microscopy.
- Myeloperoxidase negative by light microscopy but positive by electron microscopy.
- Granules stain metachromatically with toluidine blue.

- Expression of myeloid antigens.
- Poorly differentiated cases are diagnosed by electron microscopic identification of early basophil granules

Undifferentiated Leukemia.   With the advent of immunophenotyping and electron microscopy, few cases of acute leukemia are classified as undifferentiated. This number will undoubtedly continue to decline as diagnostic techniques become more refined.

Criteria for the diagnosis of undifferentiated leukemia:

- Blasts do not exhibit differentiation by morphologic or cytochemical criteria.
- No clear differentiation pattern by immunophenotyping, electron microscopy, ultracytochemistry, cytogenetics, or immunogenotypic studies.

Other Laboratory Tests

29.1 Cytochemistry

Purpose.   Cytochemical stains on blood and bone marrow smears are helpful in distinguishing AML from ALL and in subclassifying AML (Tables 29-5 and 29-6).

Principle.   Enzymatic activity in the cytoplasm is demonstrated by means of specific substrates and appropriate couplers, which provide localized color in the area of enzyme activity. The color is produced when one of the products of the enzyme action unite with the coupler.

Specimen.   Smears are made from blood and bone marrow. Capillary blood from a fingerstick or anticoagulated blood may be used. Special fixatives are recommended for some stains but most can be performed on air-dried smears. Ideally, all cytochemical stains should be made on recently prepared slides. Because this is often not practical, however, unstained

Table 29-5   Cytochemistry for Acute Leukemia

Reaction	Primary Normal Cells Manifesting Reaction	Major Diagnostic Utility
Myeloperoxidase	Neutrophil series, eosinophils (cyanide resistant), monocytes ±	Myeloid leukemia without maturation (M1), myeloid leukemia with maturation (M2), microgranular promyelocytic leukemia (M3)
Sudan black B	Neutrophil series, monocytes ±	M1, M2, microgranular M3
Chloroacetate esterase	Neutrophil series	M1, M2, microgranular M3, granulocytic sarcomas
Nonspecific esterase (alpha-naphthyl acetate or alpha-naphthyl butyrate)	Monocytes (inhibited by sodium fluoride)	Myelomonocytic leukemia (M4); monocytic leukemia, poorly differentiated (M5a); monocytic leukemia, differentiated (M5b)
Periodic acid–Schiff (PAS)		Erythroleukemia (M6), acute lymphoblastic leukemias
Terminal deoxynucleotidyl transferase (TdT)	T and B lymphocyte precursors	Acute lymphoblastic leukemias

smears can be stored away from light in a desiccator or a refrigerator for some reactions. For the myeloperoxidase stain a fresh smear is preferred.

Procedure.   A variety of cytochemical stains are available, and a specific cytochemical profile exists for each hematopoietic cell line (Table 29-5). Myeloperoxidase, which is present in primary granules, Sudan black B (SBB), and specific esterase stains (naphthol AS-D chloroacetate esterase) are reactive in cells in the neutrophil lineage, variable in other granulocytic cells, and nonreactive in lymphocytes. These stains are therefore useful in differentiating between AML and ALL. The myeloperoxidase stain appears to have the best sensitivity and specificity of the three (Image 29-13). Sudan black B stains a variety of lipids in granulocytes and is especially useful when fresh specimens are not available and in the occasional cases in which the leukemic myeloblasts have an acquired myeloperoxidase deficiency. The specific esterase stain is less sensitive than SBB and peroxidase but is useful in separating granulocytic from lymphocytic cell proliferations in paraffin-embedded tissue sections.

Table 29-6   Cytochemical Profiles of Acute Leukemias

	MPO	SBB	CAE	NSE	PAS	AP
Acute myeloid leukemia	+	+	+	+ (M4,M5) diffuse	+/– (M6,M5,M7)	+/–
Acute lymphoblastic leukemia	–	–	–	–/+ (focal)	+ (75%)	+ T-ALL focal paranuclear

Abbreviations: MPO = myeloperoxidase; SBB = Sudan black B; CAE = chloroacetate esterase; NSE = nonspecific esterase; PAS = periodic acid–Schiff; AP = acid phosphatase.

Nonspecific esterase (using alpha-naphthyl acetate or alpha-naphthyl butyrate as substrates) stains monocytes and histiocytes diffusely and is used to identify monocytic leukemias (M4 and M5) (Image 29-14). Nonspecific esterase stains with the substrates listed above do not react with myeloblasts and neutrophil precursors.

The periodic acid-Schiff (PAS) reaction is not very useful in differentiating acute leukemias. The typical block staining of lymphoblasts in ALL may occasionally be seen in AML as well. Positive reactions with PAS stain are frequently observed in acute monocytic leukemia (M5a), erythroleukemia (M6), and megakaryoblastic (M7) leukemia.

Terminal deoxynucleotidyl transferase (TdT) is a DNA polymerase present in both T- and B-lymphocyte progenitors but absent in normal myeloid cells. A TdT assay is useful in separating ALL from AML, although the myeloblasts in a small percentage of cases of AML may express TdT activity. The TdT assay is performed by immunofluorescent or immunohistochemical methods.

Interpretation.   Factors relating to the interpretation and diagnostic utility of the special stains described above are listed in Tables 29-5 and 29-6. The myeloperoxidase (MPO) reaction primarily stains normal and leukemic myeloblasts and developing neutrophils; the intensity of the reaction increases with maturation. The reaction is in a diffuse granular pattern in the cytoplasm. Monocytes stain variably positive with MPO.

When an alpha-naphthyl butyrate substrate is used, the non-specific esterase stain (NSE) produces a diffuse cytoplasmic reaction in normal monocytes and monocytic leukemias (M4 and M5). Most mature T lymphocytes react to NSE with a dot of dense, localized NSE positivity in the cytoplasm; some cases of ALL may show a similar pattern. A diffuse cytoplasmic reaction may be observed in epithelial cell malignancies. Positive staining with NSE may also be found in erythroblasts in megaloblastic anemia. In megakaryoblastic leukemia (M7), the alpha-naphthyl acetate NSE often stains the blasts in a focal pattern in the cytoplasm. This is less common with a butyrate substrate. Coarse granular PAS staining is characteristic of the blasts in ALL but is also found in erythroblasts in approximately 60% of patients with erythroleukemia (M6) and commonly in the blasts in M5a and M7. TdT is found in 95% of patients with ALL and in 5% to 10% of patients with AML. TdT positivity in ALL is uniformly strong in 80% to 100% of the blasts, while in AML the activity is weaker and present in a smaller percentage of cells.

Notes and Precautions. Many of the stains require considerable technical expertise to be performed well. Experience in interpreting cytochemical stains in acute leukemia is required, because leukemic cells may not stain the same way as their normal counterparts. For example, one may observe neutrophils from patients with AML (and myelodysplastic syndrome) that stain negatively for myeloperoxidase. Occasionally, the immature cells in AML are negative with peroxidase stains but positive with SBB. Rare cases of SBB-positive granules in ALL have also been reported.

29.2 Immunophenotyping

Purpose. Immunophenotyping leukemic blasts is important in distinguishing AML from ALL and in classifying cases of poorly differentiated AML.

Table 29-7   Antigen Expression in Acute Myeloid Leukemias

Antigen	M0, M1, M2	M3	M4, M5	M6	M7
CD13	+	+	+	+	+/−
CD33	+	+	+	+	+/−
HLA-DR	+	−	+	−/+	+/−
CD14	−	−	+	−	−
CD11b	−	−	+	−	−
CD71	−	−	−	+	−
Glycophorin	−	−	−	+	−
CD41 and CD61	−	−	−	−	+

Principle, Specimen, and Procedure.   See Test 30.2.

Interpretation.   Immunophenotype has less therapeutic and prognostic significance for AMLs than it does for ALL. It is primarily important in distinguishing cases of AML from ALL when the morphologic and cytochemical profile of the leukemic cells is not definitive. In classifying AMLs, immunophenotyping is necessary to identify M0 (minimally differentiated) and, often, M7 (megakaryoblastic) leukemias. Cases of M1 with less than 10% myeloperoxidase positive cells and the rare examples of nonspecific esterase negative M5a should also be confirmed by immunophenotyping.

　　Immunophenotypic classification of AML can be achieved by using panels of monoclonal antibodies (MoAbs) with specificity for various myeloid antigens associated with maturation and differentiation. HLA-DR (Ia) reactivity is seen in most cases of AML except for acute promyelocytic leukemia (FAB-M3). The monocytic leukemias (FAB-M4 and M5) can usually be detected by the monocyte-associated MoAbs, CD11b, and CD14. Monoclonal antibodies that recognize platelet glycoprotein determinants, CD41 and CD61, are used to identify megakaryoblasts. Table 29-7 lists antibodies commonly used in the immunophenotypic characterization of AML.

Table 29-8   Common Chromosomal Abnormalities in Acute Myeloid Leukemia

AML-M2	t(8;21)(q22;q11)
AML-M3	t(15;17)(q22;q12-21)
AML-M4 with eosinophilia	inv(16)(p13;q22)
AML-M5	t(9;11)(q22;q23; or q24)
Therapy-related leukemias	−5/5q−, −7/7q−, 20q−

Ancillary Tests

Cytogenetics. Bone marrow cytogenetic studies are increasingly important in the evaluation of patients with acute leukemia. They supplement the morphologic, cytochemical, and immunophenotypic studies in the characterization of AML and may contribute to the distinction between AML and ALL in selected cases. Most importantly, cytogenetic studies provide the most reliable independent indicator of prognosis. Chromosome abnormalities are found in most cases of acute leukemia when sensitive banding techniques are used. Structural changes are common and may involve a single rearrangement or multiple complex abnormalities. In some cases with apparently normal cytogenetic studies, molecular translocations are identified by molecular techniques.

Several specific chromosome rearrangements have been related to FAB categories of AML. These are shown in Table 29-8. Survival study data indicate that AMLs may be separated into low, intermediate-, and high-grade diseases based on bone marrow cytogenetic findings. These are shown in Table 29-9.

Electron Microscopy and Ultracytochemistry.

Electron microscopy may be useful in the characterization of acute leukemia when the leukemic blasts fail to manifest differentiating features on morphologic, cytochemical, or immunophenotypic examination. Ultracytochemical peroxidase techniques are useful in characterizing minimally differentiated (M0) and megakaryoblastic (M7) acute myeloid leukemias. Poorly differentiated basophilic leukemia may only be diagnosed by recognition of early basophil granules on ultrastructural examination. Rare cases of nonspecific esterase negative M5a (monoblastic) leukemia may be

Table 29-9 Prognostic Implications of Chromosome Findings in Acute Myeloid Leukemia*

AML	Prognostic Implications
inv 16 or t(16;16), single miscellaneous defects	Favorable
+8, t(15;17); t(6;9), t(8;21); t(9;11), t(9;22)	Intermediate
–7 or del(7q), complex defects	Unfavorable
Normal chromosomes; inv(3), del(5q); two to three miscellaneous defects	Undetermined

*From Yunis and Brunning.

recognized by electron microscopy findings or an ultracytochemical esterase reaction. The application of immunocytochemistry to electron microscopy may be useful in characterizing acute leukemias in the future.

Molecular Analysis.   Immunoglobulin and T-cell receptor gene rearrangement studies have proven useful in diagnosing various lymphoproliferative disorders, but thus far they have not been as useful in diagnosing acute leukemia. Even so, there are cases in which information provided by gene rearrangement studies contributed directly to the classification of morphologically undifferentiated leukemias. Gene rearrangement studies and polymerase chain reaction (PCR) are proving to be highly sensitive indicators of minimal residual leukemia and early relapse. The number of DNA probes available to detect specific genes associated with types of leukemia such as the PML-RARα fusion product in M3 (promyelocytic) leukemia is expanding and will continue to do so in the future. Measuring the expression of multiple drug resistance genes is another potentially important clinical application of molecular biology; such studies may prove useful in designing treatment protocols. It is likely that molecular diagnosis will play an increasingly important role in leukemia diagnosis in the future.

Coagulation Studies.   Bleeding in AML is usually caused by thrombocytopenia. In patients with severe bleeding, however, DIC should be considered. DIC is associated particularly with

Table 29-10 Differential Diagnosis of Acute Myeloid
Leukemia

FAB Category of AML	Considerations in the Differential Diagnosis	Studies Helpful in the Differential Diagnosis
M0, minimally differentiated	ALL, particularly L2	Immunophenotype
	AML-M1, M5a, M7	Cytochemistry (MPO, NSE), immunophenotype
	Poorly differentiated, basophilic leukemia	Electron microscopy
M1, without maturation	ALL, particularly L2	Cytochemistry (MPO), immunophenotype
	AML-M0, M5a, M7	Cytochemistry (MPO, NSE), immunophenotype
	Basophilic leukemia	Electron microscopy
M2, with maturation	Leukemoid reaction	Clinical history; % blasts, Auer rods, dysplasia; immunophenotypic aberrancy; cytogenetics
	Myelodysplastic syndrome	% blasts
	AML-M1, M3, M4, M6	FAB cytologic and cytochemical criteria
M3, promyelocytic		
Hypergranular	Agranulocytosis	Clinical history, cytology, Auer rods; immunophenotypic aberrancy; cytogenetics
	AML-M2	Cytology, eg, multiple Auer rods; immunophenotype cytogenetics
Microgranular	AML-M4, M5b	Cytochemistry (MPO, NSE)
M4, myelomonocytic	Leukemoid reaction	% blasts, dysplasia, Auer rods; immunophenotypic aberrancy; cytogenetics
	Myelodysplastic syndrome	% blasts
	M2, M5, microgranular M3	Cytochemistry (MPO, NSE)
M5, monocytic		
M5a	ALL-L2	Cytochemistry (NSE), immunophenotype
	AML-M0, M1, M7	Cytochemistry (MPO, NSE), immunophenotype
M5b	M4, myelodysplastic syndrome	% monoblasts and promonocytes

Table 29-10   *Continued*

FAB Category of AML	Considerations in the Differential Diagnosis	Studies Helpful in the Differential Diagnosis
M6, erythroleukemia	Megaloblastic anemia and other secondary dyserythropoiesis, eg, drug effects, arsenic	Clinical history, % blasts, type of dyserythropoiesis, B_{12} and folate, arsenic levels
	Myelodysplastic syndrome	% blasts
	AML-M2	% erythroblasts
M7, megakaryoblastic	ALL	Immunophenotype
	AML-M0, M1, M5a	Cytochemistry (MPO, NSE), immunophenotype (CD41, CD61)

acute promyelocytic leukemia (M3) and is probably caused by thromboplastic material released from leukemic promyelocytes.

Serum Biochemistry.   Serum uric acid levels are frequently elevated, especially in patients with high white blood cell counts and in patients undergoing induction chemotherapy. Uric acid is the end product of nucleic acid degeneration. Elevated serum levels of calcium and magnesium may also be seen. Similarly, serum lactate dehydrogenase (LD) levels are usually elevated.

Febrile Evaluation.   The incidence of infection in AML increases with the degree of neutropenia. Any patient with fever should be thoroughly evaluated for infection.

Differential Diagnosis

Differential diagnosis problems are often encountered in diagnosing and classifying AML. Difficulty in distinguishing AML from ALL or a myelodysplastic syndrome is most common. Other hematopoietic malignancies and, occasionally, leukemoid reactions, agranulocytosis, megaloblastic anemia, and other causes of disrupted hematopoiesis may be considerations in some cases.

Table 29-11   Studies in the Classification of Acute Leukemia*

Morphologically Differentiated		Poorly Differentiated or Undifferentiated	
Morphologic Exam Only	Cytochemical Stains or Immunophenotype are Confirmatory	Cytochemical Stains Essential to Diagnosis	Immunophenotype or EM Essential to Diagnosis
M2	Nonspecific	Myeloperoxidase:	Immunophenotype:
M3,	esterase:	M1	Some L2
hypergranular	M4 and M4e	Some M3V	Immunophenotype
M6	M5b	Nonspecific	and/or EM:
Basophilic	Immunophenotype:	esterase:	M0
differentiated	L1, some L2	M5a	M7 poorly
	L3		differentiated
	M7 differentiated		Mixed lineage
			Basophilic poorly
			differentiated

Abbreviation: EM = electron microscopy.
*From Dick.

Distinguishing AML from ALL is most difficult when the blasts are morphologically poorly differentiated (eg, M0, M1, M5a, M7). A myelodysplastic syndrome may be considered in cases with a relatively low bone marrow blast count. In such situations a diagnosis of AML will be defined by the bone marrow blast percentage, the cytologic features of the blasts, and their cytochemical profile. When a diagnosis of AML cannot be made using these techniques, immunophenotyping studies nearly always clarify the issue. Some cases require other supplementary studies (eg, cytogenetics, electron microscopy). The features that define AML and distinguish it from ALL are covered in detail above (Tables 29-2, 29-5, 29-6, 29-7; and Table 30-5). Table 29-10 lists the major differential diagnosis considerations for the individual FAB classes of AML and the studies most helpful in making a diagnosis. Table 29-11 shows the progressive complexity of diagnostic tests necessary to classify the various types of acute leukemia.

Course and Treatment

All of the categories of AML are presently treated with basically the same chemotherapy regimens. Most patients undergo three phases of chemotherapy: induction, consolidation, and maintenance. The most common induction regimens include a combination of cytosine arabinoside, an anthracycline (daunorubicin or doxorubicin), and, often, 6-thioguanine. This combination induces a complete remission in approximately 70% of patients. Duration of complete remission can be prolonged and cure rates increased by administering consolidation chemotherapy shortly after the patient achieves remission with the same agents used for induction. Maintenance chemotherapy is less important than in ALL, and its use is somewhat controversial; some studies show an improved remission duration but no apparent effect on cure rate. The median length of CR with standard chemotherapy regimens that include postinduction consolidation is about 30 months. Cure rates with chemotherapy alone are between 10% and 30%. Allogeneic bone marrow transplantation in first remission has achieved long-term disease-free survival in 45% to 60% of patients. This is presently the preferred treatment in suitable patients with a matched donor.

The most important indicators of treatment response and survival are:

- Age
- Leukocyte count
- Prior myelodysplastic syndrome
- Speed at which remission is obtained
- Cytogenetic findings

Young individuals, particularly children, have higher remission and disease-free survival rates than older individuals. Very young patients (less than 2 years old) and patients over 60 years of age have the poorest treatment responses and survival. Patients with marked leukocytosis at diagnosis respond more poorly than those with normal or mildly elevated leukocyte counts. Patients with a preceding history of a myelodysplastic syndrome have a lower complete remission rate and a shorter survival time. The rapidity of cytoreduction with chemotherapy and repopulation of the marrow with normal hematopoietic cells is a good indicator of remission duration and survival; patients who experience a rapid complete remission generally fare better than slow responders. Bone marrow cytogenetic findings are also important indicators of prognosis. The utility of cytogenetic studies in AML is discussed in the cytogenetic section above. The chromosome findings that indicate favorable and unfavorable prognosis are shown in Table 29-9.

References

Bennett JM, Catovsky D, Daniel M-T, et al. Proposals for the classification of the acute leukemias. *Br J Haematol.* 1976;33:451-458.

Bennett JM, Catovsky D, Daniel M-T, et al. Criteria for the diagnosis of acute leukemia of megakaryocyte lineage (M7). *Ann Intern Med.* 1985;103:460-462.

Bennett JM, Catovsky D, Daniel M-T, et al. Proposed revised criteria for the classification of acute myeloid leukemia. *Ann Intern Med.* 1985;103:620-625.

Bennett JM, Catovsky D, Daniel M-T, et al. Proposal for the recognition of minimally differentiated acute myeloid leukemia (AML-M0). *Br J Haematol.* 1991;78:325-329.

Bendeaux DH, Glosser L, Serokmann R, Moon T, Duric BG. Hypoplastic acute leukemia: review of 70 cases with multivariate regression analysis. *Hematol Oncol.* 1986;4:291-305.

Berger R, Bernheim A, Daniel M-T, et al. Cytologic characterization and significance of normal karyotypes in t(8;21) AML. *Blood.* 1982;59:171-178.

Bitter MA, LeBeau MM, Larson RA, et al. A morphologic and cytochemical study of acute myelomonocytic leukemia with abnormal marrow eosinophils associated with inv(16)(p13q22). *Am J Clin Pathol.* 1984;81:733-741.

Bitter MA, LeBeau MM, Rowley JD, et al. Associations between morphology, karyotype, and clinical features in myeloid leukemias. *Human Pathol.* 1987;18:211-225.

Brunning RD, McKenna RW. Tumors of the bone marrow: acute leukemias. In: Brunning RD, McKenna RW, eds. *Atlas of Tumor Pathology.* 3rd Series, Fascicle 9. Washington, DC: Armed Forces Institute of Pathology; 1994:19-142.

Cheson BD, Cassileth PA, Head D, et al. Report of the National Cancer Institute-sponsored workshop on definitions of diagnosis and response in acute myeloid leukemia. *J Clin Oncol.* 1990;8:813-819.

Dick F. Evolution of the French-American-British (FAB) proposals: is there a place for acute basophilic leukemia? *Am J Clin Pathol.* 1991;96:153-155.

Groupe Français de Morphologic Hematologique. French Registry of Acute Leukemia and Myelodysplastic Syndromes: age distribution and hemogram analysis of the 4496 cases recorded during 1982-1983 and classified according to FAB criteria. *Cancer.* 1987;50:1385-1394.

Hanson CA. Clinical applications of molecular biology in diagnostic hematopathology. *Lab Med.* 1993;24:562-573.

Holmes R, Keating M, Cork A, et al. A unique pattern of central nervous system leukemia in acute myelomonocytic leukemia associated with inv(16)(p13q22). *Blood.* 1985;65:1071-1078.

McKenna RW, Parkin J, Bloodfield C, Sundberg RD, Brunning RD. Acute promyelocytic leukemia: study of 39 cases with identification of a hyperbasophilic microgranular APL variant. *Br J Haematol.* 1982;50:201-214.

McKenna RW. A multifaceted approach to diagnosis and classification of acute leukemia. *Arch Pathol Lab Med.* 1991;115:328-330.

National Cancer Institute, Division of Cancer Prevention and Control Surveillance Program. *Cancer Statistics Review, 1973-1976.* Bethesda, Md: US Department of Health and Human Services; 1989. Publication NIH 89-2789.

Nicols J, Nimer SD. Transcription factors, translocation, and leukemia. *Blood.* 1992;80:2953-2963.

Peterson LC, Parkin JL, Arthur DC, Brunning RD. Acute basophilic leukemia: a clinical morphologic and cytogenetic study of eight cases. *Am J Clin Pathol.* 1991;96:160-170.

Second MIC Cooperative Study Group. Morphologic, immunologic and cytogenetic (MIC) working classification of AML. *Cancer Genet Cytogenet.* 1988; 30:1-15.

Stanley M, McKenna RW, Ellinger G, Brunning RD. Classification of 358 cases of acute myeloid leukemia by FAB criteria: analysis of clinical and morphologic features. In: Bloomfield CD, ed. *Chronic and Acute Leukemia in Adults.* Boston, Mass: Martinus Nijhoff; 1985:147-174.

Sultan C, Deregnaucourt J, Ko YW, et al. Distribution of 250 cases of acute myeloid leukemia (AML) according to the FAB classification and response to therapy. *Br J Haematol.* 1981;47:545-551.

Yunis JJ, Brunning RD. Prognostic significance of chromosomal abnormalities in acute leukemias and myelodysplastic syndromes. *Clin Haematol.* 1986;15:597-620.

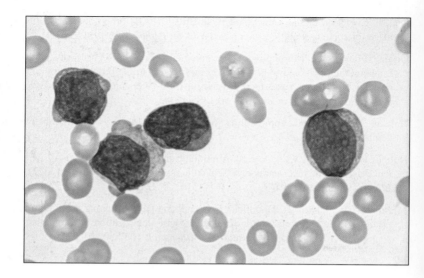

Image 29-1 AML minimally differentiated (M0). The blasts are morphologically poorly differentiated. Myeloperoxidase and nonspecific esterase stains were negative. The myeloid lineage of the blasts was identified by immunophenotyping.

Image 29-2 AML without maturation (M1). More than 90% of the bone marrow cells were myeloblasts; approximately 10% were myeloperoxidase positive. One of the myeloblasts in this field contains a small Auer rod (↑).

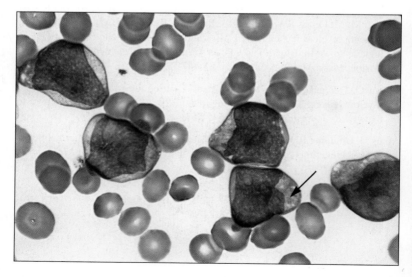

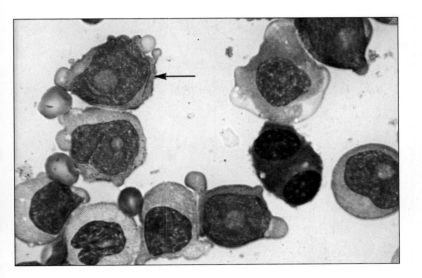

Image 29-3   AML with maturation (M2). Myeloblasts, dysplastic neutrophil precursors, and a dysplastic erythroblast are depicted. One of the myeloblasts contains a large Auer rod (↑).

Image 29-4   Acute promyelocytic leukemia (M3). Most of the cells are abnormal appearing promyelocytes with heavy granulation and reniform nuclei. Multiple Auer rods are present in the cytoplasm of one of the cells (↑).

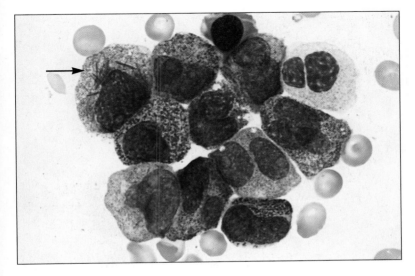

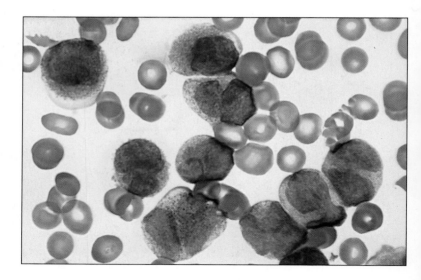

Image 29-5 Acute promyelocytic leukemia, microgranular (hypogranular) variant (M3v). The leukemic cells have smaller and fewer granules than the cells shown in Image 29-4. Most of the nuclei are folded or convoluted.

Image 29-6 Acute myelomonocytic leukemia (M4). Myeloblasts (↑) and promonocytes (↑↑) are depicted.

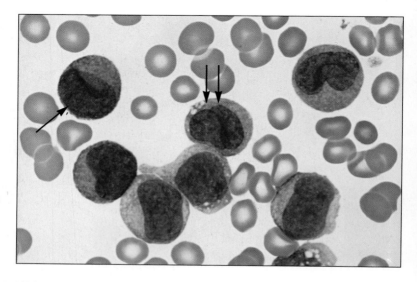

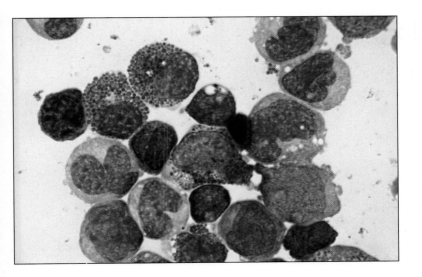

Image 29-7 Acute myelomonocytic leukemia with bone marrow eosinophilia (M4e). Increased bone marrow eosinophils with dysplastic granules characterize this M4 variant. The eosinophil precursor in the center of the field contains large and irregular dark-staining granules in addition to the eosinophil granules.

Image 29-8 Acute monocytic leukemia, poorly differentiated (M5a). The monoblasts have round nuclei and abundant cytoplasm. The lack of morphologic features typical of monocytes requires that a nonspecific esterase stain be performed to classify M5a.

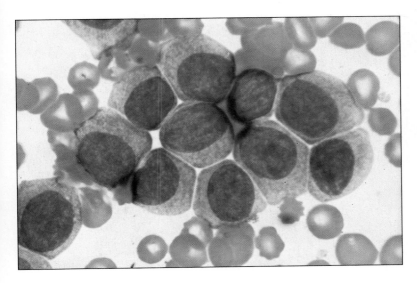

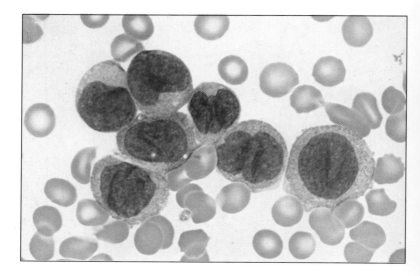

Image 29-9 Acute monocytic leukemia, differentiated (M5b). Promonocytes predominate in M5b.

Image 29-10 Erythroleukemia (M6). More than half of the bone marrow nucleated cells are erythroid. Myeloblasts constitute 30% or more of the nonerythroid cells. Markedly dysplastic changes are noted in the erythroblasts.

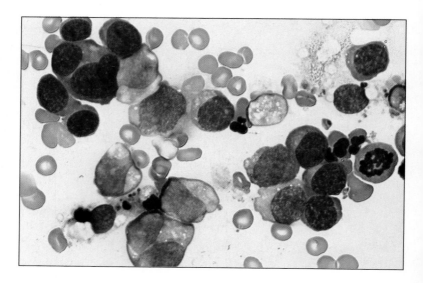

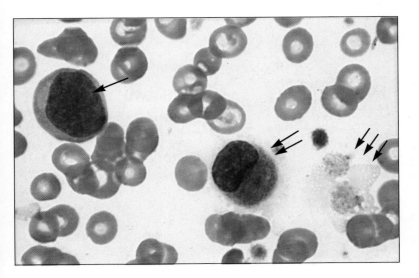

Image 29-11 Acute megakaryoblastic leukemia (M7). A megakaryoblast (↑), micromegakaryocyte (↑↑), and large atypical platelet (↑↑↑) are depicted.

Image 29-12 Acute basophilic leukemia. Blasts with coarse basophilic granules characterize this case. The granules stained metachromatically with a toluidine blue stain. Basophil granules were identified with the electron microscope.

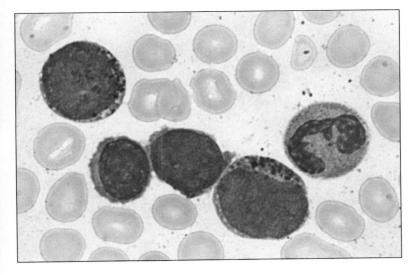

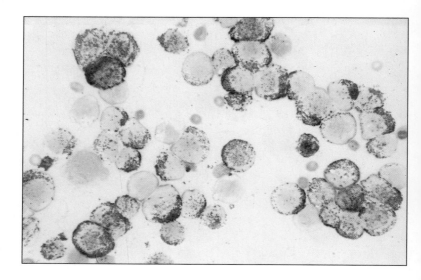

Image 29-13   Myeloperoxidase stain in a case of AML, M2. Most of the cells exhibit myeloperoxidase activity (blue granules).

Image 29-14   Nonspecific esterase stain in a case of AML, M5. The monoblasts exhibit strong alpha-naphthyl butyrate esterase reactivity (brown cytoplasm).

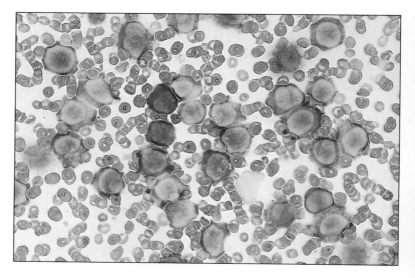

30

Acute Lymphoblastic Leukemia

Acute lymphoblastic leukemia (ALL) is a systemic, neoplastic proliferation of lymphoblasts that have their origin in lymphocyte progenitor cells of the bone marrow or thymus. About 70% of cases of ALL occur in patients less than 17 years of age. It is the most common type of leukemia in this age group, accounting for approximately 80% to 85% of cases.

Pathophysiology

The incidence of ALL is higher in developed than underdeveloped countries and higher among white than black populations. The etiology of ALL is unknown. There are little data supporting any specific environmental factor. However, children exposed to radiation in utero or at a young age appear to have an increased incidence of ALL. Genetic factors presumably play a role in some cases. The monozygotic twin of a patient with ALL has a substantially increased risk of also developing the disease. The incidence of ALL is significantly higher among individuals with certain genetic disorders such as Down syndrome and ataxia telangiectasia.

The leukemic blast cells in ALL express the immunophenotype of committed precursors of B lymphocytes (~85%) or T lymphocytes (~15%). The pattern of antigen expression varies from case to case. Although it has been established that antigen expression in ALL is similar to stages of normal B-cell and T-cell development, aberrancy of antigen expression is noted in most cases. In a minority of cases the blasts express myeloid antigens as well as lymphoid. The blasts in these cases may originate in an earlier defective hematopoietic progenitor cell.

Clinical Findings

Males are affected more commonly than females by a ratio of 1.4 to 1. ALL is most common between the ages of 2 and 10 years. The onset of clinical manifestations may be acute or insidious. The presenting signs and symptoms are similar to those of AML and are usually related to blood cytopenias. Lethargy, malaise, fever, and infection are the most common. Pain in the joints and the extremities is a typical early complaint in children. Symptoms related to bleeding occur in approximately 25% of patients. The most frequent physical findings are pallor, organomegaly, ecchymoses or petechiae, and lymphadenopathy. In a minority of patients the presenting clinical manifestations are caused by extramedullary leukemic infiltrates. Central nervous system (CNS), mediastinal, testicular, renal, and bone and joint involvement are most common but any organ system can be affected. The CNS and the testicles are the major sites of extramedullary relapse. The presenting clinical features in ALL related to pathophysiology are summarized in Table 29-1.

Approach to Diagnosis

Patients generally present with one or more of the clinical manifestations discussed above. These are indicators of a potential diagnosis of acute leukemia and dictate the types of laboratory tests that should be performed. A complete clinical history and physical examination should be followed by the studies listed below.

1. A complete blood count.

2. A blood smear examination.

3. Bone marrow aspiration and trephine biopsy morphologic examination.

4. Appropriate cytochemical studies on blood and bone marrow.

5. Immunophenotyping of leukemic blasts by flow cytometry or immunocytochemistry.

6. Bone marrow cytogenetic studies.

7. Cerebrospinal fluid examination.

8. Radiographic studies for assessment of extramedullary mass disease as indicated.

9. Other biochemical and microbiologic studies as clinically indicated.

Hematologic Findings

The diagnosis of ALL is generally made or suspected from examination of a blood smear. There is nearly always evidence of cytopenias, and in most cases lymphoblasts can be identified as well. The number of recognizable blasts varies from none to several hundred thousand/mm^3. The bone marrow is hypercellular and contains a high percentage of lymphoblasts. The three most important elements of the hematologic evaluation of ALL are:

1. Distinguishing ALL from other types of malignant lymphoproliferative disease or a nonneoplastic disorder.

2. Distinguishing ALL from AML.

3. Morphologic and immunologic classification of ALL.

The features that distinguish ALL from other disorders are discussed in the section on differential diagnosis. The cytologic features that distinguish ALL and AML are listed in Table 29-2. These cytologic features, together with cytochemical and immunophenotypic studies, facilitate correct diagnosis in nearly all cases. The classification of ALL is discussed in the sections on morphologic and immunophenotypic classifications.

Blood Cell Measurements.   Blood counts are abnormal in more than 90% of cases; there is usually bicytopenia or pancytopenia. Anemia is most common and may be mild to severe. The red blood cell indices are generally normochromic and normocytic and the reticulocyte count is decreased. Approximately 75% of patients have platelet counts below 100 x 10³/mm³ (100 x 10⁹/L), and 15% of patients have platelet counts of less than 10 x 10³/mm³ (10 x 10⁹/L). Bleeding is generally found in patients with severely depressed platelet counts.

Approximately one fourth of patients present with leukopenia or leukocyte counts in the low normal range. 50% of patients have leukocyte counts between 5 and 25 x 10³/mm³ (5 and 25 x 10⁹/L), and 10% have leukocyte counts greater than 100 x10³/mm³ (100 x 10⁹/L). Lymphoblasts are present in blood smears in the majority of cases including most of the patients who present with leukopenia. The neutrophil count is usually reduced. The rate of infection increases with the severity of neutropenia.

Blood Smear Morphology.   A decrease in normal blood cells is readily apparent from examination of blood smears. Anemia, usually normochromic-normocytic, is nearly always noted, and a variable degree of neutropenia and thrombocytopenia is observed in most cases. There is frequently a leukoerythroblastic response with variably prominent granulocyte precursors and nucleated red blood cells. Reactive lymphocytes are present in some cases; marked eosinophilia is rarely observed. In most patients lymphoblasts are easily recognized. The number of lymphoblasts varies from a few scattered about the smear to a substantial number causing a profound leukocytosis. Occasionally no lymphoblasts are observed in blood smears and the nature of the cytopenias is revealed only with a bone marrow examination.

Bone Marrow Examination.   The bone marrow smears are hypercellular and consist mostly of lymphoblasts; normal hematopoietic cells are markedly reduced. In most cases the lymphoblasts express the features of L1 ALL (see next section). They are small, approximately twice the size of normal small lymphocytes, with sparse cytoplasm and a high nuclear-cytoplasmic ratio

(Image 30-1). The nucleus is generally round or oval, but some cells have an indented or convoluted nuclear outline. Nucleoli are either not observed or are small and indistinct. The cytoplasm is sparse and variably basophilic; a few vacuoles may be present.

In L2 ALL the majority of lymphoblasts are larger than they are in L1: most exceed twice the size of a normal small lymphocyte. They have moderately abundant cytoplasm and a lower nuclear/cytoplasmic ratio than L1 lymphoblasts (Image 30-2). The nuclear outline is frequently irregular. Nucleoli vary from one to four in number and are often prominent. The cytoplasm is basophilic and may contain vacuoles. A lower nuclear/cytoplasmic ratio and prominent nucleoli are the features most useful in distinguishing L2 from L1 ALL.

The lymphoblasts in L3 ALL are medium-sized to large and morphologically homogeneous (Image 30-3). The nucleus is round to slightly oval. Two to four variably prominent nucleoli are usually observed. The cytoplasm is moderately abundant, deeply basophilic, and usually contains a large number of sharply defined, clear vacuoles. The vacuoles are often the most striking cytologic feature of L3 ALL, which is cytologically identical to small, non-cleaved cell lymphomas, Burkitt's or non-Burkitt's type.

The trephine biopsy sections in ALL are usually markedly hypercellular, though in rare cases the marrow is hypocellular. Normal hematopoietic cells are replaced by a uniform, diffuse proliferation of lymphoblasts. Scattered megakaryocytes and small collections of normoblasts or granulocytes may be present. In rare instances, part or all of the section consists of necrotic tissue.

Morphologic Classification of Acute Lymphoblastic Leukemia

The French-American-British (FAB) Cooperative Group classification system is the one most commonly used. This system separates ALL into three categories, L1, L2, and L3, and defines them according to the cytologic features of the lymphoblasts. The FAB classification criteria are detailed in Table 30-1. Cell size, the amount of cytoplasm, and the prominence of nucleoli are the char-

Table 30-1 FAB Classification of Acute Lymphoblastic Leukemias*

Cytologic Features	L1	L2	L3
Cell size	Small cells predominate	Large, heterogeneous in size	Medium to large and homogeneous
Amount of cytoplasm	Scant	Variable; often moderately abundant	Moderately abundant
Nucleoli	Not visible, or small and inconspicuous	One or more present, often large	One or more present, often prominent
Nuclear shape	Regular; occasional clefting or indentation	Irregular; clefting and indentation common	Regular; oval to round
Nuclear chromatin	Homogeneous in any one case	Variable; heterogeneous in any one case	Finely stippled and homogeneous
Basophilia of cytoplasm	Variable; usually moderate	Variable; occasionally intense	Intensely basophilic
Cytoplasmic vacuolation	Variable	Variable	Prominent

*Modified from Bennett JM, Catovsky D, Daniel M-T, et al. Proposals for the classification of the acute leukemias. French-American-British (FAB) Co-operative Group. *Br J Haematol.* 1976;33:451-458.

acteristics most important in distinguishing L1 from L2. Cytoplasmic basophilia and vacuolation are the important defining characteristics of L3.

In pediatric patients, 80% to 88% of cases of ALL are classified as FAB-L1, 8% to 18% as L2, and 1% to 3% as L3. In adults, 35% to 40% of cases are L1, approximately 60% are L2, and 1% to 3% are L3. In the past the FAB classification appeared to have important prognostic significance, because cases of L2 typically manifested earlier relapse and a shorter median survival period than cases of L1. With present day treatment protocols the distinction between these two groups appears to be less important. However, a poor prognosis is still associated with the small number of cases classified as L3.

Variant Morphologic Features of ALL

Acute Lymphoblastic Leukemia With Cytoplasmic Granules. Granules are observed in the cytoplasm of lymphoblasts in a small percentage of cases of ALL. They stain negatively for myeloperoxidase but have been reported to be Sudan black B positive in rare cases. Several cases of ALL with cytoplasmic granules have been reported in children with Down syndrome or been associated with the Philadelphia chromosome, t(9;22). The presence of cytoplasmic granules in lymphoblasts is important mainly because of the potential for confusion with myeloblasts.

Aplastic Presentation of ALL. On rare occasions, patients with ALL present with pancytopenia and a hypoplastic bone marrow. Leukemic blasts may not be identified initially. This hypocellular phase is typically followed by overt leukemia in a few weeks or months.

Acute Lymphoblastic Leukemia With Eosinophilia. Mild to marked eosinophilia is occasionally noted at diagnosis. In rare instances eosinophilia is profound and obscures a diagnosis of ALL. Some patients have clinical manifestations of the hypereosinophilic syndrome. Eosinophilia generally resolves if a complete remission is achieved but it may return with relapse.

Relapse of Lymphoblastic Leukemia. In most cases the morphology of the lymphoblasts at relapse is similar to the initial diagnostic bone marrow. In a minority of patients there is evolution from L1 to L2; the reverse is rare. Immunophenotypic and karyotypic changes may also be observed at relapse. A summary of the alterations in lymphoblasts at relapse of ALL is shown in Table 30-2.

Secondary AML. Secondary acute myeloid leukemia (therapy-related) has been reported in approximately 2% of patients treated for ALL. Secondary leukemia is presumed to result from the effect of chemotherapy on myeloid stem cells. There appears to be a specific association with the epipodophyllotoxin drugs. An 11q23 chromosome rearrangement is commonly found in secondary AML.

Table 30-2   Changes at Relapse of Acute Lymphoblastic
                   Leukemia*

Morphology
    L1 → L2 (in a minority of cases)
TdT
    Positive → negative (~25%)
Immunologic
    Major phenotype change (rare)
    Gain or loss of an antigen (more common)
        eg, CD10+ → CD10–
        HLA-DR+ → HLA-DR–
Cytogenetic
    Clonal evolution common (~75%)
    One or more new structural abnormalities
Evolution to myeloid leukemia (lineage switch)
    Therapy-related in most cases
    Often associated with 11q23 chromosome abnormality

* Modified from Brunning RD, McKenna RW. Tumors of the bone marrow. Acute lymphoblastic leukemias. *Atlas of Tumor Pathology*. 3rd Series, Fascicle 9. Washington, DC: Armed Forces Institute of Pathology; 1994:100-142.

Other Laboratory Tests

30.1 Cytochemistry

Purpose.   Cytochemical stains are used primarily to help distinguish ALL from AML (see Table 29-6).

Principle, Specimen, and Procedure.   See Test 29.1.

Interpretation.   The cytochemical characteristics of the lymphoblasts in ALL are listed in Table 30-3. Lymphoblasts are always myeloperoxidase negative but have been reported to be Sudan black B positive in rare instances. The periodic acid–Schiff (PAS) stain is positive in 70% to 75% of cases; the stain is distributed in coarse granules or clumps in the cytoplasm and generally corresponds to glycogen deposits (Image 30-4). The vacuoles in the blasts of L3 ALL stain positively

Table 30-3   Cytochemical Reactions in Acute Lymphoblastic Leukemia

	L1		L2	L3
Myeloperoxidase and Sudan black B	–		–	–
Nonspecific esterase	–/+	(focal)	–/+	–
Periodic acid–Schiff	+	(~75%)	+	–
Acid phosphatase	+	(T cell)	+	–
Oil red O	–		–	+ (vacuoles)
Methyl green pyronine	+/–		+/–	+

with the oil red O stain. The cytoplasm stains strongly with a methyl green pyronine (MGP) stain but is PAS negative.

Terminal Deoxynucleotidyl Transferase (TdT). TdT is a unique DNA polymerase found in the nuclei of cortical lymphocytes of normal human thymus and in a small number of normal bone marrow lymphoid cells. TdT is most commonly assayed by immunofluorescent or enzyme immunocytochemical microscopy techniques or by flow cytometry (Image 30-5). In more than 90% of cases of both T-cell and B-cell precursor ALL the lymphoblasts are TdT positive.

Assessment of TdT is useful in distinguishing ALL from AML and from other lymphoproliferative disorders such as adult T-cell leukemia. A positive finding does not by itself exclude AML, because in approximately 5% to 10% of cases the myeloblasts are TdT positive. However, the percentage of positive blasts and the reaction intensity are often significantly less than in ALL.

Up to 10% of the normal lymphoid progenitor cells may be TdT positive in the bone marrow of patients without hematologic malignancies, particularly young children. They are commonly observed in the bone marrow recovery phase following chemotherapy for ALL. The presence of a small number of TdT-positive cells in posttherapy marrow specimens, therefore, should not be interpreted as residual disease or relapse of ALL without supporting morphologic or immunophenotypic evidence.

Table 30-4 Common Monoclonal Antibodies Listed by
Antigen Cluster Designation (CD) for
Characterization of Hematologic Malignancies

CD	Common Names	Spectrum of Activity
CD1	Leu6, T6, OKT6	Immature thymocytes, Langerhans' cells, hairy cells
CD2	Leu5, T11, OKT11	Pan-T cells (E-rosette receptor)
CD3	Leu4, T3, OKT3	Pan-T cells
CD4	Leu3, T4, OKT4	T-helper cells
CD5	Leu1, T1, OKT1	Pan-T cells, rare B cells, B-cell CLL
CD6	T12, TU33, T411	Pan-T cell, rare B cells
CD7	Leu9, 3A1, 4A	T cells and NK cells
CD8	Leu2, T8, OKT8	T-suppressor cells
CD9	J2, BA2	T cells, B cells early myeloid, monocytes, platelets
CD10	CALLA, J5, BA3	Pre-B cells, pre-T cells, common ALL
CD11b	Leu15, Mo1, OKM1, Mo5	T-suppressor cells, monocytes, granulocytes
CD11c	LeuM5	Monocytes, activated T and B lymphocytes, granulocytes, hairy cells
CD13	My7, MCS-2	Myeloid cells, monocytes
CDw14	My4, Mo2	Monocytes, immature granulocytes
CD15	Leu M1, My1, X-hapten	Granulocytes, monocytes, RS cells
CD16	Leu11, VEP 13	Fc IgG receptor on NK cells and neutrophils
CDw17	T5A7	Granulocytes, monocytes
CD19	Leu12, B4	Pan-B cells, not plasma cells
CD20	Leu16, B1	Pan-B cells, not plasma cells
CD21	B2, CR2	Mature B cells in blood, germinal centers and mantle zone
CD22	Leu14, SHCL-1, T015	Pan-B cells
CD23	Tu1, PL13, Blast 2	B cells, not in mantle zone
CD24	BA1	Pan-B cells, granulocytes, plasma cells
CD25	Interleukin-2, Tac	Activated B and T cells, interleukin-2 receptor
CD30	Ki-1, BerH2	RS cells, activated B and T cells
CD33	My9, L4F3	Immature granulocytes
CD34	My10, B1-3C5	Hematopoietic stem cells-progenitor cells
CD38	OK10, Leu17, T16	Thymocytes, activated B and T lymphocytes, plasma cells
CDw41	J15, gpIIb/IIIa	Megakaryocytes
CD45	LCA, T200, T29/33	Leukocytes, usually not plasma cells, sometimes not lymphoblasts

Table 30-4 *Continued*

CD	Common Names	Spectrum of Activity
CD56	Leu19, NKH-1	Natural killer cells, neural adhesion molecule
CD57	Leu7, HNK-1	Natural killer cells, various carcinomas
CD68	KP-1	Monocytes-macrophages, myeloid cells
CD71	OKT9, 5E9, T9	Thymocytes, activated T and B lymphocytes (transferrin receptor)
CD74	LN2	B lymphocytes, postthymic T lymphocytes, myeloid cells
CDw75	LN1	Mature B-cell lymphomas, some postthymic T-cell lymphomas, RS cells
CD103	BLY-7	Hairy cells
—	TdT	B- and T-cell precursors, cortical thymocyte
—	HLA-DR (Ia-like)	B cells, activated T cells, monocytes, early myeloid cells
—	PCA-1	Plasma cells
—	Immunoglobulin light and heavy chains	B lymphocytes
—	HC2	Hairy cells, activated B and T lymphocytes, plasma cells

Abbreviations: CD = cluster designation; CLL = chronic lymphocytic leukemia; NK = natural killer; CALLA = common ALL antigen; ALL = acute lymphoblastic leukemia; RS = Reed-Sternberg.

The TdT assay performed on spinal fluid may be useful in identifying or excluding central nervous system (CNS) involvement in cases of ALL with relatively low spinal fluid cell counts and equivocal morphology.

30.2 Immunophenotyping

Purpose. Immunophenotyping leukemic blasts is important in distinguishing ALL from AML and other lymphoproliferative disorders. The immunophenotypic classification of ALL has prognostic significance.

Principle. The abundance of lineage restricted or associated monoclonal antibodies (MoAbs) and techniques available to immunophenotype hematopoietic cells has added an important dimension to the diagnosis of acute leukemia. In patients with morphologically and cytochemically undifferentiated leukemic blasts, immunophenotyping may be essential in distinguishing ALL from AML. Immunophenotype is also an important prognostic indicator in ALL.

The use of a TdT assay, anti-pan T-cell MoAbs, and anti-pan B-cell MoAbs facilitates identification of most cases of ALL. Anti-pan myeloid MoAbs react with the blasts in the majority of cases of AML. It is important to use panels of MoAbs that include all of the major cell lineages in order to avoid misinterpretations and to recognize phenotypic aberrancy and cases of mixed lineage leukemia. Table 30-4 lists the most common antigen cluster designations (CDs) of MoAbs used in characterizing hematologic malignancies.

Specimen.   Immunophenotyping can be performed by flow cytometry or by immunofluorescent microscopy on cell suspensions from blood, bone marrow, body fluids, or other tissues such as fresh lymph node specimens. For immunophenotyping leukemias, blood or bone marrow are preferred. If blood is the source, there must be enough circulating leukemic cells to assure valid results. Immunophenotyping can also be performed using immunohistochemical methods on blood and bone marrow smears, touch preparations, body fluid cytospin preparations, frozen sections, and paraffin-embedded sections.

Procedure.   Flow cytometry is the method of choice for immunophenotyping cell suspensions of hematopoietic tissues, because it allows a large number of cells to be phenotyped with panels of MoAbs in a relatively short time. An additional advantage of flow cytometry is that expression of two or three antigens can be simultaneously investigated on the same cell. The most common commercially available MoAbs used in characterizing leukemias are listed in Table 30-4. The list includes a spectrum of MoAbs used for detecting T-cell, B-cell, and myeloid-associated antigens.

Many of the commercially available MoAbs can also be applied to immunohistochemical stains on smears and sec-

Table 30-5 Immunologic Classification of Acute Lymphoblastic Leukemia (ALL)

	FAB Class	TdT	T-Cell Restricted Antigens	B-Cell Restricted Antigens	cIg	sIg
T-cell ALL	L1, L2	+	+	−	−	−
B-cell precursor ALL						
Early B-cell precursor ALL	L1, L2	+	−	+	−	−
Pre-B cell ALL	L1, L2	+	−	+	+	−
B-cell ALL	L3	−	−	+	−	+

Abbreviations: FAB = French-American-British; TdT = terminal deoxynucleotidyl transferase; cIg = cytoplasmic immunoglobulin; sIg = surface immunoglobulin.

tions. The immunoalkaline phosphatase techniques are preferable to immunoperoxidase methods for use on blood and bone marrow. Immunohistochemistry is particularly useful when live cell preparations are not available, which makes it impossible to perform flow cytometry.

Interpretation. Several variations of immunologic classification of ALL have been published. Table 30-5 shows a basic, clinically relevant classification system. Approximately 15% of cases of ALL type as immature T cells, and the remainder are derived from B-cell precursors.

T-Cell ALL. The lymphoblasts in T-cell ALL express one or more pan-T antigens such as CD2, CD5, and CD7. Cell surface expression of CD3, which is the most specific T-cell antigen, is lacking in the majority of T-cell ALLs. However, most of these express cytoplasmic CD3. Demonstration of clonal T-cell receptor gene rearrangements has provided additional evidence of T-cell origin in cases stemming from the earliest thymocyte stage.

T-cell ALL can be subclassified into various stages corresponding to thymocyte development by using a panel of MoAbs. Studies have shown a fairly uniform distribution of T-cell ALL at early, intermediate, and mature thymocyte stages, but phenotypic aberrancy is relatively common.

Table 30-6   Clinical Features of T-Cell Acute Lymphoblastic Leukemia (ALL)

Older median age than for non-T ALL
Male predominance
Mediastinal mass in ~50% of cases
High blood leukocyte counts
Often chromosome rearrangements involving 14q11
Earlier relapse than non-T ALL
High incidence of central nervous system relapse
Shorter disease-free survival than for non-T ALL

T-cell ALL may be either FAB-L1 or -L2, but there are distinctive morphologic and cytochemical features in many cases. A minor population of small blasts with little or no cytoplasm and markedly hyperchromatic nuclei, often with prominent nuclear convolution, may be identified in blood and bone marrow smears (Image 30-6). These contrast with a major population of larger leukemic blasts. Numerous mitotic figures are usually observed. The lymphoblasts exhibit strong focal paranuclear acid phosphatase activity in the cytoplasm. The clinical and prognostic features of T-cell ALL are summarized in Table 30-6.

B-Cell Precursor ALL.   Cases previously classified as non-T, non-B ALL are now designated B-cell precursor ALL. These leukemias are divided into subtypes based on expression of various B-associated or B-restricted surface antigens, cytoplasmic immunoglobulin (cIg), and surface immunoglobulin (sIg).

Most cases of non-T ALL lack cIg and sIg but express one or more other B-associated or B-restricted antigens, including HLA-DR, CD10, CD19, CD20, and CD22. These are often designated early B-cell precursor ALL and are the most common category (~65%) of cases. Molecular studies for immunoglobulin gene rearrangements have provided further evidence that cIg and sIg negative non-T ALLs are of early B-cell precursor lineage. Expression of cytoplasmic μ chains (cIg) in addition to other B-cell antigens is identified in the lymphoblasts in 15% to 20% of cases of ALL. These cases are designated pre-B ALL (cIg+).

Table 30-7   Clinical Features of B-Cell ALL (sIg+)

Older median age than other B-precursor ALLs
High incidence of extramedullary disease
High incidence of central nervous system disease
Chromosome translocations involving 8q24
Poor response to therapy, earlier relapse
Shorter survival than for other B-precursor ALLs

Abbreviations: ALL = acute lymphoblastic leukemia; sIg = surface immunoglobulin.

The lymphoblasts in 1% to 3% of cases of ALL express monoclonal surface immunoglobulin (sIg) and pan-B cell antigens and lack TdT. These cases are often designated B-cell ALL or sIg-positive ALL (Image 30-3). Extramedullary mass disease is usually present, often in the abdominal cavity, and is clinical evidence that a relatively high percentage of these cases represent blood and bone marrow involvement by small, noncleaved cell lymphoma. Table 30-7 lists distinctive clinical features of B-cell ALL.

Asynchronous and Mixed Phenotype Acute Leukemia.

More than half of the cases of B-cell precursor ALL involve simultaneous expression of combinations of early and late antigens not present in normal lymphocyte development. Asynchronous antigen expression is also found in T-cell ALL.

In some cases the lymphoblasts express one or more myeloid-associated antigens in addition to lymphoid antigens. This mixed phenotype expression may result from a mixed lineage leukemia in which the leukemic blasts coexpress both lymphoid and myeloid antigens, or it may result from a bilineal leukemia in which individual leukemic cells express either lymphoid or myeloid characteristics but not both (Image 30-7). In cases of the latter type the two blast populations may have different morphologic, cytochemical, and ultrastructural features as well.

In adults with ALL, the presence of myeloid antigen positive blasts indicates poor prognosis. Prognostic studies in children have been inconclusive. There is an increased incidence of chromosome translocations involving 11q23, 14q32, or a

Table 30-8 Correlation of Cytogenetic Findings With
Immunophenotype and FAB Category in Acute
Lymphoblastic Leukemia (ALL)

Most Common Cytogenetic Findings	Immunophenotypic Category	FAB Category
Translocations of 14q11; diploid chromosomes	T cell	L1, L2
Hyperploidy >50; hyperdiploidy 47-50; variable structural changes	Early B-cell precursor	L1, L2
t(1;19)	Pre B (cIg+)	L1, L2
t(8;14), t(2;8), or t(8;22)	B cell (sIg+)	L3
t(11;variable) (q23;V); t(9;22); t(14;variable) (q32;V)	Mixed phenotype ALL	L1, L2

Abbreviations: FAB = French-American-British; cIg = cytoplasmic immunoglobulin; sIg = surface immunoglobulin.

t(9;22) in mixed phenotype ALL. Translocations involving these chromosomes are associated with a poor prognosis in all age groups.

With the increase in the number of myeloid- and lymphoid-associated monoclonal antibodies and the availability of more sensitive techniques to study leukemias, an increasing number of cases exhibiting coexpression of antigens are being identified.

Phenotypic Changes at Relapse.   The consistency of major immunophenotype is generally maintained at relapse (Table 30-2). Changes from a T-cell to a B-cell precursor phenotype or vice versa have been reported only rarely. Losses or gains of individual antigens without a major evolution of immunophenotype are more common. Losses of TdT, HLA-DR, or CD10 expression are the most frequently reported alterations.

Ancillary Tests

Cytogenetics.   Bone marrow cytogenetic studies supplement the morphologic and immunophenotypic classifications of ALL. Their greatest value is in identifying prognostic groups. Tables 30-8 and 30-9 summarize the relationship between bone

Table 30-9 Correlation of Prognosis With Bone Marrow Cytogenetic Findings in Acute Lymphoblastic Leukemia*

Chromosome Findings	Prognosis
Hyperdiploidy >50 chromosomes	Good
Hyperdiploidy 47-50 chromosomes	Intermediate
Diploid chromosomes	Intermediate
Chromosome translocations	Poor
Hypodiploidy	Poor

*From Pui CH, Crist WM, Look AT. Biology and clinical significance of cytogenetic abnormalities in childhood acute lymphoblastic leukemia. *Blood.* 1990;76:1449-1463.

marrow karyotype and morphologic, immunophenotypic, and prognostic groups.

When studied with refined cytogenetic techniques, at least 80% to 90% of cases of ALL exhibit demonstrable chromosome abnormalities. Structural abnormalities are most common, either alone or in combination with numerical changes. The following discussion focuses on the most common and clinically relevant changes.

Hyperdiploidy with more than 50 chromosomes (hyperdiploidy >50) is found in approximately 25% of cases of childhood ALL. It is associated with favorable clinical features, including low leukocyte counts, white race, and patient age between 2 and 10 years. The 5-year survival rate for children with hyperdiploidy >50 is approximately 80%.

Hypodiploidy is present in 3% to 9% of cases. Most of these patients have 45 chromosomes; chromosome 20 is commonly lost. Patients with hypodiploidy are considered an intermediate to poor prognostic group, owing largely to a high percentage of cases with translocations.

Pseudodiploidy (46 chromosomes but with structural abnormalities) is found in approximately 40% of children with ALL and a higher percentage of adults. Pseudodiploidy is associated with a poor prognosis because of the high percentage of cases involving chromosome translocations. Structural changes may also be found in the other numerical groups except diploid. The most common translocations are described below.

The Philadelphia (Ph[1]) chromosome, t(9;22)(q34; q11), is identified in approximately 2% of children and 20% of adults with ALL. Ph[1]+ ALL is associated with an older age of onset, high presenting leukocyte counts, L2 morphology, B-cell precursor immunophenotype, and central nervous system (CNS) involvement. The prognosis is unfavorable in both children and adults.

Translocation (1;19) (q23; p13) is found in about 25% of cases of pre-B ALL (cIg+) and 1% of early B-cell precursor ALL (cIg–). It is the most common translocation in childhood ALL, with an overall incidence of 5% to 6%, and is particularly common in black children. The poor prognosis ascribed to pre-B ALL (cIg+) is strongly associated with t(1;19).

Reciprocal translocations involving chromosome 8q24, L3 morphology, and B-cell phenotype (sIg+) are found in 1% to 3% of cases of ALL (Image 30-3). The most common translocation is t(8;14) (p24;q32.3). The *myc* proto-oncogene on chromosome 8 assumes a position adjacent to the heavy chain gene or one of the light chain genes. A large malignant cell burden, CNS disease, and a poor prognosis are common in these cases.

Forty to fifty percent of cases of T-cell ALL involve translocations. In approximately half of them, break points are in the locations of the T-cell receptor (TCR) genes; t(11;14) (p13;q11) is the most common. The presence of these chromosome abnormalities correlates with poor prognosis.

Rearrangement of chromosome 11q23 is found in less than 5% of childhood ALL. Translocation (4;11) (q21;q23) is the most common (Image 30-7). It is associated with very young children, markedly elevated leukocyte counts, splenomegaly, and a poor prognosis. Many ALLs with an 11q23 abnormality are mixed phenotype leukemias.

Cytogenetic evolution from diagnosis to relapse is common in ALL (Table 30-2). The karyotype changes at relapse are generally related to those at diagnosis with the addition of new structural abnormalities.

Cerebrospinal Fluid (CSF) Analysis. CNS involvement is the most significant extramedullary manifestation of ALL. It is most commonly encountered at diagnosis in T-cell or B-cell (sIg+) ALL but is found in early B-cell precursor and pre-B ALL as well.

The CNS is also a common site of relapse with or without bone marrow relapse. Due to the high incidence of CNS relapse, CNS prophylactic therapy is included in ALL treatment protocols. Morphologic examination of CSF should be performed in all cases of ALL at diagnosis and periodically during the course of maintenance therapy. Cytocentrifuge preparations of CSF are preferred for morphologic examination. When the CSF is involved the cell count varies from occasional to numerous lymphoblasts. When only a few are present their identity may be difficult to establish. The TdT assay or immunophenotyping by immunofluorescent microscopy or immunocytochemical methods may assist in characterizing the leukemic cells.

Differential Diagnosis

A number of disorders may present with clinical or morphologic manifestations similar to those of ALL. Several are listed in Table 30-10. Most of these conditions can be distinguished from ALL by careful morphologic examination of blood and bone marrow. Cytochemistry, immunophenotyping, and electron microscopy or molecular studies may be required in some cases. Three of the most common and difficult considerations in the differential diagnosis are discussed below.

Acute Myeloid Leukemia.   The categories of AML that are poorly differentiated morphologically are most likely to be confused with ALL. These categories of AML—M0, M1, M5a, and M7—can be distinguished from ALL on the basis of the myeloperoxidase and nonspecific esterase stains and the profile of antigen expression by flow cytometry or immunohistochemical methods.

Increased Normal Bone Marrow Lymphocyte Progenitor Cells.   Bone marrow aspirate specimens from young children often contain increased numbers of marrow lymphocyte progenitor cells. Many of these small lymphoid cells have morphologic features in common with the lymphoblasts of ALL (Image 30-8). These cells are frequently referred to as "hematogones" in the literature. They are found in large numbers in normal

Table 30-10   Considerations in the Differential Diagnosis of
Acute Lymphoblastic Leukemia

Acute myeloid leukemia
Increased bone marrow lymphoid progenitor cells (hematogones)
Metastatic small cell tumors
Reactive lymphocytosis
Hypoplastic anemia
Chronic lymphocytic leukemia
Adult T-cell leukemia
Prolymphocytic leukemia
Non-Hodgkin's lymphoma

infants and in a number of diverse disease processes in children past infancy. When encountered in the bone marrow of children undergoing evaluation for cytopenias or organomegaly, a diagnosis of lymphoblastic leukemia or lymphoma may be considered. Regenerative marrow following chemotherapy for ALL also typically contains increased numbers of lymphoid progenitor cells. In this setting there is potential for misinterpreting them as residual or recurrent leukemic lymphoblasts.

Many marrow lymphocyte progenitor cells are TdT positive and express early and pan-B cell antigens (eg, HLA-DR, CD10, and CD19). They do not express immunophenotypic aberrancy, however, which may be helpful in distinguishing them from the lymphoblasts of B-cell precursor ALL. DNA content is also normal and there is no evidence of clonality by either cytogenetic or immunogenotypic analysis.

Metastatic Small Cell Tumors. Metastatic small cell tumors in children occasionally present with extensive marrow involvement in the absence of an identifiable primary tumor mass. Primary clinical manifestations may be related to blood cytopenias or a leukemoid reaction. In some cases the neoplastic cells in this group of tumors resemble lymphoblasts in bone marrow smears. Neuroblastoma is the most common of these; embryonal rhabdomyosarcoma, retinoblastoma, Ewing's sarcoma, and medulloblastoma may also mimic ALL. Clues to the correct diagnosis include the presence of neoplastic cells in clumps or clusters on bone marrow smears. Large numbers of bare nuclei and damaged cells may also be observed throughout the smears. The distinction between metastatic disease and ALL is usually apparent in trephine biopsy sections. In equivocal cases, TdT assays, immunopheno-typing, electron microscopy, and enzyme immunocytochemistry using appropriate antibodies for the characterization of small cell tumors facilitate the correct diagnosis.

Course and Treatment

The prognosis for children with ALL has improved dramatically during the past three decades. For B-cell precursor ALL, standard induction chemotherapy protocols that include vincristine, pred-nisone, L-asparaginase, and daunorubicin produce a complete remission in more than 95% of cases. With central nervous system prophylaxis and maintenance chemotherapy, more than half of children with ALL will achieve long-term disease-free survival and presumably be cured. With additional postinduction intensive chemotherapy, overall cure rates may soon improve to 70%.

For high-risk types of ALL, treatment results are less favor-able. More aggressive therapy with higher doses of standard chemotherapy agents plus additional drugs has improved long-term disease-free survival in children with T-cell ALL to 40% to 50% in some cancer treatment centers. Allogeneic bone marrow transplantation for children with high-risk ALL and patients who relapse after standard chemotherapy provides another potentially curative treatment. Adults with ALL fare more poor-ly than children. This is partly because of the higher frequency of bad prognostic features such as the t(9;22) chromosome rearrangement.

Several clinical, morphologic, immunophenotypic, and cyto-genetic parameters have been identified as indicators of prognosis. Table 30-11 lists some of the most commonly considered factors. The significance of these factors varies in different studies. Some indicators of poor prognosis presently have less significance in predicting survival because management of high-risk ALL has recently improved.

Table 30-11   Prognostic Indicators in Acute Lymphoblastic Leukemia (ALL)*

	Favorable	Less Favorable
Clinical		
Age	1 to 10 yrs	<1 and >10 yrs
Sex	Female	Male
Race	White	Black
WBC count	$<10 \times 10^3/mm^3$ ($10 \times 10^9/L$)	$>50 \times 10^3/mm^3$ ($50 \times 10^9/L$)
Rapidity of cytoreduction	Bone marrow free of disease by day 14	Residual disease at day 14
Relapse	No relapse	Relapse
Morphologic	L1	L2, L3
Immunophenotypic	Early B-cell precursor, CD10+	Pre-B (cIg+), CD10–, T-ALL, B-ALL
Cytogenetic	Hyperdiploidy >50 chromosomes	Translocations [especially t(9;22) and t(4;11)]

*From Brunning RD, McKenna RW. Tumors of the bone marrow. Acute lymphoblastic leukemias *Atlas of Tumor Pathology*. 3rd Series, Fascicle 9. Washington, DC: Armed Forces Institute of Pathology; 1994:100-142.

References

Behm FG. Morphologic and cytochemical characteristics of childhood lymphoblastic leukemia. *Hematol Oncol Clin North Am.* 1990;4:715-741.

Bennett JM, Catovsky D, Daniel M-T, et al. Proposals for the classification of the acute leukemias. French-American-British (FAB) Co-operative Group. *Br J Haematol.* 1976;33:451-458.

Bennett JM, Catovsky D, Daniel M-T, et al. The morphological classification of acute lymphoblastic leukemia: concordance among observers and clinical correlations. *Br J Haematol.* 1981;47:553-561.

Bleyer WH. Acute lymphoblastic leukemia in children. *Cancer.* 1990;65:689-695.

Borowitz MJ. Immunological markers in childhood acute lymphoblastic leukemia. *Hematol Oncol Clin North Am.* 1990;4:743-765.

Brunning RD, McKenna RW. Tumors of the bone marrow. Acute lymphoblastic leukemias. *Atlas of Tumor Pathology*. 3rd Series, Fascicle 9. Washington, DC: Armed Forces Institute of Pathology; 1994:100-142.

National Cancer Institute, Division of Cancer Prevention and Control Surveillance Program. *Cancer Statistics Review 1973–1986.* Bethesda, Md: US Department of Health and Human Services, 1989; publication NIH 89-2789.

Crist W, Boyett J, Pullen J, et al. Clinical and biological features predict poor prognosis in acute lymphoid leukemias in children and adolescents: a pediatric oncology group review. *Med Pediatr Oncol.* 1986;14:135-143.

Gaynon PS. Primary treatment of childhood acute lymphoblastic leukemia of non-T cell lineage (including infants). *Hematol Oncol Clin North Am.* 1990;4:915-936.

Hammond D, Sather H, Nesbit M, et al. Analysis of prognostic factors in acute lymphoblastic leukemia. *Med Pediatr Oncol.* 1986;14:1240-1254.

Homans AC, Barker BE, Forman EN, Cornell CJ, Dickerman JP, Truman JT. Immunophenotypic characteristics of cerebral spinal fluid cells in children with acute lymphoblastic leukemia at diagnosis. *Blood.* 1990;76:1807-1811.

Hurwitz CA, Mirro J. Mixed lineage leukemia and asynchronous antigen expression. *Hematol Oncol Clin North Am.* 1990;4:767-794.

Kurec AS, Belair P, Stefanu C, Barrett DM, Dubowy RL, Davey FR. Significance of aberrant lymphophenotypes in childhood acute lymphoid leukemia. *Cancer.* 1991;67:3081-3086.

Leitenberg D, Rappeport JM, Smith BR. B-cell precursor bone marrow reconstitution after bone marrow transplantation. *Am J Clin Pathol.* 1994;102:231-236.

Lilleyman JS, Hann IM, Stevens RF, et al. Cytomorphology of childhood acute lymphoblastic leukemia: a prospective study of 2000 patients. *Br J Haematol.* 1992;81:52-57.

Longacre TA, Foucar K, Crago S, et al. Hematogones: a multiparameter analysis of bone marrow precursor cells. *Blood.* 1989;73:543-552.

Pui CH, Ribeiro PC, Hancock ML, et al. Acute myeloid leukemia in children treated with epipodophyllotoxins for acute lymphoblastic leukemia. *N Engl J Med.* 1991;325:1682-1687.

Pui CH, Crist WM, Look AT. Biology and clinical significance of cytogenetic abnormalities in childhood acute lymphoblastic leukemia. *Blood.* 1990; 76:1449-1463.

Pui CH, Raimondi SC, Behm FG, et al. Shifts in blast phenotype and karyotype at relapse of childhood lymphoblastic leukemia. *Blood.* 1986;68:1306-1310.

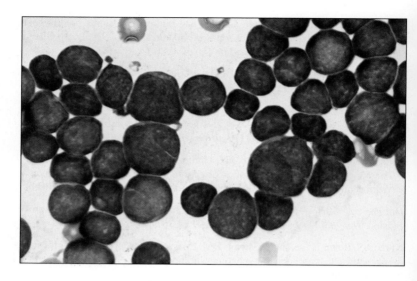

Image 30-1 L1 ALL. The lymphoblasts are small with little cytoplasm and lack nucleoli.

Image 30-2 L2 ALL. The lymphoblasts are larger than L1 blasts, have more cytoplasm, and contain distinct nucleoli.

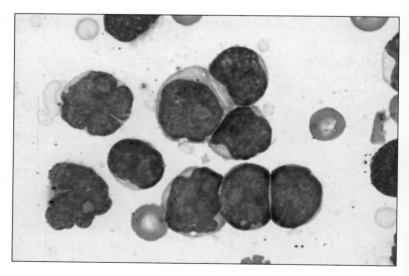

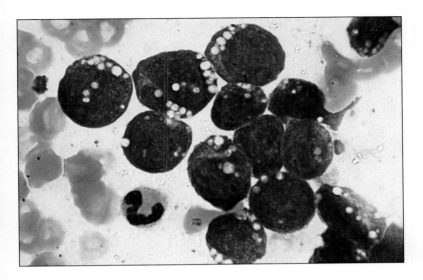

Image 30-3   L3 ALL. The lymphoblasts are large and have a moderate amount of deeply basophilic cytoplasm that contains numerous sharply defined clear vacuoles. The nuclei are round with relatively coarse chromatin; nucleoli are observed in some of the cells.

Image 30-4   A PAS stain on a bone marrow smear from a child with ALL. The lymphoblasts exhibit coarse granular and block PAS positivity.

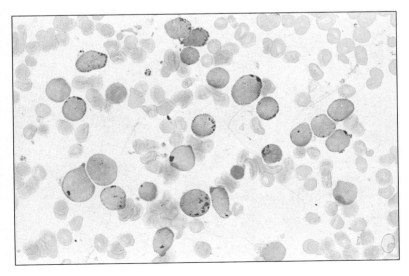

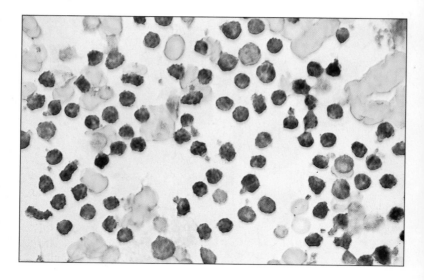

Image 30-5 Immunohistochemical (immunoperoxidase) reaction for TdT on a bone marrow smear from a child with ALL. The lymphoblasts show a nuclear distribution of reactivity for TdT.

Image 30-6 A blood smear from a young man with T-cell ALL and a markedly elevated leukocyte count. The lymphoblasts are heteromorphous. The minor population consists of small lymphoblasts with hyperchromatic, convoluted nuclei.

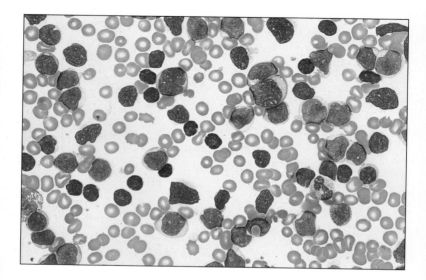

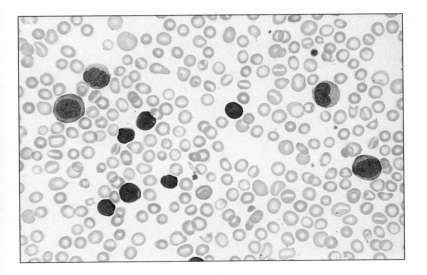

Image 30-7 Bilineal leukemia. A blood smear from a neonate with congenital leukemia. The leukemic blast population expresses morphologic, cytochemical, and immunophenotypic markers of two separate lineages; lymphoblasts (small); and monoblasts-promonocytes (large).

Image 30-8 A bone marrow aspirate smear from a 3-year-old healthy child who was a bone marrow transplant donor for a sibling with aplastic anemia. There are several lymphoid progenitor cells (hematogones) (↑) in the field. These normal cells may resemble leukemic lymphoblasts morphologically and immunophenotypically.

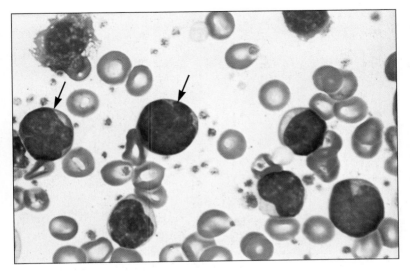

Myeloproliferative Disorders

PART
III

Myeloproliferative Disorders

31

Myelofibrosis

The term "myeloproliferative disorder" (MPD) was introduced to describe a group of closely related syndromes—chronic myelogenous leukemia (CML), polycythemia vera, myelofibrosis (MF) with myeloid metaplasia, and essential thrombocythemia (Table 31-1). These disorders have similar clinical and hematologic manifestations at some stage in the disease processes (Table 31-2). Polycythemia vera, essential thrombocythemia, and CML are described in Chapters 32, 33, and 34, respectively, and this chapter will be confined to a discussion of MF with myeloid metaplasia, a clinical and pathological state common to all of these disorders and to other hematologic and nonhematologic disorders as well.

Pathophysiology

A large number of synonyms have been used for MF with myeloid metaplasia, including idiopathic MF, chronic myelosclerosis, agnogenic myeloid metaplasia, aleukemic megakaryocytic myelosis, and leukoerythroblastic anemia. These names usually indicate the feature of the disease most striking to the observer. The disorder is clonal in nature, arising from an abnormal multipotent hematopoietic stem cell. Unlike CML, no specific cytogenetic abnormality

Table 31-1   Classification of Myeloproliferative Disorders

Polycythemia vera
Chronic myelogenous leukemia
Myelofibrosis with myeloid metaplasia
Essential thrombocythemia

Table 31-2   Common Features of Myeloproliferative Disorders

Similar clinical manifestations
    Asymptomatic, or fatigue, bleeding, splenomegaly
Peripheral blood
    Anemia with variable red blood cell changes
    Variable degrees of leukocytosis with immature cells
    Variable degrees of eosinophilia and basophilia
    Qualitative and quantitative platelet abnormalities
Bone marrow
    Panmyelosis with variable degrees of myelofibrosis
Spleen
    Extramedullary hematopoiesis
Apparent "transitional" forms between various types
Accelerated phase or "blastic" crisis common in terminal stages

has been described. There are variable degrees of fibrosis in the bone marrow and a variable proliferation of the granulocytic, erythrocytic, and megakaryocytic series in the bone marrow, spleen, liver, and lymph nodes. It is thought that abnormal megakaryocyte precursors release growth factors (platelet factor IV and platelet-derived growth factor) that stimulate fibroblasts, causing the fibrosis in the marrow. MF may be secondary to a known cause, such as metastatic carcinoma (Figure 31-1). Patients suffering from MF characteristically have an enlarged spleen, the degree of which may be considerable. The cause of the splenomegaly is a combination of vascular expansion, tremendous red cell pooling, hematopoietic hyperplasia, and fibrosis.

Recent studies have not demonstrated a correlation between the extent of marrow fibrosis and duration of disease, splenic weight, or degree of splenic myeloid metaplasia. Likewise, studies have been unable to document a progression of marrow fibrosis as a cause for the increase in splenomegaly.

Several theories have been postulated to explain extramedullary hematopoiesis in MF. One states that circulating hematopoi-

Figure 31-1   Conditions associated with myelofibrosis.

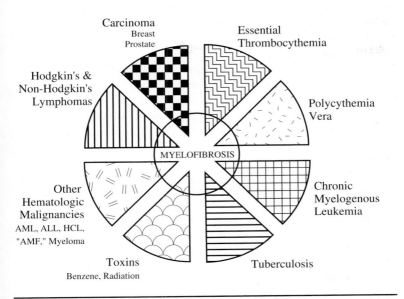

etic precursors are filtered from the peripheral blood by the spleen and accumulate there. If not phagocytosed, these cells proliferate and are released, resulting in the leukoerythroblastosis characteristic of this disorder. Autonomous hematopoiesis may occur later in the course of the disease. The characteristic features of this disorder are listed in Table 31-3.

Clinical Findings

The MPDs usually have an insidious onset. The patient may present with a long history of weakness or may be relatively asymptomatic. In MF with myeloid metaplasia, patients develop a variety of symptoms, including malaise, weight loss, bleeding, diarrhea, and fever. Splenomegaly is the main physical finding and may be associated with abdominal discomfort, pain, indigestion, or dyspnea. Other features that may be present include hepatomegaly, petechiae and bleeding (usually secondary to thrombocytopenia or abnormal platelet function, or both), ascites, jaundice, portal hypertension, cirrhosis, and rarely, lymphadenopathy.

Table 31-3   Characteristics of Idiopathic Myelofibrosis

Insidious onset with weakness, weight loss, pallor
Splenomegaly
Normochromic anemia
Red blood cell morphology
    Prominent poikilocytosis (teardrop forms) and anisocytosis
Nucleated red blood cells common in peripheral blood
White blood cell count
    Elevated ($<30 \times 10^3$/mm^3 [30×10^9/L]), normal or rarely decreased,
        immature granulocytes, occasional myeloblasts, mild eosinophilia, and
        basophilia
Platelet count
    Increased, normal or decreased; giant platelets, micromegakaryocytes, and
        megakaryocytic fragments
Bone marrow
    Panmyelosis with increasing myelofibrosis

Approach to Diagnosis

Following a clinical history and physical examination with attention to the presence of splenomegaly, the laboratory diagnosis of MF with myeloid metaplasia proceeds in the following sequence:

1. A complete blood count.
2. Examination of the peripheral blood smear.
3. Examination of the bone marrow.
4. Cytogenetic studies.

See Figure 32-1 for an algorithm for the differential diagnosis of MF and the other chronic MPDs.

Hematologic Findings

The hematologic findings in MF are variable and depend on the stage of the disease. As expected, there is considerable overlap among the different chronic MPDs. Myelodysplastic syndrome may be extremely difficult to differentiate from MF with myeloid metaplasia. The former usually does not have significant splenomegaly or the teardrop red blood cell morphology typically

Table 31-4 Conditions Associated With Myelofibrosis and/or Leukoerythroblastosis

Nonmalignant	Malignant
Tuberculosis	Myeloproliferative disorders
Gaucher's disease	Acute and chronic leukemias
Radiation	Hodgkin's disease
Renal osteodystrophy	Non-Hodgkin's lymphomas
Paget's disease of bone	Plasma cell myeloma
Benzene	Metastatic carcinomas
Congenital syphilis	

present in MF. In the differential diagnosis of MF with myeloid metaplasia, other conditions associated with bone marrow fibrosis and leukoerythroblastosis must be considered (Table 31-4).

Blood Cell Measurements. In MF with myeloid metaplasia, initially there is a mild normochromic, normocytic anemia, which becomes progressively more severe. The leukocyte count may be slightly increased, usually less than 30 x 10^3/mm³ (30 x 10^9/L), or decreased. The platelet count is initially normal or high. As the disease progresses, thrombocytopenia and leukopenia are common.

Peripheral Blood Smear Morphology. In MF, the whole spectrum of granulocytic precursors may be seen, and the blood smear resembles a granulocytic leukemoid reaction. The percentage of blasts varies from 0% to 10%, and the presence of blasts in the peripheral blood does not necessarily indicate an accelerated phase or blast crisis. Eosinophilia and basophilia may be present but are usually less marked than in CML. In addition to immature granulocytes, there is usually a small number of nucleated red blood cells, which, together with the immature granulocytes, constitute the so-called leukoerythroblastic picture (Image 31-1). The red blood cell morphology usually includes a significant degree of anisocytosis, poikilocytosis, and polychromasia. Teardrop forms (dacryocysts) and ovalocytes are common in MF. Hypochromic microcytic cells may be present in patients who have developed iron deficiency caused by bleeding. Platelets will often exhibit abnormal morphology and may be extremely large. Fragments of megakaryocytes or micromegakaryocytes may also be seen.

Bone Marrow Examination. In MF, aspiration of the bone marrow often results in a dry tap. A bone marrow biopsy must always be performed in patients in whom a diagnosis of chronic MPD is being considered. Early in the course of MF, the bone marrow may not show striking abnormalities except for hypercellularity with an increased number of all cell lines. All stages of maturation are represented. This is the so-called cellular phase of MF (Image 31-2). Usually an increased proportion of neutrophilic precursors and megakaryocytes are seen. The megakaryocytes occur in clusters, are frequently abnormal in size and shape, and may be difficult to recognize as megakaryocytes. The marrow sinusoids are characteristically distended.

A reticulin stain is necessary to detect early fibrosis. The amount of fibrosis increases as the disease progresses (Image 31-3). The marrow gradually becomes less cellular, and the megakaryocytes persist until fibrosis is the predominant feature (Image 31-4). Formation of collagen in the marrow is associated with the appearance of extramedullary hematopoiesis of spleen, liver, and sometimes lymph nodes. The degree of marrow fibrosis does not, however, necessarily correlate with the duration of the disease and splenic myeloid metaplasia. In addition to MF, increasing osteosclerosis may be seen.

Other Laboratory Tests

31.1 Leukocyte Alkaline Phosphatase (LAP)

Purpose. The LAP score may be useful in differentiating CML from other MPDs.

Principle, Specimen, and Procedure. See Test 16.1.

Interpretation. In CML, the LAP score is characteristically zero or markedly decreased, although it is usually elevated in the other MPDs. In MF with myeloid metaplasia, however, the LAP score may be high, normal, or low. Low scores are particularly common in patients with low white blood cell counts. Therefore, a low LAP score does not rule out MF with myeloid metaplasia.

31.2 Cytogenetic Studies

Purpose. Cytogenetic studies may be useful in distinguishing CML from the other MPDs.

Principle, Specimen, and Procedure.   See Test 34.2.

Interpretation.   The Philadelphia (Ph^1) chromosome, which is present in most cases of CML, is absent in MF. Several chromosome changes have been observed in the MPDs, but none is specific, except for the Ph^1 chromosome.

Ancillary Tests

Platelet Aggregation Studies.   Bleeding problems occur in all of the MPDs. The bleeding may be caused by thrombocytopenia or by a defect in platelet function. The latter is manifest as impairment of in vitro platelet aggregation, most typically impaired responses to epinephrine and collagen.

Blood Biochemistry.   Serum uric acid level is frequently elevated and may lead to gouty arthritis, urate stones, and nephropathy, particularly in patients with a high leukocyte count. In addition, the serum alkaline phosphatase level may be elevated, which may be a reflection of extramedullary hematopoiesis in the liver. Increased lactic dehydrogenase levels are also seen.

Radiology.   Osteosclerosis has been demonstrated in approximately 50% of patients with MF and myeloid metaplasia. The bones most frequently affected are (in order of frequency) femur, pelvis, vertebrae, radius, tibia, and sternum. Foci of rarefaction may also be seen.

Biopsy of Tissue Other Than Bone Marrow.   Extra-medullary hematopoiesis may be associated with lymph node enlargement. Biopsy of a lymph node usually reveals normal architecture and a mixed proliferation of hematopoietic cells in the sinuses. Atypical megakaryocytes may predominate. This

Table 31-5   Differential Characteristics of Chronic Myeloproliferative Syndromes

Variable	Myelofibrosis Myeloid Metaplasia	Essential Thrombocythemia
Hemoglobin	Decreased	Normal or decreased
Leukocyte count	Usually <30 x 10³/mm³ (30 x 10⁹/L)	Usually <20 x 10³/mm³ (20 x 10⁹/L)
Differential count	Moderate number of immature granulocytes	Usually normal
Eosinophilia and/or basophilia	Usually present	May be present
Red blood cell morphology	Anisocytosis and teardrop poikilocytosis	Normal or hypochromic, microcytic
Nucleated red blood cells in blood	Common	Rare
Platelet count	Normal, increased, or decreased	Increased
Bone marrow	Hypercellular with increasing fibrosis	Hypercellular with megakaryocytosis
LAP	Variable, usually increased	Usually normal
Ph¹	Absent	Absent
Splenomegaly	Marked	Absent or mild

Abbreviations: CML = chronic myelogenous leukemia; LAP = leukocyte alkaline phosphatase; Ph1 = Philadelphia chromosome.

extramedullary hematopoiesis can exhibit such bizarre morphology that it may be mistaken for a malignant lymphoma or metastatic carcinoma. A chloroacetate esterase stain is helpful in confirming the presence of granulocytic precursors.

Course and Treatment

Patients exhibiting MF with myeloid metaplasia usually show a gradual, progressive deterioration that is associated with increasing splenomegaly and fibrosis of the marrow. Anemia becomes progressively more severe, requiring blood transfusions. The median survival is 4 to 5 years, but some patients live 10 years or longer. In 10% to 12% of patients, there is an expansion of the malignant clone in the form of an accelerated phase (blast crisis). The clinical and laboratory picture may then be indistinguishable from acute myelogenous leukemia.

Table 31-5 *Continued*

CML	Polycythemia Vera
Decreased	Normal or increased
Usually <50 x 10^3/mm³ (50 x 10^9/L)	Usually <20 x 10^3/mm³ (20 x 10^9/L)
Many immature granulocytes	Usually normal
Present	May be present
Usually normal	Normal or hypochromic, microcytic
Rare	Rare
Normal, increased, or decreased	Normal or increased
Marked myeloid hyperplasia	Hypercellular with decreased iron stores
Decreased	Usually increased
Present	Absent
Moderate	Absent or mild

Therapy for MF with myeloid metaplasia is mainly sympto-matic. Androgen therapy has been used in patients who are markedly anemic and/or thrombocytopenic. In patients who have painful splenomegaly, splenectomy or local radiation may be ben-eficial. Allopurinol may be indicated in patients with high serum uric acid levels.

Special Diagnostic Considerations

Acute Myelofibrosis (Myelosclerosis). Acute or malig-nant MF is a rare disease characterized by pancytopenia, minimal poikilocytosis and anisocytosis (in contrast to MF with myeloid metaplasia), bone marrow fibrosis, and panmyelosis. Most of the cells present are immature, and megakaryocytes or megakary-oblasts are prominent. Also, in contrast to MF with myeloid meta-plasia, splenomegaly is minimal or absent. The disease is fulminant and usually fatal. It may be impossible to distinguish acute megakaryocytic leukemia (AML, M7 [see Chapter 29 for classification schema]) from acute MF; indeed, they may be variants of the same disease process.

Undifferentiated or Atypical Myeloproliferative Syndrome.   Approximately one third of the patients are classified as having so-called undifferentiated or atypical myeloproliferative syndrome. Their clinical and laboratory findings do not fit precisely into a specific disease category. Thus, some patients exhibit myeloid metaplasia in the spleen and liver with a classic leukoerythroblastic blood smear, but the bone marrow shows only panmyelosis with minimal fibrosis. This may closely resemble CML; however, in contrast to CML, these patients have normal or elevated LAP scores and lack the Ph[1] chromosome. To exclude polycythemia vera, the red blood cell mass must be normal. Still other patients may have severe MF but only minimal myeloid metaplasia. A summary of the differential characteristics of the various myeloproliferative syndromes is shown in Table 31-5.

References

Frisch B, Bartl R. Histology of myelofibrosis and osteomyelosclerosis. In: Lewis SM, ed. *Myelofibrosis: Pathophysiology and Clinical Management.* New York, NY: Marcel Dekker Inc; 1985:51-86.

Hasselbalch H. Idiopathic myelofibrosis: a clinical study of 80 patients. *Am J Hematol.* 1990;34:291-300.

Lichtman MA. Agnogenic myeloid metaplasia. In: Williams WJ, Beutler E, Erslev AJ, Lichtman MA, eds. *Hematology.* New York, NY: McGraw Hill; 1990:223-232.

Thiele J, Zankovich R, Steinberg T, et al. Agnogenic myeloid metaplasia (AMM)—correlation of bone marrow lesions with laboratory data: a longitudinal study of 114 patients. *Hematol Oncol.* 1989;7:327-343.

Visani G, Finelli C, Castelli U, et al. Myelofibrosis with myeloid metaplasia: clinical and haematological parameters predicting survival in a series of 133 patients. *Br J Haematol.* 1990;75:4-9.

Wolf BC, Neiman RS. Hypothesis-splenic infiltration and the pathogenesis of extramedullary hematopoiesis in agnogenic myeloid metaplasia. *Hematol Pathol.* 1987;1:77-80.

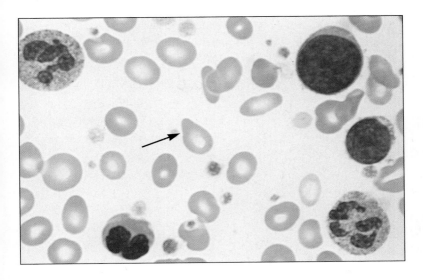

Image 31-1 Peripheral blood smear from a patient with myelofibrosis showing a myeloblast, a dysplastic nucleated red blood cell, and a rare teardrop form red blood cell (↑).

Image 31-2 Bone marrow biopsy section from a patient with early myelofibrosis showing panhyperplasia.

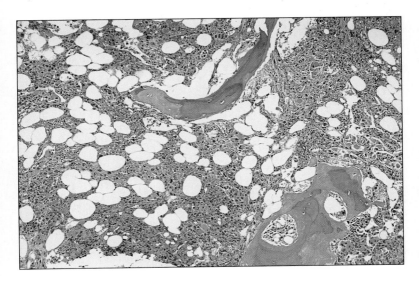

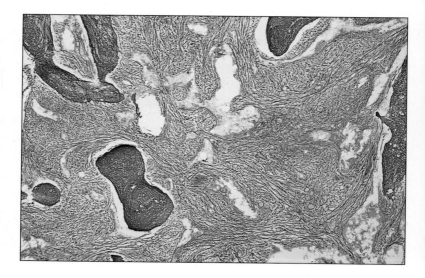

Image 31-3   Reticulin stain of marrow biopsy in advanced myelofibrosis showing marked (4+) reticulin fibrosis.

Image 31-4   Prominent fibrosis, osteosclerosis, and dilated sinuses are seen in this bone marrow biopsy section from a patient with advanced myelofibrosis.

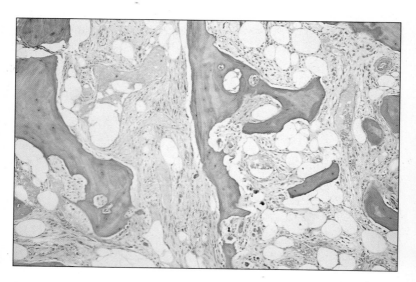

32

Polycythemia: Primary and Secondary

Erythrocytosis (polycythemia) is defined as an increase in the concentration of red blood cells in the peripheral blood measured by the red blood cell count, the hemoglobin, or the hematocrit, and is due to an increase in the total number of red blood cells or a decrease in plasma volume. The terms "erythrocytosis" and "polycythemia" are often used interchangeably, although the latter term implies an increase in multiple hematopoietic cell lines. For simplicity, however, the terms will be used interchangeably in this chapter. Erythrocytosis can result from an intrinsic bone marrow defect, altered erythropoietin regulatory activity, or decreased plasma volume (Table 32-1).

Types of Erythrocytosis

Polycythemia Vera (Primary Erythrocytosis).   Primary erythrocytosis, or polycythemia vera (PV), is a chronic myeloproliferative disorder that occurs when all hematopoietic cell lines undergo uncontrolled proliferation with intact maturation. By definition, the erythroid proliferation is dominant. The abnormal cells are derived from a single parent cell and the proliferation is erythropoietin-independent. The disease has an estimated annual incidence of one case per 100,000 population; there is a slight male predominance; and most patients are older than 50 years. The diagnostic features of PV are separated into major and minor criteria, as shown below.

Major criteria:
1. Elevated red blood cell mass.
2. Normal arterial oxygen saturation ($\geq 92\%$).
3. Splenomegaly.

Minor criteria:
1. Platelet count > 400 x10^3/mm^3 (400 x 10^9/L).
2. White blood cell count >12 x 10^3/mm^3 (12 x 10^9/L).
3. Elevated leukocyte alkaline phosphatase level.
4. Elevated vitamin B_{12} level or vitamin B_{12}–binding capacity.

A diagnosis of PV can be made when all three major criteria are present or when the first two major criteria plus any two minor criteria are identified.

Secondary Erythrocytosis. Patients with secondary erythrocytosis have an erythropoietin-mediated and absolute increase in red blood cell mass that may be either physiologically appropriate or inappropriate. Physiologically appropriate erythrocytosis results from a hypoxic stimulus, such as residence at high altitude, chronic pulmonary or cardiac diseases, high oxygen-affinity hemoglobinopathies, or increased carboxyhemoglobin levels. Patients with secondary polycythemia that is physiologically inappropriate do not have tissue hypoxia but have excess production of either erythropoietin or anabolic steroids. Disorders associated with this type of secondary erythrocytosis include renal disorders such as cystic disease and hydronephrosis; various erythropoietin-producing tumors such as uterine, liver, and cerebellar tumors; and adrenal cortical hypersecretion.

Relative Erythrocytosis. In patients with relative or stress erythrocytosis, the primary disorder is one of decreased plas-

Table 32-1   Differential Diagnosis of Polycythemia*

Nonneoplastic
    Increased erythropoietin production, appropriate response
        High altitude
        Chronic obstructive pulmonary disease
        Left-to-right cardiovascular shunt
        High-oxygen affinity hemoglobinopathy
        Congenital deficiency of red blood cell diphosphoglycerate
    Increased erythropoietin production, inappropriate response
        Tumor
            Uterine leiomyoma
            Adenocarcinoma of kidney
            Cerebellar hemangioblastoma
            Hepatocellular carcinoma
        Renal disease
    Increased plasma volume or relative (stress) polycythemia
Neoplastic: polycythemia vera

*Modified with permission from Berlin NI. Diagnosis and classification of the polycythemias. *Semin Hematol.* 1975;12:340.

---

ma volume rather than true or absolute erythrocytosis. Although the hematocrit is elevated, the red blood cell mass is normal or decreased. This is sometimes known as stress polycythemia.

Pathophysiology

Bone marrow production of red blood cells is regulated by erythropoietin, a glycoprotein hormone that induces committed bone marrow stem cells to mature into red blood cells. The erythropoietin precursor substance is produced in the kidneys in response to tissue hypoxia. Once oxygen delivery to the tissues is increased, erythropoietin production is suppressed.

In patients with PV, a stem cell defect results in unregulated production of all hematopoietic elements. The production of red blood cells in this disorder is not regulated by erythropoietin.

The excess red blood cell production in secondary erythrocytosis is erythropoietin-mediated. In patients with physiologically appropriate secondary erythrocytosis, the tissue hypoxia responsible for erythropoietin production can result from decreased oxygen in the atmosphere, impaired oxygen–carbon dioxide exchange in the lungs, or decreased delivery of oxygen to tissues (Table 32-1). In all of the disorders associated with secondary erythrocytosis, the erythropoietin production will decrease if the tissue hypoxia is alleviated.

Physiologically inappropriate erythrocytosis occurs when high levels of erythropoietin, erythropoietin-like substances, or anabolic steroids drive the bone marrow to produce excessive numbers of red blood cells in the absence of tissue hypoxia. The disorders associated with this type of secondary erythrocytosis are listed in Table 32-2 and include a variety of neoplasms from the kidney, liver, uterus, ovary, adrenal gland, and brain. The nonneoplastic disorders associated with physiologically inappropriate erythrocytosis are by and large renal diseases.

The relative or stress erythrocytosis present in patients with decreased plasma volume can be secondary to either dehydration or excess water loss (renal or gastrointestinal abnormalities). Decreased plasma volume is also a contributing factor to the erythrocytosis frequently observed in heavy smokers.

Clinical Findings

Patients with PV are generally middle-aged and present with symptoms related to increased blood volume or thromboembolic or hemorrhagic phenomena. These patients often experience fatigue, malaise, headache, light-headedness, and pruritus. The pruritus is thought to be secondary to excessive histamine release by basophils, which may also help explain the increased frequency of peptic ulcer disease in these patients.

The thromboembolic and hemorrhagic episodes seen both at presentation and during the disease course in patients with PV are secondary to thrombocytosis, platelet functional defects, and hyperviscosity. The uric acid level is also often increased and is associated with gout in approximately 10% of patients. Some patients present with erythromelalgia, a vaso-occlusive process localized to the distal extremities, although this finding is probably more common in essential or primary thrombocythemia (see Chapter 33).

Table 32-2   Disorders Associated With Physiologically Inappropriate Erythrocytosis

Organ	Disorder
Kidney	Cystic renal disease
	Hydronephrosis
	Adenocarcinoma
	Transplant rejection
Liver	Hepatocellular carcinoma
Uterus	Leiomyoma
Ovary	Ovarian carcinoma
Adrenal Glands	Pheochromocytoma
	Adrenal cortical hyperplasia
Brain	Cerebellar hemangioblastoma

On physical examination, patients with PV almost invariably have splenomegaly; they may be plethoric, with conjunctival and retinal venous engorgement.

The clinical findings in patients with secondary erythrocytosis vary greatly depending on the underlying cause. For instance, patients with physiologically appropriate secondary erythrocytosis may have manifestations of cardiopulmonary disease, such as cyanosis, clubbing, and increased respiratory rate. Many other patients with secondary erythrocytosis, however, may have no specific clinical findings. Splenomegaly is not a clinical manifestation of secondary erythrocytosis.

In patients with relative erythrocytosis, the underlying cause of the decreased plasma volume is usually apparent and includes such disorders as diarrhea, vomiting, dehydration, and renal disease. Splenomegaly, the physical finding that is the hallmark of the chronic myeloproliferative disorders, is not present in patients with relative erythrocytosis.

Approach to Diagnosis

Patients should be evaluated for possible primary or secondary erythrocytosis when there is an elevated hemoglobin level in the absence of an obvious clinical cause. An algorithm to encompass all possible diagnostic explanations for erythrocytosis is very complex and includes tests rarely performed in routine clinical or laboratory practice. A simplified approach to the diagnosis of erythrocytosis, however, allows classification of most patients' diseases. Figure 32-1 is an algorithm for the diagnosis of the chronic myeloproliferative disorders, including PV.

1. Eliminate cases of relative erythrocytosis by careful clinical evaluation for disorders associated with loss of plasma volume.

2. If the patient has an established diagnosis of renal disease or of a neoplasm associated with erythrocytosis, consider it a possible cause of erythrocytosis.

3. Assess other hematologic features for abnormalities not explained by the clinical setting, notably leukocytosis and thrombocytosis.

4. Proceed to evaluate for diagnostic criteria of PV in patients in whom these other unexplained hematologic abnormalities are identified. This includes measurements of arterial oxygen saturation and red blood cell mass.

5. In patients with no other unexplained hematologic abnormalities, distinguish between physiologic and nonphysiologic secondary erythrocytosis. Most of the physiologically appropriate cases of erythrocytosis will be secondary to pulmonary or cardiovascular disorders or to smoking. Causes such as high oxygen-affinity hemoglobinopathy, however, require more extensive laboratory investigation.

6. In the absence of PV or a physiologic cause for the erythrocytosis, a diverse group of disorders, including occult tumors and renal diseases, should be considered (see Table 32-2).

Hematologic Findings

The hematologic findings of PV differ from those of secondary and relative erythrocytoses. In PV, abnormalities are detected in all three cell lines in the blood, while secondary and relative erythrocytoses are generally associated with red blood cell changes only.

Figure 32-1 Algorithm for diagnosis of chronic myeloproliferative disorders.

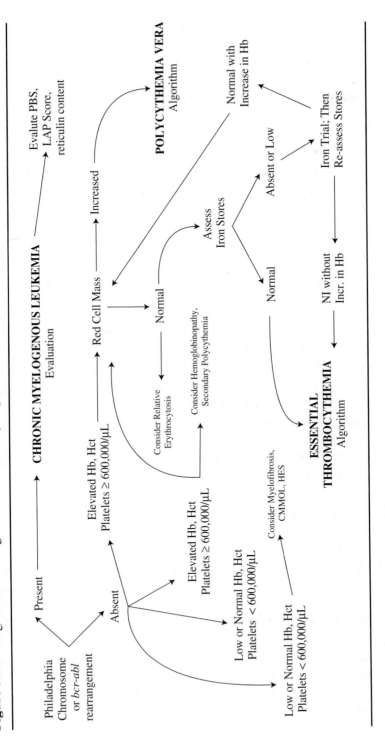

Blood Cell Measurements.   In PV, the hemoglobin level, hematocrit, white blood cell count, and platelet count are all characteristically elevated. The red blood cell indices and red cell distribution width are generally normal but may be abnormal in patients with concurrent iron deficiency. Since more than 90% of patients with PV are iron deficient at diagnosis, the mean corpuscular volume in particular may be misleading. The percentage of reticulocytes is within normal limits.

Patients with secondary erythrocytosis have elevated hemoglobin and hematocrit levels with normal white blood cell and platelet counts. The red blood cell indices and red cell distribution width are generally normal. The absolute reticulocyte count is often elevated.

The elevated hematocrit value noted in patients with relative erythrocytosis is almost always less than 60% (0.60) and is not associated with an increased reticulocyte count.

Peripheral Blood Smear Morphology.   In PV, the erythrocytes are generally normocytic and normochromic, except when there is concurrent iron deficiency. Increased numbers of platelets and megakaryocyte fragments may be present. The white blood cell differential count occasionally shows basophilia and/or eosinophilia.

The peripheral blood smear morphology in secondary erythrocytosis is normal, except for the increase in normal-appearing red blood cells. Polychromasia may be present.

No specific morphologic abnormalities are present in blood smears from patients with relative erythrocytosis.

Bone Marrow Examination.   In PV, the bone marrow is characteristically hypercellular with a panhyperplasia involving all cell lines. Although an increase in reticulin fibers can be present at diagnosis, there is generally a progressive increase in the amount of reticulin fibrosis throughout the patient's disease course. As this fibrosis increases, there is an associated progressive decrease in the cellularity, which is sometimes referred to as the "spent phase" of PV. This occurs in 10% of patients with PV. Storage iron is often markedly decreased because of increased red blood cell production, bleeding, and the periodic phlebotomy that is sometimes used for treatment.

Bone marrow examination is generally not necessary to establish a diagnosis of secondary erythrocytosis. If bone marrow is obtained, erythroid hyperplasia will be the major finding. In patients with relative erythrocytosis, bone marrow examination is not indicated.

Other Laboratory Tests

Laboratory tests that can be utilized to distinguish PV, secondary polycythemia, and relative polycythemia are shown in Table 32-3.

32.1 Red Blood Cell Mass

Purpose.   Measurement of the red blood cell mass can be used to distinguish true from a relative erythrocytosis.

Principle.   Erythrocyte mass is measured by a dilution technique using radiolabeled red blood cells, with the degree of dilution directly proportional to red blood cell mass.

Specimen.   Anticoagulated venous blood is used.

Procedure.   A fixed number of the patient's erythrocytes are radiolabeled in vitro and intravenously injected back into the patient. After a 10- to 20-minute equilibrium period, a second sample of venous blood is drawn from the opposite arm. A scintillation counter is used to measure the radioactivity of the injected sample and the second venous sample. Red blood cell mass is calculated using the formula:

$$\text{Red Blood Cell Mass} = \frac{\text{Injected Radioactivity}}{\text{Radioactivity of Erythrocytes After Mixing}}$$

Interpretation.   An elevated erythrocyte mass is seen in primary and secondary erythrocytosis but not in relative erythrocytosis.

Notes and Precautions.   Because red blood cell mass is related to lean body mass, spuriously low values can occur in patients with marked obesity. When ^{51}chromium is used to radiolabel the patient's erythrocytes, the patient should not have previously received antibiotics or ascorbic acid because these substances impair the labeling process, yielding spuriously low results.

32.2   Arterial Oxygen Saturation

Purpose.   Arterial oxygen saturation is performed to determine whether or not there is hypoxemia.

Principle, Procedure.   The standard nomogram and spectrophotometric techniques used to measure arterial oxygen saturation are detailed in clinical pathology texts.

Specimen.   Arterial blood specimens for blood gas determinations are collected with a minimum amount of heparin, maintained under anaerobic conditions, and analyzed promptly.

Interpretation.   When the arterial oxygen saturation is less than the established normal range, hypoxia is present.

Notes and Precautions.   Proper and prompt specimen handling is necessary to ensure the accuracy of the result. Normal range values are affected by altitude and need to be established for each laboratory.

Ancillary Tests

Other laboratory tests that can be utilized on a selected basis to distinguish the three types of erythrocytosis are listed in Table 32-3. The characteristic test result for each type of erythrocytosis is also included in this table.

Platelet Aggregation Studies. Bleeding problems may occur in myeloproliferative disorders, particularly in PV. The bleeding may be caused by a defect in platelet function. This is most commonly manifested in vitro as a defect in aggregation in response to epinephrine and collagen. Some patients will also display aggregation defects in response to adenosine diphosphate.

Course and Treatment

The increased blood viscosity associated with erythrocytosis causes a significant morbidity and even mortality in these patients. Blood viscosity increases dramatically as the patient's hematocrit value rises from 50% to 60% (0.50-0.60). As viscosity increases, the oxygen-carrying ability of erythrocytes actually decreases. In patients with physiologically appropriate secondary erythrocytosis, this decrease in oxygen delivery leads to further erythropoietin release and greater erythrocytosis. In addition to impaired oxygen delivery, patients with increased blood viscosity are at risk for thrombosis, especially in slow flow rate venous channels.

Polycythemia Vera. PV typically follows an indolent, slowly progressive course with gradual evolution from a hypercellular bone marrow picture to bone marrow fibrosis, with associated decline in peripheral blood counts (spent phase). Thrombosis and hemorrhage caused by increased blood viscosity, thrombocytosis, and platelet function abnormalities are causes of increased morbidity and mortality in patients with PV. With proper management, risks from these complications can be substantially reduced. Without treatment, patients with PV have a median survival of about 18 months. With treatment, however, these patients can have survival times equal to those of age- and sex-matched control populations. Treatment modalities that have been utilized successfully in patients with PV include periodic phlebotomy to reduce the viscosity and alkylating agent or radioactive phosphorus (^{32}P) therapy to reduce bone marrow production of all hematopoietic elements. Alkylating agent therapy has been associated with an increased incidence of both acute leukemia and non-Hodgkin's lymphoma.

Table 32-3 Laboratory Tests Used to Distinguish Types of Erythrocytosis

Laboratory Test	Polycythemia Vera	Secondary Erythrocytosis*	Relative Erythrocytosis
Red blood cell mass	Increased	Increased	Normal
Erythropoietin	Usually decreased	Normal to increased	Usually normal
PO_2	Usually normal	Decreased in some cases	Normal
Leukocyte alkaline phosphatase	Increased	Usually normal†	Usually normal
Vitamin B_{12}	Increased	Normal	Normal
Vitamin B_{12}–binding proteins	Increased	Normal	Normal
Carboxyhemoglobin‡	Usually normal	May be increased	May be increased
Uric acid	Increased	Normal	Normal
Serum iron	Decreased	Normal	Normal
Marrow iron stores	Decreased	Normal	Normal
Hemoglobinopathy	Absent	Present in some cases	Absent
Platelet aggregation	Abnormal	Normal	Normal
Marrow chromosome abnormalities	May be present	Absent	Absent

*Includes both physiologically appropriate and inappropriate causes of erythrocytosis.
†Can be elevated during pregnancy or with oral contraceptive drugs; also may be elevated in inflammatory/infectious disorders.
‡Increased in patients who smoke.

Therapy with ^{32}P also increases the risk of acute leukemia and so is generally reserved for patients older than 70 years.

Newer agents—theoretically less leukemogenic—include hydroxyurea and the interferons. Patients undergoing periodic phlebotomy should be monitored for the development of iron deficiency, because hypochromic erythrocytes have increased internal viscosity and decreased deformability, which enhances blood viscosity and further compromises tissue oxygen delivery.

Secondary Erythrocytosis. The clinical course and proper management of patients with secondary erythrocytosis depends on the specific cause of the excessive red blood cell production. While there is no curative treatment for some cases such as high oxygen-affinity hemoglobinopathies, others such as certain cardiopulmonary disorders can be alleviated with proper treatment. To reduce blood viscosity, periodic phlebotomy may be indicated for some patients with physiologically appropriate secondary erythrocytosis.

Management of the neoplasm is the primary treatment goal in patients with excessive erythropoietin production caused by the tumor. In a small proportion of patients with tumors of the kidney, adrenal gland, liver, or brain, erythropoietin production is the first sign that the patient has a neoplasm. Identification of these tumors before they are clinically obvious may be associated with improved survival. Management of nonneoplastic renal disease is necessary to reduce erythropoietin production in this group of patients with physiologically inappropriate erythrocytosis.

Relative Erythrocytosis. In these patients, the primary cause of the decreased plasma volume is often apparent and can usually be properly treated. Other factors that could aggravate the erythrocytosis, such as hypertension and smoking, should be addressed. The course of the disease and treatment vary with the underlying cause of the reduced plasma volume.

References

Berk PD, Goldberg JD, Donovan PB, et al. Therapeutic recommendations in polycythemia vera based on Polycythemia Vera Study Group Protocols. *Semin Hematol.* 1986;23:132-143.

Berlin NI. Diagnosis and classification of the polycythemias. *Semin Hematol.* 1975;12:339-351.

Ellis JT, Peterson P, Geller SA, et al. Studies of the bone marrow in polycythemia vera and the evolution of myelofibrosis and second hematologic malignancies. *Semin Hematol.* 1986;23:144-155.

Golde DW, Hocking WG, Koeffler HP, et al. Polycythemia: mechanisms and management. *Ann Intern Med.* 1981;95:71-87.

Murphy S. Polycythemia vera. In: Williams WJ, Beutler E, Erslev AJ, Lichtman MA, eds. *Hematology*. New York, NY: McGraw-Hill International Book Co; 1990:193-202.

Nand S, Messmore H, Fischer SG, et al. Leukemic transformation in polycythemia vera: analysis of risk factors. *Am J Hematol*. 1990;34:32-36.

Wasserman LR, Berk PD, Berlin NI, eds. *Polycythemia Vera*. Philadelphia, Pa: WB Saunders Co; 1994:348.

33

Thrombocytosis: Primary and Secondary

Thrombocytosis (thrombocythemia) is defined as an increase in the number of platelets in the peripheral blood and is usually due to an increase in the total number of megakaryocytes. The terms "thrombocytosis" and "thrombocythemia" are often used interchangeably, although the latter term implies a hematopoietic stem cell disorder. For simplicity, however, the terms will be used interchangeably in this chapter. Thrombocytosis can be due to an intrinsic stem cell defect or may be a reaction to hemorrhage or other clinical states (Table 33-1).

Essential Thrombocythemia (Primary Thrombocytosis)

Primary thrombocytosis, or essential thrombocythemia (ET), is a chronic myeloproliferative disorder (MPD) that occurs when all hematopoietic cell lines undergo uncontrolled proliferation with intact maturation. By definition, megakaryocytic proliferation is dominant. The abnormal cells are derived from a single parent cell. This disease is the least common of the chronic MPDs; there is no

Table 33-1 Classification of Thrombocytosis

Type	Examples
Primary	Essential thrombocythemia
	Polycythemia vera
	Chronic myelogenous leukemia
	Myelofibrosis with myeloid metaplasia
Secondary (reactive)	Hemorrhage
	Chronic iron deficiency
	Postsplenectomy
	Chronic inflammatory/infectious states
	Collagen vascular disorders
	Ulcerative colitis
	Tuberculosis
	Malignancies
	Drugs: vincristine, high-dose erythropoietin

sex predominance; and patients range from 25 to 70 years of age. The diagnostic features of ET are shown below.

1. Sustained platelet count >600,000/mm^3 (600 x 10^9/L).

2. Normal hemoglobin level or normal red blood cell mass.

3. Stainable iron in the marrow or failure of hemoglobin to rise 1.0 g/dL (10 g/L) after 1 month of iron therapy.

4. Absence of the Philadelphia (Ph^1) chromosome or *bcr* rearrangement.

5. Collagen fibrosis of marrow either absent or less than one third of marrow area without both splenomegaly and leuko-erythroblastic reaction.

6. No known cause for reactive thrombocytosis.

An algorithm for the differential diagnosis of thrombocytosis is shown in Figure 33-1; see Figure 32-1 for the differential diagnosis of ET and the other chronic MPDs.

Secondary Thrombocytosis

Patients with secondary thrombocytosis have an increase in platelet number that results from a hemorrhagic stimulus, such as bleed-

Figure 33-1   Algorithm for the evaluation of thrombocytosis.*

Thrombocytosis and Megakaryocytic Hyperplasia

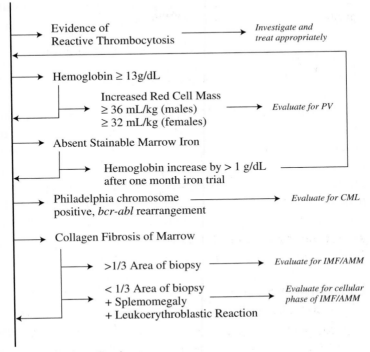

Essential Thrombocythemia

*Adapted with permission from Iland HJ, Laszlo J, Peterson P, et al. Essential thrombocythemia: clinical and laboratory characteristics at presentation. *Trans Assoc Am Physicians.* 1983;96:167..

ing, or that is in response to chronic inflammatory or infectious states, a postsplenectomy state, certain medications, or a rebound phenomenon from a thrombocytopenic state (See Table 33-1).

Pathophysiology

ET (primary, idiopathic thrombocythemia), the least common of the chronic MPDs, is marked by megakaryocyte proliferation. Overproduction of the platelets is the predominant feature. The recurrent thrombosis and hemorrhage observed in patients suffering from this disorder are caused by the marked elevation in the platelet count associated with distinctly abnormal platelet function. Hence, this entity has also been called "hemorrhagic thrombocythemia." Iron deficiency anemia may develop as a result of chronic gastrointestinal hemorrhage. Between hemorrhages, there may be a tendency toward polycythemia. As with other MPDs, ET has been shown to be a clonal abnormality of the multipotential stem cell. The main features of this disorder are listed in Table 33-2.

Patients with ET may be asymptomatic or may complain of weakness, headache, paresthesias, and dizziness. Bleeding may occur in the gastrointestinal tract and, less commonly, in the urinary tract or the skin. Other features include thrombosis and peptic ulceration. Splenomegaly is present in approximately 60% of patients but is usually not as prominent as in myelofibrosis with myeloid metaplasia. The liver may be slightly enlarged, but only rarely is there lymph node enlargement.

Hematologic Findings

In ET, the hemoglobin level is usually normal. Microcytic hypochromic anemia may develop if the patient has chronic bleeding. Almost one third of patients, however, show an elevated hematocrit value, in which case the patient may be misdiagnosed as having polycythemia vera. The leukocyte count may be normal but is usually moderately increased. The striking feature in ET is the markedly elevated platelet count, by definition exceeding $600 \times 10^3/\text{mm}^3$ ($600 \times 10^9/\text{L}$) and very often greater than $1,000 \times 10^3/\text{mm}^3$ ($1,000 \times 10^9/\text{L}$).

Peripheral Blood Smear Morphology. In ET, large clumps or swarms of platelets are usually seen (Image 33-1). In addition, the platelets show a marked variation in size and shape, including giant platelets, microplatelets, and platelets showing abnormal granularity. The leukocytes are slightly increased in number and may show metamyelocytes, but promyelocytes are unusual. As with myelofibrosis, mild eosinophilia may be seen. The red blood cells are usually normochromic and normocytic, but

Table 33-2 Characteristic Features of Essential Thrombocythemia

Insidious onset
Splenomegaly
Bleeding and thromboembolic phenomena
Sustained elevation of platelet count >600 x 10^3/mm^3 (600 x 10^9/L)
Normal hemoglobin level (unless iron-deficient from bleeding)
Slight neutrophilic leukocytosis
Marrow megakaryocytic hyperplasia and dysplasia

microcytic hypochromic red blood cells can be found in patients who have chronic blood loss.

Bone Marrow Examination. In ET, the bone marrow also shows panmyelosis. There is a preponderance of megakaryocytes showing extensive platelet production. Megakaryocytes frequently occur in clusters and vary considerably in size and shape (Image 33-2). In general, the bone marrow findings in ET are difficult to separate from those of polycythemia vera. As the disease progresses, a transition to acute myelogenous leukemia and/or myelofibrosis can occur.

Other Laboratory Tests

33.1 Red Blood Cell Mass

Purpose. The red blood cell mass may be useful in differentiating polycythemia vera from ET. The test should be performed only when the patient's iron stores are replete.

Principle, Specimen, and Procedure. See Test 32.1.

Interpretation. In ET, the red blood cell mass is normal; it is elevated in polycythemia vera.

33.2 Leukocyte Alkaline Phosphatase (LAP)

Purpose. The LAP score may be useful in differentiating CML from ET and the other chronic MPDs.

Principle, Specimen, and Procedure. See Test 16.1.

Interpretation. In CML, the LAP score is characteristically 0 or markedly decreased. In ET the LAP score is usually normal or elevated.

33.3 Cytogenetic Studies

Purpose. Cytogenetic studies may be useful in distinguishing CML from ET and the other chronic MPDs.

Principle, Specimen, and Procedure. See Test 34.2.

Interpretation. The Ph[1] chromosome, present in most cases of CML, is absent in ET. Several chromosome changes have been observed in patients with ET, but none is specific.

Ancillary Tests

Platelet Aggregation Studies. Bleeding problems occur in MPDs, particularly in ET. The cause of bleeding in ET however, is poorly understood. In part the bleeding is caused by a defect in platelet function. This is most commonly manifested in vitro as a defect in aggregation in response to epinephrine and collagen. Many patients will also display aggregation defects in response to ADP.

Blood Biochemistry. Serum potassium levels may be artifactually elevated because of release from platelets during clotting. Plasma potassium levels, however, will be accurate. In addition, serum uric acid, alkaline phosphatase, and lactate dehydrogenase levels will be elevated in over half of patients.

Course and Treatment

In essential thrombocythemia, a number of patients, especially younger ones, may not require therapy for years. Other patients may experience repeated hemorrhagic and thromboembolic episodes. In a small percentage of patients, blastic crisis or myelofibrosis develops.

Therapy may not be needed in ET, especially in younger patients. When a patient develops a thrombotic or bleeding episode, however, treatment is probably indicated and usually consists of the antimetabolite hydroxyurea to reduce the platelet count. Occasionally, vaso-occlusive events may require drugs that interfere with normal platelet function, such as aspirin. The use of aspirin may increase the incidence of hemorrhage, especially gastrointestinal.

References

Buss DH, O'Connor ML, Woodruff RD, et al. Bone marrow and peripheral blood findings in patients with extreme thrombocytosis. *Arch Pathol Lab Med.* 1991; 115:475-480.

Hehlman R, Jahn M, Baumann B, Kopcke W. Essential thrombocythemia: clinical characteristics and course of 61 cases. *Cancer.* 1988;61:2487-2496.

Iland HJ, Laszlo J, Case DC, et al. Differentiation between essential thrombocythemia and polycythemia vera with marked thrombocytosis. *Am J Hematol.* 1987;25:191-201.

Iland HJ, Laszlo J, Peterson P, et al. Essential thrombocythemia: clinical and laboratory characteristics at presentation. *Trans Assoc Am Physicians.* 1983; 96:165-174.

McIntyre KJ, Hoagland HC, Silverstein MN, Pettitt RM. Essential thrombocythemia in young adults. *Mayo Clin Proc.* 1991;66:149-154.

Murphy S. Primary thrombocythemia. In: Williams WJ, Beutler E, Erslev AJ, Lichtman MA, eds. *Hematology.* New York, NY: McGraw Hill; 1990:232-236.

Stoll DB, Peterson P, Exten R, et al. Clinical presentation and natural history of patients with essential thrombocythemia and the Philadelphia chromosome. *Am J Hematol.* 1988;27:77-83.

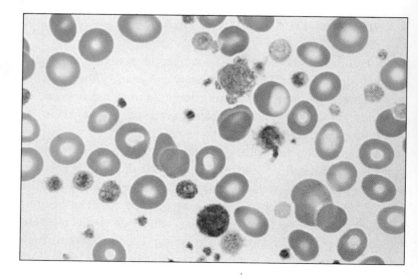

Image 33-1   Peripheral blood smear from patient with essential thrombocythemia showing increased numbers of platelets, many of which are enlarged.

Image 33-2   Bone marrow biopsy from patient with thrombocythemia showing increased megakaryocytes that vary in size and shape.

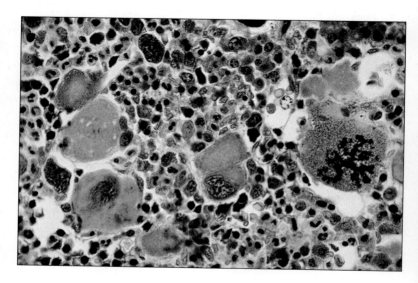

34

Chronic
Myelogenous
Leukemia

Chronic myelogenous leukemia (CML), once known as chronic granulocytic leukemia, is a chronic myeloproliferative disorder characterized by a clonal proliferation of myelogenous cells that results in a large increase in total body granulocyte mass. In the majority of patients, there is a terminal blastic metamorphosis. CML comprises approximately 20% of all adult leukemias and is seen most frequently in the middle-aged and rarely in children.

Pathophysiology

CML is a clonal disorder originating from the multipotential hematopoietic stem cell. More than 95% of patients with CML have a translocation of one of the long arms of chromosome 22, usually to one of the nine chromosomes [t(9;22)]. Variant chromosomal translocations have also been identified. The presence of this abnormal chromosome, the Philadelphia chromosome (Ph[1]), in a patient with leukocytosis and granulocytic hyperplasia in the bone marrow is diagnostic of CML. In CML, reciprocal chromosomal rearrangements are associated with translocation and activation of cellular oncogenes. The proto-oncogene *c-abl* is located on chromosome 9. This oncogene is translocated to chromosome 22. The breakpoint on chromosome 22 occurs within the *bcr* (breakpoint cluster region) gene. The final result is a chimeric gene *bcr-abl*. This fusion gene is expressed as a protein with enhanced tyrosine kinase activity. The clonal nature of CML has also been confirmed by isoenzyme studies of G6PD.

The granulocytic hyperplasia, at all stages of maturation within the bone marrow, is explained by a combination of stem cell expansion and a delay in cell cycle, maturation-division, and compartmental transit time. The average half-life of granulocytes in the blood in patients with CML is five to 10 times longer than normal. At the same time, the granulocyte turnover rate may be increased 10-fold. Thus, CML is characterized by major regulatory defects that are probably due to abnormalities in the multipotential stem cells.

Clinical Findings

CML is most frequent in patients between 50 and 60 years of age and usually develops insidiously. The initial symptoms may include malaise, fatigue, weight loss, and upper abdominal fullness or discomfort. Physical examination usually reveals splenomegaly. Hepatomegaly is less common and lymphadenopathy is very unusual; when present, it is often associated with the accelerated phase of the disease. As the disease progresses, the spleen may become markedly · enlarged, and in general the magnitude of splenomegaly correlates with the magnitude of the leukocyte count.

Approach to Diagnosis

Following clinical history and physical examination, the laboratory diagnosis of CML proceeds in the following sequence:

1. A complete blood count.
2. Examination of the peripheral blood smear.
3. A leukocyte alkaline phosphatase (LAP) score.

4. Examination of the bone marrow aspirate smear and biopsy.
5. Cytogenetic studies for the Philadelphia chromosome or molecular studies for the *bcr-abl* rearrangement.

See Figure 32-1 for an algorithm of the differential diagnosis of CML and the other myeloproliferative disorders. Table 34-1 compares the major findings in chronic and acute leukemias.

Hematologic Findings

The hematologic findings in CML are characteristic but not diagnostic. Severe leukemoid reactions—due to infections, for example—can mimic CML. Other myeloproliferative disorders such as myelofibrosis may have similar blood and bone marrow findings.

Blood Cell Measurements. The majority of patients have mild normochromic, normocytic anemia at the time of diagnosis. The anemia becomes more severe as the leukocyte count increases. The rise in leukocyte count is gradual, the majority of patients having counts ranging between 50 x 10^3/mm^3 and 400 x 10^3/mm^3 (50-4,000 x 10^9/L) at the time of diagnosis. In contrast to acute myelocytic leukemia, the platelet count is normal or often elevated.

Peripheral Blood Smear Morphology. The diagnosis of CML can usually be suspected from an examination of the peripheral blood. The striking feature is granulocytosis, with the entire spectrum of granulocytic precursors being present (Image 34-1). Mature granulocytes and metamyelocytes predominate. Promyelocytes and myeloblasts do not exceed 10% in the chronic phase. An absolute increase in basophils is characteristic of CML and may be useful in distinguishing CML from a leukemoid reaction. There are also increased numbers of eosinophils. Nucleated red blood cells are infrequent. Thrombocytosis may result in megakaryocyte nuclei and giant platelets.

Bone Marrow Examination. The bone marrow is markedly hypercellular with a large increase in the myeloid:ery-

Table 34-1   Comparison of Acute and Chronic Leukemia

Variable	Acute	Chronic
Age	All ages	Adults
Clinical onset	Sudden	Insidious
Lymphadenopathy	Mild	Moderate
Splenomegaly	Mild	Moderate to prominent
Anemia and thrombocytopenia	Prominent	Mild
Leukemic cells	Immature	Mature
Course (untreated)	6 months or less	2-6 years

throid ratio—as much as 10:1 to 40:1. As in the peripheral blood, all stages of maturation of the granulocytic series are present and there is usually an increased number of basophils and eosinophils. The number of erythroid precursors appears decreased. The megakaryocytes are usually increased in number and frequently show dysplastic features. Megakaryocytic hyperplasia and platelet clumping can obscure the changes in the granulocytic line. Increased numbers of dysplastic megakaryocytes is a feature common to the chronic myeloproliferative disorders (see Chapters 31-33). The bone marrow biopsy specimen may reveal reticulin fibrosis, which may become more severe as the disease progresses. Bone marrow fibrosis is associated with a higher incidence of splenomegaly and with a poorer prognosis. Marked fibrosis is often associated with the accelerated or blastic phases of the disease.

Bone marrow examination per se is often of little help in making the diagnosis of CML. It is indicated, however, to obtain material for cytogenetic or molecular studies (Ph[1] chromosome, *bcr* rearrangement) and to evaluate the degree of marrow fibrosis.

Other Laboratory Tests

34.1 Leukocyte Alkaline Phosphatase (LAP)

Purpose. Together with cytogenetic studies, LAP is the most useful confirmatory test in CML.

Principle, Specimen, and Procedure. See Test 16.1.

Interpretation. In CML, the LAP score is 0 or markedly decreased. The diagnostic value of a low score in patients with CML is increased by the fact that the LAP scores are usually elevated in the conditions with which CML is most commonly mistaken, such as leukemoid reactions, polycythemia vera, and myelofibrosis with myeloid metaplasia (Table 34-2). However, the LAP score in CML may be normal or increased in the presence of infection, during pregnancy, and after splenectomy. Also, during the accelerated blastic phase, the LAP score may be normal or elevated.

34.2 Cytogenetics

Purpose. The Philadelphia chromosome (Ph[1]) is present in 95% of patients with CML. In the presence of granulocytic hyperplasia and absolute basophilia in the peripheral blood and bone marrow, it is diagnostic of CML.

Principle. Ph[1] chromosome abnormality results from translocation of the greater part of the long arm of chromosome 22 to another chromosome, most usually chromosome 9 (Image 34-2). This is an acquired somatic mutation of a common stem cell of granulocytic-monocytic, erythroid, megakaryocytic, and B-lymphoid precursors. The Ph[1] chromosome persists throughout the course of the disease although treatment with α-interferon may reduce its frequency to levels undetectable by conventional means.

Specimen. Bone marrow is the tissue of choice. A buffy coat preparation of peripheral blood contains an adequate number of cells of the myelocytic stage or earlier. Bone marrow is aspirated directly into a syringe that has been rinsed with heparin. An aliquot of 0.5 to 1.0 mL of bone marrow is transferred immediately into (1) a sterile screw-top vial containing 2 mL of sterile tissue culture medium, or (2) a sterile small (2- to 3-mL) plain

Table 34-2 Conditions Associated with Abnormal LAP

Decreased	Increased
Chronic myelogenous leukemia	Leukemoid reactions
PNH	Pregnancy; oral contraceptive use
Hypophosphatemia	Polycythemia vera
ITP	Myelofibrosis
Infectious mononucleosis	Hodgkin's disease
Pernicious anemia	Essential thrombocythemia
Myelodysplastic syndromes	G-CSF administration
	Plasma cell myeloma

Abbreviations: LAP = leukocyte alkaline phosphatase; PNH = paroxysmal nocturnal hemoglobinuria; ITP = idiopathic thrombocytopenic purpura; G-CSF = granulocyte colony-stimulating factor.

(red top) vacuum tube. This specimen should not be refrigerated. The sample can be transported to a reference laboratory with satisfactory results if the specimen arrives within 24 hours. In special circumstances, lymph node biopsy specimen and splenic tissue may also be subjected to chromosome analysis.

Procedure. Chromosome charts are prepared by examining metaphase spreads of leukocytes from blood or bone marrow or both. Chromosome analysis is performed following 24 to 48 hours of incubation at 37°C without phytohemagglutinin stimulation. Many techniques are available by which chromosomes can be studied. The simplest type is termed a "direct study." A cell suspension is made of leukocytes from blood or bone marrow and incubated with colchicine to arrest cell division at the metaphase stage. The cells are swollen by hypotonic saline treatment and fixed. The fixed cells are placed on a slide, flattened, and dried. The metaphase spreads are then stained, examined under the microscope, and photographed.

Cell culture techniques are employed when the cells have a low mitotic index. Malignant leukocytes grow in vitro without stimulation, and peak cell division occurs 24 to 48 hours after onset of cell culture. G and Q banding is utilized for detailed karyotypic analysis.

Interpretation. Ph[1] chromosome is present in more than 95% of patients with CML, both in relapse and during apparent remission of the disease. During accelerated phase or blast crisis, additional chromosome abnormalities are frequently found, often a duplication of the Ph[1] chromosome, isochromosome 17q, or loss of the Y chromosome. A small number of patients lack the Ph[1] chromosome. These patients may have a disease different from classic CML (see below).

Although the Ph[1] chromosome translocation is the cytogenetic hallmark of CML, molecular detection of rearrangement of the genes involved in the translocation break point (the *bcr* locus on chromosome 9 and the *c-abl* proto-oncogene on chromosome 22) is a more sensitive marker for CML. The *bcr-abl* rearrangements may be present in cytogenetically normal cases of CML. Nonetheless, cytogenetic studies remain the gold standard.

34.3 Molecular Diagnostic Studies

34.3.1 Southern Blot Hybridization

Purpose. The *bcr-abl* rearrangement is present in most patients with CML. In the absence of the Ph[1] chromosome and in the appropriate clinical setting, it is diagnostic of CML.

Principle. The *bcr-abl* rearrangement results from a translocation in a very narrow region of the long arm of chromosome 22. Translocation of the *c-abl* oncogene into the *bcr* region alters a restriction enzyme site on the normal chromosome 22 and changes the normal germline configuration (banding pattern) of the *bcr* locus.

Specimen. Bone marrow is the tissue of choice.

Procedure. Cellular DNA is extracted and digested into varying length fragments by restriction endonucleases. These DNA fragments are separated according to length by agarose gel electrophoresis. A nitrocellulose film is then placed in contact with the gel surface, and the DNA in the gel is transferred ("blotted") onto the nitrocellulose film by either capillary action or vacuum force. The presence or absence of the *bcr-abl* rearrangement in the cellular DNA is then analyzed by DNA-DNA hybridization to a radioactive, usually ^{32}P-labeled, nucleotide probe. *HindIII/BgII* DNA fragment corresponding to *bcr-abl* junction is the most commonly used probe to detect this rearrangement in CML.

Interpretation. The *bcr-abl* rearrangement is present in 90% to 95% of patients with CML.

34.3.2 Polymerase Chain Reaction (PCR)

Purpose. Same as Southern blot.

Principle. Same as Southern blot.

Specimen. Bone marrow is the tissue of choice.

Procedure. PCR is a technique using a DNA polymerase to amplify short segments of either genomic DNA or cDNA. In CML, the presence of t(9;22) leads to the synthesis of *bcr-abl* mRNA. This aberrant mRNA product can be reversely transcribed into cDNA, which then serves as the template for PCR. The presence of an amplification product by gel electrophoresis thus documents the presence of *bcr* and *abl* gene sequences in a continuous gene segment, ie, the *bcr-abl* rearrangement.

Interpretation. The *bcr-abl* rearrangement is present in 90% to 95% of patients with CML.

Ancillary Tests

Terminal Deoxynucleotidyl Transferase (TdT). TdT is a marker for early lymphoid cells (see Chapter 30). In approximately one third of patients with CML in blast crisis, TdT is present. The reason to perform a TdT test in patients with CML is that TdT-positive patients respond more frequently to vincristine and prednisone, drugs normally used for treatment of acute lymphoblastic leukemia. Identification of TdT can be done on blasts in peripheral blood (if an adequate number of blast lymphocytes are present), on bone marrow aspirate material, or on imprints from a biopsy specimen. With the use of an immunoperoxidase technique, TdT can also be demonstrated in histologic sections.

Course and Treatment

CML has a constant, predictable course during the chronic phase with a median survival of 3.5 to 4 years. Approximately 20% of the patients survive 7 years or more from initial diagnosis. The majority of patients die of complications associated with blast crisis, usually infection or hemorrhage or both.

The principle of therapy in CML is to reduce the total granulocyte mass and relieve symptoms of hyperleukocytosis, thrombocytosis, and splenomegaly. The most commonly used therapeutic agents at present are the antimetabolite hydroxyurea and α-interferon (IFN-α). The alkylating agent busulphan is also an effective drug during the chronic phase of the disease, but it is less used now because of concerns regarding its leukemogenicity. No effective therapy is available yet for blast crisis. The only definitive prospect for curing CML appears to be high-dose chemotherapy followed by marrow transplantation.

Table 34-3 is a summary of the characteristic features in CML.

Special Diagnostic Considerations

Accelerated Phase and Blast Crisis in CML. There are three phases in the natural history of CML: the chronic phase,

Table 34-3 Characteristics of Chronic Myelogenous Leukemia

Age	35-50 years; rarely in children
Physical examination	Splenomegaly
Leukocyte count	50-200 x 10^3/mm^3 (50-200 x 10^9/L)
Blood findings	Granulocytosis with entire spectrum of precursors from myeloblasts (<2%) to polymorphonuclear neutrophils; absolute basophilia; eosinophilia; normal or increased platelet count
Bone marrow findings	Granulocytic hyperplasia; basophilia and eosinophilia; megakaryocytic hyperplasia; variable degree of fibrosis
Leukocyte alkaline phosphatase	Markedly decreased or zero
Chromosome analysis	Philadelphia chromosome (Ph^1)
Molecular studies	*bcr* rearrangement
Clinical course (untreated)	Chronic phase: 2-4 years
	Accelerated phase: weeks to months
	Blast phase: days to weeks

the accelerated phase, and the terminal blastic phase (blast crisis). The metamorphosis from the chronic phase to blast crisis can occur very rapidly or gradually over several months. The less fulminant transition is referred to as the accelerated phase or acute transformation. The development of blast crisis occurs in the majority of patients between 2 and 6 years from the time of diagnosis. The accelerated phase and blast crisis are associated with a maturation block similar to that in AML. Features associated with the accelerated phase include increased number of basophils, additional chromosomal abnormalities, and myelofibrosis.

Blast crisis is usually myeloid (60% of cases) (Images 34-3, 34-4), but lymphoid blast crisis (approximately 30% of cases) also occurs. In some instances, myeloid-lymphoid hybrid blasts or granulocytic blast mixtures may be present. This mixture of blast crises is not surprising, as CML represents a lesion of the multipotential stem cell. Blast crisis is associated with a clonal expansion of any of several potential progeny. The type of blast crisis (myeloid vs lymphoid) influences therapy in that TdT-positive blasts dictate therapy normally used for acute lymphocytic leukemia. In addition to TdT-positivity, lymphoid blasts usually have a lymphoblastic morphology and are CALLA-positive.

Clinically the accelerated phase and blastic crisis are associated with marked malaise, fatigue, anorexia, bone pain, and weight loss. Lymphadenopathy may develop, and biopsy of such lymph nodes reveals a predominance of blasts (granulocytic sarcoma or chloroma), which may be mistaken for large cell lymphoma. Increasing anemia and thrombocytopenia are other common features.

Atypical CML. In 5% to 10% of the patients who initially show a CML-like picture, the Ph[1] chromosome is absent. Some of these patients have the *bcr-abl* gene and can be reclassified as typical CML. Compared to classic CML, the Ph[1]-, *bcr-abl*–negative patients are usually older and have a higher incidence of anemia, thrombocytopenia, and marrow blasts; they also have decreased megakaryocytes and a lower incidence of basophilia and thrombocytosis. Atypical CML may actually be a group of disorders, including myelodysplastic syndrome and chronic myelomonocytic leukemia, as well as true atypical CML.

References

Bennett JM, Catovsky D, Daniel MT, et al. The chronic myeloid leukaemias: guidelines for distinguishing chronic granulocytic, atypical chronic myeloid, and chronic myelomonocytic leukaemia. Proposals by the French-American-British Cooperative Leukaemia Group. *Br J Haematol.* 1994;87:746-754.

Dekmezian R, Kantarjian HP, Keating MJ, et al. The relevance of reticulin stain-measured fibrosis at diagnosis in chronic myelogenous leukemia. *Cancer.* 1987;59:1739-1743.

Dexter TM, Chang J. New strategies for the treatment of chronic myelogenous leukemia. *Blood.* 1994;84:673-675.

Epner DE, Koeffler HP. Molecular genetic advances in chronic myelogenous leukemia. *Ann Intern Med.* 1990;113:3-6.

Foti A, Ahuja HG, Allen P, et al. Correlation between molecular and clinical events in the evolution of chronic myelocytic leukemia to blast crisis. *Blood.* 1991;77:2441-2444.

Hyun BH, Gulati GL, Ashton JK. Myeloproliferative disorders: classification and diagnostic features with special emphasis on chronic myelogenous leukemia and agnogenic myeloid metaplasia. *Clin Lab Med.* 1990;10:825-838.

Kantarjian HM, Deisseroth A, Kurzrock R, et al. Chronic myelogenous leukemia: a concise update. *Blood.* 1993;82:691-703.

Kantarjian HM, Keating MJ, Walters RS, et al. Clinical and prognostic features of Philadelphia chromosome–negative chronic myelogenous leukemia. *Cancer.* 1986;58:2023-2030.

Kurzrock R, Gutterman JU, Talpaz M. The molecular genetics of Philadelphia chromosome–positive leukemias. *N Engl J Med.* 1988;319:990-998.

Rowley JD. The Philadelphia chromosome translocation: a paradigm for understanding leukemia. *Cancer.* 1990;65:2178-2184.

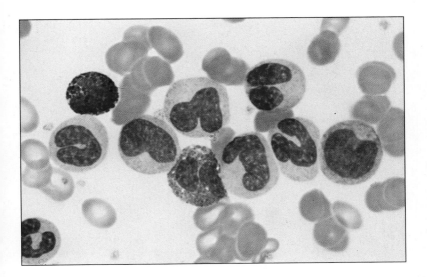

Image 34-1 CML. A spectrum of granulocytes, from immature to mature, together with one basophil and one eosinophil, are seen in a peripheral blood smear.

Image 34-2 CML karyotype: 46, XY t(9;22). The classic Philadelphia chromosome is a translocation from the long arm of chromosome 22 to the long arm of chromosome 9.

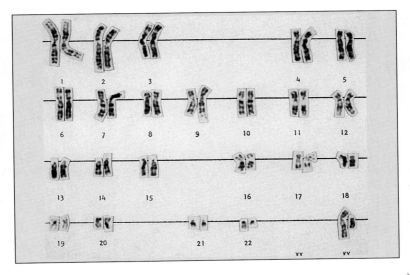

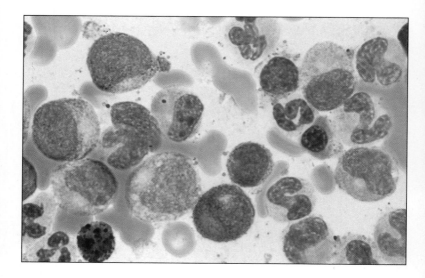

Image 34-3 Marrow aspirate in CML. As in the peripheral smear, granulocytic cells at all stages of differentiation are present.

Image 34-4 CML in blast crisis (transformation). Two blasts (in the center), several basophils, and enlarged platelets are present in this peripheral smear.

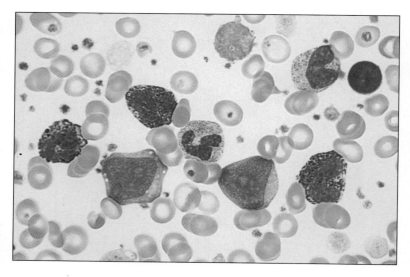

PART IX

Chronic Lymphoid
Leukemias

35

Chronic Lymphocytic Leukemia and Other Lymphoid Leukemias

Chronic lymphocytic leukemia (CLL) is an acquired chronic lymphoproliferative disorder almost always of B-cell lineage. The hallmark of CLL is an absolute lymphocytosis in both the peripheral blood and bone marrow; lymphadenopathy and splenomegaly may also be present. CLL is the most common leukemia in the United States and Europe, but it is rare in the Orient. It typically occurs in middle-aged and elderly individuals.

Pathophysiology

CLL is a clonal disorder of B lymphocytes that express pan B-cell surface antigens, including CD19, CD20, and CD24. The cells display surface immunoglobulin that is restricted to one or two classes of heavy chains, usually IgM or IgM and IgD. Since the lymphocytes are clonal, only a single light chain, either kappa or lambda, is expressed. Intracytoplasmic immunoglobulin is also present. Cells from patients with CLL show clonal immunoglobulin gene rearrangements. In most cases, the CLL lymphocytes react with antibodies against the CD5 antigen. This antigen was initially thought to be a specific pan T-cell antigen, but it is now known that a subset of normal lymphocytes coexpress B-cell antigens and CD5. Current evidence suggests that even though CLL lymphocytes are morphologically mature, immunologically they are immature cells arrested at an early stage of development.

Abnormalities of T cells have also been identified in patients with CLL. Increased absolute numbers of T lymphocytes have been reported in untreated patients with CLL, although the level fluctuates during the course of the disease. Inversion of the normal T helper-to-suppressor ratio in the blood with decreased T-helper function is usually present. Natural killer (NK) function is often decreased or absent, even though the absolute number of NK cells in the blood may be increased in CLL.

Almost all patients with CLL eventually develop hypogamma-globulinemia. The hypogammaglobulinemia probably results from impaired B cell function, but abnormalities of T cell regulation may also be important. Related to the hypogammaglobulinemia and T cell abnormalities, patients with CLL have impaired antibody and cell-mediated immunity to recall antigens. Many patients develop autoantibodies; most are directed against mature hematopoietic cells. Autoimmune hemolytic anemia occurs during the course of disease in about 15% of patients, while immune thrombocytopenia and granulocytopenia are less common.

Clonal chromosome alterations are detected in about 50% to 60% of patients with CLL. The most common abnormality is trisomy 12, present in 20% to 30% of the patients. The most common structural abnormality involves the long arm of chromosome 13 at chromosome band 13q14. Abnormalities of chromosomes 14q, 6q, 11, and others also occur in CLL.

Clinical Findings

Most patients with CLL are over 50 years of age; the disease is unusual before 30 years of age. There is a higher incidence of CLL among men: the ratio of affected men to women is approximately 2:1. Many patients are asymptomatic when the disease is diagnosed. Symptoms, when present, usually include weakness, easy fatigability, and weight loss. Fever, night sweats, or frequent viral and bacterial infections are more common as the disease progresses, but may be present at diagnosis. The most frequent abnormality on physical examination is the presence of lymphadenopathy that varies from enlargement of only a single node or node group to enlargement of virtually all lymph nodes. Hepatomegaly or splenomegaly occurs at diagnosis, but is less common.

The most widely used clinical staging system for CLL in the United States is the Rai system (Table 35-1). Patients with minimal evidence of disease, ie, lymphocytosis only, are considered to be in the earliest stage of disease, while those demonstrating compromise of bone marrow function such as anemia and thrombocytopenia are in advanced stages. The Rai system has been modified according to degree of risk, with stage 0 being low risk; stages I and II intermediate risk; and stages III and IV high risk. The survival times correlate inversely with the clinical stage. Survival times in these three categories are greater than 10, 6, and 2 years, respectively.

Approach to Diagnosis

Following a clinical history and physical examination, the laboratory diagnosis of CLL includes the following:

1. A complete blood cell count.
2. Examination of the peripheral blood smear.
3. Examination of bone marrow.
4. Immunologic cell marker studies.
5. Ancillary studies such as immunoglobulin analysis, antiglobulin tests, and cytogenetic studies.

Hematologic Findings

CLL is characterized by a sustained peripheral blood lymphocytosis. Morphologically, the lymphocytes appear mature, even though immunologic studies indicate that they are immature at an early stage of B-cell differentiation. Immunophenotypic analysis is useful in the diagnostic workup of CLL to confirm monoclonality of the lymphocytes and is especially important when the lymphocy-

Table 35-1   Rai's Clinical Staging System for Chronic
Lymphocytic Leukemia

Stage 0:	Lymphocytosis in blood and bone marrow only
Stage I:	Lymphocytosis plus enlarged lymph nodes
Stage II:	Lymphocytosis plus enlarged liver and/or spleen; lymphadenopathy may be present
Stage III:	Lymphocytosis plus anemia (hemoglobin <11 g/dL [110 g/L]); lymph nodes, spleen, or liver may be enlarged
Stage IV:	Lymphocytosis and thrombocytopenia (platelet count <100 x 10^3/mm^3 [100 x 10^9/L]); anemia and organomegaly may be present

tosis is mild. A bone marrow aspirate and core biopsy are often performed to confirm the diagnosis and to provide prognostic information. Cytogenetic analysis is occasionally performed since the karyotype also gives information about prognosis.

Several benign diseases such as infectious mononucleosis and acute cytomegalovirus infection are also accompanied by a peripheral lymphocytosis (see Chapters 23 and 24). These entities are usually readily distinguishable from CLL since they generally occur in younger patients, are characterized by fever and other acute symptoms, and exhibit a lymphocytosis that differs morphologically and immunologically from that of CLL. Several malignant lymphoproliferative disorders, such as prolymphocytic leukemia, hairy cell leukemia, leukemic lymphoma, and large granular lymphocyte leukemia, may closely resemble CLL and are discussed later in this chapter.

Blood Cell Measurements. Anemia (hemoglobin less than 11.0 g/dL [110 g/L]) is present in about 15% to 20% and thrombocytopenia (less than 100 x 10^3/mm^3 [100 x 10^9/L]) is present in about 10% of patients at diagnosis. Bone marrow replacement and hypersplenism contribute to the cytopenias. The anemia is typically normochromic and normocytic. The reticulocyte count is usually normal unless the patient has an autoimmune hemolytic anemia, in which case it is elevated.

Usually the absolute peripheral lymphocyte count is greater than 10 x 10^3/mm^3 (10 x 10^9/L), but the degree of lymphocytosis is sometimes milder (in the range of 5-10 x 10^3/mm^3 [5-10 x

10^9/L]). Extreme lymphocytosis over 500 x 10^3/mm^3 (500 x 10^9/L) occurs only late in the disease.

Peripheral Blood Smear Morphology. The red blood cells are usually normochromic and normocytic. If an autoimmune hemolytic anemia is present, spherocytes and increased numbers of polychromatophilic cells may be present in the blood smear. In most cases of CLL, the lymphocytes are small with condensed chromatin patterns and narrow rims of cytoplasm (Image 35-1). The lymphocytes tend to resemble one another and look monotonous in appearance, although in some cases variable numbers of larger lymphocytes may also be present. Smudged or damaged lymphocytes are often prominent in the smear. Lymphocytes having the appearance of prolymphocytes may also be present. Prolymphocytes are identified by their larger size, loosely condensed chromatin, nucleoli, and small-to-moderate amounts of basophilic cytoplasm. In a typical case of CLL, prolymphocytes represent less than 10% of the total lymphocyte population.

Bone Marrow Examination. The bone marrow is usually hypercellular; greater than 20% to 30% of the nucleated cells are lymphocytes. The lymphocytes are morphologically similar to those in the blood. Histologic sections of core biopsy specimens have revealed four possible morphologic patterns of bone marrow infiltration in CLL: (1) interstitial, with preservation of the marrow architecture and fat cells; (2) nodular (focal); (3) mixed interstitial and nodular (Image 35-2); and (4) diffuse with replacement of the bone marrow space by CLL cells. The nodular infiltrates are not paratrabecular. Bone marrow histopathologic features in CLL have emerged as prognostic indicators independent of clinical stage. Patients with a diffuse pattern of involvement have a poorer prognosis than those with a nondiffuse pattern.

Other Laboratory Tests

35.1 Cell Surface Markers

Purpose. Immunophenotypic analysis is used to confirm a diagnosis of CLL in a patient with a peripheral blood lymphocytosis that is morphologically consistent with CLL. It documents that the disease is a monoclonal B cell disorder by identifying light chain restriction (Figure 35-1). This is especially important in patients with a low-grade lymphocytosis, ie, less than $10 \times 10^3/mm^3$ ($10 \times 10^9/L$). Coexpression of B-cell antigens and CD5, positivity for CD23 (Figure 35-1) and the low intensity of expression of both CD20 and surface immunoglobulin are characteristic of CLL lymphocytes. Immunophenotypic evidence of these findings not only aids in confirming the diagnosis, but may also help to differentiate it from other chronic lymphoproliferative disorders and lymphoma.

Principle.   Labeled lineage-restricted or associated monoclonal antibodies combine with determinants on B lymphocytes, T lymphocytes, their subsets, and other hematopoietic cells (see Table 30-4). Labeled cells in suspension can then be characterized by flow cytometry.

Specimen.   Fresh peripheral blood anticoagulated with heparin is the usual specimen for immunophenotypic analysis of the lymphocytes in CLL. Cell suspensions from bone marrow or other tissues such as fresh lymph node can also be used.

Procedure.   Flow cytometry involves a fluid system that delivers the cell sample past an excitation light beam in a single-file stream. The scattered light and any fluorescence emitted from this interaction (from dyes used to stain specific cell molecules) are collected and converted to electrical signals. These can then be analyzed to give quantitative information about specific cell characteristics. With flow cytometry, the expression of two or more antigens can be simultaneously investigated on the same cell. The most common commercially available monoclonal antibodies used for characterization of leukemias, including CLL, are shown in Table 30-4. Many of the available monoclonal antibodies are also applicable to immunohistochemical methods for use on smears, touch preparations, and sections.

Figure 35-1   Dual parameter flow cytometric analysis of lymphocytes from a patient with chronic lymphocytic leukemia. The lymphocytes coexpress CD19 and CD5, are positive for CD19 and CD23, and exhibit light chain (kappa) restriction; these findings are characteristic of B-cell chronic lymphocytic leukemia.

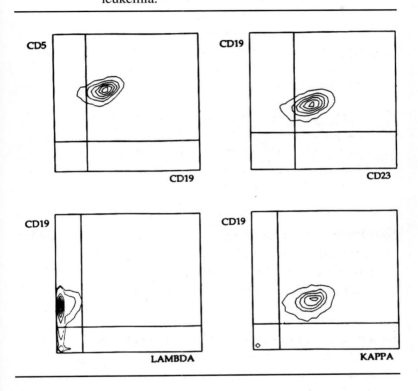

Interpretation.   The lymphocytes in CLL are positive for the pan B-cell antigens, CD19, CD20, and CD24. The cells express surface immunoglobulin that is restricted to a single light chain, either kappa or lambda, but not both (Figure 35-1). In addition, the lymphocytes usually have IgM or IgM and IgD heavy chains on their surface; IgG or IgA is much less common. Concentration of the monoclonal surface immunoglobulin is usually low, with dim immunofluorescence intensity on flow cytometry. The intensity of the positivity for the pan B-antigen, CD20, is also dim. This contrasts with the strong intensity seen with other B-cell chronic lymphoproliferative disorders or non-Hodgkin's lymphomas. In most cases of CLL, the cells coexpress CD5 along with the pan B-cell antigens (Figure 35-1). This finding is characteristic of CLL, but is not specific for CLL since it is also present on cells from most cases of mantle cell lymphoma. CLL lymphocytes are usually positive for HLA-DR, CD21, and CD23. They are negative for CD10.

Ancillary Tests

Antiglobulin Test.   Autoimmune hemolytic anemia develops in approximately 15% of patients with CLL at some time during the disease course. The hemolysis is mediated by a warm-reacting IgG antibody and the direct antiglobulin test is usually positive. The direct antiglobulin test may be positive in approximately 25% of patients with CLL, but autoimmune hemolysis occurs only about half as frequently. Autoimmune thrombocytopenia and neutropenia may also occur in CLL, but laboratory demonstration of these antibodies is difficult.

Serum Immunoglobulin.   Hypogammaglobulinemia occurs initially or during the course of the disease in most patients with CLL. All immunoglobulin classes—IgG, IgM, and IgA—are depressed. In about 5% of patients, a monoclonal protein, usually IgM, may be present.

Cytogenetic Analysis.   Clonal chromosome abnormalities can be detected in 50% to 60% of patients with CLL, and the karyotype of the malignant cells is useful in predicting the prognosis of patients with CLL. The most common numerical chromosome abnormality in CLL is trisomy 12. The most common structural abnormality involves the long arm of chromosome 13 at band 13q14. Abnormalities of chromosomes 14q, 6q, 11, and others have also been identified. Patients with trisomy 12 or abnormalities of chromosome 14q appear to have a poorer prognosis than patients with normal karyotypes or those with abnormalities of 13q. Patients with 13q abnormalities appear to have a similar prognosis to those patients with normal karyotypes.

Lymph Node Biopsy. A lymph node biopsy is not necessary for the diagnosis of CLL, but may be performed to evaluate enlarged lymph nodes for evidence of transformation of the CLL to a more aggressive lymphoma such as Richter's syndrome (see below). Lymph nodes involved with chronic phase CLL (Image 35-3) typically exhibit diffuse effacement by a monotonous infiltrate of small lymphocytes with round nuclear contours, inconspicuous nucleoli, and scant cytoplasm. Pseudonodules, also referred to as proliferation or growth centers, are frequently present. These areas consist of larger cells with more prominent nucleoli and more readily apparent mitotic activity. Occasionally, the larger cells are diffusely mixed with the smaller lymphocytes but usually account for less than 30% of the total cells.

Course and Treatment

The clinical course of CLL is extremely variable. Many patients have an indolent, almost benign course and live for over 10 or 20 years without major complications from CLL. Others have a rapid downhill course and die within 1 to 2 years after diagnosis. Most patients with CLL, however, have a disease course somewhere in between these two extremes, with a median survival rate of 3 to 4 years. Since CLL tends to occur in elderly patients, death often results from other unrelated illnesses in this age group. Patients younger than 60 years of age almost always die as a result of CLL or one of its complications, usually infections. Gram-positive organisms usually cause infections that occur early in the disease, but most deaths are due to infections by gram-negative bacteria or fungal infections. Infections by other organisms such as viruses, *Pneumocystis carinii*, or *Mycobacterium tuberculosis* may also contribute to death in CLL.

Some patients with CLL (about 15%) develop what has been called prolymphocytoid transformation. Prolymphocytoid transformation occurs following a chronic phase of CLL and is associated with progressive anemia, thrombocytopenia, increasing lymphadenopathy and splenomegaly, and resistance to therapy. The blood contains two distinct cell populations, typical CLL cells and an increasing number of prolymphocytes. The latter express the same immunoglobulin isotype as the CLL cells, and it appears that pro-lymphocyte transformation evolves from the original CLL clone.

Richter's syndrome occurs in about 5% of patients with CLL and is characterized by the abrupt onset of fever, weight loss, increasing organomegaly, and poor prognosis. Rapidly enlarging tumor masses often develop in nodes and other sites. Biopsy specimens of these masses reveal a large cell lymphoma. Other morphologic types of lymphoma, including Hodgkin's disease, have also been reported in patients with CLL.

Since patients with CLL are usually late in life and the disease may be stable for many years, it is traditional to delay treatment of early stage CLL until the disease progresses. Signs for progressive disease often include cytopenias, organ enlargement, and increased susceptibility to infections. Treatment of CLL has usually involved alkylating agents such as chlorambucil or cyclophosphamide, often combined with prednisone. A number of newer agents now appear to be active against CLL, including fludarabine, 2-chloro-deoxyadenosine, and deoxycoformycin. Biologic agents such as alpha interferon, interleukin-2, and monoclonal antibodies directed against CLL are also being studied. Bone marrow transplantation is being attempted in some younger patients with CLL.

Other Chronic Lymphoid Leukemias

Chronic Lymphocytic Leukemia/PL. In a minority of cases of CLL, the percentage of the prolymphocytes in the blood falls somewhere between that found in typical chronic phase CLL (less than 10%) and that found in prolymphocytic leukemia (PLL) (greater than 55%) (Image 35-4). These have been designated as CLL/PL. Some of these patients have a progressive increase in the proportion and absolute number of prolymphocytes, which may represent prolymphocytoid transformation. In many cases, however-er, the proportion of prolymphocytes remains stable and the patients have a clinical course similar to that of typical CLL. Surface marker studies of CLL/PL are similar to those found in CLL and suggest a close relationship of these two disorders.

Prolymphocytic Leukemia. PLL is a rare variant of CLL that occurs predominantly in older men and is characterized by leukocytosis, prominent splenomegaly, and minimal or absent lymphadenopathy. The leukocyte count is frequently markedly elevated, often greater than 100,000 x 10^3/mm^3 (100,000 x 10^9/L). Prolymphocytes are the predominant cell in the blood, representing more than 55% of the lymphocytes. Prolymphocytes are characterized by large size, moderate rims of basophilic cytoplasm, moderately condensed chromatin patterns, and prominent nucleoli (Image 35-5). Anemia, thrombocytopenia, and neutropenia are common at diagnosis. The bone marrow is usually extensively infiltrated in a diffuse or mixed interstitial and nodular pattern. The spleen shows both white and red pulp infiltration. Sections of lymph nodes show a diffuse pattern of infiltration with or without a pseudonodular pattern. Patients with PLL have an aggressive clinical course with shorter survival times than those with CLL.

About 80% of cases of PLL are of B-cell origin (Table 35-2) and express several pan B-cell antigens such as CD19, CD20, and CD22. Prolymphocytes exhibit surface immunoglobulin that is more intense than the cells in CLL. Unlike CLL, prolymphocytes are negative for CD5. The most common cytogenetic abnormality in B-cell PLL appears to be a 14q+ chromosome with the break point at the heavy-chain immunoglobulin gene locus. About 20% of cases of PLL are T cell in origin and express CD2, CD5, and CD7. Most have a CD4+, CD8– phenotype; a minority coexpress CD4 and CD8 or are CD4–, CD8+. Cytogenetic abnormalities of chromosome 14 with break points at q11 and q32 are common in T-PLL.

Hairy Cell Leukemia. Hairy cell leukemia (HCL) is a rare type of leukemia characterized by pancytopenia or other combinations of cytopenias, splenomegaly, minimal lymphadenopathy, and the presence of hairy cells in both the blood and bone marrow. The disease affects adults with a mean age of about 50 years and is more common in men than in women. Patients often present with systemic symptoms such as weakness, weight loss, recurrent bacterial infections, or abdominal discomfort.

On peripheral blood films, hairy cells are one to two times the size of small lymphocytes and have round, oval, or kidney-shaped nuclei (Image 35-6). The chromatin patterns are stippled and nucleoli are usually single, small, and inconspicuous. The cytoplasm is moderate to abundant, pale blue, and has poorly defined borders or

Table 35-2   Immunophenotype of Chronic Lymphoproliferative Disorders

Antigen	CLL	B-PLL	T-PLL	HCL	FCL	T-LGLL*	ATLL	SS
SIg	+(dim)	+	−	+	+	−	−	−
CD19	+	+	−	+	+	−	−	−
CD20	+(dim)	+	−	+	+	−	−	−
CD22	+/−	+	−	+	+	−	−	−
CD11c	+/−	−	−	+	−	−	−	−
CD25	+/−	+/−	−	+	−	−	+	−
CD2	−	−	+	−	−	+	+	+
CD3	−	−	+	−	−	+	+	+
CD4	−	−	+	−	−	−	+	+
CD8	−	−	+/−	−	−	+	−	−
CD5	+	−	+	−	−	+/−	+	+
CD7	−	−	+	−	−	+/−	−	−
CD10	−	−	−	−	+	−	−	−

Abbbreviations: + = most cases are positive for this antigen; − = most cases are negative; +/− = cases are variably positive; CLL = chronic lymphocytic leukemia; PLL = prolymphocytic leukemia; HCL = hairy cell leukemia; FCL = follicle cell leukemia; LGLL= large granular lymphocyte leukemia; ATLL = adult T-cell leukemia/lymphoma; SS = Sézary syndrome; SIg = surface immunoglobulin.
*Also CD57+.

hairy projections. Although these cells are present in the blood of most patients with HCL, they may be rare and difficult to find.

Bone marrow examination is essential for a diagnosis of hairy cell leukemia. The bone marrow is often inaspirable, but the core biopsy specimen reveals variable degrees of focal or diffuse infiltration by hairy cells. The hairy cells can be identified in sections by their abundant, clear cytoplasm, and well-spaced nuclei that do not touch one another (Image 35-7). On high power, the hairy cell nuclei appear bland with round, oval, or indented nuclei. Bone marrow reticulin fibrosis is almost always present. The histologic sections of the spleen show red pulp infiltration by hairy cells with widening of the pulp cords and frequent blood-filled pseudosinuses lined by hairy cells.

A cytochemical stain detecting the presence of tartrate-resistant acid phosphatase (TRAP) is the most widely used test to confirm the diagnosis of HCL. This stain is usually performed on blood smears and bone marrow aspirate smears or touch preparations of bone marrow.

Hairy cells are of B-cell lineage and display immunopheno-typic features that suggest they are mid to late stage in differentiation. They express pan B-cell antigens such as CD19, CD20, and CD22. They are also almost always positive for CD25 (the p55 receptor for interleukin-2) and CD11c (a leukocyte adhesion molecule). Coexpression of a pan B-cell marker, CD11c, and CD25, although not entirely specific, strongly suggests the diagnosis of HCL. Hairy cells in fixed sections react with several monoclonal antibodies directed against B cells, including L26 and DBA.44.

HCL is an indolent, slowly progressive disease with median survival times of about 5 years. Until recently, the mainstay of therapy was splenectomy. In the past few years, however, effective medical therapies have become available that control the disease in most patients. These include the interferons, the adenosine deaminase inhibitor deoxycoformycin, and more recently 2-chlorodeoxyadenosine (2-CdA).

Leukemic Manifestations of Follicle Cell Lymphoma.

Approximately 55% to 70% of patients with follicle cell lymphoma (FCL) have bone marrow involvement. About 50% of the patients with bone marrow involvement have peripheral manifestations of the lymphoma. In most cases, the number of morphologically recognizable lymphoma cells is small and does not alter the differential count significantly. Occasionally, however, the involvement of the blood is characterized by a striking lymphocytosis that mimics CLL. The presence of small cleaved lymphocytes in the blood smear aids in the morphologic distinction of this disease from CLL.

The circulating cells in FCL are small- to medium-sized with a smooth, evenly staining nucleus that is frequently cleaved or folded (Image 35-8). Nucleoli are absent or inconspicuous. The cytoplasm is very sparse and pale blue. Bone marrow involvement is characterized by a focal, paratrabecular location of the lymphoma. This is in contrast to CLL in which the marrow lesions are randomly focal or diffuse.

FCL is a clonal B-cell malignancy, but membrane surface marker studies show some immunophenotypic differences between FCL and CLL (Table 35-2). Surface membrane immunoglobulin in FCL is intense; the cells are CD5 negative and frequently CD10 positive. Follicle lymphomas are positive for the t(14;18) chromosome translocation and/or its molecular counterpart, the BCL-2/IgH gene fusion.

Large Granular Lymphocyte Leukemia. Large granular lymphocyte leukemia (LGLL) is a rare disorder characterized by circulating large granular lymphocytes and neutropenia. Many terms have been used to describe this entity, including T-γ-lymphoproliferative disorder, large granular lymphocytosis, granulated T-cell lymphocytosis with neutropenia, and T-cell CLL. LGLL is a chronic disorder characterized by mild to moderate blood lymphocytosis (4-40 x 10³/mm³ [4-40 x 10⁹/L]), bone marrow infiltration, absence of lymphadenopathy, and mild to moderate splenomegaly. The disease occurs in adults with a median age of about 60 years; occasionally, patients are affected in their teenage years. Patients usually present with recurrent bacterial infections. Rheumatoid arthritis is also associated with this disease.

The lymphocyte in this disorder is a large granular lymphocyte, medium to large in size, with coarse chromatin, moderate pale cytoplasm, and prominent azurophilic granules (Image 35-9). The bone marrow in this disorder generally shows a mild to moderate increase in lymphocytes that are morphologically similar to those in the blood. Patients with LGLL usually have neutropenia, which is often severe. An anemia and/or mild thrombocytopenia is present in some cases. The involvement of the core biopsy sections is usually diffuse, with focal accentuation in some cases.

In most cases of LGLL, the cells have a mature postthymic phenotype and are CD3 positive; most are CD8 positive and CD4 negative. They also express CD16, the gamma Fc receptor, and sometimes CD56. A subset of LGLL marks as true NK cells. The usual phenotype of these cases is CD3–, CD8–, CD4–, CD16+, and CD56+.

Most patients with LGLL have a prolonged clinical course with little progression of symptoms. Although the neoplastic nature of this disorder was originally uncertain, the demonstration of clonal cytogenetic abnormalities and/or T-cell receptor gene rearrangements indicate that this is a clonal, neoplastic disorder. Reactive proliferations of large granular lymphocytes also exist but are rare.

Adult T-Cell Leukemia/Lymphoma.   Adult T-cell leukemia/lymphoma (ATLL) was first described in individuals from southwestern Japan, but now has been identified in other areas including the Caribbean and the United States. This disorder occurs in adults and is characterized by a proliferation of multilobated T lymphocytes in the blood, lymphadenopathy, splenomegaly, and skin lesions. Many patients have osteolytic lesions and hypercalcemia. ATLL is caused by a retrovirus, human T-cell leukemia virus–1 (HTLV-1). Most patients have a subacute or acute course that is refractory to therapy.

Leukocytosis is present and ranges from 25 to 500 x 10^3/mm^3 (25-500 x 10^9/L). The malignant cells vary from small to large and possess nuclei that are markedly irregular in outline with deep nuclear indentations or lobulation (Image 35-10). Nucleoli are usually inconspicuous in the smaller cells but may be prominent in the larger cells. Cytoplasm is scant. The bone marrow, lymph nodes, skin, liver, and spleen are frequently infiltrated by these cells.

The immunophenotype of the leukemic cells in ATLL is predominantly that of helper T cells that are CD2+, CD3+, and CD4+. They also express CD25.

Sézary Syndrome.   Mycosis fungoides (MF) is a primary T-cell lymphoma of the skin. A small percentage of patients with MF develop Sézary syndrome (SS), which is characterized by a generalized exfoliative erythroderma and a peripheral blood lymphocytosis. The lymphocytosis is caused by circulating abnormal lymphocytes called Sézary cells. Sézary cells may be small or large with a small-to-moderate amount of cytoplasm; the nuclei have marked convolutions that give them a cerebriform appearance (Image 35-11). Nucleoli are usually absent or inconspicuous. Many of the Sézary cells will show periodic acid–Schiff–positive cytoplasmic vacuoles around the nuclei.

The membrane immunophenotype of Sézary cells is that of a mature helper T lymphocyte, CD3+, CD4+, and CD8–. Patients with Sézary syndrome have a poorer prognosis than those with classic MF and frequently exhibit hepatosplenomegaly and lymphadenopathy. The bone marrow may be normal or show minimal infiltration, but is often involved, especially when the white blood cell count is high.

References

Anastasi J, LeBeau MM, Vardiman JW, et al. Detection of trisomy 12 in chronic lymphocytic leukemia by fluorescence in situ hybridization to interphase cells: a simple and sensitive method. *Blood.* 1992;79:1796-1801.

Bennett JM, Catovsky D, Daniel M-T, et al. Proposals for the classification of chronic (mature) B and T lymphoid leukemias. *J Clin Pathol.* 1989;42:567-584.

Bitter MA. Hairy-cell leukemia. In: Knowles DM, ed. *Neoplastic Hematopathology.* Baltimore, Md: Williams and Wilkins; 1992: 1209-1234.

Brunning RD, McKenna RW. Small lymphocytic leukemia and related disorders. In: *Atlas of Tumor Pathology: Tumors of the Bone Marrow.* Washington, DC: Armed Forces Institute of Pathology; 1994:255-312.

Carey JL, Hanson CA. Flow cytometric analysis of leukemia and lymphoma. In: Keren DF, Hanson CA, Hurtubise PE, eds. *Flow Cytometry and Clinical Diagnosis.* Chicago, Ill: ASCP Press; 1994:197-308.

Dighiero G, Travade P, Chevret S, et al. B-cell chronic lymphocytic leukemia: present status and future directions. *Blood.* 1991; 78:1901-1914.

Foon KA, Thiruvengadam R, Saven A, et al. Genetic relatedness of lymphoid malignancies: transformation of chronic lymphocytic leukemia as a model. *Ann Intern Med.* 1993;119:63-73.

Hakimian D, Tallman MS, Kiley C, Peterson L. Detection of minimal residual disease by immunostaining of bone marrow biopsies after 2-chlorodeoxyadenosine of hairy cell leukemia. *Blood.* 1993;82:1798-1802.

Jaffe E, Blattner WA, Blayney DW. The pathologic spectrum of adult T-cell leukemia/lymphoma in the United States. *Am J Surg Pathol.* 1984;8:263-275.

Juliusson G, Oscier DG, Fitchett M, et al. Prognostic subgroups in B-cell chronic lymphocytic leukemia defined by specific chromosomal abnormalities. *N Engl J Med.* 1990;323:720-724.

Loughran TP Jr. Clonal diseases of large granular lymphocytes. *Blood.* 1993;82:1-14.

Matutes E, Brito-Babapulle V, Swanbury J, et al. Clinical and laboratory features of 78 cases of T-prolymphocytic leukemia. *Blood.* 1991;78:3269-3274.

Melo JV, Catovsky D, Galton DAG. The relationship between chronic lymphocytic leukemia and prolymphocytic leukemia, I: clinical and laboratory features of 300 patients and characterisation of an intermediate group. *Br J Haematol.* 1986;63:377-387.

Peterson LC, Lindquist LL, Church S, et al. Frequent clonal abnormalities of chromosome band 13q14 in B-cell chronic lymphocytic leukemia: multiple clones, subclones and nonclonal alterations in 82 midwestern patients. *Genes Chromosomes Cancer.* 1992;4:273-280.

Rozman C, Montserrat E, Rodriquez-Fernandez JM, et al. Bone marrow histologic pattern—the best single prognostic parameter in chronic lymphocytic leukemia: a multivariate survival analysis of 329 cases. *Blood.* 1984;64:642-648.

Wood GS. Benign and malignant cutaneous lymphoproliferative disorders including mycosis fungoides. In: Knowles DM, ed. *Neoplastic Hematopathology.* Baltimore, Md: Williams and Wilkins; 1992:917-952.

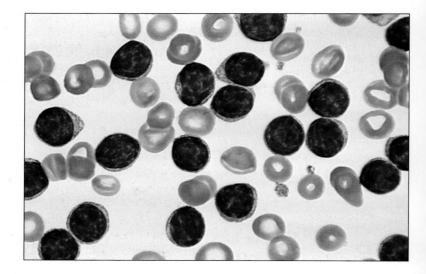

Image 35-1 Blood smear from a patient with chronic lymphocytic leukemia. The lymphocytes have scant cytoplasm and condensed chromatin patterns.

Image 35-2 Bone marrow core biopsy specimen from a patient with chronic lymphocytic leukemia shows a mixed interstitial and nodular pattern of infiltration.

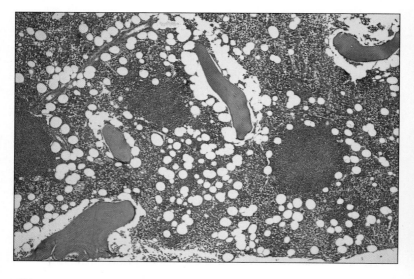

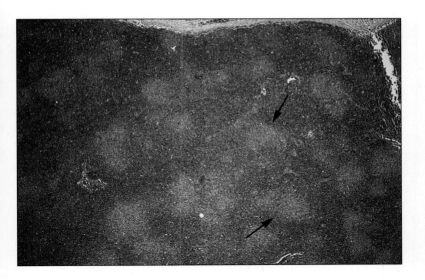

Image 35-3 Lymph node biopsy specimen from a patient with chronic lymphocytic leukemia shows diffuse effacement with proliferation centers (↑).

Image 35-4 Blood smear from a patient with CLL/PL shows two morphologic types of lymphocytes: those with scant cytoplasm and condensed chromatin, which is typical for CLL; and larger prolymphocytes with moderately condensed chromatin and nucleoli.

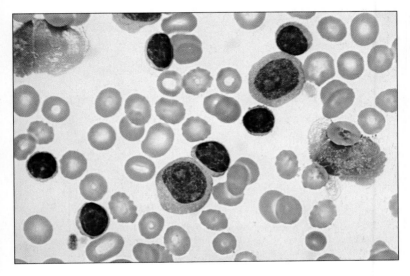

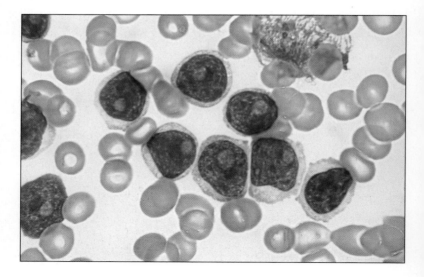

Image 35-5 Blood smear from a patient with prolymphocytic leukemia.

Image 35-6 Blood smear shows pancytopenia and a hairy cell with stippled chromatin pattern and an indistinct cytoplasmic border.

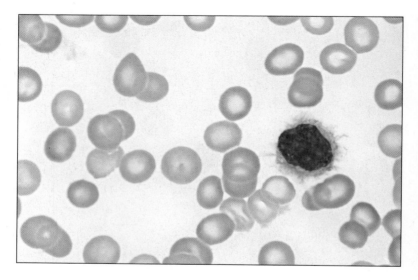

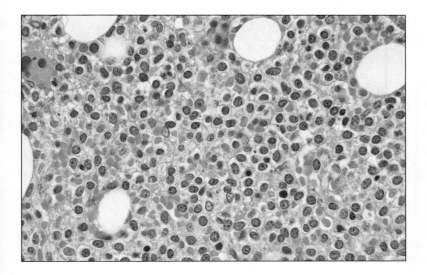

Image 35-7 Bone marrow core biopsy specimen shows diffuse infiltration by hairy cells with well-spaced nuclei.

Image 35-8 Blood smear from a patient with follicle cell lymphoma with circulating small cleaved lymphocyte.

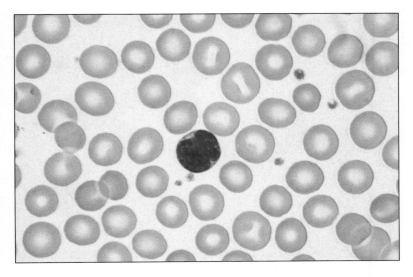

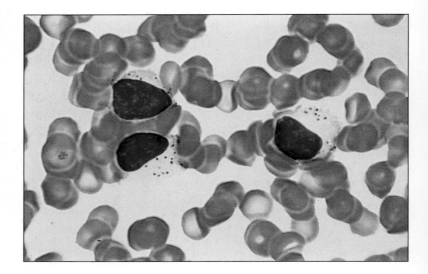

Image 35-9   Blood smear from a patient with large granular lympho-cyte leukemia.

Image 35-10   Blood smear from a patient with adult T-cell leukemia/lymphoma shows multilobated lymphocytes.

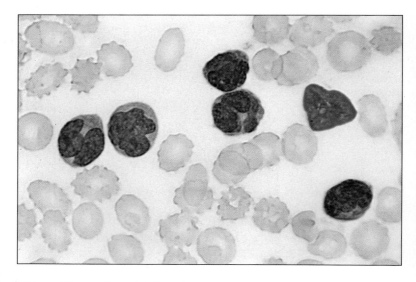

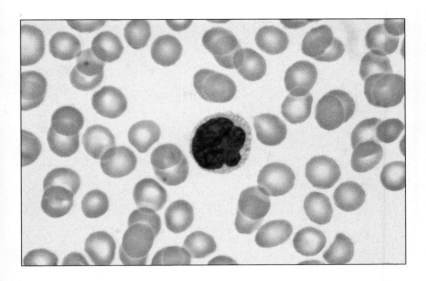

Image 35-11   Blood smear shows Sézary cell with convoluted nuclei.

PART
X

Lymphomas

36

Non-Hodgkin's Lymphoma

Malignant lymphoma is the generic term for malignant neoplasms of the lymphoid tissue. The two major subgroups of malignant lymphoma are Hodgkin's disease and non-Hodgkin's lymphoma (NHL). Malignant lymphomas are increasing in frequency, and in 1992 approximately 41,000 new cases were diagnosed in the United States. Between 1973 and 1988, there was a 50% increase in the incidence of NHLs; a significant portion of this increase is a strong association with NHL in patients with AIDS. There is, however, also a significant increase in non-AIDS–related cases. NHL affects patients of all ages, with an increasing incidence from childhood to old age. The ratio of affected men to women is approximately 2 to 1.5.

NHLs are a group of disorders with varying histopathologic features, clinical presentations, responses to therapy, and prognoses. Most NHLs originate in lymph nodes, but the disease also frequently begins in extranodal sites (especially in children and immunosuppressed patients). In some patients, the lymphoma involves bone marrow with or without circulating malignant cells similar to that seen in leukemias (eg, small lymphocytic lymphoma/chronic lymphocytic leukemia, lymphoblastic lymphoma/-

acute lymphoblastic leukemia). There is also considerable diversity in the clinical behavior with some lymphomas being relatively indolent (small lymphocytic lymphoma and follicular lymphomas), while others are very aggressive and fast-growing (immunoblastic lymphoma and Burkitt's lymphoma). Paradoxically, the current therapies are able to cure many patients with the most aggressive lymphomas, while the indolent (low grade) lymphomas are at this time usually not curable.

There is considerable difference in the geographic distribution of NHL. Follicular lymphomas are primarily tumors of adults and are common in the United States and in Europe. They are uncommon in Japan, Latin America, and Africa. Burkitt's lymphoma occurs more frequently in tropical Africa and adult T-cell leukemia lymphoma is seen particularly in southwestern Japan and the Caribbean countries.

Pathophysiology

NHLs are neoplasms of the immune system characterized by monoclonal proliferations of malignant B or T lymphocytes. The tumors arise from their normal cell counterparts within the lymphoreticular system and are probably caused by the repression of lymphocyte transformation as a consequence of molecular genetic changes. The cause of most cases of NHLs remains unknown. Immunologic studies indicate that multiple factors are involved. Some of these factors include oncogenic viruses, oncogene transformation with chromosomal aberrations, congenital or iatrogenic immunosuppression, exposure to pesticides, and ionizing radiation. Table 36-1 lists some of the predisposing conditions and factors in the development of NHLs.

Clinical Findings

Clinical manifestations of NHL are varied and are to a large extent dependent on histologic features. More than two thirds of patients with NHL present with painless peripheral lymph node enlargement, most commonly in the cervical region. Patients with follicu-

Table 36-1 Possible Predisposing Conditions and Factors in Development of Non-Hodgkin's Lymphoma

Congenital
    Ataxia telangiectasia
    Wiskott-Aldrich syndrome
    Chédiak-Higashi syndrome
    X-linked lymphoproliferative syndrome
Acquired
    Organ transplantation
    Sjögren's syndrome
    Hashimoto's thyroiditis
Viruses
    Human immunodeficiency virus
    Epstein-Barr virus (Burkitt's lymphoma)
    Retrovirus human T-cell leukemia virus
Bacteria
    Helicobacter pylori (MALT lymphoma of stomach)
Physical and chemical agents
    Chemotherapy
    Ionizing radiation
    Phenoxyherbicides
    Benzene
    Phenytoin

lar lymphoma usually have multiple sites of involvement, including extranodal disease within bone marrow, liver, or spleen. Large cell lymphomas are more frequently localized at presentation. Although most patients are asymptomatic at presentation, about 20% of the patients have so-called B symptoms, manifested by fevers, night sweats, weight loss, pruritus, and pain. B symptoms are more commonly seen in the aggressive type of lymphomas.

In addition to lymph nodes, NHLs can present in almost any organ system. Such extranodal lymphomas can present great diagnostic difficulties and unusual clinical problems because of the variable clinical features. The most common sites of extranodal lymphomas are gastrointestinal tract, lung, brain, thyroid, salivary gland, orbit, the gonads, central nervous system, bone, and skin. A comparison of characteristic features in NHL and Hodgkin's disease is presented in Table 36-2.

Table 36-2 Comparison of Non-Hodgkin's Lymphoma and Hodgkin's Disease

Feature	Non-Hodgkin's Lymphoma	Hodgkin's Disease
B symptoms	20%	40%
Presentation	Often extranodal	Predominantly nodal
Involvement	Rarely localized	Usually localized
Peripheral blood	Affected in 20%-30%	Not affected
Bone marrow involvement	Frequent	Uncommon
Mediastinal involvement	Uncommon except for lymphoblastic and mediastinal large B-cell lymphoma	Common
Gastrointestinal involvement	Common	Extremely rare
Skin involvement	Common	Extremely rare
Central nervous system involvement	Occasionally	Extremely rare

Staging

The purpose of staging a patient with lymphoma is to identify the extent of the disease to choose the optimal therapy for each patient (Table 36-3). The extent of staging studies depends on the histopathologic features of the biopsy specimen, the age of the patient, clinical symptoms, and the physical examination. The Ann Arbor staging classification for Hodgkin's disease may also be used in NHL, but it is less prognostically helpful in NHL compared with Hodgkin's disease. A National Cancer Institute modified staging system exists for intermediate- and high-grade lymphomas (Table 36-4).

The most important part of the clinical history is to determine the presence or absence of systemic B symptoms and whether there are symptoms related to extranodal involvement such as bone pain or gastrointestinal disorders. It is also helpful to assess the duration of the disease to determine the growth rate of the tumor. The physical examination should include examination of all nodal areas, including Waldeyer's ring, periauricular, epitrochlear, and popliteal lymph nodes, and the presence or absence of hepatosplenomegaly.

Table 36-3 Stages of Lymphoma

Stage I:	Disease limited to one anatomic region or two contiguous regions on the same side of the diaphragm
Stage II:	Disease in more than two anatomic regions or in noncontiguous regions on the same side of the diaphragm
Stage III:	Disease on both sides of the diaphragm, but limited to involvement of lymph nodes and spleen
Stage IV:	Disease of any lymph node region with involvement of liver, lung, or bone marrow

Table 36-4 National Cancer Institute Modified Staging for Intermediate- and High-Grade Lymphomas

Stage	Characteristics
I	Localized nodal or extranodal disease (Ann Arbor stage I or IE)
II	Two or more nodal sites of disease or a localized extranodal site plus draining nodes with one of the following: performance status ≤ 70, B symptoms, any mass >10 cm in diameter (particularly gastrointestinal), serum lactate dehydrogenase >500, three or more extranodal sites ofdisease
III	Stage II plus any poor prognostic factor

The skin, breasts, testicles, central nervous system, and lungs should be examined for possible extranodal involvement. Other staging studies usually include complete blood cell count, evaluation of renal and liver function, radiologic studies including chest radiograph, bilateral lower extremity lymphangiogram, abdominal pelvic computed tomography scan, and bilateral bone marrow needle biopsies and aspirate. Cerebrospinal fluid cytologic studies are indicated in intermediate- or high-grade lymphomas. The clinical staging procedures are summarized in Table 36-5.

Classification of Non-Hodgkin's Lymphoma

The diagnosis and classification of NHL are based primarily on the morphologic features of the tissue biopsy specimen and on immunologic characteristics, cytogenetic studies, and biologic behavior (Table 36-6). Many classification systems of NHL have

Table 36-5 Staging Procedures for Non-Hodgkin's Lymphoma

1. Clinical history with special attention to duration and specific symptoms
2. Physical examination including all lymph node–bearing areas, liver, and spleen
3. Surgical biopsy
4. Complete blood cell count, including examination of peripheral blood smear
5. Bilateral bone marrow aspirate and biopsy
6. Liver and renal function tests
7. Serum lactate dehydrogenase and β_2-microglobulin levels
8. Serum protein electrophoresis
9. Radiologic studies including chest radiograph, bilateral lower extremity lymphogram, and abdominal-pelvic computed tomography
10. Cytologic examination of any effusions
11. Lumbar puncture for cerebrospinal fluid cytologic studies in intermediate and high-grade lymphomas

been used through the years. In the past 10 years, the Working Formulation in the United States and the Kiel classification in Europe have been used successfully. The classification system used in this chapter is the one recently proposed by the International Lymphoma Study Group (Table 36-7). This classification is based on the Lukes and Collins and Kiel classifications and includes the more recently described subtypes of NHL. Although several of the entities listed are considered provisional, it appears to be a practical classification system. Undoubtedly, several modifications will take place when the system has been tested in clinical trials. Such studies are also needed to define prognostic groups valuable to clinicians. Comparison of this classification with the Working Formulation and the Kiel classification is illustrated in Tables 36-8 and 36-9, respectively.

This classification is based on current knowledge of histologic, immunologic, and genetic features; the clinical presentation and course of the disease; and the postulated normal cell counterparts. The classification is divided into B-cell and T-cell lymphomas; this distinction should be made whenever possible. In this classification, the term "grade" refers to morphologic features such as cell size, density of chromatin, and proliferation rate, and for clinical behavior of tumor the terms "prognostic group" or

Table 36-6   Principles of Classification of Non-Hodgkin's Lymphoma

Morphology
    Pattern
        Follicular
        Diffuse
        Interfollicular
        Sinusoidal
    Cytology
        Cell size
            Small (small lymphocytic lymphoma)
            Small to intermediate (mantle cell lymphoma, marginal zone B-cell lymphoma)
            Intermediate (follicular small cleaved cell, Burkitt's and lymphoblastic lymphoma)
            Large (large-cell lymphoma)
    Nuclear contour
        Round—small lymphocytes, noncleaved cells (Burkitt's lymphoma, centroblastic lymphoma)
        Irregular—mantle cell lymphoma
        Cleaved—follicle center lymphoma
        Convoluted—lymphoblastic lymphoma
        Multilobated—some large cell lymphomas
        Pleomorphic—anaplastic large cell lymphoma
        Monocytoid—marginal zone B-cell lymphoma
        Cerebriform—mycosis fungoides
    Chromatin pattern
        Clumped—small lymphocytic, centrocytic (small cleaved cell), mantle cell, marginal zone B cell
        Fine—lymphoblastic cells
        Vesicular—centroblasts
    Nucleoli
        Burkitt's lymphoma, immunoblastic large-cell lymphoma

Immunologic characteristics
    Determination of B- and T-cell immunophenotype, and monoclonality using immunohistochemistry or flow cytometry and sometimes gene rearrangement studies

Cytogenetics and oncogenes

Biologic behavior

Table 36-7   List of Lymphoid Neoplasms Recognized by the
International Lymphoma Study Group*

B-Cell Neoplasms
  I. Precursor B-cell neoplasm: Precursor B-lymphoblastic
      leukemia/lymphoma
 II. Peripheral B-cell neoplasms
      1. B-cell chronic lymphocytic leukemia/prolymphocytic leukemia/small
          lymphocytic lymphoma
      2. Lymphoplasmacytoid lymphoma/immunocytoma
      3. Mantle cell lymphoma
      4. Follicle center lymphoma, follicular
          Provisional cytologic grades: I (small cell), II (mixed small and large
          cell), III (large cell)
          Provisional subtype: diffuse, predominantly small cell type
      5. Marginal zone B-cell lymphoma
          Extranodal (MALT type ± monocytoid B cells)
          Provisional subtype: nodal (± monocytoid B cells)
      6. Provisional entity: splenic marginal zone lymphoma (± villous
          lymphocytes)
      7. Hairy cell leukemia
      8. Plasmacytoma/plasma cell myeloma
      9. Diffuse large B-cell lymphoma[†]
          Subtype: primary mediastinal (thymic) B-cell lymphoma
     10. Burkitt's lymphoma
     11. Provisional entity: high-grade B-cell lymphoma, Burkitt-like[†]

T-Cell and Putative NK-Cell Neoplasms
  I. Precursor T-cell neoplasm: precursor T-lymphoblastic
      lymphoma/leukemia
 II. Peripheral T-cell and NK-cell neoplasms
      1. T-cell chronic lymphocytic leukemia/prolymphocytic leukemia
      2. Large granular lymphocyte leukemia (LGL)
          T-cell type
          NK-cell type
      3. Mycosis fungoides/Sézary syndrome
      4. Peripheral T-cell lymphomas, unspecified[†]
          Provisional cytologic categories: medium-sized cell, mixed medium
          and large cell, large cell, lymphoepithelioid cell
          Provisional subtype: hepatosplenic $\gamma\delta$ T-cell lymphoma
          Provisional subtype: subcutaneous panniculitic T-cell lymphoma
      5. Angioimmunoblastic T-cell lymphoma (AILD)
      6. Angiocentric lymphoma
      7. Intestinal T-cell lymphoma (± enteropathy-associated)
      8. Adult T-cell lymphoma/leukemia (ATL/L)
      9. Anaplastic large cell lymphoma (ALCL), CD30+, T- and null-cell types
     10. Provisional entity: anaplastic large cell lymphoma, Hodgkin's-like

Table 36-7 *Continued*

Hodgkin's Disease
  I. Lymphocyte predominance
  II. Nodular sclerosis
  III. Mixed cellularity
  IV. Lymphocyte depletion
  V. Provisional entity: lymphocyte-rich classic Hodgkin's disease

Abbreviations: MALT = mucosa-associated lymphoid tissue; NK = natural killer.
*From Harris NL, Jaffe ES, Stein H, et al. A revised European-American classification of lymphoid neoplasms: a proposal from the International Lymphoma Study Group. *Blood.* 1994;84:1361-1392.
†These categories are thought likely to include more than one disease entity.

"aggressiveness" is used. It is recognized that a number of the entities described in this classification have a range of morphologic grade and clinical aggressiveness.

B-Cell Neoplasms

Precursor B-Cell Neoplasms: B-Precursor (B-Lymphoblastic Lymphoma/Leukemia [B-LBL]). The morphologic features of B-precursor lymphoblastic lymphoma are identical to the more common T-precursor lymphoblastic lymphoma (T-LBL). The cells are intermediate in size between small lymphocytes and large-cell lymphoma with convoluted or round nuclei, delicate chromatin, indistinct nucleoli, and scant cytoplasm. Mitoses are frequently seen and starry sky pattern may be present. The differential diagnosis based on morphologic features includes Burkitt's lymphoma, granulocytic sarcoma, and lymphoblastic or lymphoblastoid variant of mantle cell lymphoma.

Immunophenotyping of this tumor shows the following features: TdT+, CD19+, CD20–/+, CD22+, CD10+/–, SIg–, and CD34+/–. The tumor may coexpress myeloid markers CD13 and/or CD33. The cytogenetic changes are variable.

The majority of patients who have precursor B-cell neoplasms are children and the disease represents 80% of acute lymphoblastic leukemia. B-LBL probably represents less than 20% of lymphoblastic lymphomas, the majority being of T-cell phenotype. This tumor is highly aggressive but is often curable with chemotherapy.

Table 36-8   Comparison of the Proposed Classification With
the Working Formulation*

Revised European-American Lymphoma Classification	Working Formulation
Precursor B-lymphoblastic lymphoma/leukemia	Lymphoblastic
B-cell CLL/prolymphocytic leukemia/SLL	Small lymphocytic, consistent with CLL[†]; small lymphocytic, plasmacytoid
Lymphoplasmacytoid lymphoma	Small lymphocytic, plasmacytoid[†]; diffuse, mixed small and large cell
Mantle cell lymphoma	Small lymphocytic; diffuse, small cleaved cell[†]; follicular, small cleaved cell; diffuse, mixed small and large cell; diffuse, large cleaved cell
Follicular center lymphoma, follicular Grade I	Follicular, predominantly small cleaved cell[†]
Grade II	Follicular, mixed small and large cell[†]
Grade III	Follicular, predominantly large cell
Follicular center lymphoma, diffuse, small cell [provisional]	Diffuse, small cleaved cell[†]; diffuse, mixed small and large cell
Extranodal marginal zone B-cell lymphoma (low-grade B-cell lymphoma of MALT type)	Small lymphocytic[†]; diffuse, small cleaved cell; diffuse, mixed small and large cell
Nodal marginal zone B-cell lymphoma [provisional]	Small lymphocytic[†]; diffuse, small cleaved cell; diffuse, mixed small and large cell; unclassifiable
Splenic marginal zone B-cell lymphoma [provisional]	Small lymphocytic[†]; diffuse, small cleaved cell
Hairy cell leukemia	—
Plasmacytoma/myeloma	Extramedullary plasmacytoma
Diffuse large B-cell lymphoma	Diffuse, large cell[†]; large cell immunoblastic; diffuse, mixed small and large cell
Primary mediastinal large B-cell lymphoma	Diffuse, large cell[†]; large cell immunoblastic
Burkitt's lymphoma	Small noncleaved cell, Burkitt's
High-grade B-cell lymphoma, Burkitt-like [provisional]	Small noncleaved cell, non-Burkitt's[†]; diffuse, large cell; large cell immunoblastic
Precursor T-lymphoblastic lymphoma/leukemia	Lymphoblastic
T-cell CLL/prolymphocytic leukemia	Small lymphocytic[†]; diffuse, small cleaved cell
Large granular lymphocytic leukemia (T-cell type, NK-cell type)	Small lymphocytic[†]; diffuse, small cleaved cell
Mycosis fungoides/Sézary syndrome	Mycosis fungoides

Table 36-8   *Continued*

Revised European-American Lymphoma Classification	Working Formulation
Peripheral T-cell lymphomas, unspecified [including provisional subtype: subcutaneous panniculitic T-cell lymphoma]	Diffuse, small cleaved cell; diffuse, mixed small and large cell[†]; diffuse, large cell; large cell immunoblastic[†]
Hepatosplenic γδ T-cell lymphoma [provisional]	—
Angioimmunoblastic T-cell lymphoma	Diffuse, mixed small and large cell[†]; diffuse, large cell; large cell immunoblastic[†]
Angiocentric lymphoma	Diffuse, small cleaved cell; diffuse mixed small and large cell[†]; diffuse, large cell; large cell immunoblastic[†]
Intestinal T-cell lymphoma	Diffuse, small cleaved cell; diffuse, mixed small and large cell[†]; diffuse, large cell; large cell immunoblastic[†]
Adult T-cell lymphoma/leukemia	Diffuse, small cleaved cell; diffuse, mixed small and large cell[†]; diffuse, large cell; large cell immunoblastic[†]
Anaplastic large cell lymphoma, T- and null-cell types	Large cell immunoblastic

Abbreviations: CLL = chronic lymphocytic leukemia; MALT = mucosa-associated lymphoid tissue; NK = natural killer.
*From Harris NL, Jaffe ES, Stein H, et al. A revised European-American classification of lymphoid neoplasms: a proposal from the International Lymphoma Study Group. *Blood.* 1994;84:1361-1392.
[†]When more than one Working Formulation category is listed, these comprise the majority of the cases.

Peripheral B-Cell Neoplasms: B-Cell Chronic Lymphocytic Leukemia (B-CLL)/Prolymphocytic Leukemia (B-PLL)/Small Lymphocytic Lymphoma (B-SLL). This tumor is made up of small lymphocytes, which may be somewhat larger than normal lymphocytes (Image 36-1). A helpful diagnostic feature is the presence of proliferation centers consisting of larger lymphoid cells (prolymphocytes and paraimmunoblasts) that may produce a nodular (pseudofollicular) pattern. The morphologic features of B-cell chronic lymphocytic leukemia and small lymphocytic lymphoma are identical. In B-prolymphocytic leukemia,

Table 36-9 Comparison of the Proposed Classification With the Kiel Classification*

Kiel Classification	Revised European-American Lymphoma Classification
B-lymphoblastic	Precursor B-lymphoblastic lymphoma/leukemia
B-lymphocytic, CLL†; B-lymphocytic, prolymphocytic leukemia; lymphoplasmacytoid immunocytoma	B-cell CLL/prolymphocytic leukemia/small lymphocytic lymphoma
Lymphoplasmacytic immunocytoma	Lymphoplasmacytoid lymphoma
Centrocytic†; centroblastic, centrocytoid subtype	Mantle cell lymphoma
Centroblastic-centrocytic, follicular†; centroblastic, follicular	Follicular center lymphoma, follicular (grade I, grade II, grade III)
Centroblastic-centrocytic, diffuse	Follicular center lymphoma, diffuse, small cell [provisional]
—	Extranodal marginal zone B-cell lymphoma (low-grade B-cell lymphoma of MALT type)
Monocytoid, including marginal zone†; immunocytoma	Nodal marginal zone B-cell lymphoma [provisional]
—	Splenic marginal zone B-cell lymphoma [provisional]
Hairy cell leukemia	Hairy cell leukemia
Plasmacytic	Plasmacytoma/myeloma
Centroblastic† (monomorphic, polymorphic, and multilobated subtypes); B-immunoblastic†; B-large cell anaplastic (Ki-1+)	Diffuse large B-cell lymphoma
—‡	Primary mediastinal large B-cell lymphoma
Burkitt's lymphoma	Burkitt's lymphoma
—	High-grade B-cell lymphoma, Burkitt-like [provisional]
? Some cases of centroblastic and immunoblastic	
T-lymphoblastic	Precursor T-lymphoblastic lymphoma/leukemia
T-lymphocytic, CLL type†; T-lymphocytic, prolymphocytic leukemia	T-cell chronic lymphocytic leukemia/prolymphocytic leukemia
T-lymphocytic, CLL type	Large granular lymphocytic leukemia
—	T-cell type
—	NK-cell type
Small cell cerebriform (mycosis fungoides, Sézary syndrome)	Mycosis fungoides/Sézary syndrome

Table 36-9 *Continued*

Kiel Classification	Revised European-American Lymphoma Classification
T-zone Lymphoepithelioid Pleomorphic, small T-cell Pleomorphic, medium-sized and large T-cell[†] T-immunoblastic	Peripheral T-cell lymphomas, unspecified [including provisional subtype: subcutaneous panniculitic T-cell lymphoma]
—	Hepatosplenic γδ T-cell lymphoma [provisional]
Angioimmunoblastic (AILD, LgX)	Angioimmunoblastic T-cell lymphoma
—[‡]	Angiocentric lymphoma
—	Intestinal T-cell lymphoma
Pleomorphic small T-cell, HTLV1[+] Pleomorphic medium-sized and large T-cell, HTLV1[+†]	Adult T-cell lymphoma/leukemia
T-large cell anaplastic (Ki-1[+])	Anaplastic large cell lymphoma, T-and null-cell types

Abbreviations: CLL = chronic lymphocytic leukemia; MALT = mucosa-associated lymphoid tissue; NK = natural killer; HTLV = human T-cell leukemia virus.
*From Harris NL, Jaffe ES, Stein H, et al. A revised European-American classification of lymphoid neoplasms: a proposal from the International Lymphoma Study Group. *Blood*. 1994;84:1361-1392.
[†]When more than one Kiel category is listed, these comprise the majority of the cases.
[‡]Not listed in classification, but discussed as rare or ambiguous type.

the cells are larger with clumped chromatin, prominent centrally placed nucleolus, and abundant cytoplasm. These cells comprise more than 50% of the tumor. Tumors that have plasmacytoid differentiation are considered a variant of B-CLL and are not considered a separate diagnostic category.

Immunophenotypic studies of B-CLL/B-SLL are as follows: faint SIgM, SIgD+/–, CD19+, CD20+, CD23+, CD5+, CD43+, CD11c–/+ (faint), and CD10–. CD23 is especially useful in distinguishing this tumor from mantle cell lymphomas, which are often CD23–. B-prolymphocytic leukemia cells have dense surface immunoglobulin and are often CD5–. CD22 is more often seen in B-PLL than in B-CLL. Cytogenetic studies have shown trisomy 12 in 30% of cases and abnormalities of 13q have been seen in 25% of the cases. The majority of patients are older adults, with involvement of multiple lymph nodes, spleen, and liver. Bone marrow and peripheral blood involvement is usually present at diagnosis. B-PLL is characterized by a very high white blood cell count, prominent spleno-megaly, and a more aggressive clinical course than B-CLL.

Lymphoplasmacytoid Lymphoma/Immunocytoma.

This lymphoma is characterized by proliferation of small lympho-cytes, plasmacytoid lymphocytes, and plasma cells. However, it lacks the histologic features seen in B-CLL, mantle cell, or mar-ginal zone lymphomas. The growth pattern of this lymphoma is often interfollicular.

Immunophenotypic studies reveal the following features: IgM+, IgD usually negative; CD19+, CD20+, CD22+, CD5–, CD10–, CD43+/–, CD25, or CD11c may be weakly positive in some cases. This tumor is distinguished from B-CLL by lack of CD5 and the presence of strong cytoplasmic immunoglobulin. Clinically, this lymphoma occurs in an older age group similar to B-CLL. Lymph nodes, spleen, and bone marrow are usually involved while periph-eral blood or extranodal sites are less frequently involved. Most of the patients have monoclonal IgM, and when hyperviscosity symp-toms are present, the findings are consistent with Waldenström's macroglobulinemia. As with B-CLL/small lymphocytic lymphomas, the lymphoplasmacytoid lymphomas have an indolent course and the disease is usually not curable with chemotherapy.

Mantle Cell Lymphoma.

This type of lymphoma com-prises cells that are usually slightly larger than normal lymphocytes, and have more dispersed chromatin, scant cytoplasm, and indistinct nucleoli. The nuclear contours are slightly irregular (Image 36-2). Variable morphologic features may, however, be seen in this lym-phoma. A blastic or lymphoblastoid variant and an anaplastic or large cell type has also been seen. Typically in mantle cell lym-phomas, transformed cells are rare or absent. The morphologic pat-tern of this lymphoma is vaguely nodular or usually diffuse.

Immunophenotypic studies reveal the following: SIgM+, SIgD+, CD19+, CD20+, CD22+, CD5+, CD10–/+, CD23–, CD43+, CD11c–. In contrast to B-CLL/small lymphocytic lym-phoma, mantle cell lymphoma shows stronger CD20 vs CD19 expression with flow cytometry. The absence of CD23 is a useful marker in distinguishing mantle cell lymphoma from B-CLL. The presence of CD5 in mantle cell lymphomas is useful in distinguishing it from marginal zone lymphoma. The reciprocal chromosome translocation t(11;14) (q13;q32), the putative proto-oncogene bcl-1, has been found in 30% to 70% of cases. The chromosome translocation t(11;14) results in overexpression of a gene called PRAD1, which encodes for cyclin D1.

The majority of patients with mantle cell lymphomas are over the age of 60 years and have stage 3 or 4 disease. There is frequent involvement of the gastrointestinal tract and Waldeyer's ring. Mantle cell lymphomas have a moderately aggressive course and at this time are incurable with chemotherapy. The median survival time ranges from 3 to 5 years. A diffuse morphologic pattern (particularly lymphoblastoid variant) is associated with a poor prognosis (median survival time, 3 years). In contrast to small lymphocytic lymphoma there is absence of progression to large cell lymphoma.

Follicle Center Lymphoma, Follicular (Provisional Cytologic Grade: Predominantly Small Cell, Mixed Small and Large Cell, Predominantly Large Cell). The follicle center lymphomas are composed of a mixture of centrocytes (cleaved follicle center cells) and centroblasts (large noncleaved follicle center cells). In addition to the follicular pattern (Image 36-3), diffuse areas may also be present. In the majority of cases, centrocytes (small cleaved follicle center cells) predominate, but variable numbers of centroblasts (large noncleaved cells) are always present. Of the follicle center lymphomas, the least common are those composed predominantly of centroblasts. Results of recent studies suggest that the small, mixed small and large, and predominantly large cell categories have a similar prognosis and the grading of the follicle center lymphomas may not be clinically important.

Immunophenotypic studies reveal the following features: CD19+, CD20+, CD10+/–, CD5–, CD23–/+, CD43–, CD11c–. The absence of CD5 and CD43 is helpful in differentiating follicle center lymphoma from mantle cell lymphoma and the presence of CD10 may be helpful in the differential diagnosis from marginal zone cell lymphoma. bcl-2 protein expression is present in the majority of follicle center lymphomas but is absent from reactive follicles. The expression of bcl-2 protein is not useful in distinguishing follicle center lymphomas from other lymphomas since bcl-2 is also frequently present in other types of indolent (low-grade) lymphomas.

The majority of patients with follicle center lymphoma have stage III or IV disease at diagnosis with involvement of lymph node, spleen, bone marrow, and frequently peripheral blood. It is the most indolent type of NHL, but is usually not curable with current chemotherapy. Progression to diffuse large cell lymphomas is seen in some patients.

Follicle Center Lymphoma, Diffuse (Predominantly Small Cell). These are extremely rare lymphomas that are composed of small cleaved cells resembling centrocytes. It is assumed that most of these cases represent a sampling problem and are a diffuse counterpart of a follicle center lymphoma. When larger biopsy specimens have been obtained, follicular areas are frequently seen.

Marginal Zone B-Cell Lymphoma. With this classification, the low-grade B-cell lymphoma mucosa–associated lymphoid tissue (MALT type), monocytoid B-cell lymphoma, and splenic marginal zone lymphoma has been combined under the term marginal zone lymphoma. These tumors are characterized by an infiltrate of marginal zone cells. These cells have also been referred to as centrocyte-like, which may be described as small atypical cells resembling small cleaved follicle center cells, except that they have more abundant cytoplasm (Image 36-4). In addition to the marginal zone cells, monocytoid B-cells, small lymphocytes, and plasma cells are seen. Reactive follicles are frequently present and the neoplastic marginal zone or monocytoid B cells occupy the marginal zone and/or the interfollicular region. So-called follicular colonization by the neoplastic cells may also be present. When the tumor involves epithelial tissues, the marginal zone cells infiltrate the epithelium, forming lymphoepithelial lesions (Image 36-5). A perisinusoidal, perifollicular, or marginal zone pattern of involvement may be seen in lymph nodes, and when the spleen is involved the tumor is usually seen within the marginal zone and the red pulp.

Immunophenotypic studies reveal the following: CD19+, CD20+, CD22+, CD5–, CD23–, CD43–/+, CD11c+/–. Rearrangement of *bcl*-2 or *bcl*-1 have not been seen in these tumors.

Extranodal Marginal Zone Lymphoma (Low-Grade B-Cell Lymphoma MALT Type). These tumors usually occur in adults, with a slight predominance of affected women. There is often a history of autoimmune disease such as Sjögren's syndrome or Hashimoto's thyroiditis, and infection with *Helicobactor pylori,* which may cause gastritis, is seen in many patients. At presentation, the majority of patients have stage I or II extranodal disease with involvement of glandular epithelial tissue at various sites. The most frequently involved organ is the stomach. Other affected organs include salivary glands, thyroid gland, lung, and orbit. This lymphoma often remains localized to the primary extranodal site, but dissemination may be seen in up to 30% of the cases involving sometimes two or more MALT sites synchronously or asynchronously. Transformation to large-cell lymphoma occurs in some patients. When the disease is localized, it may be cured with local treatment, and when disseminated the course is usually indolent and not curable with current chemotherapy.

Nodal Monocytoid B-Cell Lymphomas. Most of the so-called nodal monocytoid B-cell lymphomas are seen in patients with Sjögren's syndrome and are thought to represent nodal spread of a MALT type lymphoma. There are, however, also cases where the disease appears to be confined to the lymph nodes, and the morphologic features are similar to those of extranodal MALT type or monocytoid B-cell (Image 36-6). Such lesions are also seen accompanying other NHLs, particularly follicle center lymphomas. As with the extranodal marginal zone lymphoma, the nodal marginal zone lymphoma has an indolent course and when disseminated it is usually not curable with current therapy. The nodal marginal zone lymphomas appear to have a longer survival time than the extranodal marginal zone lymphomas.

Splenic Marginal Zone Lymphoma. The splenic marginal zone lymphoma represents cases where the lymphoma involves the marginal zone of the splenic white pulp. In some cases splenic marginal zone lymphoma may overlap with a type of chronic B-lymphocytic leukemia called splenic lymphoma with villous lymphocytes.

Tables 36-10 and 36-11 summarize the morphologic, immunophenotypic, and cytogenetic features of the indolent or low-grade B-cell lymphomas discussed above.

Table 36-10   Low-Grade B-Cell Lymphomas: Characteristic Morphologic Features in Differential Diagnostics*

Lymphoma	Pattern	Small Cells	Large Cells
B-CLL/SLL	Diffuse with pseudofollicles	Round (may be cleaved)	Prolymphocytes, paraimmunoblasts
Lympho-plasmacytoid lymphoma	Diffuse	Round (may be cleaved), plasma cells	Centroblasts, immunoblasts
Mantle cell lymphoma	Diffuse, vaguely nodular, mantle zone, rarely follicular	Cleaved (may be round or oval)	Rare
Follicle center lymphoma	Follicular with or without diffuse areas, rarely diffuse	Cleaved (centrocytes)	Centroblasts
Marginal zone B-cell lymphoma	Diffuse, interfollicular, marginal zone, occasionally follicular (colonization)	Heterogeneous: round (small lymphocytes), cleaved (marginal zone/monocytoid B cells), plasma cells	Centroblasts, immunoblasts

*From Harris NL, Jaffe ES, Stein H, et al. A revised European-American classification of lymphoid neoplasms: a proposal from the International Lymphoma Study Group. *Blood.* 1994;84:1361-1392.

Diffuse Large B-Cell Lymphoma.   Because of the difficulty in subclassifying large cell lymphomas, it is proposed in this classification system that they all be in one group of large B-cell lymphomas. In the majority of cases, the predominant cell is either centroblast (large noncleaved cell) (Image 36-7) or an immunoblast (Image 36-8). Frequently there is a mixture of centroblast-like and immunoblast-like cells. Also in this group of lymphomas are large cleaved or multilobated cell lymphomas and anaplastic large cell lymphomas of B-cell phenotype. The so-called T-cell–rich B-cell lymphomas (Image 36-9) also belong to this group of diffuse large B-cell lymphomas.

Immunophenotypic studies reveal the following: CD19+, CD20+, CD45+/–, CD5–/+, CD10–/+. The *bcl-2* gene is rearranged in about 30% of cases.

Table 36-11 Low-Grade B-Cell Lymphomas: Immunophenotypic and Genetic Features*

Lymphoma Type	SIg	CIg	CD5	CD10	CD23	CD43†	Chromosome Abnormality	Oncogene Rearranged
B-CLL/SLL	+†	-/+	+	-	+	+	Trisomy 12 (30%)	NA
Lymphoplasmacytoid	+	+	-	-	-	-/+	NA	NA
Mantle cell	+	-	+	-/+	-	+	t(11;14)	bcl-1
Follicle center	+	-	-	+/-	-/+	-	t(14;18)	bcl-2
Marginal zone	+	40%+	-	-	-/+	-/+	Trisomy 3 (extranodal)	NA

Abbreviations: SIg = surface immunoglobulin; CIg = cytoplasmic immunoglobulin; CLL = chronic lymphocytic leukemia; SLL = small lymphocytic leukemia; NA = not applicable.
+ = 90% positive; +/- = over 50% positive; -/+ less than 50% positive; - = <10% positive.
*From Harris NL, Jaffe ES, Stein H, et al. A revised European-American classification of lymphoid neoplasms: a proposal from the International Lymphoma Study Group. *Blood.* 1994;84:1361-1392.
†Positivity may vary depending on antibody used.

Large B-cell lymphomas are seen at all ages, but are more common in the older age group. The typical clinical presentation is that of a rapidly enlarging single node. In approximately 40% of cases the disease is extranodal.

B Large Cell Lymphoma Subtype: Primary Mediastinal (Thymic) Large B-Cell Lymphoma. These tumors are composed of centroblasts, multilobated cells, or immunoblasts. A variable degree of compartmentalizing sclerosis is seen. The thymus is often involved. This can be best demonstrated with stain for cytokeratin.

Immunophenotypic studies reveal: CD19+, CD20+, CD22+, CD45+/–, CD30–/+, CD15–.

B large cell lymphomas involving the mediastinum appear to represent a distinct clinical pathologic entity with a higher incidence in women than men and a median age in the fourth decade. Table 36-12 lists features useful in the differential diagnosis of mediastinal lymphomas.

Burkitt's Lymphoma. This lymphoma is characterized by an infiltrate composed of monomorphic, medium-sized cells with round nuclei (small noncleaved cells), moderately clumped chromatin, multiple nucleoli, and moderately abundant, basophilic cytoplasm. Imprints of tumor tissue are helpful in demonstrating cytoplasmic lipid vacuoles (Image 36-10). A high mitotic index is seen and starry sky pattern is usually present.

Immunophenotypic studies reveal: CD19+, CD20+, CD22+, CD10+, CD5–, and CD23–. *c-myc* oncogene rearrangement is usually present.

Burkitt's lymphoma accounts for approximately 30% of childhood lymphomas. In adults the tumor is often associated with immunodeficiency. In African cases, the jaw and other facial bones are particularly commonly involved, while in other cases the most common site is in the abdomen, usually in the distal ileum, cecum, and/or mesentery. The tumor is highly aggressive but is curable in approximately 60% of cases with aggressive therapy.

Provisional Category: High-Grade B-Cell Lymphoma, Burkitt-like. In these cases, the size and nuclear mor-

Table 36-12 Useful Features in the Differential Diagnosis of Mediastinal Lymphomas*

Characteristic	PMLCL	LBL	HD
Histopathologic Findings			
Cell morphology	Large cells	Blasts	Reed-Sternberg cells
Sclerosis	Present	Usually absent	Present
Immunophenotype			
CD20 (B cell)	Present	Usually absent	Usually absent
CD3 (T cell)	Absent	Usually present	Absent
CD15	Absent	Absent	Present
CD30	Absent	Absent	Present
TdT	Absent	Present	Absent

Abbreviations: PMLCL = primary mediastinal large cell lymphoma; LBL = lymphoblastic lymphoma; HD = Hodgkin's disease; TdT = terminal deoxynucleotidyl transferase.
*From Piira T, Perkins SL, Anderson JR, et al. Primary mediastinal large cell lymphoma in children: a recent report from the Children Cancer Group. *Pediatr Pathol*. In press.

phologic features of these tumors are intermediate between those of Burkitt's lymphoma and large cell lymphoma. There is a high proliferation rate with or without the starry sky pattern. This category is not thought to be reproducible and may not be a single disease entity, but it may represent cases that are borderline between large B-cell lymphoma and Burkitt's lymphoma.

Immunophenotypic studies reveal: CD19+, CD20+, CD5–, and CD10–. *c-myc* rearrangement is unusual.

The majority of these cases appear to occur in adults. In children the survival times in the typical Burkitt's lymphomas and Burkitt-like lymphomas appear to be similar.

T-Cell and Putative Natural Killer (NK) Cell Neoplasms

Precursor T-Cell Neoplasm: T-Precursor Lymphoblastic Lymphoma/Leukemia (LBL). The morphologic features in this tumor are identical to those previously described for B-precursor LBL-ALL. The infiltrating lymphoblasts have convoluted or round nuclei, delicate chromatin pattern, indistinct nucleoli, and scant cytoplasm. Frequent mitotic figures are seen (Image 36-11). In the differential diagnosis, one should consider Burkitt's lymphoma, granulocytic sarcoma, and lymphoblastoid variant of mantle cell lymphoma.

Immunophenotypic studies reveal CD3+, CD7+, and variable expression of other T-cell–associated antigens. Many of the cases show the presence of both CD4 and CD8 antigens. B-cell–associated antigens CD19 and CD20 are negative. Terminal deoxynucleotidyl transferase (TdT) is typically positive. A few cases express NK antigen CD16 and CD57.

This tumor is most commonly seen in adolescent and young adult men, and it constitutes 40% of childhood lymphomas and 15% of acute lymphoblastic leukemias when leukemia is defined as more than 25% bone marrow lymphoblasts. The most common presentation is that of a mediastinal mass. If left untreated, this tumor terminates in acute leukemia, and central nervous system involvement is common. Although this tumor is highly aggressive, it is curable in approximately 60% of the cases with intensive chemotherapy.

Peripheral T-Cell Neoplasms. T-cell lymphomas account for less than 20% of lymphomas in the United States and Europe but are considerably more common in Asia.

T-Cell Chronic Lymphocytic Leukemia (T-CLL)/ T-Prolymphocytic Leukemia (T-PLL). In the majority of cases, the morphologic features of prolymphocytic leukemia are characterized by cells with prominent nucleoli, abundant cytoplasm, and nuclear irregularities.

Immunophenotypic studies reveal CD2+, CD3+, CD5+, CD7+, and CD25–. CD4 is seen in approximately 60% of the cases. TdT is negative. Cytogenetic studies show 75% of the cases with inv 14 (q11;q32).

As with B-cell prolymphocytic leukemia, the patients have a high white blood cell count, but in addition the T-cell type have cutaneous or mucosal involvement. This is usually an aggressive disease and not curable with current chemotherapy.

Large Granular Lymphocytic (LGL) Leukemia, T-Cell and NK/Cell Types. The morphologic features in the peripheral blood are lymphocytosis with a predominant cell having round nuclei with moderately condensed chromatin and characteristically azurophilic granules in abundant blue cytoplasm. The bone marrow infiltration is usually mild. Focal aggregates are often present.

Immunophenotypic studies reveal two types of LGL leukemia: (1) T-cell: CD2+, CD3+, CD5–, CD7–, CD4–, CD8+, CD16+, CD56–, CD57+/–, CD25–, and T-cell gene rearrangement is present; and (2) NK cell: CD2+, CD3–, CD4–, CD8+/–, CD16+, CD56+/–, CD57+/–, and T-cell gene rearrangement is usually not present.

Patients with this disease usually have mild-to-moderate lymphocytosis, often associated with neutropenia and mild anemia. In the majority of patients the clinical course is indolent, but in some patients who have both T-cell and NK-cell type the disease is aggressive. At this time there are no reliable markers for predicting the clinical course.

Mycosis Fungoides/ Sézary Syndrome. Mycosis fungoides is the most common of the cutaneous T-cell lymphomas. Skin biopsies show an infiltrate composed of small and large cells with cerebriform nuclei in the upper dermis, frequently with infiltrates in the epidermis (Pautrier's abscesses) (Image 36-12). Involvement of the peripheral blood and pericortex of the lymph nodes may also be seen.

Immunophenotypic studies reveal CD2+, CD3+, CD4+, CD5+, CD8–.

Clinically, mycosis fungoides presents as a scaly exematous lesion that progresses through a plaque stage to eventually form tumors in the skin. Sézary syndrome is characterized by exfoliated erythroderma and malignant cells (Sézary cells) in the peripheral blood. The initial diagnosis of mycosis fungoides may be difficult to make. Frequently, several skin biopsies over time are necessary. Blood smears for detection of Sézary cells should be obtained from fingersticks and should be technically perfect. Usually more than 20% of the total lymphocytes in the peripheral blood smear should have cerebriform nuclei before a confident determination can be made that the cells are true Sézary cells. The presence of large Sézary cells appears to be particularly significant and is often associated with progressive disease. Large-cell lymphomas that are CD30+, similar to anaplastic large-cell lymphoma, have been reported as a terminal event. There also appears to be an association with Hodgkin's disease and lymphomatoid papulosis.

Peripheral T-Cell Lymphomas (Provisional Subtypes: Medium-Sized Cell, Mixed Medium and Large Cell, Large Cell). The nonlymphoblastic and non-CLL T-cell lymphomas have been placed into one group in this classification system. The morphologic features of the peripheral T-cell lymphomas are that of an infiltrate with atypical small cells to medium-sized or large cells. The majority of cases contain a mixture of small and large cells. Occasional Reed-Sternberg–like cells may be present. A variable number of eosinophils and/or epithelioid histiocytes are present. Lymphoepithelioid lymphoma (Lennert's lymphoma) is thought to belong to this category of lymphomas.

Immunophenotypic studies reveal that the T-cell–associated antigens are variably expressed: CD2+, CD3+, CD5+/–, CD7–/+; CD4 is more frequently seen than CD8. Aberrant loss of T-cell–associated antigens is a characteristic feature. T-cell gene rearrangement is usually seen.

The majority of patients are adults with stage III or IV disease. The skin and lungs appear to be frequently involved. The clinical course is usually more aggressive than that of corresponding B-cell lymphomas.

Peripheral T-Cell Lymphoma Variants. Angioimmunoblastic T-cell lymphoma, angiocentric lymphoma, intestinal T-cell lymphoma, and adult T-cell lymphoma leukemia have been separated from the peripheral T-cell lymphomas because of their characteristic histopathologic, immunologic, genetic, and clinical features.

Angioimmunoblastic T-Cell Lymphoma. The majority of cases of angioimmunoblastic lymphadenopathy with dysproteinemia (AILD) or immunoblastic lymphadenopathy (IBL) show clonal rearrangement of T-cell receptor genes and are thought to be malignant lymphomas.

Immunophenotypic studies reveal tumor cells to express T-cell–associated antigens with the predominance of cases being CD4+. T-cell gene rearrangement is seen in 75% of the cases.

The clinical features in this disorder are fairly typical with generalized lymphadenopathy, fever, weight loss, skin rash, and polyclonal hypergammaglobulinemia. The disease process is moderately aggressive, but occasional spontaneous responses to steroids may be seen. In some patients, progression to large cell T- or sometimes B-cell type lymphomas is seen.

Angiocentric Lymphoma. This tumor corresponds to polymorphic reticulosis, lethal midline granuloma, nasal T-cell lymphoma, and many cases of lymphomatoid granulomatosis. The morphologic features include angiocentric and angioinvasive infiltrate composed of a variable number of atypical lymphoid cells with irregular nuclear contours and immunoblasts together with variable number of plasma cells, eosinophils, and histiocytes.

Immunophenotypic studies reveal CD2+, CD3–, CD5+, CD7+. The atypical cells may be CD4 or CD8 positive and are frequently CD56 positive. The atypical cells may express B-cell lineage in some cases, especially those involving the lung, but the majority of cells present are T cells. Results of studies for T- and B-cell rearrangement are usually negative.

A number of affected extranodal sites have been described including nose, palate, lungs, skin, and central nervous system. The clinical course is variable. In some cases, the disease appears to be indolent, while in others it is aggressive.

Intestinal T-Cell Lymphoma (With or Without Enteropathy). A variable mixture of small, medium, and large cells is seen. There are frequently intraepithelial T cells in adjacent mucosa.

Immunophenotypic studies reveal CD3+, CD7+, CD8+/–, CD4–, CD103+. T-cell receptor (TCR) beta genes are clonally rearranged.

This disease is often associated with a history of gluten-sensitive enteropathy. The jejunum is most frequently involved, but the stomach and colon may also be affected. The disease is aggressive and characterized by multiple jejunal ulcers often associated with perforation.

Adult T-Cell Lymphoma/Leukemia (ATL/L). A diffuse infiltrate is seen in lymph nodes consisting of a mixture of small and large atypical cells with prominent nuclear pleomorphism. Reed-Sternberg–like cells are present. In the peripheral blood, cells with hyperlobated nuclei (cloverleaf or flower cells) are a characteristic feature. Bone marrow infiltration may be focal or diffuse.

Immunophenotyping studies reveal CD2+, CD3+, CD4+, CD5+, CD7–, CD25+. TCR genes are clonally rearranged. Human T-cell leukemia virus I (HTLV-I) genomes are found in most cases.

This disease is most commonly seen in Japan but has also been described in the Caribbean, with occasional cases seen in the United States. Several clinical forms of disease have been described. The acute form appears to be most common, characterized by high white blood cell count, hepatosplenomegaly hypercalcemia, and a median survival of less than 1 year. Other cases appear to be more chronic or smoldering in nature.

Anaplastic Large Cell Lymphoma (T and Null Cell Types). The morphologic features in this lymphoma are characterized by an infiltrate of large pleomorphic cells frequently with horseshoe shaped (wreath-like) nuclei and prominent nucleoli (Image 36-13). Reed-Sternberg–like cells are often seen. The tumor cells often have a cohesive pattern and involve the lymph node sinuses similar to metastatic carcinoma. In a small number of patients the tumor cells are much smaller than the typical anaplastic large cell lymphoma cells, and this has been referred to as a small cell variant. Immunophenotypic studies usually reveal CD3+/–, CD15–, CD30+/–, CD43+/–, CD45+/–, EMA+/–. Sixty percent of the patients described have TCR rearrangement and 40% have no rearrangement of TCR or Ig genes.

This lymphoma has been reported in all age groups. There appears to be two distinct forms of primary anaplastic large cell lymphoma: a systemic form, which involves lymph nodes and extranodal sites including skin; and a primary cutaneous form, without extracutaneous spread at the time of diagnosis. The primary cutaneous lymphomas occur predominantly in adults and may spontaneously regress, similar to what is seen in lymphomatoid papulosis type A.

Provisional Category: Anaplastic Large-Cell Lymphoma Hodgkin's-like (Hodgkin's Related). In this tumor, the cellular morphologic features are similar to those of classic anaplastic large cell lymphoma, but the architectural features on low power are similar to those of Hodgkin's disease and nodular sclerosis. The morphologic features are what many pathologists will call nodular sclerosing Hodgkin's syncytial type or lymphocyte-depleted subtype of nodular sclerosis.

Immunophenotypic studies reveal findings identical to those seen in classical anaplastic large-cell lymphoma.

The clinical features include a large mediastinal mass usually seen in young women. At this time, it is uncertain whether this represents a defined entity.

This concludes the discussion of the newly proposed classification system for NHL by the International Lymphoma Study Group. Clinical trials utilizing this classification have not yet taken place, and it is likely that a number of modifications will be made as more information is obtained about each entity.

Non-Hodgkin's Lymphoma in Children

Lymph node enlargement is a frequent finding in children, usually representing a transient response to localized infection. No single clinical feature allows one to predict whether one is dealing with a benign or malignant lymphadenopathy. When supraclavicular or generalized lymphadenopathy with systemic symptoms are present, however, a lymph node biopsy is strongly recommended.

Children respond to antigenic stimuli with more pronounced lymph node hyperplasia than adults. Pathologists who have little experience in evaluating lymph node biopsy specimens from children may mistake florid immunoblastic proliferations, often seen in viral infections (such as infectious mononucleosis), for large cell lymphoma (see Chapter 26). A

Table 36-13   Comparison of Non-Hodgkin's Lymphoma Features in Children and Adults

Children	Adults
Predominantly extranodal	Predominantly nodal
Rapidly proliferative (aggressive, high grade)	Often slowly proliferative (indolent, low grade)
Rarely follicular	Often follicular
Often leukemic	Rarely leukemic

Table 36-14   Classification of Non-Hodgkin's Lymphoma in Children

Lymphoblastic lymphoma (precursor T and B cell)
Burkitt's lymphoma
Burkitt's-like lymphoma
Large-cell lymphoma (B and T cell, anaplastic large-cell lymphoma)
Others

diagnosis of large cell immunoblastic lymphoma in a child or young adult should not be made without first considering the possibility of a viral infection.

Malignant lymphoma in children differs in many ways from that in adults and deserves separate attention. Table 36-13 outlines the major differences between NHL in children and adults. Lymphomas with a follicular pattern, which in adults account for about 50% of all NHLs, are very unusual in children. The majority of children have aggressive, disseminated disease at the time of diagnosis. Peripheral B-cell lymphomas such as small lymphocytic lymphoma, mantle cell lymphoma, follicle center lymphoma, and marginal zone lymphoma are very rare in children. As seen in Table 36-14, the classification of NHL in children is much more limited than that in adults and mainly confined to lymphoblastic lymphoma (35%-47%), Burkitt's and Burkitt's-like lymphoma (20%-35%), and large cell lymphoma (30%-35%). Table 36-15 presents a comparison of the major morphologic, cytochemical, and immunophenotypic features of childhood NHL.

There is a strong propensity for extranodal involvement in children, and a close relationship exists between the histologic types and the anatomic site of involvement. Thus, the lymphoblastic lymphomas are predominantly supradiaphragmatic, presenting with a mediastinal mass. Burkitt's lymphomas usually occur in the abdomen, particularly in the ileocecal region.

Posttransplantation Lymphoproliferative Disorders

Immunosuppression following bone marrow transplantation (0.6%), renal transplantation (1%-5%), and cardiac transplantation (2%-20%) have been associated with an increase in NHLs. The lymphoproliferative disorders associated with transplantation immunosuppression are unique and have many features in common, including predilection for extranodal sites, variable morphologic features, an association with Epstein-Barr virus infection, frequent absence of immunophenotypic or genotypic proof of monoclonality, poor response to standard chemotherapeutic or irradiation treatment protocols, and potential remission with reduction in immunosuppression.

The onset of disease may vary from 1 to 12 months after transplantation. It is important that these lymphoproliferative disorders be identified immediately since they may be cured with appropriate management. The most common sites of involvement are the gastrointestinal tract, followed by lung, kidney, prostate, and the engrafted organ.

The histopathologic diagnosis of this disorder is difficult because of the range of morphologic features that may be present, ranging from B-cell polymorphic hyperplasia (a mixture of small lymphocytes, small cleaved lymphocytes, large transformed cells, and immunoblasts admixed with plasma cells) to frank immunoblastic large cell lymphoma. Unfortunately, there does not appear to be a good correlation between the morphologic features, demonstration of monoclonality, and biologic behavior. Because of this, the term posttransplantation lymphoproliferative disorder (PTLD) is recommended. This disorder may be divided into two morphologic types, polymorphic PTLD and monomorphic PTLD.

Table 36-15 Comparison of Morphologic, Cytochemical, and Immunophenotypic Features of Childhood Non-Hodgkin's Lymphomas

Feature	Lymphoblastic	Burkitt's
Imprint cytology, Wright's stain	FAB L1 or FAB L2 blasts	FAB L3 blasts
Nuclear size	Smaller than macrophage nucleus	Approximates macrophage nucleus; nuclear monotony
Nuclear chromatin	Delicate	Coarsely reticulated
Nucleoli	Small, inconspicuous	Prominent
Mitotic index	High	High
Cytoplasm	Scant	Moderate
Cytoplasmic vacuoles	Inconspicuous	Prominent
Periodic acid–Schiff stain	Often positive	Negative
Methyl green pyronine stain	Negative or focally positive	Strongly positive
TdT	Positive	Negative
Immunologic markers	Precursor T or B cell	B cell

Abbreviations: FAB = French-American-British acute leukemia classification; TdT = terminal deoxynucleotidyl transferase.

The polymorphic form responds more often to reduction in immunosuppression than does the monomorphic form, which is composed of a uniform population of immunoblasts.

Immunophenotyping will almost always show a B-cell proliferation. Genotyping may reveal polyclonal, oligoclonal, and monoclonal rearrangements. However, gene rearrangement studies are of limited value in the treatment of an individual patient. In situ hybridization studies usually reveal evidence of Epstein-Barr virus, and acyclovir is often used in combination with reduced immunosuppression. The monomorphic type of PTLD is more frequently associated with *c-myc* oncogene rearrangement. It would appear that the clinical progression of the disease is the most important prognostic factor. In general, a diagnosis of malignant lymphoma should be considered if PTLD progresses despite a trial of reduced immunosuppression.

Table 36-15 *Continued*

Burkitt's-like	Large Cell
FAB L3 blasts	Variable, large transformed lymphocytes
Sometimes larger than macrophage nucleus; nuclear variability	Larger than macrophage nucleus
Coarsely reticulated	Clumped, vesicular
Prominent	Variable, often prominent
High	Variable
Moderate	Moderate to abundant
Variable	Inconspicuous
Negative	Occasionally positive
Strongly positive	Variable, usually positive
Negative	Negative
Usually B cell	Usually B cell; 20% T cell

Approach to Diagnosis

Management of a patient with NHL requires a team approach between the clinician, the oncologist, the radiotherapist, the surgeon, the radiologist, and the pathologist. Good communication should be established between these specialists in planning the evaluation and therapy of the patient.

Following a clinical history and physical examination, the workup of a patient with possible malignant lymphoma should proceed in the following fashion: (1) a tissue biopsy (required to diagnose malignant lymphoma); (2) complete blood cell count including evaluation of peripheral blood smear for circulating lymphoma cells; (3) bone marrow aspirate and biopsy examination; (4) radiologic studies; (5) liver and renal function assessment; and (6) cytologic examination of effusions if present.

Figure 36-1 Schematic outline illustrating the handling of a tissue biopsy specimen of suspected malignant lymphoma.

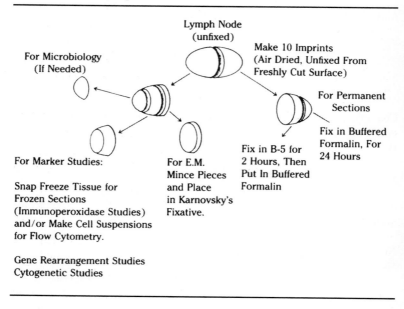

Lymph Node (unfixed)

For Microbiology (If Needed)

Make 10 Imprints (Air Dried, Unfixed From Freshly Cut Surface)

For Permanent Sections

Fix in Buffered Formalin, For 24 Hours

Fix in B-5 for 2 Hours, Then Put In Buffered Formalin

For Marker Studies:

Snap Freeze Tissue for Frozen Sections (Immunoperoxidase Studies) and/or Make Cell Suspensions for Flow Cytometry.

Gene Rearrangement Studies Cytogenetic Studies

For E.M. Mince Pieces and Place in Karnovsky's Fixative.

Tissue Biopsy

A tissue biopsy is required for the diagnosis of NHL and is the most important part of the diagnostic evaluation; it is therefore discussed separately.

Histopathologic evaluation of a lymph node biopsy specimen is one of the more difficult problems in surgical pathology, and consultation from a hematopathologist is often desirable. The major reason for difficulties in interpretation of lymph node biopsy specimens, unfortunately, is still technical in nature and results from improper handling of the biopsy specimen. An adequate lymph node biopsy specimen must be delivered to the pathologist intact immediately following removal. Before fixation, the tissue should be divided into multiple sections, as outlined in Figure 36-1, allowing a variety of studies to be performed. Not all of the procedures indicated in Figure 36-1 may be necessary to make a correct diagnosis; however, samples for immunologic and possibly genotypic studies should be obtained routinely. A section of the tissue should be routinely snap-frozen for immunophenotypic and genotypic studies in case histopathologic evaluation or immunophenotypic studies of paraffin sections are not conclusive.

When immunologic procedures cannot be performed in the hospital where the biopsy is performed, the specimen can be sent to reference laboratories without compromising the immunologic and cytochemical investigations. Frozen tissue must be sent in dry ice, or sections of frozen tissue may be sent. Another method that is simpler, but may not work for all tumors, is to send tissue left intact in refrigerated saline solution that is placed in a Styrofoam container with cold packs and immediately sent to the reference laboratory.

A diagnosis should never be made on the basis of immunologic or cytochemical studies alone, but always be correlated with clinical and histopathologic features of the biopsy specimen. To provide the best morphologic features, the specimen to be used for histopathologic studies should be fixed in a mercury-containing fixative, such as B5 as well as in buffered formalin fixative. For adequate fixation in buffered formalin, the tissue should be fixed for at least 12 hours, but not more than 24 hours. Postfixation in B5 after the tissue has been fixed in formalin often provides better morphologic results than formalin alone. The sections of the biopsy specimen must be thin (one cell thickness) and well stained.

The diagnosis and subclassification of malignant lymphoma should be made on the basis of the histopathologic features in the lymph node biopsy specimen before any treatment is initiated. The initial diagnosis should not be made on the basis of results of a bone marrow or liver biopsy alone unless this is the only tissue involved. In true extranodal lymphomas, the diagnosis will, of course, have to be made from a biopsy specimen from the organ involved; however, every attempt should be made to find a suitable lymph node for biopsy.

Fine-needle aspiration or true cut needle biopsy or both are proven methods for obtaining samples of malignant tissue in the appropriate clinical setting. These techniques should probably not be used alone for the initial diagnosis unless it is impossible to obtain a lymph node biopsy specimen or appropriate extranodal biopsy specimen. Such procedures may be very helpful in follow-up diagnosis. A liver biopsy specimen may be used to document the relatively common liver involvement of NHLs.

Hematologic Findings

The hematologic findings in NHLs are variable and depend on the type of lymphoma present. In some lymphomas, such as small lymphocytic lymphoma and follicle center lymphomas, blood and bone marrow involvement are frequently present. On the other hand, in large cell lymphomas the peripheral blood and bone marrow are usually not involved.

Blood Cell Measurements. The majority of patients who present with NHLs have normal blood counts. Anemia develops during the course of the disease in about 50% of patients. One or several of the following may be the cause of anemia: bone marrow insufficiency caused by bone marrow replacement by lymphoma; therapy-induced bone marrow hypoplasia; hypersplenism; autoimmune hemolytic anemia; and bleeding from lymphoma in the gastrointestinal tract or from low platelet count.

Peripheral Blood Smear Morphology. Circulating lymphoma cells have in the past been referred to as lymphosarcoma cell leukemia (see Chapter 35). This is not a specific clinical pathologic entity and may be found in many subtypes of NHL. The overall incidence is 10% to 25%. In follicle center lymphomas, especially the small and mixed small and large, the circulating lymphoma cells have scant cytoplasm with a characteristic notched or clefted nucleus (Image 36-14). In small lymphocytic lymphoma, the circulating cells are morphologically indistinguishable from those in chronic lymphocytic leukemia. Confirmation that the circulating cells are malignant can usually be made by the demonstration of light chain restriction using flow cytometric techniques. The presence of circulating lymphoma cells in indolent NHL usually does not significantly affect the prognosis. In aggressive NHL, circulating lymphoma cells may be associated with poor prognosis.

Circulating lymphoma cells can also be detected in the peripheral blood of patients where the morphologic evaluation of the peripheral blood smear is negative. With sensitive methods, such as Southern blot hybridization studies for rearranged immunoglobulin genes or polymerase chain reaction (PCR) analysis, occult disease may be detected frequently. At this time, however, such findings do not influence therapy.

Bone Marrow Examination. Bone marrow aspiration and bone marrow biopsy should be done routinely in the staging of malignant lymphoma. A biopsy is usually more useful than an aspirate. A bilateral, posterior iliac crest biopsy will increase the chance of detecting lymphoma. The overall incidence of bone marrow involvement in NHL is 30% to 50% and varies with different subtypes.

The bone marrow is involved at the time of diagnosis in 60% of patients with follicle center cell lymphoma. The bone marrow involvement is seen in less than 25% of patients with diffuse large cell lymphomas. In large cell lymphomas, bone marrow involvement is associated with spread to the central nervous system in up to 35% of cases. So-called bone marrow discordance is not infrequently seen in patients with diffuse large cell lymphomas, where the bone marrow is infiltrated by a more indolent lesion, especially small cleaved follicle center cells. Survival times in these patients are similar to those seen in patients with no bone marrow involvement and are better than those in patients with concordant (lymphoma in lymph node and bone marrow have same histologic features) bone marrow involvement.

The pattern of bone marrow involvement in NHL is usually focal (nodular) rather than diffuse. In small lymphocytic and lymphoplasmacytoid NHL, the incidence of involvement is 80% to 90% and the pattern is random focal or interstitial. In follicle center NHL, the pattern is characteristically focal and paratrabecular (Image 36-14). In lymphoblastic and Burkitt's lymphoma, the pattern is interstitial or diffuse. It is important that nodules of lymphoma in the bone marrow be differentiated from benign lymphoid nodules, which are commonly seen in older patients. Nodules of malignant lymphoma are usually less well circumscribed than benign lymphoid nodules; in lymphoma, the infiltrate is frequently located adjacent to bone trabeculae (paratrabecular position). In addition, in benign lymphoid nodules, the lymphocytes are usually small and normal-appearing, and germinal centers may be seen.

Other Laboratory Tests

36.1 Radiologic Studies

Purpose. Various radiologic techniques are used to depict NHL in the mediastinum, peritoneum, and bones. Mediastinal and hilar lymph nodes are demonstrated primarily with standard posterior-anterior and lateral chest roentgenograms. Computed tomographic (CT) scans of the thorax may be helpful if abnormalities are found on the routine chest roentgenogram. Bipedal lymphangiography is the standard procedure for assessment for periaortic and pelvic lymph nodes with an overall accuracy of 90%. CT is considered to be the technique of choice in the diagnosis of mesenteric, portahepatic, and splenic hilar nodal involvement.

36.2 Renal and Liver Function Tests

Purpose. The evaluation of renal and liver function with routine serum chemistries and urine analysis should be performed in every patient. The results may help detect disease in those organs and must be done as part of the workup before giving the patient chemotherapy or radiotherapy or both. An elevated serum creatinine level indicates renal insufficiency, suggesting obstruction from a retroperitoneal NHL. Abnormal liver enzymes, bilirubin, and alkaline phosphatase may be an indication of liver or bone involvement.

36.3 Laparotomy

Purpose. Exploratory laparotomy and splenectomy are occasionally performed if management decision depends on the identification of abdominal involvement. If a laparotomy is performed, a preoperative lymphangiogram should be done as a guide to direct surgical sampling of the lymph nodes.

36.4 Cytology of Cerebrospinal Fluid and Serous Effusions

Purpose. Of the NHLs, the most common types to involve the central nervous system (CNS) are lymphoblastic lymphoma, Burkitt's lymphoma, and large cell immunoblastic lymphoma. Indolent lymphomas such as follicle center lymphomas and small lymphocytic lymphomas rarely involve the CNS. Morphologically, lymphoblastic lymphomas affecting cerebrospinal fluid have a similar appearance to acute lymphoblastic leukemia. There appears to be an increase in primary CNS lymphomas, which are particularly common in patients with cellular immune dysfunction, as seen in transplant patients and in patients with AIDS. Immunoblastic lymphoma and Burkitt's lymphoma are the most common types of lymphomas in these patients.

Pleural and peritoneal effusions are not uncommon in NHLs, and cytologic examination of fluid specimens is an essential part of the clinical evaluation in such situations. Immunocytologic marker studies either by immunoperoxidase studies on cell suspensions or with flow cytometry may be helpful in differentiating reactive from malignant effusions and in making the diagnosis. Such studies are especially helpful in peritoneal effusions in patients who may have Burkitt's lymphoma, or in a pleural effusion in a patient with lymphoblastic lymphoma involving the mediastinum.

36.5 Fine-Needle Aspiration (FNA)

Purpose. FNA of lymph nodes may be used to document recurrent disease, to demonstrate transformation to another type of lymphoma, or to obtain cells for immunophenotypic analysis in patients who are referred for treatment of NHL previously diagnosed with a tissue biopsy specimen. Most pathologists are reluctant to utilize FNA as the primary evaluation of lymphadenopathy, partly because of problems with sampling errors if the lymph node is only partially involved with NHL, or if the malignant lymphoid cells are small in number. It has been shown that FNA immunohistochemistry using cytospin specimens and flow cytometry give equally reliable results.

Ancillary Tests

Cytochemistry.   Cytochemical studies, such as using the specific esterase stain (chloroacetate esterase), may be helpful in identifying immature granulocytic cells in granulocytic sarcomas to differentiate such tumors from malignant lymphoma or undifferentiated carcinoma. Immunoperoxidase studies using antibody to myeloperoxidase, however, is a more sensitive and reliable method for identifying granulocytic sarcomas. The identification of TdT is very helpful in the diagnosis of lymphoblastic lymphoma (Image 36-11), since this enzyme is not present in other malignant lymphomas. Identification of TdT can be done on imprints of tissue biopsy specimens, on cytocentrifuge preparations made from cell suspension of the biopsy specimen, on frozen sections, and more recently on paraffin sections using an immunoperoxidase procedure. The periodic acid–Schiff and methyl green pyronine stains are sometimes helpful in separating lymphoblastic lymphoma from Burkitt's lymphoma, as noted in Table 36-15.

Immunophenotypic Analysis.   Immunohistochemistry has become available in most major pathology laboratories. A wide spectrum of immunologic markers are being used in surgical pathology to aid the pathologist in the diagnosis of difficult cases. With the classification system used in this chapter, the diagnosis is made on the basis of histopathology and immunophenotypic analysis. Immunophenotypic studies may be used to rule out nonhematopoietic tumors, to determine whether the lymphoid lesion is benign or malignant, to determine cell lineage (Images 36-9, 36-15), to indicate stage of differentiation of the tumor, to subclassify lymphoma (Image 36-13), and sometimes to detect minimal residual disease.

Several approaches may be used for the immunophenotypic analysis of lymphoproliferative disorders. Such approaches include flow cytometric analysis of cell suspensions from the tissue biopsy specimen, immunohistochemical studies of frozen tissue sections, immunohistochemical studies of paraffin-embedded tissue sections, and immunohistochemical analysis of cytocentrifuge smears prepared from cell suspensions of the biopsy specimen. Each of these procedures has its advantages and disadvantages. The flow cytometric analysis and immunohistochemical analysis of frozen tissue sections and/or cytocentrifuge smears give the most information because the number of antibodies that are available for such procedures is considerably greater than what is available for paraffin sections. Immunohistochemical analysis on paraffin-embedded tissue has several advantages because of superior morphologic characteristics, allowing better analysis of immunoreactivity in both malignant and reactive cell populations, and paraffin sections are much more readily available. In recent years, a large number of excellent antibodies have been introduced that can be used in paraffin-embedded tissue sections. When good techniques are applied in appropriately fixed tissue, reliable immunophenotypic analysis can be performed in more than 80% of cases utilizing paraffin-embedded tissue sections. Unsuitable fixation of tissue is probably the most common cause of unsatisfactory results.

B5 appears to be the fixative of choice for most hematopoietic antigens, but properly fixed buffered formalin tissue also often gives satisfactory results. The immunoreactivity may be improved in some cases by protease digestion with pepsin, pronase, or trypsin. Antigen retrieval from formalin-fixed, paraffin-embedded tissues with microwave irradiation is frequently very helpful and decreases the dependence of staining quality on the fixative used. This may be very helpful in consultation cases where the type of fixative used is unknown.

When using paraffin-embedded tissue sections for immunophenotypic analysis of lymphoproliferative disorders, it is important to recognize that many of the antibodies lack specificity, and knowledge of the immunoreactivity profile of each antibody is essential to avoid making incorrect diagnoses. A panel of antibodies should always be used and the results should be correlated with the histologic appearance and clinical history before a diagnosis is rendered. A diagnosis should never be made on the basis of immunostaining alone. Also, attempts should always be made to obtain fresh or frozen tissue that may be needed for more detailed immunophenotypic analysis and immunogenotypic analysis.

Table 36-16 Major Reactivities of Antibodies Used in Immunophenotyping of Malignant Lymphomas in Paraffin Sections*

Antibody	Reactivity	Comments†
CD45 (LCA)	Leukocytes	Immunoblastic plasmacytoid and lymphoblastic NHL, Ki-1 ALCL, and multiple myeloma are often negative; Reed-Sternberg cells and variants (except for L&H cells) are usually negative
B-Cell Associated		
CD20 (L26)	B cells	Reacts with 90% of B-cell NHL, rarely with T-cell NHL; reacts with 40% of precursor B-cell ALL/LBL; reacts with 80% of LPHD (L&H cells) and 10%-20% of HDNS and HDMC; no reactivity with nonhematopoietic tumors
CD45R (4KB5)	B cells	Reacts with 80% of B-cell NHL and 10% of T-cell NHL; immunoblastic B-cell NHL and plasma cell tumors are often negative; reacts with 20% myeloid tumors
Antihuman light chain Ig	B cells, plasma cells, immunoblasts	Used to identify light chain restriction in plasma cells and immunoblasts; with proteolytic digestion and microwave light chains, may also be identified in small and intermediate NHL and in L&H cells in LPHD
Antihuman heavy chain Ig	B cells, plasma cells, immunoblasts	Used to identify heavy chain Ig in plasma cell tumors and immunoblastic NHL
DBA-44	Hairy cell leukemia, B cells, mantle zone, monocytoid B cells	Useful in detecting hairy cell leukemia in bone marrow sections; CLL is usually unreactive; may react with follicle center lymphomas and high grade B-cell NHL
T-Cell Associated		
UCHL-1 (CD45RO)	T cells, some B cells, monocytes,	Reacts with 75% of T-cell NHL and <5% of B-cell NHL (large cell); myeloid cells reacts with <50% of T-cell ALL/LBL and 25% of AML; rarely positive in carcinomas
CD3 (anti-CD3)	T cells	Most specific T-cell antibody; reacts with 80% of T-cell NHL; unreactive with most B-cell NHL

Table 36-16 *Continued*

Antibody	Reactivity	Comments†
CD43	T cells, some B cells, myeloid cells, monocytes	Reacts with >80% of T-cell NHL; shows coexpression with CD20 in most small lymphoid NHL; such coexpression is usually not seen in benign proliferations; reacts with megakaryoblasts, granulocytic sarcomas, AML, most ALLs, plasmacytomas, and some nonhematopoietic tumors

Myeloid/Macrophage Associated

Antibody	Reactivity	Comments†
Myelo-peroxidase (MPO)	Granulocytes	Most sensitive and specific antibody for myeloid leukemias and granulocytic sarcoma
CD68 (KP1)	Monocytes, macrophages, mast cells	Reacts with 50% of AML; positive with most FAB M4, M5; reacts with some B-cell NHL, hairy cell leukemia, Langerhans cell histiocytosis, mastocytosis, and SHML; occasionally reacts with nonhematopoietic tumors (melanoma)
S100	Macrophages, melanocytes, glial cells, Schwann cells, Langerhans cells	Reactive in Langerhans cell histiocytosis, SHML, melanomas, brain tumors, some carcinomas; stains blast cells in AML in 50% of cases, and in granulocytic sarcoma; rare reactivity in HD and NHL (ALCL)

Others

Antibody	Reactivity	Comments†
CD15 (Leu M1)	Granulocytes, Reed-Sternberg cells	Reacts with Reed-Sternberg cells in 85% of HDNS and HDMC, and 20% of LPHD; reacts with 20% of T-cell NHL, 5% of B-cell NHL (large cell), and 50% of carcinomas
CD30 (Ber-H2)	Activated B and T cells, Reed-Sternberg cells, granulocytes	Reacts with 90% of NHL, ALCL (Ki-1 lymphoma), Reed-Sternberg cells in 90% of HDNS and HDMC, and 10% of LPHD; reactivity may be seen in several low-, intermediate-, and high grade NHL; reactivity may also be seen in benign immunoblastic proliferations (infectious mononucleosis); reacts with 20% of plasma cell tumors, and rarely with nonhematopoietic tumors (germ cell)

Table 36-16   *Continued*

Antibody	Reactivity	Comments†
Bauhinia purpurea (BPA)	Reed-Sternberg cells, granulocytes, macrophages, germinal center lymphocytes	Reacts with Reed-Sternberg cells in >90% of HDNS and HDMC, and 75% of LPHD
CD34	Hematopoietic progenitor cells, leukemic blasts, vascular endothelial cells	Reacts with 30%-60% blasts in AML and ALL; nonreactive with NHL and HD; reacts with neoplasms of vascular origin, hemangiopericytomas, epithelioid sarcoma, dermatofibrosarcoma protuberans
CD61 (GPIIIa)	Platelets, megakaryocytes	Reacts with AML M7 and with erythroblasts in some cases of erythroleukemia
Factor VIIIR	Megakaryocytes, endothelial cells	Reacts with megakaryocyte proliferations and 70% of vascular tumors
Glyco-phorin A	Erythroid cells	Reacts with erythroid precursors; AML M6.
Epithelial membrane antigen (EMA)	Epithelial cells	Reacts with 20%-30% of LPHD (L&H cells), 50% of Ki-1 ALCL, and most plasmacytic tumors; reacts with most epithelial cell tumors
bcl-2	*bcl*-2 proto-oncogene	Serves as a marker of t(14;18) associated overexpression, seen in 60% of follicular lymphomas; also seen in some large cell lymphomas and in HD
bcl-1	*bcl*-1 (cyclin D1) proto-oncogene	Marker of t(11;14); reactivity seen in mantle cell lymphoma
MIB-1	Ki-67 nuclear antigen	Indicator of proliferation rate in NHL
TdT	B- and T-cell precursors	Reactive with 90% of lymphoblastic lymphoma; negative in other NHL

Abbreviations: NHL = non-Hodgkin's lymphoma; ALCL = anaplastic large cell lymphoma; L&H = lymphocyte and histiocyte; ALL = acute lymphoblastic leukemia; LBL = lymphoblastic lymphoma; LPHD = lymphocyte-predominant Hodgkin's disease; HDNS = Hodgkin's disease (nodular sclerosing); HDMC = Hodgkin's disease (mixed cellularity); CLL = chronic lymphoblastic leukemia; AML = acute myelogenous leukemia; FAB = French-American-British classification; SHML = sinus histiocytosis with massive lymphadenopathy; HD = Hodgkin's disease; TdT = terminal deoxynucleotidyl transferase.
* Modified from Perkins SL, Kjeldsberg CR. Immunophenotyping of lymphomas and leukemias in paraffin-embedded tissues. Am J Clin Pathol. 1993;99:362-373.
† The reactivity percentages listed are approximate and depend on many technical factors.

Table 36-17 Applications of Immunophenotypic Analysis

Disorder	Antibody Panel
Rule out nonhematopoietic tumors (cell lineage determination)	CD45, keratin, S100, HMB45, vimentin, MPO, CD20, CD3
Reactive hyperplasia vs NHL	Light chains, CD5, CD43,* CD20,* bcl-2
Subclassification of NHL	CD45, CD20, CD43, CD3, CD30, EMA, TdT
NHL vs HD	CD45, CD20, CD43, CD3, CD30, CD15, EMA
NHL proliferation rate	MIB1 (Ki67), topoisomerase II

Abbreviations: CD45 = leukocyte common antigen; MPO = myeloperoxidase; CD20 = B-cell antigen; CD3, CD5, CD43 = T-cell antigen; NHL = non-Hodgkin's lymphoma; CD30 = (Ki-1); EMA = epithelial membrane antigen; TdT = terminal deoxynucleotidyl transferase; HD = Hodgkin's disease.
*Coexpression of CD20 and CD43 favors a malignant lymphoma.

In addition to phenotyping of paraffin and frozen sections, similar studies can successfully be performed on touch preparations (imprints) of the tumor.

Establishing monoclonality of a B-lymphocyte proliferation is usually accomplished by the demonstration of light chain restriction. Within the tumor this can usually be established with frozen tissue sections, although the interpretation at times may be difficult. In small and medium malignant lymphoid cell populations, it is difficult to demonstrate surface immunoglobulin in paraffin sections. Microwave techniques are being improved so that light chain restriction may now be demonstrated also in the majority of paraffin-embedded tissues. In difficult cases, immunogenotypic analysis is necessary. For T-lymphocyte proliferations, clonality can be conclusively shown only by T-lymphocyte receptor gene rearrangement studies. For frozen section immunophenotypic analysis, the most useful criteria in the diagnosis of T-cell neoplasia is the deletion of one or more of the pan T-cell antigens.

Table 36-16 presents a list of major reactivities of antibodies used in immunophenotyping malignant lymphomas in paraffin-embedded tissue sections. Tables 36-17, 36-18, and 36-19 present the usefulness of immunophenotypic analysis in a number of NHLs.

In general, the T-cell NHLs appear to be more aggressive than B-cell types. High proliferative rates in NHL correlate with poor prognosis. Immunohistochemical methods using antibody

Table 36-18 Undifferentiated Large Cell Neoplasm Antibody Panel for Paraffin Sections*

Disease	CD45	CD3	CD20	CD15	CD30	S100	Myeloperoxidase	Keratin	Vimentin
NHL	+	±	±	–	–/+	–	–	–	–
Hodgkin's disease	–	–	–	+	+	–	–	–	–
Carcinoma	–	–	–	–	–	–/+	–	+	–
Melanoma	–	–	–	–	–	+	–	–	+
Granulocytic sarcoma	–/+	–	–	–/+	–	–	+	–	–
Sarcoma	–	–	–	–	–	–	–	–	+

Abbreviations: ± = may be positive or negative depending on cell lineage (B or T); –/+ = less than 50% of cases positive; NHL = non-Hodgkin's lymphoma.
*CD45 may be negative in NHL, especially in immunoblastic and anaplastic large cell lymphoma. Rare carcinomas may express CD30. Keratin may be focally present in anaplastic large cell lymphoma. Myelomas are often CD45–, CD20–, CD43+, epithelial membrane antigen positive, and sometimes keratin positive.

Table 36-19   Immunophenotyping of Non-Hodgkin's Lymphoma (NHL) and Hodgkin's Disease (HD) in Paraffin Sections*

Lymphoma	CD45[†]	CD20	CD43[‡]	CD3	CD30[§]	CD15
NHL						
B cell	+	+	−	−	+ALCL	−
T cell	+	−	+	+	+ALCL	−
HD						
LPHD	+	+	−	−	−/+	−
HD (NS-MC)[‖]	−	−	−	−	+	+

Abbreviations: ALCL, anaplastic large cell lymphoma; LPHD, lymphocyte-predominant Hodgkin's disease; HD (NS-MC), Hodgkin's disease (nodular sclerosing and mixed cellularity).
*Modified from Perkins SL, Kjeldsberg CR. Immunophenotyping of lymphomas and leukemias in paraffin-embedded tissues. Am J Clin Pathol. 1993;99:362-373.
[†]CD45 is often negative in large cell lymphoma immunoblastic type, ALCL, lymphoblastic lymphoma, and in Reed-Sternberg cells in HDMC and HDNS.
[‡]Coexpression of CD43 and CD20 is common in low-grade small lymphoid neoplasms (small lymphocytic lymphoma, mantle cell lymphoma). This coexpression is usually not seen in reactive proliferations.
[§]CD30 is often positive in immunoblasts in infectious mononucleosis.
[‖]CD20 or CD3 may be present occasionally in malignant cells in HD (NS, MC).

Ki-67 (frozen sections) or MIB1 (paraffin sections) may be used to determine the proliferative index. A proliferative index greater than 80% has been shown to be associated with very poor prognosis in aggressive NHL. Another marker that may prove to be useful is topoisomerase II.

Immunogenotypic Analysis.   B and T lymphocytes have surface membrane antigen receptor proteins, immunoglobulins, and TCRs that are essential to the function of these cells. Monomeric immunoglobulins consist of two identical heavy chains adjoined with two identical light chains of either kappa or lambda type. T-cell receptors exist in two forms: alpha-beta or gamma-delta heterodimers. The purpose of antigen receptor gene rearrangement analysis is to determine whether a proportion of B or T lymphoid cells in the biopsy specimen contain identical antigen receptor gene rearrangement. The presence of uniform antigen receptor gene rearrangement indicates the presence of a clonal lymphoid cell population. The majority of malignant lymphoproliferative disorders are clonal proliferations, representing a single cell that has undergone malignant transformation. Benign proliferations represent progeny of multiple cell clones and are thus polyclonal. Therefore, gene rearrangement studies are used to distinguish between malignant monoclonal cell populations and polyclonal benign proliferations.

Gene rearrangement may be determined with the Southern blot hybridization analysis or with polymerase chain reaction techniques. Unfixed cells in suspension or unfixed fresh or frozen tissue are the specimens of choice for such studies. Formalin-fixed tissue may also be used, but such tissue is not a good source of DNA for such studies. B5-fixed tissue cannot be used. Almost all B-cell NHLs have clonal Ig heavy chain gene rearrangement. The vast majority of NHLs of T-cell lineage derivation have clonal TCR beta gene rearrangements.

Gene rearrangement studies with Southern blot hybridization is a very sensitive method capable of detecting clonal populations comprising only 1% or 2% of the total DNA in a specimen. This may be used to advantage in detecting a small number of neoplastic cells in specimens where histopathologic and immunophenotypic analysis is difficult. The major disadvantage of the Southern blot hybridization method is that the assay takes 1 to 2 weeks to complete and is generally not available except for in reference laboratories.

Recently, immunogenotypic analysis has become available with PCR, which may not be as sensitive for detecting gene rearrangements; if the study is negative, Southern blot hybridization studies should be performed. The advantages of PCR, however, are that the method requires only very small amounts of DNA and the results are available within 1 to 2 days. PCR is especially valuable when the biopsy specimen contains only small amounts of lymphoid infiltrates (eg, cutaneous lymphoid infiltrates).

It is important to recognize that although clonal lymphoid proliferations are usually malignant, clonality cannot be equated with malignancy. It should also be recognized that not all NHLs contain clonal antigen receptor gene rearrangement. One third of anaplastic large cell, CD30+ lymphomas appear to lack clonal antigen receptor gene rearrangement. Also, only a small number of T-cell angiocentric lymphomas show TCR gene rearrangement. Thus, the results of immunogenotypic analysis should always be interpreted together with the clinical, histopathologic, and immunophenotypic findings.

Oncogenes. Specific chromosome translocations are associated with certain types of NHL. Three well-known oncogenes are thought to be important in the genesis of human lymphoma: *bcl*-1, *bcl*-2, and *c-myc*. The reciprocal chromosome translocation t(11;14)(q13;q32) is characterized by the reposition of the putative proto-oncogene *bcl*-1 from its normal location on chromosome 11 to a site adjacent to one of the joining segments of the Ig heavy chain gene on chromosome 14. Mantle cell lymphoma and rarely B-cell chronic lymphocytic leukemia show chromosome translocation t(11;14) involving rearrangement of the *bcl*-1 oncogene. *bcl*-1 may be detected with Southern hybridization analysis and polymerase chain reaction. The *bcl*-1 oncogene encodes cyclin D1 (PRAD 1). Cyclin D1 protein expression may be identified with immunoperoxidase stains on paraffin sections. *bcl*-1 rearrangement has been found in up to 70% of mantle cell lymphomas. Thus the detection of *bcl*-1 may be useful in the diagnosis of mantle cell lymphoma.

The t(14;18) translocation brings the proto-oncogene *bcl*-2 from chromosome 18 into the immunoglobulin heavy chain joining region on chromosome 14. Overexpression of *bcl*-2 protein prevents programmed cell depth. *bcl*-2 may be analyzed with Southern blot hybridization studies, polymerase chain reaction, and immunohistochemical studies (Image 36-16). *bcl*-2 is rearranged in the majority of follicle center lymphomas and in about one third of diffuse large cell lymphomas. There is some evidence suggesting that large cell lymphomas that express *bcl*-2 are indolent and are incurable. Immunohistochemical staining for Bcl-2 oncoprotein may be useful in distinguishing follicular lymphoma from reactive hyperplasia. In follicular lymphomas, overexpression of *bcl*-2 is seen in the malignant follicle center cells. In reactive hyperplasia there is an absence of germinal center staining and weak staining of the mantle zone and interfollicular areas. Staining bone marrow biopsy specimens with an antibody to *bcl*-2 oncogene may also be useful in differentiating benign lymphoid aggregates from follicular lymphomas. Follicular lymphomas stain positive while benign lymphoid nodules are usually negative.

The t(8;14) translocation moves the *c-myc* oncogene into the immunoglobulin heavy chain locus. *c-myc* rearrangement occurs in Burkitt's lymphoma, also frequently in AIDS-related lymphoma, diffuse large-cell lymphomas, and posttransplant lymphoprolifera-tive disease.

Although *c-myc* rearrangement has been found in almost all cases of Burkitt's lymphoma, in Burkitt's-like lymphoma *c-myc* rearrangement is not present.

The breakpoints of the t(2,5) translocation, seen in approximately 40% of anaplastic large cell lymphomas, involve a tyrosine kinase gene, anaplastic lymphoma kinase (ALK), and the nucleophosmin (NPM) gene. Reverse transcriptase polymerase chain reaction using nucleophosmin and anaplastic lymphoma kinase primers detects a fusion product in anaplastic large cell lymphomas with the translocation, but not in Hodgkin's disease.

Cytogenetics. Although more than 90% of NHLs have cytogenetic abnormalities, cytogenetic analysis at this time has limited clinical value. Since cytogenetic studies depend on viable cells, it is essential that the biopsy specimen be transported to the cytogenetic laboratory without delay. For cytogenetic analysis, a portion of the fresh biopsy material is mixed into a cell suspension. Chromosomes are harvested from direct preparations and short-term cultures.

In more than 90% of Burkitt's lymphomas, t(8;14)(q24;q32) or one of its variants, t(8;22)(q24;q11) and t(2;8)(p11;q24), has been observed. Follicular center lymphomas have t(14;18)(q32;q21) in 80% of cases. As mentioned previously, the t(11;14)(q13;q32) translocation has been found in 70% of mantle cell lymphomas. In anaplastic large cell lymphoma, CD30+ (Ki-1) t(2;5)(p23;q35) is frequently seen. In small lymphocytic lymphoma, trisomy 12 is seen in 30% of cases.

Serum and Urine Protein Electrophoresis and Immunoelectrophoresis. The NHLs may be associated with polyclonal or monoclonal gammopathy (usually IgM), and occasionally hypogammaglobulinemia.

Serum Chemistry. Serum lactate dehydrogenase (LDH) and serum β_2-microglobulin can be used as indirect indicators of tumor burdens and are independent prognostic factors. Serum calcium levels may be elevated in NHL, particularly in some of the peripheral T-cell lymphomas (adult T-cell leukemia/lymphoma),

Table 36-20 Causes of Lymph Node Enlargement Simulating
Malignant Lymphoma

Nonspecific reactive follicular hyperplasia
Infectious mononucleosis
Toxoplasmosis
Viral lymphadenitis (herpes, cytomegalovirus)
AIDS
Cat-scratch disease
Syphilis
Phenytoin lymph node hyperplasia
Rheumatoid arthritis
Dermatopathic lymphadenopathy
Giant lymph node hyperplasia (Castleman's disease)
Sinus histiocytosis with massive lymphadenopathy
Leukemia
Metastatic carcinoma
Metastatic melanoma

---

and uric acid levels may increase dramatically during treatment of fast-growing lymphomas such as Burkitt's lymphoma. Elevated liver enzymes, bilirubin level, and alkaline phosphatase level may be a sign of liver or bone involvement.

Diseases Simulating Malignant Lymphoma

A variety of disorders other than NHLs may not only cause enlargement of lymph nodes, but may be mistaken on histologic examination for lymphoma (Table 36-20). These disorders are described in Chapter 26. It is important that the pathologist have an accurate clinical history and strong familiarity with the lymph node changes that may occur in a variety of benign reactive lymphadenopathies.

Course and Treatment

Treatment of patients with NHL is based on the histopathologic features, the stage of the disease, and the clinical features (age and functional status of patient). The types of treatments utilized include surgery (rarely curative), cytotoxic chemotherapy, radiotherapy, biologic modifiers, and bone marrow transplantation. In general, patients with aggressive disease (intermediate and high-grade) are treated with the intent of curing the patient, while patients with indolent disease (low-grade) can usually not be cured. The patients with indolent NHLs, however, have a long median survival.

Most patients with indolent NHL (follicle center lymphomas and small lymphocytic lymphoma) survive for 5 or more years, with patients with the follicle center lymphomas having considerably longer survival times than those with small lymphocytic lymphomas. The optimal method of treatment for localized, indolent NHL is radiotherapy, and many of these patients are long-term, disease-free survivors. Unfortunately, the majority of patients with indolent (low-grade) NHL have stage (III or IV) disease, and treatment for these patients remains controversial. A variety of chemotherapeutic approaches have been utilized and many appear to be associated with complete remission; however, there is a very high relapse rate. Over a period of years a number of patients with indolent disseminated NHL have their disease transform to an aggressive NHL—usually diffuse large cell lymphoma or immunoblastic lymphoma. This transformation is usually manifested as a rapidly growing tumor in one or several sites.

In the aggressive (intermediate and high-grade) NHLs that are localized, intensive therapy (chemotherapy and radiotherapy) is curable in approximately 60% of the patients. In patients with disseminated aggressive NHL, combination chemotherapy is utilized, and patients with diffuse large cell or immunoblastic lymphoma who achieve remission may be cured in 60% to 80% of cases. However, the prognosis is very poor in patients with aggressive NHL that relapses after combination chemotherapy.

Patients with lymphoblastic lymphoma are usually treated with intensive multiagent chemotherapy, similar to acute lymphoblastic leukemia. In patients with Burkitt's lymphoma, surgical debulking of abdominal tumors, combination chemotherapy, and intensive metabolic support often provide remission. Approximately 60% of children with lymphoblastic lymphoma and Burkitt's lymphoma are curable. The prognosis is less favorable in adults.

Recently, bone marrow transplantation with peripheral blood stem cell or allogenic bone marrow has improved the prognosis of patients with relapsed aggressive NHL from being fatal to potentially curable.

Radiotherapy, especially combined with chemotherapy, and chemotherapy alone, is associated with a number of serious side effects. The most common is myelosuppression associated with infection and/or hemorrhage. Other complications that occur later include infertility, second malignancies (especially myelodysplasia), and secondary leukemia. Elderly patients are more prone to develop these serious side effects than younger patients.

References

Brunning RD, McKenna RW. Tumors of the bone marrow. *Atlas of Tumor Pathology*. 3rd series, fascicle 9. Washington, DC: Armed Forces Institute of Pathology; 1994.

Craig FE, Gulley ML, Banks PM. Post-transplantation lymphoproliferative disorders. *Am J Clin Pathol*. 1993;99:265-276.

Harris NL, Jaffe ES, Stein H, et al. A revised European-American classification of lymphoid neoplasms: a proposal from the International Lymphoma Study Group. *Blood*. 1994;84:1361-1392.

Joachim HL. *Lymph Node Pathology*. 2nd ed. Philadelphia, Pa: JB Lippincott Co; 1994.

Jaffe ES. *Surgical Pathology of the Lymph Nodes and Related Organs*. 2nd ed. Philadelphia, Pa: WB Saunders Co; 1994.

Knowles DM. *Neoplastic Hematopathology*. Baltimore, Md: Williams & Wilkins; 1992.

Knowles DM. Immunophenotypic and immunogenotypic approaches useful in distinguishing benign and malignant lymphoid proliferations. *Semin Oncol*. 1993;20:583-610.

Lennert A, Feller A. *Histopathology of Non-Hodgkin's Lymphoma*. 2nd ed. New York, NY: Springer-Verlag NY Inc; 1992.

Longo DL, DeVita VT, Jaffe ES, et al. Lymphocytic lymphomas. In: DeVita VT, Helman S, Rosenberg SA, eds. *Cancer: Principles and Practice of Oncology*. 4th ed. Philadelphia, Pa: JB Lippincott Co; 1993.

Lukes RJ, Collins RD. Tumors of the hematopoietic system. In: *Atlas of Tumor Pathology*. 2d series, fascicle 28. Washington, DC: Armed Forces Institute of Pathology; 1992.

Morris SW, Kirstein MN, Valentine BM. Fusion of a kinase gene, ALK, to a nucleolar protein gene, NPM, in non-Hodgkin's lymphoma. *Science*. 1994;263:1281-1284.

Perkins SL, Kjeldsberg CR. Immunophenotyping of lymphomas and leukemias in paraffin-embedded tissues. *Am J Clin Pathol*. 1993;99:362-373.

Willemze R, Beljaards RC, Meijer CJLM. Classification of primary cutaneous T-cell lymphomas. *Histopathology*. 1994;405-415.

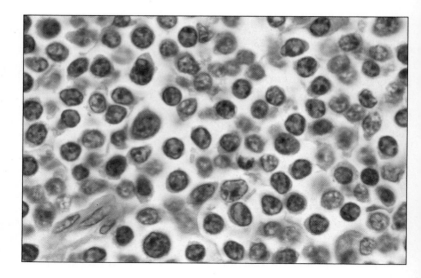

Image 36-1   Small lymphocytic lymphoma. There is a diffuse infiltrate of small lymphocytes.

Image 36-2   Mantle cell lymphoma. The cells have more dispersed chromatin than those seen in Image 36-1, and the nuclear contours are slightly irregular.

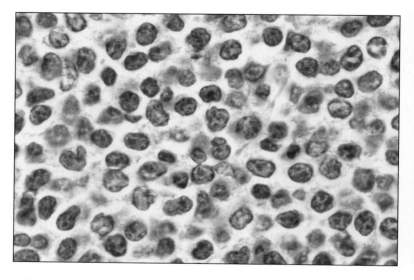

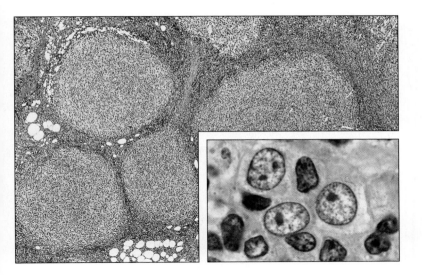

Image 36-3 Low-power view of follicle center lymphoma shows the follicular pattern. Inset shows high-power view of centrocytes (cleaved follicle center cells) and a smaller number of centroblasts (large noncleaved cells).

Image 36-4 Section of intestine from a patient with marginal zone B-cell lymphoma or low-grade B-cell lymphoma of mucosa-associated lymphoid tissue (MALT). Inset shows high-power view of lymphoma cells with centrocyte-like features.

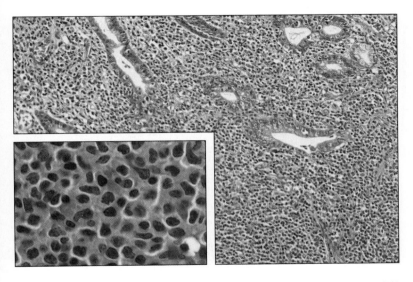

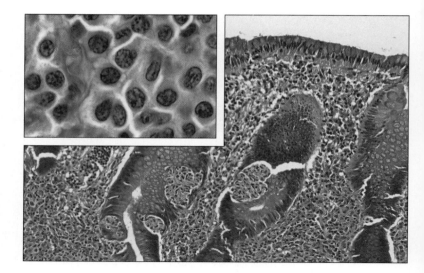

Image 36-5   Section of stomach from a patient with extranodal marginal zone B-cell lymphoma or low-grade B-cell lymphoma of mucosa-associated lymphoid tissue (MALT). Lymphoma cells are seen to infiltrate epithelial structures (↑) forming lymphoepithelial lesions. Inset shows high-power view of cellular infiltrate to have monocytoid B-cell–like features.

Image 36-6   Lymph node section showing nodal monocytoid B-cell lymphoma. As noted, the monocytoid B cells (upper half) are slightly larger than small lymphocytes and have moderately abundant cytoplasm. Inset shows high-power view of the monocytoid B cells.

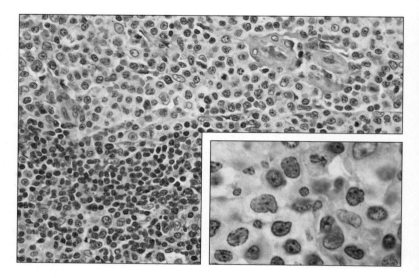

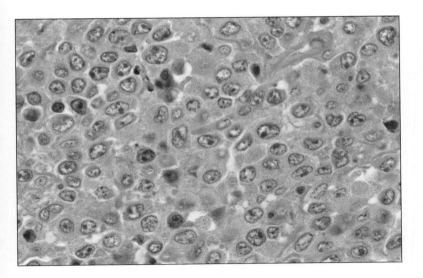

Image 36-7 Section of lymph node biopsy with diffuse large B-cell lymphoma. The majority of the cells are centroblasts (large non-cleaved cells).

Image 36-8 Diffuse large B-cell lymphoma in the stomach. Section shows a predominance of immunoblasts characterized by a prominent centrally placed nucleolus and abundant cytoplasm.

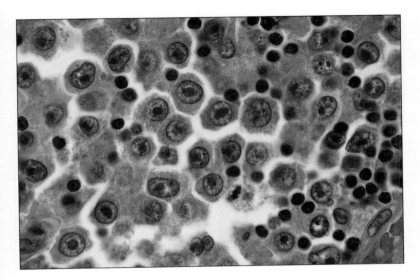

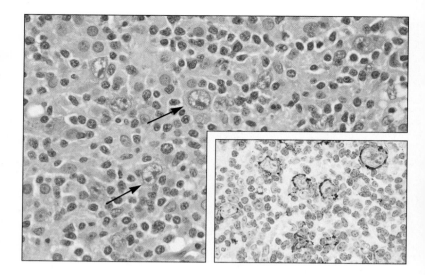

Image 36-9 Lymph node section showing the morphologic features of T-cell–rich B-cell lymphoma. The majority of the cells present are reactive, small T-lymphoid cells. The malignant cells (↑) are much larger but fewer in number. Inset shows an immunoperoxidase study, with the large cells showing immunoreactivity with CD20 (B-cell antigen).

Image 36-10 Burkitt's lymphoma in the distal ileum. Section shows an infiltrate of monomorphic, medium-sized cells with moderately abundant cytoplasm, moderately clumped chromatin, and several nucleoli. Inset shows imprint of tumor cells having characteristic cytoplasmic vacuoles.

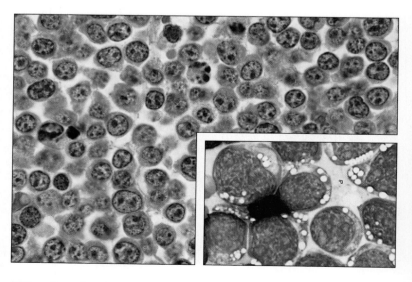

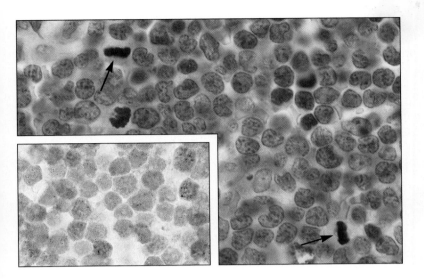

Image 36-11   Mediastinal mass in a child with lymphoblastic lymphoma. Medium-sized lymphoid cells have scant cytoplasm, convoluted nuclei with delicate chromatin pattern, and indistinct nucleoli. Several mitotic figures (↑) are present. Inset shows immunoperoxidase study utilizing antibody to terminal deoxynucleotidyl transferase.

Image 36-12   Section of skin biopsy showing mycosis fungoides. A cellular infiltrate is seen in the upper dermis and epidermis. Several of Pautrier's abscesses are present (↑). Inset shows a Sézary cell in the peripheral blood.

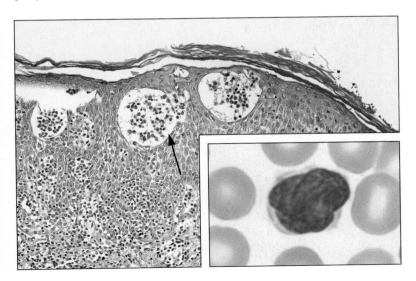

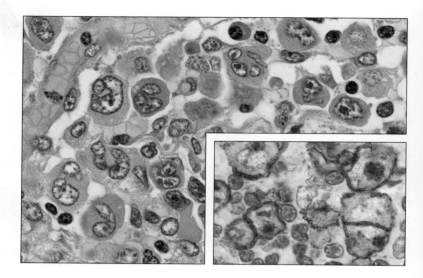

Image 36-13   Anaplastic large cell lymphoma on a lymph node biopsy section shows a sinusoidal infiltrate of pleomorphic, large cells. Inset shows an immunoperoxidase study, with the malignant cells expressing CD30 (Ki-1).

Image 36-14   Bone marrow biopsy section shows characteristic paratrabecular location of follicle center lymphoma. Inset shows peripheral blood with two circulating lymphoma cells having characteristic cleaved nuclei.

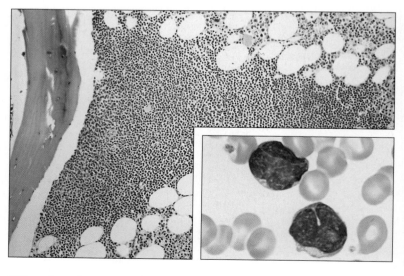

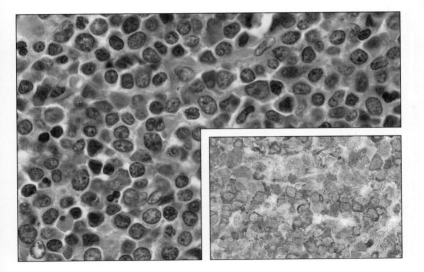

Image 36-15 Section of an orbital tumor shows a diffuse infiltrate of large cells. Inset shows immunoperoxidase study with the malignant cells expressing myeloperoxidase. The diagnosis is granulocytic sarcoma.

Image 36-16 Section of lymph node with follicle center lymphoma. Corresponding section shows immunoperoxidase study with the cells expressing *bcl*-2.

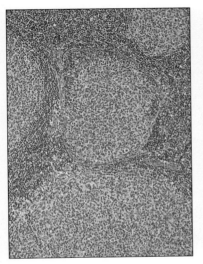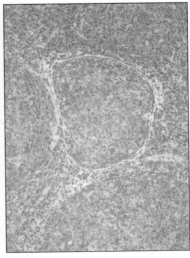

37

Hodgkin's Disease

The malignant lymphomas are a group of diseases divided into Hodgkin's disease and non-Hodgkin's lymphoma. In both disorders, normal lymphoid architecture is replaced by collections of one or several cell types. Hodgkin's disease is characterized by the presence of multinucleated giant cells called Reed-Sternberg cells.

Pathophysiology

Hodgkin's disease is a complex disorder of the immune system and comprises neoplastic mononuclear cells that are admixed with variable numbers of presumably reactive small lymphocytes, plasma cells, eosinophils, and histiocytes. The exact nature of the malignant cell population is still unknown. Controversy continues to exist as to whether the neoplastic cells are transformed lymphocytes (B or T) or histiocytes; this may vary depending on the type of Hodgkin's disease. The different histologic types vary both in clinical findings and in the cell line involved. Thus, the lymphocyte-predominance type of Hodgkin's disease may be a B-cell, germinal center cell proliferation, while mixed cellularity Hodgkin's disease may involve primarily T lymphocytes. Gene rearrangement analyses in Hodgkin's disease have been contradictory. A few studies have shown immunoglobulin gene rearrangement, others have shown a pattern consistent with polyclonal or monoclonal T cells, and most have shown only a germline pattern. Hodgkin's disease may be a clinical syndrome rather than a specific disease. The cause of the disease is still unknown.

Clinical Findings

There are approximately 8,000 new cases of Hodgkin's disease in the United States each year. Hodgkin's disease has a bimodal age-specific incidence curve, with one mode in the 15- to 45-year-old age group and another after the age of 50 years. The overall incidence of Hodgkin's disease in economically underdeveloped countries is lower than that in developed countries, but the incidence before the age of 15 is higher.

The clinical presentation of Hodgkin's disease is usually a progressive, painless enlargement of one or more lymph nodes in the neck. Occasionally, patients present with a mediastinal mass that may be discovered on a routine chest radiograph or on a radiograph obtained because of respiratory symptoms. Hodgkin's disease is more frequently associated with constitutional symptoms (so-called B symptoms), such as fever, night sweats, pruritus, and weight loss, than is non-Hodgkin's lymphoma. Physical examination may reveal splenomegaly and hepatomegaly in addition to enlarged lymph nodes. In contrast to non-Hodgkin's lymphoma, primary extranodal disease is very unusual.

Classification

In contrast to the non-Hodgkin's lymphomas, one histopathologic classification is generally accepted, ie, the one proposed by Lukes and Butler and modified at the Rye symposium into four subcategories (Table 37-1). Three of the types (lymphocyte predominance, mixed cellularity, and lymphocyte depletion) differ mainly in the relative proportions of malignant mononuclear and Reed-Sternberg cells to the presumed reactive cells. Correlation

Table 37-1 Classification Schema for Hodgkin's Disease

Luke's and Butler	Rye Modification
Lymphocyte and/or histiocyte predominance	Lymphocyte predominance
Nodular	
Diffuse	
Nodular sclerosis	Nodular sclerosis
Mixed cellularity	Mixed cellularity
Lymphocyte depletion	Lymphocyte depletion
Diffuse fibrosis	
Reticular type	

is good between the ratio of reactive lymphocytes to neoplastic cells in the lymph node biopsy specimen and the biologic behavior of the tumor. Thus, when lymphocyte proliferation is prominent, Reed-Sternberg cells are rare, the disease is more likely to be localized, and the prognosis is better. It should be recognized, however, that with the marked improvement in therapy for Hodgkin's disease, the prognosis is mainly dependent on the stage of the disease and is becoming independent of the histologic subclassification. The pathologist must be able to accurately make the initial diagnosis and be able to identify Hodgkin's disease in laparotomy specimens and biopsy specimens if relapse occurs.

The Reed-Sternberg cell, which is required for the pathologic diagnosis of Hodgkin's disease, is a large binucleated or multinucleated cell. It has moderately abundant cytoplasm with a characteristic clear halo around a large, prominent eosinophilic or amphophilic nucleolus. Mononuclear variants with the nuclear features of Reed-Sternberg cells, thought to be the actively proliferating component, are called Hodgkin's cells. Even though the presence of Reed-Sternberg cells is required for a pathologic diagnosis of Hodgkin's disease, similar, if not identical, cells may be observed in a variety of other disorders, including non-Hodgkin's lymphoma, infectious mononucleosis, and metastatic carcinoma. Therefore, to make a diagnosis of Hodgkin's disease, both the appropriate architectural and cellular environment and the presence of Reed-Sternberg cells are necessary.

Lymphocyte Predominance Type. This type is characterized by complete or partial obliteration of the lymph node by
small, mature-appearing lymphocytes and varying numbers of histiocytes. The pattern is usually vaguely nodular (Image 37-1) and is
rarely diffuse. Classic Reed-Sternberg cells are usually not found.
Reed-Sternberg cell variants, called L&H cells, that feature multilobated (popcorn) nuclei and small nucleoli are, however, often
plentiful (Image 37-1). Progressively transformed germinal centers
are often seen, and some degree of sclerosis may be present.

The main differential diagnosis includes atypical lymphoid
hyperplasia and non-Hodgkin's lymphoma, small lymphocytic
type. The nodular variant may also be mistaken for non-Hodgkin's
lymphoma, follicular, mixed cell type, and a benign lesion called
progressive transformation of germinal centers (Table 37-2).

Most patients with lymphocyte predominance Hodgkin's disease are young, have clinical stage I or II disease, and are asymptomatic. The disease pursues an indolent course, and despite a relatively high rate of late relapses, the patients respond well to therapy, and the prognosis is good.

The nodular lymphocyte predominance type of Hodgkin's disease appears to be a B-cell, germinal center cell proliferation.
Further evidence that Hodgkin's disease, lymphocyte predominance, is related to B-cell lymphomas is the simultaneous presence,
in some cases (2%), of large B-cell lymphoma. However, this may
represent a monomorphic proliferation of L&H cells rather than
large cell lymphoma, and most patients have an indolent course.

Occasionally, cases are seen where rare, classic Reed-
Sternberg cells are present in a background of predominantly small
lymphocytes, rare eosinophils, and plasma cells. The terms *lymphocyte-rich classical Hodgkin's disease* or *lymphocyte predominant mixed cellularity* have been proposed for such cases.

Mixed Cellularity Type. This type is characterized by a
greater number of abnormal mononuclear cells (Hodgkin's cells)
and readily found classic Reed-Sternberg cells (Image 37-2). The
infiltrate is diffuse or vaguely nodular. A variable number of
eosinophils, plasma cells, and histiocytes are usually present. This
type of Hodgkin's disease must be differentiated from various reactive lymphadenopathies (eg, infectious mononucleosis) and from

Table 37-2 Differential Diagnosis of Hodgkin's Disease

Nodular sclerosis
    Anaplastic large cell lymphoma (Ki-1 lymphoma)
    Peripheral T-cell lymphoma
    Mediastinal large B-cell lymphoma with sclerosis
    Metastatic carcinoma
Lymphocyte predominance
    Progressive transformation of germinal centers
    Follicular hyperplasia
    Non-Hodgkin's, follicular lymphoma
    Non-Hodgkin's, T-cell–rich, B-cell lymphoma
    Non-Hodgkin's lymphoma, small lymphocytic
    Chronic lymphocytic lymphoma
Mixed cellularity
    Non-Hodgkin's, T-cell–rich, B-cell lymphoma
    Peripheral T-cell lymphoma
    Infectious mononucleosis
    Angioimmunoblastic lymphadenopathy
Lymphocyte depletion
    Nodular sclerosis, syncytial type
    Anaplastic large cell lymphoma (Ki-1 lymphoma)
    Peripheral T-cell lymphoma

certain types of non-Hodgkin's lymphoma, particularly the peripheral or node-based T-cell lymphomas (including so-called Lennert's lymphoma), and T-cell rich B-cell lymphoma (Table 37-2). As mentioned in Chapter 36, it may sometimes be difficult, even with immunologic markers, to distinguish certain T-cell lymphomas from this type of Hodgkin's disease. Patients with mixed cellularity Hodgkin's disease usually have stage III or IV disease and are symptomatic.

Lymphocyte Depletion Type. This is rare in the United States and Europe and reveals a paucity of lymphocytes with increased numbers of abnormal mononuclear cells. Reed-Sternberg cells are often numerous. Fibrosis and necrosis may be prominent. The patient is usually older, has stage III or IV disease, and is symptomatic. There is some doubt as to whether this entity exists. Most of the cases reported as lymphocyte depletion appear to have been non-Hodgkin's lymphoma (especially anaplastic large cell lymphoma, Ki-1), or nodular sclerosis, Hodgkin's disease, syncytial variant.

Nodular Sclerosis, Hodgkin's Disease. This has two distinct histologic features: the lymph node is divided into nodules by thick bands of collagen extending from the capsule, and Reed-Sternberg cell variants are present in lacunar spaces (so-called lacunar cells) (Image 37-3). Extensive sheets of lacunar cells and atypical mononuclear cells are frequently present. Necrosis is not uncommon. A variant of nodular sclerosis, called syncytial, sarcomatous, or monomorphic type, is characterized by sheets of lacunar cells and atypical mononuclear cells (Image 37-4). When a small biopsy specimen is obtained and fibrosis is evident, it may be extremely difficult to differentiate this type of Hodgkin's disease from non-Hodgkin's large cell lymphoma, metastatic carcinoma, melanoma, or seminoma. Immunologic markers may be helpful in such instances; one must recognize, however, that we still have no specific marker for Hodgkin's disease. The presence of a high mitotic rate, extension through the capsule, prominent irregularity of the nucleus of small lymphocytes, absence of eosinophilia, and prominence of immunoblasts would favor a diagnosis of non-Hodgkin's lymphoma over Hodgkin's disease.

Nodular sclerosis, Hodgkin's disease, is by far the most common type of Hodgkin's disease in the United States and Europe and occurs with equal frequency in both sexes, while in all the other types, men predominate. It is unusual in patients more than 50 years of age. Nodular sclerosis is usually associated with lower cervical, supraclavicular, and mediastinal lymph node involvement. It is the type most commonly affecting the lungs. The majority of patients have clinical stage II disease.

Table 37-3 presents a summary of the histopathologic features and the frequency of the different subtypes of Hodgkin's disease.

Approach to Diagnosis

Successful treatment of Hodgkin's disease depends on accurate identification of all disease-bearing sites in the body. Compared to non-Hodgkin's lymphoma, patients with Hodgkin's disease have

Table 37-3 Histopathologic Features of Hodgkin's Disease

Classification	Histopathologic Features	Relative Frequency (%)
Nodular sclerosis	Bands of collagen extending from capsule surrounding cellular areas, lacunar cell variants of RS cells	70
Mixed cellularity	Mixture of lymphocytes, plasma cells, eosinophils, histiocytes, and many classic RS cells	10
Lymphocyte predominance	Usually nodular pattern of many small lymphocytes, and variable number of L&H cells	15
Lymphocyte depletion	Few lymphocytes, many RS cells, fibrosis	<5

Abbreviations: RS = Reed-Sternberg.

less frequent involvement of Waldeyer's ring, the gastrointestinal tract, mesenteric lymph nodes, bone marrow, and skin. Generally, Hodgkin's disease is in a less advanced stage than non-Hodgkin's lymphoma when initially detected. In addition, patients with Hodgkin's disease have more frequent involvement of the mediastinal lymph nodes than patients with non-Hodgkin's lymphoma. The procedures required to stage Hodgkin's disease are outlined in Table 37-4. Once all these pretreatment evaluation data are collected, the patient's disease is assigned a Roman numeral stage according to the criteria in Table 37-5. The stage is also assigned a substage designation depending on the presence (B) or absence (A) of significant systemic symptoms.

Following a clinical history and physical examination, the workup of a patient with possible Hodgkin's disease proceeds in the following fashion:

1. Tissue biopsy. The diagnosis and subclassification of Hodgkin's disease should be made on the basis of histopathologic features in a lymph node biopsy specimen before initiating therapy. The initial diagnosis should not be made on the basis of a bone marrow biopsy or liver biopsy specimen alone.

2. Complete blood cell count.

Table 37-4 Staging Procedures in Hodgkin's Disease

Required procedures
  Clinical history and physical examination
  Lymph node biopsy
  Radiologic studies: chest roentgenogram; computed tomographic scan of chest and whole abdomen, including the pelvis; lymphangiography
  Laboratory tests: complete blood cell count; serum alkaline phosphatase and lactate dehydrogenase; liver and renal function tests, including uric acid and urinalysis; erythrocyte sedimentation rate
  Bilateral iliac crest bone marrow biopsy
Ancillary studies (when clinically indicated)
  Skeletal radiographic examination
  Gallium whole body scanning
  Laparotomy to include splenectomy, liver biopsy, and intra-abdominal lymph node biopsy (celiac, porta hepatis, mesenteric, para-aortic, iliac nodes), if information is likely to affect therapy

3. Bone marrow aspirate and biopsy specimen examination.

4. Radiologic studies.

5. Liver and renal function studies.

6. Laparotomy. Staging laparotomy may be of value in distinguishing patients eligible for treatment with radiation therapy alone from those requiring combination chemotherapy. Clinical staging of abdominal disease is inaccurate in approximately 25% of patients.

Hematologic Findings

In contrast to non-Hodgkin's lymphomas, significant abnormal hematologic findings are uncommon in Hodgkin's disease. Despite this fact, examination of the peripheral blood and bone marrow should be done routinely as part of the staging procedure.

Blood Cell Measurements. A mild to moderate anemia is frequently present in patients with Hodgkin's disease. It is usually normochromic, normocytic, with a low or normal reticulocyte count. In a small percentage of patients, autoimmune hemolytic anemia develops. One third of the patients have leukocytosis caused by neutrophilia. The platelet count is normal or increased. Rarely,

Table 37-5 The Cotswald Staging Classification for Hodgkin's Disease*

Stage I:	Involvement of a single lymph node region or a lymphoid structure (eg, spleen, thymus)
Stage II:	Involvement of two or more lymph node regions on the same side of the diaphragm (ie, the mediastinum is a single site, hilar lymph nodes are lateralized). The number of anatomic sites should be indicated by a subscript (eg, II_2).
Stage III:	Involvement of lymph node regions or structures on both sides of the diaphragm
	III_1: With or without splenic hilar, celiac, or portal nodes
	III_2: With para-aortic, iliac, mesenteric nodes
Stage IV:	Involvement of extranodal site(s) beyond that designated E:
	A: No symptoms
	B: Fever, drenching sweats, weight loss
	X: Bulky disease: >1/3 the width of the mediastinum >10 cm maximal dimension of nodal mass
	E: Involvement of a single extranodal site, contiguous or proximal to a known nodal site
	CS: Clinical stage
	PS: Pathologic stage

*From Lister TA, Crowther D, Sutcliffe SB, et al. Report of a committee convened to discuss the evaluation and staging of patients with Hodgkin's disease: Cotswald meeting. *J Clin Oncol.* 1989;7:1630-1636; *J Clin Oncol.* [erratum] 1990;8:1602.

severe anemia or pancytopenia resulting from extensive involvement of the bone marrow or hypersplenism may be observed.

Peripheral Blood Smear Morphology. Neutrophilia, monocytosis, or eosinophilia are seen in 10% to 20% of patients, and lymphopenia may be present in patients with extensive disease.

Bone Marrow. A bilateral posterior iliac crest bone marrow biopsy should be performed routinely in the staging procedure in patients with Hodgkin's disease. Bone marrow involvement is unusual (less than 10% of patients) at time of diagnosis, especially in lymphocyte predominance type and nodular sclerosis. When the bone marrow is affected, the lesion is usually focal, is often associated with fibrosis, and may resemble a granuloma. Reed-Sternberg cells may be difficult to identify. The presence of mononuclear cells, with nuclear features of Reed-Sternberg cells, in the characteristic cellular environment of Hodgkin's disease should be regarded as consistent with bone marrow involvement, provided that a diagnosis of Hodgkin's disease has been made from a lymph node biopsy specimen.

Other Laboratory Tests

37.1 Tissue Biopsy

A lymph node biopsy is required for the diagnosis of Hodgkin's disease. Proper handling of the biopsy specimen is extremely important to make a correct diagnosis. The reader is referred to Chapter 36 for a detailed description of the handling of a tissue biopsy specimen of a suspected malignant lymphoma. The histopathologic features observed in different types of Hodgkin's disease have been described earlier in this chapter.

37.2 Radiologic Studies

The radiologic evaluation plays a crucial role in determining the extent of disease. It should start with routine chest radiographs. Computed tomography (CT) of the chest provides better definition of mediastinal, hilar, and paravertebral lymphadenopathy and pulmonary involvement. It should be done in all patients.

A bilateral lower extremity lymphangiogram is essential in detecting disease in the retroperitoneal lymph nodes. It should be noted that splenic, hilar, celiac, porta hepatis, and mesenteric nodes are not demonstrated by lymphangiography. The CT scan is particularly useful in the delineation of lymphadenopathy, which is not revealed on lymphangiography. A CT scan may also reveal tumor nodules in the spleen. Skeletal surveys or bone scans may be included in search of lytic or, less commonly, osteoblastic lesions in patients with bone pain. A gallium scan may be helpful in detecting disease in a variety of sites and may be used in patients unable to undergo lymphangiography, and is especially useful in evaluating response to therapy and in detecting recurrence after therapy.

37.3 Laparotomy

Exploratory laparotomy is primarily a diagnostic procedure, and includes splenectomy and open liver biopsy. It is not a routine procedure in staging Hodgkin's disease and should only be done if the outcome will significantly alter therapy. It is occasionally used in patients considered to have stage I, II, or IIIA disease after clinical examination and radiologic tests. At surgery, the surgeon should obtain a biopsy specimen of all major lymph node groups regardless of the size and gross appearance of the nodes. Application of radiopaque clips at biopsy sites will later assist the radiotherapist in port design. The spleen and splenic hilar lymph nodes should be removed, and a wedge biopsy specimen should be taken from the liver.

The pathologist must carefully examine the removed spleen because excellent correlation exists between splenic involvement and the probability of hepatic involvement. It is extremely rare to have Hodgkin's disease in the liver without splenic involvement. The spleen must be cut into thin sections and carefully inspected; multiple sections should be examined microscopically.

Approximately 30% of patients thought to have stage I or II disease will be reclassified as having stage III disease after laparotomy.

Ancillary Tests

Immunophenotypic Analysis. Immunophenotyping and occasionally genotyping may facilitate the diagnosis of Hodgkin's disease and help differentiate this disease from non-Hodgkin's lymphoma and metastatic nonhematopoietic neoplasms. Of the non-Hodgkin's lymphomas that may simulate Hodgkin's disease, one should especially consider anaplastic large cell lymphoma (Ki-1 lymphoma), peripheral T-cell lymphoma, T-cell–rich B-cell lymphoma, and primary mediastinal large B-cell lymphoma with sclerosis.

In the majority of cases, satisfactory immunophenotypic analysis can be done on paraffin sections, but fresh tissue should always be set aside (frozen) for possible gene rearrangement studies. This may be especially helpful when dealing with small medi-

Table 37-6 Immunophenotypic Features in Hodgkin's Disease

Type of Disease	CD15	CD30	CD45	CD20 (B cell)*
HDNS	+	+	–	–
HDMC	+	+	–	–
HDLP	–	–/+	+	+/–

Abbreviations: HDNS = Hodgkin's disease, nodular sclerosis; HDMC = Hodgkin's disease, mixed cellularity; HDLP = Hodgkin's disease, lymphocyte predominance;
–/+ = less than 50% of cases; +/– = more than 50% of cases.
*CD20 is occasionally positive in HDNS.

astinal biopsy specimens, where the diagnosis may be uncertain.

Table 37-6 shows the common immunophenotypic findings in paraffin sections of different subtypes of Hodgkin's disease. Nodular sclerosis and mixed cellularity have similar immunophenotype (CD15+, CD30+, CD45–), while lymphocyte predominance type is usually distinctly different (CD15–, CD30–/+, CD45+, CD20+/–). Table 37-7 illustrates how immunophenotyping can be useful in distinguishing Hodgkin's disease from non-Hodgkin's, anaplastic large cell lymphoma (Ki-1 lymphoma).

Epstein-Barr Virus. Epstein-Barr virus (EBV) can be shown to be associated with Reed-Sternberg cells in approximately one half of the cases of Hodgkin's disease, especially mixed cellularity type. It is rarely seen in lymphocyte predominance type. The presence of EBV can be demonstrated with polymerase chain reaction technique, with in situ hybridization for the detection of EBV RNA in tissue section, and with immunohistochemistry studies identifying the EBV latent membrane protein. These studies are of interest related to the pathogenesis of Hodgkin's disease, but they are not useful in the diagnosis of this disease.

Another interesting observation, but not diagnostically useful, is the expression of bcl-2 oncoprotein by Hodgkin's cells in approximately one half the cases studied.

Gene Rearrangement Studies. Gene rearrangement studies may be helpful in difficult cases of distinguishing Hodgkin's disease from non-Hodgkin's lymphoma when the

Table 37-7   Immunophenotypic Features Useful in the
Differential Diagnosis of Hodgkin's Disease vs
Anaplastic Large Cell Lymphoma

Disease	CD15[*]	CD30[†]	CD45	CD43 (T cell)	CD20[‡] (B cell)	EMA
HD	+	+	–	–	–	–
ALCL	–	+	+/–	+/–	–/+	+/–

Abbreviations: EMA = epithelial membrane antigen; HD = Hodgkin's disease; ALCL = anaplastic large cell lymphoma; –/+ = less than 50% of cases; +/– = more than 50% of cases.
*CD15+ is occasionally (<10%) present in ALCL.
†CD30 in ALCL shows membranous and Golgi staining.
‡CD20 is occasionally expressed in HD, nodular sclerosing type. T-cell' or less commonly, B-cell gene rearrangement, is present in two thirds of cases of ALCL, but is usually absent in HD. With polymerase chain reaction, B-cell gene rearrangement may be seen in HD, lymphocyte-predominant type.

immunophenotypic studies are equivocal. For the classic technique of Southern blot analysis, fresh or frozen tissue is required. Recently, polymerase chain reaction techniques have been developed that can also utilize tissue from paraffin sections. The presence of B- or T-cell gene rearrangement would favor a diagnosis of non-Hodgkin's lymphoma rather than Hodgkin's disease. The failure to identify clonal gene rearrangement of immunoglobulin or T-cell receptor genes in Hodgkin's disease may, however, be due to the fact that Reed-Sternberg cells often account for a very small part of the DNA extracted from the tissue biopsy specimen. Recently, supersensitive polymerase chain reaction techniques have demonstrated B-cell gene rearrangement in many cases of Hodgkin's disease, lymphocyte-predominant type.

Cytogenetics.   Karyotypic analysis of tissue with Hodgkin's disease frequently (50% of cases) shows clonal abnormalities of hyperdiploid nature. However, chromosome abnormalities specific for Hodgkin's disease have not been described.

Course and Treatment

Approximately 75% of patients with Hodgkin's disease can be cured. Factors that adversely affect the prognosis include stage III disease with involvement of lower abdominal lymph nodes, stage IV disease, old age, constitutional B symptoms, bulky disease, and extensive splenic involvement (>4 nodules).

The primary treatment of Hodgkin's disease that is confined to lymph nodes (stages I and II) is extended-field radiation therapy. Patients with stage III or IV disease are treated with combination chemotherapy. Selected patients may be treated with combined radiotherapy and chemotherapy.

References

Banks PM. The distinction of Hodgkin's disease from T-cell lymphoma. *Semin Diagn Pathol.* 1992;9:279-283.

Burke JS. Hodgkin's disease: histopathology and differential diagnosis. In: Knowles DM, ed. *Neoplastic Hematopathology.* Baltimore, Md: Williams & Wilkins; 1992:497-534.

Butler JJ. The histologic diagnosis of Hodgkin's disease. *Semin Diagn Pathol.* 1992;9:252-256.

Harris NL. The relationship between Hodgkin's disease and non-Hodgkin's lymphoma. *Semin Diagn Pathol.* 1992;9:304-310.

Harris NL, Jaffe ES, Stein H, et al. A revised European-American classification of lymphoid neoplasms: a proposal from the International Lymphoma Study Group. *Blood.* 1994;84:1361-1392.

Kadin ME. Hodgkin's disease: immunobiology and pathogenesis. In: Knowles DM, ed. *Neoplastic Hematopathology.* Baltimore, Md: Williams & Wilkins; 1992:535-554.

Lukes RJ, Collins RJ. Tumors of the hematopoietic system. In: *Atlas of Tumor Pathology.* 2d series, fascicle 28. Washington, DC: Armed Forces Institute of Pathology; 1992.

Said JW. The immunohistochemistry of Hodgkin's disease. *Semin Diagn Pathol.* 1992;9:265-271.

Warnke RA. The distinction between Hodgkin's disease from B-cell lymphoma. *Semin Diagn Pathol.* 1992;9:284-290.

Weiss LM, Chang KL. Molecular biologic studies of Hodgkin's disease. *Semin Diagn Pathol.* 1992;9:272-278.

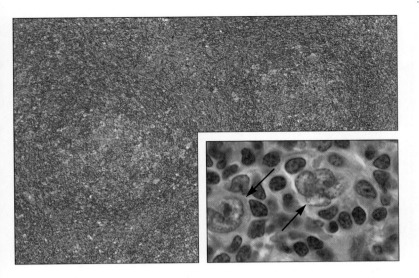

Image 37-1 Hodgkin's disease, lymphocyte predominance type. Low-power view shows the nodular pattern frequently present. Inset shows high-power view of many small lymphocytes and two L&H cells (↑).

Image 37-2 Hodgkin's disease, mixed cellularity type. A classic binucleated Reed-Sternberg cell is seen in the center (↑) surrounded by many small lymphocytes and occasional plasma cells.

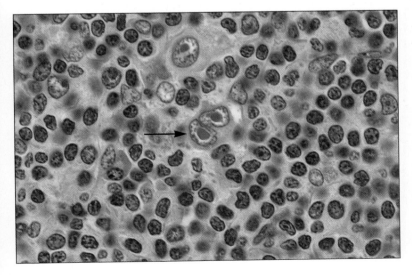

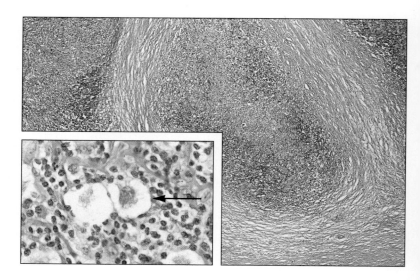

Image 37-3 Hodgkin's disease, nodular sclerosis type. Low-power view shows a nodule of lymphoid tissue surrounded by a thick band of collagen. Inset shows high-power view of the typical lacunar cells (↑).

Image 37-4 Hodgkin's disease, nodular sclerosis type, syncytial variant. A sheet of large, monomorphic cells is seen surrounded by collagen. The morphologic features resemble non-Hodgkin's, large cell lymphoma. Inset shows an immunoperoxidase study of same tissue utilizing antibody to CD15.

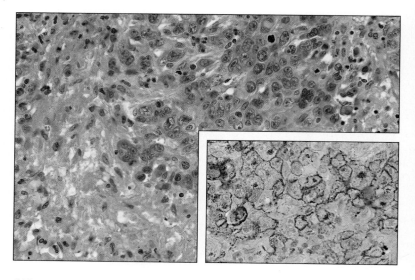

PART XI

Immunoproliferative
Disorders

38

Multiple Myeloma and Related Disorders

The plasma cell dyscrasias comprise a group of diseases characterized by the proliferation of a single clone of immunoglobulin-producing cells usually recognized as either plasma cells or lymphocytes. In these disorders a single class or subunit of immunoglobulin is secreted and can be detected as a monoclonal peak on electrophoresis of either serum or urine. The plasma cell dyscrasias include the following entities: multiple myeloma, Waldenström's macroglobulinemia, the heavy-chain diseases, monoclonal gammopathy of undetermined significance, primary amyloidosis, and cryoglobulinemia (Table 38-1). Multiple myeloma will be the focus of this chapter. Waldenström's macroglobulinemia and the heavy-chain diseases will also be discussed. Monoclonal gammopathy of undetermined significance, primary amyloidosis, and cryoglobulinemia will be presented in Chapter 39.

Pathophysiology

Multiple myeloma (plasma cell myeloma) is characterized by a neoplastic proliferation of plasma cells. The plasma cells prolifer-

Table 38-1 Classification of Plasma Cell Dyscrasias

Multiple myeloma
Waldenström's macroglobulinemia
Heavy chain disease
Monoclonal gammopathies of undetermined significance
Primary amyloidosis
Cryoglobulinemia

ate throughout the bone marrow and frequently invade adjacent bone, causing widespread skeletal destruction. Other organs may be involved secondarily.

One of the major features of multiple myeloma is the secretion of monoclonal proteins (Table 38-2). The protein is usually a complete immunoglobulin molecule with immunoelectrophoresis of serum revealing monoclonal IgG or IgA heavy chains combined with either kappa or lambda light chains. Monoclonal immunoglobulins of the IgG type are approximately two to three times more frequent than IgA. Monoclonal proteins of IgD or IgE type occur but are rare. In about 20% of patients, only the light chain portion of the immunoglobulin molecule is present. Because light chains are excreted in the urine, they are usually detected as a monoclonal peak on urine electrophoresis.

Clinical Findings

Bone pain, particularly in the back or chest, is the most common symptom of patients with multiple myeloma. Typically the pain is well localized and aggravated by movement. It is often associated with pathologic compression fractures of the thoracic or lumbar spine. Weakness and fatigue, often related to anemia, are also common.

Pallor is the most common physical finding. Hepatosplenomegaly is present in 20% and splenomegaly in 5% of patients. Palpable plasmacytomas may also be noted.

Table 38-2   Monoclonal Immunoglobulins in Malignant
Plasma Cell Dyscrasias

Disease Process	Monoclonal Immunoglobulin	Percentage of Cases
Multiple myeloma*	IgG	55
	IgA	22
	Light chain only	18
	IgD	2
	Biclonal	2
	Nonsecretory	1
	IgE	<1
	IgM	<1
Waldenström's macroglobulinemia	IgM	100
Heavy chain (HC) diseases†	γ-HC fragment	25
	α-HC fragment	75
	μ-HC fragment	<5

*Kappa light chains are more common than lambda in all immunoglobulin types
of myeloma except IgD.
†Percentages are approximate; reliable statistics are not available.

Approach to Diagnosis

The laboratory studies used to diagnose multiple myeloma are listed below. The extent to which these evaluations are done depends on the level of suspicion of the diagnosis.

1. Complete blood cell count with leukocyte differential.
2. Blood and bone marrow examination.
3. Serum protein electrophoresis.
4. Serum immunoelectrophoresis or immunofixation.
5. Quantitation of serum immunoglobulins.
6. Urine protein quantitation.
7. Urine protein electrophoresis.
8. Immunoelectrophoresis or immunofixation of a concentrated 24-hour urine specimen.
9. Radiographic skeletal survey.

Hematologic Findings

The minimal criteria for diagnosis of multiple myeloma require at least 10% plasma cells in the bone marrow or the presence of a plasmacytoma plus one or more of the following:

1. Monoclonal protein in the serum (usually >30 g/L [3 g/dL]).
2. Monoclonal protein in the urine.
3. Lytic bone lesions.

Blood Cell Measurements. A normochromic, normocytic anemia is present in most patients with multiple myeloma at presentation. Leukopenia and thrombocytopenia are present in less than 20% of patients at diagnosis but are common in the later stages of the disease.

Peripheral Blood Smear Morphology. Rouleaux formation (Image 38-1) may be striking in the peripheral blood. The degree of rouleaux formation correlates with the magnitude of the monoclonal immunoglobulin and parallels the erythrocyte sedimentation rate. Occasional circulating plasma cells may be present. Plasma cell leukemia is a rare type of multiple myeloma in which plasma cells in the blood exceed greater than 20% of the total leukocytes, or the absolute plasma cell count is greater than 2.0 x 10^3/mm^3 (2.0 x 10^9/L).

Bone Marrow Examination. Bone marrow aspirate smears and core biopsy sections are essential for adequate evaluation for multiple myeloma. The plasma cells comprise greater than 10% of the nucleated cells in the aspirate and usually average about 20% to 40%. The plasma cells vary from mature-appearing cells to those resembling blasts (Image 38-2). They vary in size with moderate to abundant basophilic cytoplasm. The nuclei are often larger than normal and the chromatin less condensed. Multinucleation may be present. Nucleoli are often prominent and intranuclear inclusions may be apparent. In rare myelomas, the nuclei may have a monocytoid appearance. Several types of cytoplasmic inclusions have been described in the plasma cells including hyaline inclusions, crystalline inclusions, vacuoles, and granules. Patients with IgA myeloma tend to have strikingly pleomorphic plasma cells, including multinucleated cells, flaming plasma cells, and frequent intranuclear inclusions.

In core biopsy specimens, the plasma cell infiltrate is either interstitial, focal, or diffuse. With diffuse involvement, large areas of normal hematopoietic tissue are replaced.

Intracytoplasmic immunoglobulin within plasma cells reacts strongly to antibodies against kappa or lambda light chains. This property allows plasma cells in sections to be studied with immunohistochemical techniques (Image 38-3). Using these methods, the plasma cells in myeloma exhibit a monoclonal pattern of reactivity with antibodies against kappa and lambda light chains. The ratio of the predominant light chain to the normal light chain is usually greater than 16:1. In reactive plasma cell proliferations, there is a mixture of kappa- and lambda-positive cells. This technique is especially useful when the percentage of plasma cells is low and in those rare cases where no monoclonal protein is identified in either serum or urine.

Other Laboratory Tests

38.1 Serum Protein Electrophoresis

Purpose.   Serum protein electrophoresis is a screening test for monoclonal proteins and should be done when multiple myeloma or another plasma cell dyscrasia is suspected.

Principle.   Proteins migrate in an electrical field. A monoclonal protein migrates to a single location creating a dense, discrete band on the cellulose acetate membrane or the agarose gel (Figure 38-1) or a narrow spike in the densitometric tracing (Figure 38-2).

Specimen.   Serum is usually used but plasma is acceptable.

Procedure.   Electrophoresis with cellulose acetate membrane is satisfactory for screening, but high-resolution agarose gel elec-

Figure 38-1   Serum protein electrophoresis reveals a dense, discrete band (M) in the gamma region. Control (C) specimen is below patient (P) specimen.

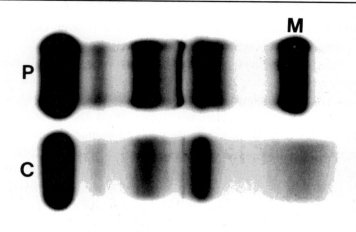

trophoresis is more sensitive for detection of small monoclonal proteins. Electrophoresis is usually performed at a pH of 8.6. The proteins are separated into albumin and α_1, α_2, β, and γ globulins. The membranes or gels are then fixed and stained. The patterns can be evaluated visually and the protein fractions quantitated with densitometry.

Interpretation.   Monoclonal immunoglobulins usually appear in the γ region but can also be found in the β or α_2 globulin area. Immunoelectrophoresis or immunofixation should be performed when a band or peak is seen to confirm the presence of a monoclonal protein and to determine the heavy chain class and light chain type. Hypogammaglobulinemia is characterized by a decrease in the γ component and is seen in about 15% of patients with multiple myeloma. In this situation, light chains may be present in the urine, and immunoelectrophoresis or immunofixation of the urine and serum is necessary for identification. Polyclonal increases in immunoglobulins produce broad bands or peaks and are usually limited to the γ region.

Figure 38-2   Scan of serum protein electrophoresis demonstrating a monoclonal spike (M) in the gamma
region.

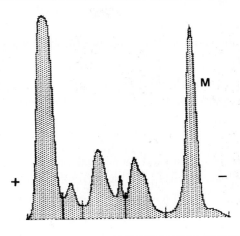

Small monoclonal proteins may be missed with this technique. Monoclonal light chains are rarely detected in cellulose
acetate tracings. In addition, in IgD myeloma the monoclonal
peak is small or not detected at all. Often, the monoclonal
protein in heavy chain diseases is not detected with this
method. Therefore, immunoelectrophoresis or immunofixation should be done whenever multiple myeloma or a
related disorder is suspected.

Serum protein electrophoresis can also be used to monitor
changes in the amount of monoclonal protein after diagnosis.

38.2 Urine Electrophoresis

Purpose.   Urine electrophoresis is done to determine the presence or absence of a monoclonal protein in patients suspected
of having multiple myeloma or other plasma cell dyscrasia.
Classic heat precipitation tests for Bence-Jones protein are not
reliable and should be abandoned.

Principle. As in serum, a monoclonal protein migrates as a band on zone electrophoresis and can be quantitated.

Specimen. A 24-hour collection of urine should be done from which the total protein excreted is determined. Then an aliquot of the urine is concentrated for electrophoresis.

Procedure. Urine is applied on cellulose membranes and electrophoresis is performed at a pH of 8.6. Proteins are quantitated with densitometry.

Interpretation. A urine monoclonal protein is seen on electrophoresis as a dense band on the cellulose strip or a narrow peak on the densitometer tracing. The protein should be further characterized by immunoelectrophoresis or immunofixation.

38.3 Serum and Urine Immunoelectrophoresis

Purpose. Immunoelectrophoresis is useful for identification of a monoclonal protein. It should be done whenever a dense band or sharp peak is noted with serum protein electrophoresis or when multiple myeloma or other plasma cell dyscrasia is suspected. It also reliably detects the presence of light chains in a concentrated 24-hour urine specimen.

Principle. An initial protein electrophoretic separation is followed by application of antiserum along the path of migration. Individual protein molecules diffuse toward the antibody, forming immune precipitin arcs whenever antigen meets specific antibody.

Specimen. Serum or urine. A concentrated 24-hour urine specimen may be needed to detect the monoclonal protein.

Procedure. Immunoelectrophoresis uses agar gel or cellulose as the support medium. Serum or urine is applied into a well and electrophoresed at a pH of 8.6 to separate component proteins. Monospecific antisera to IgG, IgA, IgM, IgD, and IgE as well as kappa and lambda light chains are inoculated along the path of migration. The electrophoretically separated albumin and globulins diffuse toward the antiserum. Whenever antigen and antibody specificity correspond, a precipitin arc is deposited.

Interpretation. Monoclonal proteins have a characteristic thickening or bowing of the precipitin arcs rather than the smooth symmetric appearance of a heterogeneous population of molecules.

About 90% of patients with multiple myeloma have a serum monoclonal protein at diagnosis. Approximately 80% have a urine monoclonal protein at diagnosis. Ninety-nine percent of patients with multiple myeloma have a monoclonal protein in either serum or urine at diagnosis. The incidence of the various monoclonal immunoglobulins in multiple myeloma is shown in Table 38-2.

38.4 Serum and Urine Immunofixation

Purpose. Immunofixation gives similar information to that obtained with immunoelectrophoresis but is more sensitive than immunoelectrophoresis. It can be used if the results obtained with immunoelectrophoresis are equivocal or when a small monoclonal protein is suspected.

Principle. The patient's serum or urine sample is subjected to electrophoresis to separate protein zones. The migration path is overlaid with membrane, and specific antibody for each immunoglobulin is added. Immune precipitates occur at the sites of antigen-antibody reaction.

Specimen. Serum or concentrated urine.

Procedure. Serum or urine is inoculated into a series of wells in a supporting thin layer gel or a cellulose acetate membrane and electrophoresed. Strips of cellulose acetate impregnated with monospecific antibody are applied over the separate migration paths and allowed to diffuse. Antigen-antibody recognition results in immune precipitates on the supporting membrane.

Interpretation.   A sharp, narrow band indicates a monoclonal protein (Figure 38-3), whereas a broad blurred band is consistent with polyclonality.

Notes.   The concentration of antigen to antibody is critical in this technique. Technical and interpretation expertise are essential for correct results.

38.5 Serum Immunoglobulin Quantitation

Purpose.   This procedure is used to measure the concentration of immunoglobulin. It is more useful than either immunoelectrophoresis or immunofixation for identification of hypogammaglobulinemia.

Principle.   Rate nephelometry is the preferred method of immunoglobulin quantitation. The degree of turbidity produced by antigen-antibody interactions is measured with nephelometry.

Specimen.   Serum.

Procedure.   Specific antisera are mixed with serum at a series of fixed dilutions. A background measurement is taken when the patient's specimen is added, and the rate of increase in light scattered is measured. A microprocessor calculates the concentration of immunoglobulin.

Interpretation.   Immunoglobulin concentration is age-dependent. Reference values in adults are: IgG, 800 to 1,200 mg/dL (8.00-12.00 g/L); IgA, 180 to 480 mg/dL (1.80-4.80 g/L); IgM, 50 to 150 mg/dL (0.50-1.50 g/L); IgD, 3 mg/dL (30 mg/L); and IgE, 0.3 mg/dL (3,000 µg/L).

Figure 38-3 Immunofixation of serum documenting that the monoclonal protein is IgG kappa.

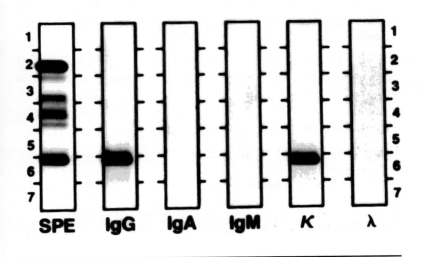

Levels of monoclonal protein greater than 3 g/dL (30 g/L) usually indicate an overt multiple myeloma or macroglobulinemia. Levels of the uninvolved immunoglobulin classes are often reduced in multiple myeloma or Waldenström's macroglobulinemia.

It should be emphasized that a monoclonal protein can be present even when the quantitative immunoglobulin levels are all within normal limits. In addition, about 15% of patients with multiple myeloma have a hypogammaglobulinemia.

Ancillary Tests

β_2-**Microglobulin.** β_2-microglobulin is synthesized by all nucleated cells. Serum levels of β_2-microglobulin increase in proportion to the tumor burden in multiple myeloma and may be helpful in predicting prognosis. Levels above 6 μg/mL (508 nmol/L) indicate a poor prognosis.

Tests of Renal Function.   Proteinuria is present in about 90% of patients with multiple myeloma. Immunofixation or immunoelectrophoresis detects light chains in the urine in 80% of patients. Serum creatinine is elevated in 50% of patients at diagnosis. The two major causes of renal insufficiency are myeloma kidney and hypercalcemia. Myeloma kidney is characterized by waxy, laminated casts in the distal and collecting tubules and correlates with the amount of free light chain in the urine and the severity of the renal insufficiency. Amyloidosis (see Chapter 39) occurs in 10% to 15% of patients with multiple myeloma and may produce renal insufficiency or nephrotic syndrome.

Bone Radiographs.   Bone radiographs show osteolytic lesions, osteoporosis, or fractures in 80% of patients at diagnosis. The skull, ribs, vertebrae, and long bones are the most frequently involved (Figure 38-4). Bone scans do not demonstrate lytic lesions well, but computed tomographic scans may identify myeloma infiltrates when radiographs are normal in patients with severe bone pain.

Serum Viscosity.   Serum viscosity should be done when IgG or IgA levels are greater than 4.0 g/dL or if IgM is greater than 3.0 g/dL and in any patient where symptoms suggest a hyperviscosity syndrome. Symptoms of hyperviscosity are rare unless the value is greater than 4 centipoises.

Course and Treatment

Most patients with multiple myeloma have a progressive course with a median survival of about 3 years. Survival is overall related to extent of disease at diagnosis. About 10% of patients with multiple myeloma, however, have a chronic course and survive greater than 10 years; many of these patients have a smoldering or indolent myeloma.

Patients who are asymptomatic are usually followed without therapy. The standard therapy for symptomatic patients is alkylating agent chemotherapy. Melphalan or cyclophosphamide are used as single agents, combined with steroids, or as components of mul-

Figure 38-4 Osteolytic lesions in the skull of a patient with multiple myeloma.

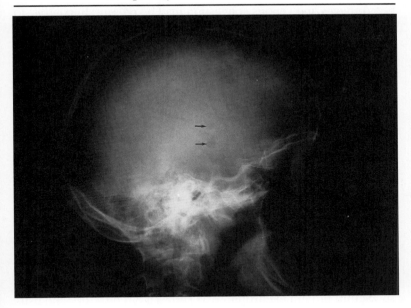

tidrug chemotherapeutic regimens. Alpha-interferon is sometimes added to the chemotherapeutic regimen and has been associated with increased response rates. Autologous and allogeneic bone marrow transplantation is being performed in an increasing number of patients.

The most common cause of death is infection. Renal failure contributes to death in many patients.

Other Plasma Cell Dyscrasias

Waldenström's Macroglobulinemia. Waldenström's macroglobulinemia is a lymphoplasmacytoid lymphoma associated with the production of monoclonal IgM. The bone marrow is involved with the lymphoma in most patients, and lymphadenopathy and hepatosplenomegaly are common. The median age at diagnosis is about 60 years, and over half of the patients are men. The most frequent symptoms include weakness, fatigue, and bleeding. Some patients suffer from hyperviscosity syndrome related to increased levels of the monoclonal proteins. Physical findings include pallor, lymphadenopathy, and hepatosplenomegaly. Retinal hemorrhages and venous congestion may be present. In contrast to multiple myeloma, lytic bone lesions are usually absent.

Most patients have a moderate to severe normochromic, normocytic anemia with marked rouleaux formation. About 30% of patients have a leukemic blood picture consisting of lymphocytes, lymphoplasmacytoid lymphocytes, and occasional plasma cells. Leukopenia and thrombocytopenia may be present.

The bone marrow aspirate specimen shows increased numbers of well-differentiated lymphocytes and plasmacytoid lymphocytes. Plasma cells, mast cells, and histiocytes are almost always increased. The extent of involvement in the biopsy specimens varies from small focal lesions to extensive bone marrow replacement. The pattern of infiltration is interstitial, focal, or diffuse. The infiltrating cells range from lymphocytes to plasma cells. Intranuclear inclusions (Dutcher bodies) are commonly observed but are not specific for this disease.

Serum protein electrophoresis shows a tall peak or band usually in the gamma region. Immunoelectrophoresis characterizes the peak as IgM; 75% of IgM proteins have a kappa light chain. Uninvolved immunoglobulins are decreased in half the patients. A small amount of light chain is often present in the urine. Serum viscosity is increased in 90% of patients. Defects in platelet function and inhibition of coagulation factors are often related to the elevation in IgM and may be associated with a bleeding diathesis.

The median survival for patients with macroglobulinemia is 5 years. Treatment is aimed at ameliorating the hyperviscosity syndrome and treating the underlying lymphoma. Plasmapheresis is often used in patients who have symptoms from hyperviscosity syndrome.

Heavy Chain Diseases. Heavy chain diseases are rare malignant disorders characterized by the production of a monoclonal protein that is composed of a portion of the immunoglobulin heavy chain molecule in the serum, urine, or both. The heavy chains are devoid of light chains and are usually associated with a lymphocyte or plasma cell proliferation. There are three types of heavy chain diseases: γ heavy chain disease, α heavy chain disease, and μ heavy chain disease.

The median age of patients with γ heavy chain disease is about 60 years. Weakness, fatigue, and fever are common presenting symptoms. The clinical picture resembles a lymphoma. Hepatomegaly, splenomegaly, and lymphadenopathy are each found in 60% of patients. The bone marrow is involved in two thirds of patients. Anemia is usually present and leukopenia and thrombocytopenia are common. The proliferating cells consist of lymphocytes, plasma cells, or plasmacytoid lymphocytes. The histologic picture is variable, and in some cases there is no evidence of a lymphoproliferative disorder. The prognosis of patients ranges from a rapid downhill course to a stable course.

α *heavy chain disease* is the most common heavy chain disease and affects individuals in the second and third decades of life. Usually the gastrointestinal tract is involved, resulting in malabsorption, diarrhea, abdominal pain, and weight loss. The small intestine and mesenteric lymph nodes are infiltrated with plasma cells. Hepatosplenomegaly and lymphadenopathy are rare and the bone marrow is typically normal. Patients with this disorder tend to have a progressive downhill course but may respond to chemotherapy or even antibiotic therapy.

μ *heavy chain disease* is very rare. Most patients have a history of chronic lymphocytic leukemia. Hepatosplenomegaly is common but lymphadenopathy is rare. Two thirds of patients have vacuolated plasma cells in the bone marrow. In some patients, monoclonal light chains that do not bind with heavy chains are excreted in the urine.

References

Barlogie B, Epstein J, Selvanayagam P, et al. Plasma cell myeloma—new biological insights and advances in therapy. *Blood.* 1989;73:865-879.

Brunning RD, McKenna RW. Plasma cell dyscrasias and related disorders. In: *Atlas of Tumor Pathology: Tumors of the Bone Marrow.* Washington, DC: Armed Forces Institute of Pathology; 1994:323-367.

Crawford J. Protein electrophoresis and immunofixation. In: Koepke JA, ed. *Practical Laboratory Hematology.* New York, NY: Churchill Livingstone Inc; 1991:237-250.

Dimopoulos MA, Alexanian R. Waldenstrom's macroglobulinemia. *Blood*. 1994; 83:1452-1459.

Farhangi M, Merlini G. The clinical implications of monoclonal proteins. *Semin Oncol*. 1986;13:366-379.

Greipp PR, Kyle RA. Clinical, morphological and cell kinetic differences among multiple myeloma, monoclonal gammopathy of undetermined significance, and smoldering multiple myeloma. *Blood*. 1983;62:166-171.

Greipp PR, Lust JA, O'Fallon MO, et al. Plasma cell labeling index and β_2-microglobulin predict survival independent of thymidine kinase and c-reactive protein in multiple myeloma. *Blood*. 1993;81:3382-3387.

Grogan TM, Spier CM. The B cell immunoproliferative disorders, including multiple myeloma and amyloidosis. In: Knowles DM, ed. *Neoplastic Hematopathology*. Baltimore, Md: Williams and Wilkins; 1992:1235-1265.

Kyle RA. Plasma cell disorders. In: Wyngaarden JB, Smith LH, Bennett JC, ed. *Cecil Textbook of Medicine*. Philadelphia, Pa: WB Saunders Co; 1992:967-978.

Kyle RA, Garton JP. Laboratory monitoring of myeloma proteins. *Semin Oncol*. 1986;13:310-317.

Kyle RA, Greipp PR. Smoldering multiple myeloma. *N Engl J Med*. 1980; 302:1347-1349.

Kyle RA, Greipp PR. Plasma cell dyscrasias: current status. *CRC Crit Rev Oncol Hematol*. 1988;9:93-152.

Oken MM. Multiple myeloma. *Med Clin North Am*. 1984;68:757-787.

Peterson LC, Brown BA, Crosson JT, et al. Application of the immunoperoxidase technique to bone marrow trephine biopsies in the classification of patients with monoclonal gammopathies. *Am J Clin Pathol*. 1986;85:688-693.

Reed M, McKenna RW, Bridges R, Parkin J, Frizzera G, Brunning RD. Morphologic manifestations of monoclonal gammopathies. *Am J Clin Pathol*. 1981;76:8-23.

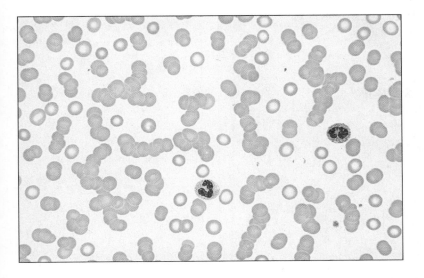

Image 38-1   Blood smear shows marked rouleaux formation.

Image 38-2   Bone marrow aspirate from a patient with multiple myeloma shows numerous plasma cells, many of which have nucleoli.

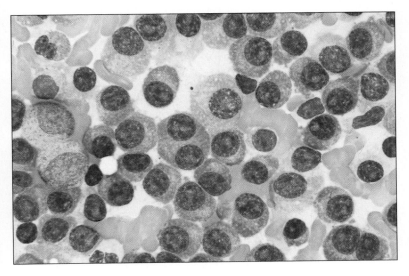

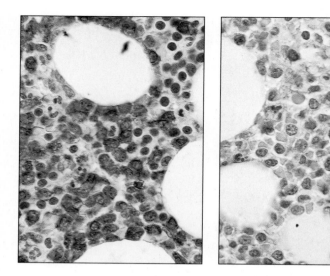

Image 38-3 Bone marrow biopsy specimen from a patient with multiple myeloma. Plasma cells are positive for kappa light chains and negative for lambda light chains, confirming that they are monoclonal.

39

Monoclonal Gammopathy of Undetermined Significance and Other Disorders Associated With Monoclonal Immunoglobulins

The malignant plasma cell dyscrasias, multiple myeloma, Waldenström's macroglobulinemia, and the heavy chain diseases were discussed in Chapter 38. Monoclonal gammopathy of undetermined significance (MGUS) will be the focus of this chapter. Primary amyloidosis and cryoglobulinemia will also be discussed.

Pathophysiology

MGUS is the term used to describe the presence of a monoclonal immunoglobulin in serum, urine, or both without any evidence of multiple myeloma, macroglobulinemia, or other related diseases. MGUS is the most frequent type of monoclonal gammopathy, occurring in two thirds of patients with monoclonal immunoglobulins. MGUS is rare before the age of 40 years but increases with each succeeding decade. MGUS is present in 1% of patients who are more than 50 years old and in 3% over 70 years old. Most patients have stable or benign disease, but in a significant number of patients a malignant plasma cell dyscrasia such as multiple myeloma may evolve. The paraprotein is usually IgG but may be

IgA or IgM. It is usually less than 3 g/dL (30 g/L). Monoclonal proteins in the urine are rare in this disorder.

Clinical Findings

The median age of patients with MGUS is 64 years; 60% of the patients are men. Because of the advanced age of the patients, they frequently have underlying disorders seemingly unrelated to this gammopathy. No specific symptoms or physical findings are related to MGUS.

Approach to Diagnosis

It is important to differentiate MGUS from malignant plasma cell dyscrasias, usually multiple myeloma. In most cases, this is not difficult since the criteria used to diagnose multiple myeloma (see Chapter 38) are absent in MGUS. Patients with MGUS usually have less than 3 g/dL (30 g/L) of monoclonal protein and no monoclonal immunoglobulin in the urine. Plasma cells are less than 5% in the bone marrow. In addition, lytic bone lesions are absent. The diagnostic workup includes the following:

1. Complete blood cell count with differential.
2. Blood and bone marrow examination.
3. Serum protein electrophoresis.
4. Serum immunoelectrophoresis or immunofixation.
5. Quantitation of serum immunoglobulins.
6. Immunoelectrophoresis or immunofixation of a concentrated 24-hour urine specimen.
7. Radiographic skeletal survey.

Hematologic Findings

No specific hematologic findings are associated with MGUS.

Blood Cell Measurements. When blood cell abnormalities such as anemia, leukopenia, or thrombocytopenia are present, they are unrelated to the MGUS.

Peripheral Blood Smear Morphology. Rouleaux formation may be increased in patients with high levels of monoclonal immunoglobulin.

Bone Marrow Examination. Plasma cells may be increased in the bone marrow, ranging from 1% to 10%. Usually they are less than 5%. The appearance of the plasma cells is usually normal, but mild abnormalities including nucleoli may be present in some cases. The bone marrow core biopsy specimens are generally normocellular with plasma cells scattered throughout the bone marrow or in small groups, often around blood vessels.

Immunostaining for kappa and light chains in the cytoplasm of plasma cells can aid in distinguishing MGUS from multiple myeloma. In most cases of multiple myeloma, the abnormal light chain is present in a ratio to the other light chain exceeding 16:1. In MGUS, the ratio is usually less than 16:1.

Other Laboratory Tests

39.1 Serum and Urine Protein Electrophoresis

Purpose, Principle, Specimen, and Procedure.
See Tests 38.1 and 38.2.

Interpretation. A monoclonal spike is found on serum protein electrophoresis in most cases of MGUS. The monoclonal protein in MGUS is usually less than 3 g/dL (30 g/L). It has been suggested that if the serum protein is less than 2 g/dL (20 g/L), it should be repeated 6 months later and if stable, checked annually. If the monoclonal protein is 2 g/dL (20g/L) or greater without evidence of multiple myeloma or related disorders, electrophoresis should be repeated in 3 months, and if stable, repeated at 6 months. If there is no progression, it is appropriate to repeat the electrophoresis annually thereafter. In MGUS, monoclonal proteins in the urine are usually absent.

39.2 Urine and Serum Immunoelectrophoresis

Purpose, Principle, Specimen, and Procedure.
See Test 38.3.

Interpretation. The most common monoclonal protein in MGUS is IgG (74%), followed by IgM (16%) and IgA (10%). Monoclonal proteins in the urine are rare but may be present. If a monoclonal protein is identified in the urine, the patient should be followed up more closely.

39.3 Serum Immunoglobulin Quantitation

Purpose, Principle, Specimen, and Procedure.
See Test 38.5.

Interpretation. The monoclonal immunoglobulin in MGUS ranges from less than 0.3 g/dL (3 g/L) to more than 3 g/dL (30 g/L), with a median of 1.7 g/dL (17 g/L). In greater than 95% of cases, it is less than 3 g/dL (30 g/L). Uninvolved immunoglobulins are decreased in about 30% of cases.

Course and Treatment

Treatment for MGUS is not necessary. In most patients with MGUS, the monoclonal protein is stable with no evidence to progression of a malignant plasma cell dyscrasia. A minority, however, do experience progression to an overt malignant plasma cell disorder. In a long-term follow-up study (range, 11-32 years) of 241 patients with MGUS, the patients were placed into four groups (Table 39-1). About 25% of the patients were stable with no significant increase in the monoclonal protein and appeared to have a benign monoclonal gammopathy. In a small number of patients (3%), the monoclonal protein increased to more than 3 g/dL (30 g/L), but multiple myeloma, macroglobulinemia, or a related disorder did not develop. Approximately 50% of the patients died of seemingly unrelated causes without the occurrence of a malignant

Table 39-1   Course of 241 Patients With Monoclonal
Gammopathy of Undetermined Significance*

Group	Outcome†	Percentage of Patients
1	No significant increase in monoclonal protein	24
2	Increase of monoclonal protein to >3 g/dL (30 g/L)	3
3	Died of unrelated causes	51
4	Developed multiple myeloma (15%), macroglobulinemia (3%), related diseases (4%)	22

*Modified from Kyle RA. Plasma cell disorders. In: Wyngaarden JB, Smith LH, Bennett JC, eds. *Cecil Textbook of Medicine*. Philadelphia, Pa: WB Saunders Co; 1992:967-978.
†Median follow-up was 19 years.

plasma cell dyscrasia. Finally, about 25% of the patients did develop an overt malignant plasma cell dyscrasia. The majority developed multiple myeloma, but macroglobulinemia and other related disorders were also observed. The time from the identification of the monoclonal protein to the diagnosis of the serious disorders ranged from 2 to 22 years with a median of 8 years. An increasing level of the serum monoclonal protein was the most reliable prediction of progression to a malignant plasma cell dyscrasia.

Primary Amyloidosis

Amyloid is a fibrillary protein that is deposited in various tissues and may cause damage to involved vital organs such as the heart and kidneys. Systemic amyloidosis consists of three major types: primary amyloidosis (AL), secondary amyloidosis (AA), and familial amyloidosis (AF). Local amyloidosis associated with aging, hemodialysis, or endocrinopathy also occurs. Primary amyloidosis is the only one of these disorders associated with plasma cell dyscrasias and is discussed in this section. In primary amyloidosis, the amyloid is derived from all or part of a monoclonal immunoglobulin light chain. About 20% of patients with primary amyloidosis have multiple myeloma; most of the remaining cases have a plasmacytosis in the bone marrow, even though the diagnostic criteria for myeloma are lacking.

Primary amyloidosis is rare. Most patients are between 60 and 70 years of age at diagnosis. Two thirds of patients are men. Weight loss and fatigue are the most common presenting features. Symptoms related to congestive heart failure, peripheral neuropathy, nephrotic syndrome, and bleeding tendency are also relatively common.

A monoclonal protein can be identified in urine or serum in 80% to 90% of patients with primary amyloidosis. A monoclonal protein is found in serum in about two thirds of patients. Two thirds of patients have a monoclonal protein in urine, with lambda chains being more common than kappa at a ratio of about 3:1. The monoclonal spike is often small. It manifests as light chains only in the urine in about 20% of patients. The protein may be missed by screening with serum or urine protein electrophoresis; therefore, immunoelectrophoresis or immunofixation of serum or urine should be done whenever an amyloidosis is suspected. Evidence of nephrotic syndrome is present in about 35% of patients. The serum creatinine level is elevated in 20% to 25% of patients. Coagulation factor X deficiency may be present secondary to binding of the factor to amyloid protein.

A diagnosis of amyloidosis is made by demonstration of amyloid in a biopsy specimen of an affected organ such as the kidney or heart. Subcutaneous fat aspirate samples and rectal biopsy specimens are each diagnostic in about 80% of cases. Results of bone marrow biopsy specimens are positive in about 50% of cases. Amyloid stains a pale pink with hematoxylin-eosin stain (Image 39-1). Its presence is confirmed with a Congo red stain that produces a characteristic apple-green birefringence when viewed with polarized light microscopy. Ultrastructurally, the amyloid consists of fine, linear, nonbranching fibrils.

Peripheral blood counts are often normal in patients with primary amyloidosis at diagnosis, but cytopenias are common in patients having concurrent multiple myeloma. Rouleaux formation may be increased in patients with a large monoclonal spike. About 20% of patients with primary amyloidosis have bone marrow findings that are diagnostic of multiple myeloma. In these patients, amyloid can usually be demonstrated in the bone marrow core biopsy section. Patients with primary amyloidosis but without myeloma frequently have increased plasma cells, but they are usually less than 10% of the bone marrow cells. Immunostaining for kappa and lambda light chains reveals that the plasma cells are often clonal, even if the diagnostic criteria for myeloma are not present. In patients without multiple myeloma, amyloidosis is demonstrated in the bone marrow in less than 50% of the cases. When present in the bone marrow core biopsy section, the amyloid is frequently localized to the walls of blood vessels (Image 39-1). Rarely, the entire bone marrow core biopsy specimen is replaced with amyloid.

Treatment of primary amyloidosis is directed at controlling amyloid production. Alkylating agent therapy in combination with steroids is the standard chemotherapeutic regimen. The overall survival rate for patients with amyloidosis, however, is poor. The median survival times range from 12 to 24 months from diagnosis. The most frequent causes of death include cardiac disease, renal failure, infection, and hemorrhage.

Cryoglobulinemia

Cryoimmunoglobulins are proteins that precipitate on cooling and redissolve upon rewarming. Cryoglobulins have been classified into three types: type I (monoclonal), type II (mixed), and type III (polyclonal).

Type I cryoglobulins are composed of IgM, IgG, IgA, or Bence-Jones (monoclonal light chains) proteins. Type I cryoglobulinemia is associated with multiple myeloma, Waldenström's macroglobulinemia, MGUS, chronic cold agglutinin disease, and other lymphoproliferative disorders. Type II cryoglobulins consists of a monoclonal immunoglobulin (usually IgM) and polyclonal IgG. Type II cryoglobulinemia is associated with chronic infections including hepatitis C. Patients with type II cryoglobulinemia have an increased incidence of B-cell lymphoproliferative disorders. The protein levels are usually high (1-30 mg/dL) in type I and type II cryoglobulinemia, and cryoprecipitation occurs easily. Some patients have no symptoms related to the cryoglobulinemia, while others have cutaneous manifestations such as purpura, pain, Raynaud's phenomenon, or ulceration. Arthralgias, nephritis, or neurologic symptoms may also be observed in patients with cryoglobulinemia. Corticosteroid administration is the usual therapy for cryoglobulinemia, although alkylating agents, plasmapheresis, and alpha-interferon have also been of benefit.

In type III cryoglobulinemia, one or more classes of polyclonal immunoglobulins are present. The concentration of the protein is low, usually in the range of 0.1 to 1.0 mg/dL, and cryoprecipitation does not occur readily. This type is found in many patients with inflammatory or infectious diseases.

References

Brunning RD, McKenna RW. Plasma cell dyscrasias and related disorders. In: *Atlas of Tumor Pathology: Tumors of the Bone Marrow.* Washington, DC: Armed Forces Institute of Pathology; 1994:323-367.

Farhangi M, Merlini G. The clinical implications of monoclonal immunoglobulins. *Semin Oncol.* 1986;13:366-379.

Gertz MA, Kyle RA. How to recognize, evaluate and treat amyloidosis. *Contemp Oncol.* 1993;3:346-352.

Gertz MA, Kyle RA, Greipp PR. Response rates and survival in primary systemic amyloidosis. *Blood.* 1991;77:257-262.

Kyle RA. Plasma cell disorders. In: Wyngaarden JB, Smith LH, Bennett JC, eds. *Cecil Textbook of Medicine.* Philadelphia, Pa: WB Saunders Co; 1992:967-978.

Kyle RA. Benign monoclonal gammopathy—after 20 to 35 years of follow-up. *Mayo Clin Proc.* 1993;68:26-36.

Kyle RA, Greipp PR. Amyloidosis (AL): clinical and laboratory features in 229 cases. *Mayo Clin Proc.* 1983;58:665-683.

Orfila C, Giraud P, Modesto A, et al. Abdominal fat tissue aspirate in human amyloidosis: light, electron, and immunofluorescence microscopic studies. *Hum Pathol.* 1986;17:366-369.

Peterson LC, Brown BA, Crosson JT, et al. Application of the immunoperoxidase technique to bone marrow trephine biopsies in the classification of patients with monoclonal gammopathies. *Am J Clin Pathol.* 1986;85:688-693.

Reed M, McKenna RW, Bridges R, et al. Morphologic manifestations of monoclonal gammopathies. *Am J Clin Pathol.* 1981;76:8-23.

Solomon A. Clinical implications of monoclonal light chains. *Semin Oncol.* 1986; 13:341-349.

Stone MJ. Amyloidosis: a final common pathway for protein deposition in tissues. *Blood.* 1990;75:531-545.

Wolf BC, Kumar A, Vera JC, et al. Bone marrow morphology and immunology in systemic amyloidosis. *Am J Clin Pathol.* 1986;86:84-88.

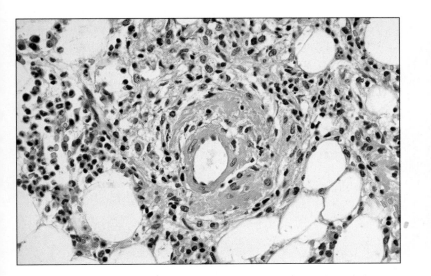

Image 39-1   Bone marrow biopsy specimen from a patient with primary amyloidosis shows amyloid associated with a small vessel.

PART
XII

Bleeding Disorders

40

Diagnosis of Bleeding Disorders

Hemostatic Mechanisms

Hemostasis can be defined as that property of the circulation that maintains blood in the fluid state within the blood vessels and prevents excessive blood loss after vascular injury. Hemostasis depends on reciprocal and balanced interactions between three anatomic compartments—the tissues, especially vascular endothelium; blood cells, especially platelets; and blood plasma containing the coagulation proteins. Other important factors are the size and blood flow of the affected blood vessel.

In response to vascular damage, blood clots to seal vascular leakage. There are three major events involved in blood coagulation—vascular constriction, platelet aggregation, and fibrin formation—which are intimately related and occur virtually simultaneously. Once the clot has formed and tissue repair has begun, digestion of the clot (fibrinolysis) begins, eventually leading to vascular patency.

The sequence of events leading to clotting is initiated by trauma to the vessel. Reflex vasoconstriction occurs, resulting in reduced blood flow. With damage to the vascular endothelium, platelets adhere to subendothelial collagen fibers and microfibrils.

Tissue factor is exposed in the vessel wall to initiate clotting. The result of the coagulation mechanism is generation of thrombin. In addition to aggregating platelets, thrombin converts fibrinogen to fibrin, which becomes incorporated into the platelet plug. With cross-linking of fibrin strands by factor XIIIa and contraction of the platelet mass, a stable clot (thrombus) is formed. Thrombi formed in the arterial system are called white thrombi and are composed primarily of platelets. Red thrombi, found in the venous circulation, are composed of erythrocytes trapped in fibrin; red thrombi contain few platelets.

Physiology and Biochemistry of Hemostasis

Platelets. Platelets are anucleate disc-shaped cells, 2 to 4 μm in diameter, normally found in the peripheral blood. In a Wright-stained blood smear, they are identified by their blue-gray cytoplasm and purplish granules. Platelets are formed in the bone marrow from giant (40-60 μm) polyploid cells called megakaryocytes. Megakaryocytes mature by a series of nuclear replications within a common cytoplasm (endomitosis), leading to multilobed nuclei, and by differentiation of specific cytoplasmic granules. Following maturation, the megakaryocyte cytoplasm becomes demarcated into platelet subunits, and the platelets are released into the circulation through the marrow sinusoids. Image 40-1 illustrates platelet and megakaryocyte morphology as seen in a Wright-stained blood smear and marrow aspirate, respectively. Ordinarily, each megakaryocyte produces approximately 1,000 platelets. Platelets normally circulate for 9 to 10 days, and one third of the platelet mass is sequestered in a splenic pool that exchanges freely with the circulatory pool.

Platelets contain three types of secretory granules—lysosomes, containing acid hydrolases; α-granules that contain proteins; and (electron)-dense bodies (δ-granules) that contain adenosine triphosphate, adenosine diphosphate, calcium, and serotonin. The α-granules contain platelet-specific proteins (platelet factor-4, β-thromboglobulin), as well as other proteins, such as platelet-derived growth factor (a mitogen for fibroblasts and smooth muscle cells), and coagulation proteins also found in plasma (fibrinogen, von Willebrand's factor).

Adhesion of platelets to subendothelium initiates the platelet phase of hemostasis (primary hemostasis). von Willebrand's factor mediates platelet adhesion by binding to subendothelial receptors, as well as glycoprotein 1b on platelets. Collagen fibers then induce platelets to aggregate by stimulating them to secrete intracellular granular contents (adenosine diphosphate) and to synthesize thromboxane A_2. These secreted substances mediate and further amplify aggregation. Thrombin formed by the soluble coagulation system also activates platelets.

Vasoconstriction is enhanced by release of serotonin and thromboxane A_2. Platelet activation induces expression of binding sites for coagulation proteins; this activity has been termed platelet factor 3. In addition to platelet–vessel wall interactions (adhesion), platelet-platelet interactions (aggregation) occur; the latter are mediated by fibrinogen, which links two platelets together by the fibrinogen receptor, glycoprotein IIb-IIIa. The platelet plug formed is provisional and will not remain hemostatically effective unless a firm fibrin clot forms around it. Platelet actomyosin provides for clot retraction and consolidation.

Blood Coagulation. The process of blood coagulation represents the second phase of hemostasis in which the soluble plasma protein, fibrinogen, is converted to an insoluble fibrin clot as a result of a series of enzymatic interactions leading to the formation of thrombin. These enzymatic interactions involve conversion of a zymogen (enzyme precursor) to a corresponding protease (active enzyme), which is responsible for activation of a subsequent zymogen.

Initiation of the enzymatic pathways leading to fibrin formation can occur by two mechanisms (Figure 40-1). There is in vivo interdependence between the pathways, and important feedback-activation mechanisms occur. Formation of a normal blood clot requires several plasma coagulation proteins. There are four general categories of coagulation factors.

Serine proteases: Factors II (prothrombin), VII, IX, X, XI, XII, and prekallikrein circulate in the zymogen form. Initiation of coagulation results in the activation of each factor. The subscript "a" indicates the active factor, ie, factor X_a. Prothrombin and factors VII, IX, and X are vitamin K–dependent, in that vitamin K is

Figure 40-1 The blood coagulation mechanism. In vivo coagulation is initiated by tissue factor expression; the tissue factor–factor VII_a complex activates factors IX and X. When small amounts of factor X_a are generated, tissue factor pathway inhibitor inhibits subsequent tissue factor activity. Thrombin generated by initial tissue factor activates factor XI to initiate intrinsic coagulation and additional thrombin formation. Thrombin generation is amplified by thrombin feedback-activation of factors V and VIII. Factor XII initiation of coagulation is important in the presence of artificial surfaces, but not for in vivo coagulation. The initial fibrin generated by thrombin action on fibrinogen is soluble ($fibrin_s$); hemostatically effective insoluble fibrin ($fibrin_i$) is generated by action of factor XIII_a.

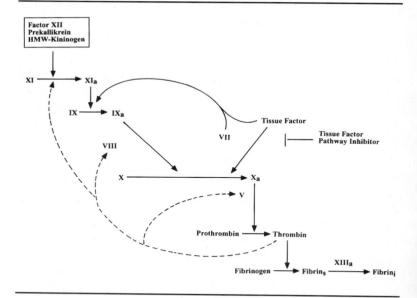

required for a posttranslational modification to synthesize fully active coagulation proteins (Table 40-1).

Cofactors required for activation of some of the above enzymes include high-molecular-weight kininogen and factors V

Table 40-1   The Vitamin K–Dependent Procoagulant Proteins[*]

Prothrombin
Factor VII
Factor IX
Factor X

*Following synthesis of these proteins by the liver, a posttranslational modification (γ-carboxylation of certain glutamic acid residues) occurs, resulting in functional coagulation proteins. This posttranslational modification requires vitamin K. In the absence of vitamin K (vitamin K deficiency), nonfunctional coagulation proteins are synthesized.

and VIII. The latter two proteins have minimal activity until activated. Tissue factor may also be considered a cofactor, since factor VII is inactive unless complexed with tissue factor.

Fibrinogen (factor I) is a soluble protein that becomes the insoluble clot (fibrin) following cleavage by thrombin.

Factor XIII is a plasma transglutaminase, which, when activated to factor XIII_a, stabilizes the fibrin clot.

Activation of coagulation occurs by two mechanisms (Figure 40-1). Tissue factor initiates the extrinsic pathway of clotting. High concentrations of tissue factor are present in skin, brain, lung, and placenta, as well as in monocytes and the adventitia of large blood vessels. In the basal, unperturbed state, blood is not in contact with tissue factor. Clotting is initiated only by induction of normally latent tissue factor, or by exposure of blood to extravascular tissues containing tissue factor.

Tissue factor initiates clotting by forming a complex with factor VII_a. Factor VII_a–tissue factor complex activates factor X; factor X_a in the presence of the cofactor, factor V_a, activates prothrombin, forming thrombin. Excessive activity of the factor VII_a–tissue factor complex is regulated by tissue factor pathway inhibitor. Prothrombin activation occurs on cellular surfaces of platelets, endothelial cells, smooth muscle cells, and monocytes, and requires calcium and factor V_a. Prothrombin activation and thrombin cleavage of fibrinogen constitute the common pathway of coagulation.

Once thrombin is formed, clotting occurs. Thrombin cleavage of fibrinogen results in fibrin monomer formation. Polymerization of fibrin monomers and cross-linking of fibrin by thrombin-activated factor XIII_a lead to generation of the insoluble fibrin clot.

A variety of feedback-activation mechanisms are important in the amplification of coagulation. For example, thrombin activates factors V and VIII, markedly enhancing thrombin generation. Factor X_a can also activate factor VII to enhance factor X activation by the tissue factor (factor VIIa) complex.

An alternative mechanism for initiating coagulation is the intrinsic pathway (Figure 40-1). In the past, it was thought that exposure of subendothelial connective tissue, presumably collagen, activates factor XII; factor XII_a then converts prekallikrein to kallikrein, which then converts more factor XII to factor XII_a, which in turn then activates factor XI. The above reactions require a cofactor protein, high-molecular-weight kininogen. Factor XI_a then converts factor IX to factor IX_a. Factor XII, prekallikrein, and high-molecular-weight kininogen are referred to as the contact proteins, since their activation occurs on contact with an abnormal surface (glass or kaolin).

Interdependence between the extrinsic and intrinsic pathways has been demonstrated, in that the factor VII_a–tissue factor complex can activate factor IX, providing a mechanism for bypassing the initial steps of the intrinsic pathway (Figure 40-1). Factor IX_a activates factor X in a reaction that requires a cofactor (factor VIII_a). Like factor V, factor VIII must be activated by thrombin to participate in factor X activation.

It is unclear how the intrinsic pathway of coagulation is actually initiated in vivo. Because patients with a deficiency of factor XII, prekallikrein, or high-molecular-weight kininogen do not have abnormal bleeding, the importance of these factors in hemostasis is in question. However, the physiologic importance of both pathways is indicated by the fact that patients lacking components of either the extrinsic (factor VII) or intrinsic (factors VIII, IX, and XI) pathways have hemorrhagic disease.

Thrombin feedback-activation of factor XI has been proposed as a mechanism to explain how intrinsic coagulation might begin in the absence of the contact factors (ie, to explain why patients with contact factor deficiency do not have a bleeding disorder). A current model for blood coagulation would involve the following steps. First, tissue factor is expressed following vascular injury; complex formation with factor VII_a would initiate clotting by activation of both factors X and IX. Tissue factor pathway inhibitor then prevents subsequent extrinsic activation of factor X. Thrombin formation is further amplified by feedback activation of factors V, VIII, and XI, leading to persistent activation of intrinsic coagulation. This model has the advantages of explaining why patients with hemophilia (deficiencies of factors VIII, IX, or XI) bleed, as well as why patients with contact factor deficiency do not bleed.

A summary of the hemostatic events that occur immediately after vascular injury is presented in Figure 40-2. In the normal hemostatic response to vascular trauma, the processes of platelet function and blood coagulation are intimately related.

Fibrinolysis. Following hemostatic plug formation and cessation of hemorrhage, vascular repair begins with lysis of the fibrin clot (Figure 40-3). Local thrombin formation stimulates secretion of vascular endothelial cell tissue–plasminogen activator (t-PA). Plasminogen and t-PA diffuse within the thrombus, where t-PA activates plasminogen to plasmin, a protease capable of degrading fibrin in a process called physiologic fibrinolysis. Fibrinolysis is restricted to the clot because inhibitors to t-PA and plasmin are present in blood (plasminogen activator inhibitors and alpha$_2$-antiplasmin, respectively).

Approach to the Bleeding Patient

In evaluating a patient with a putative bleeding disorder, information should be obtained for the following questions.

History. What is the duration of the bleeding tendency, ie, is it inherited or acquired? Is there a family history of bleeding? If so, is it transmitted in a dominant or recessive fashion? Is bleeding spontaneous, or is surgery or trauma required to elicit bleeding? What is the location and type of bleeding?

Physical Examination. Is bleeding represented by petechiae or large soft tissue bruises? Are hemarthroses present? Are there telangiectasias?

Table 40-2 distinguishes the two major classes of bleeding disorders—platelet-vascular type vs coagulation type—based on

Figure 40-2 Summary of hemostatic events immediately following vascular injury. (1) Thromboresistant properties of the blood vessel wall (discussed in Chapter 47) maintain blood in a fluid state. Platelets circulate in a nonadhesive state. (2) Immediately after vascular injury, exposure of subendothelial components, including collagen fibrils, induces platelet adhesion, mediated by the adhesive plasma protein, von Willebrand's factor, and its platelet receptor, glycoprotein I_b. (3) Platelet activation results from exposure to collagen, leading to thromboxane A_2 generation, platelet secretion (release reaction), and formation of thrombin. These events lead to additional platelet recruitment into the platelet plug (aggregation). The platelet-platelet interaction results from fibrinogen binding to its platelet receptor, glycoprotein II_b III_a. (4) Tissue factor expressed by the subendothelium or by adventitial tissues generates thrombin; thrombin activity results in cross-linked fibrin strands that reinforce the platelet plug. Platelet actomyosin mediates clot retraction.

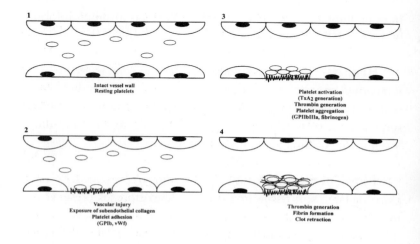

1 — Intact vessel wall
Resting platelets

2 — Vascular injury
Exposure of subendothelial collagen
Platelet adhesion
(GPIb, vWf)

3 — Platelet activation
(TxA$_2$ generation)
Thrombin generation
Platelet aggregation
(GPIIbIIIa, fibrinogen)

4 — Thrombin generation
Fibrin formation
Clot retraction

Figure 40-3 Physiologic fibrinolysis is shown. Fibrin formation (shaded area) initiates secretion of vascular endothelial cell tissue plasminogen activator (t-PA). Plasminogen and t-PA assemble on fibrin to generate plasmin, an enzyme that degrades fibrin to fibrin degradation products (FDP). t-PA and plasmin activity are inhibited by plasminogen activator inhibitor and alpha$_2$-antiplasmin, respectively, if the active enzymes escape the confines of the clot.

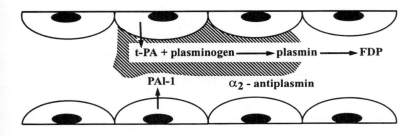

information obtained from the patient. Inherited bleeding disorders can be differentiated from acquired disorders by family history, age, and the presence or absence of an underlying disorder. Factors VIII and IX deficiency (hemophilia A and B, respectively) are both X-linked recessive disorders among men. von Willebrand's disease is the most common bleeding disorder and is transmitted in an autosomal dominant fashion. Other inherited bleeding disorders are usually transmitted in an autosomal recessive manner (factor VII deficiency, factor XI deficiency).

Acquired bleeding disorders usually result from systemic disease, such as leukemia, sepsis, uremia, and liver disease. It is important to remember that certain vascular disorders (ie, abnormalities in blood vessels or their supportive tissues) may result in inherited or acquired bleeding (hereditary hemorrhagic telangiectasia, scurvy).

Table 40-2   Clinical Manifestations in Patients With Bleeding Disorders

Findings	Disorders of Coagulation	Disorders of Platelets or Vessels
Petechiae	Rare	Characteristic
Deep hematomas	Characteristic	Rare
Hemarthroses	Characteristic	Rare
Delayed bleeding	Common	Rare
Bleeding from superficial cuts	Minimal	Persistent
Sex of patient	Most inherited disorders occur in men	Most inherited disorders occur in women
Mucosal bleeding	Minimal	Typical

Laboratory Screening Tests of Coagulation

Coagulation tests are conducted primarily on plasma, which is the anticoagulated, acellular portion of the blood. Trisodium citrate (3.2% or 3.8%), which inhibits clotting by complexing free calcium, is used to anticoagulate the blood for coagulation tests. Most laboratories use silicone-coated glass tubes for collection. Unlike many clinical pathology laboratory tests, sample quality is extremely important for coagulation testing. A correct ratio of citrate to plasma and the quality of venipuncture are important factors in the sample collection. Details of coagulation screening tests are given below, and Table 40-3 summarizes test results in common bleeding disorders.

40.1 Prothrombin Time Assay

Purpose.   The prothrombin time (PT) assay is used to screen for inherited or acquired abnormalities in the extrinsic (factor VII) and common (factors V, X, prothrombin, and fibrinogen) pathways (Table 40-4). The PT assay is also used to monitor the effect of oral anticoagulant therapy.

Table 40-3 Screening Laboratory Tests in Common Bleeding Disorders

Disorder	PT	aPTT	Platelet Count	Bleeding Time
von Willebrand's disease	Normal	Normal or increased	Normal	Normal or increased
Hemophilia A or B	Normal	Usually increased	Normal	Normal
Thrombocytopenia	Normal	Normal	Decreased	Usually increased (test not usually indicated)
Vitamin K deficiency	Increased	Normal or increased	Normal	Normal

Abbreviations: PT = prothrombin time; aPTT = activated partial thromboplastin time.

Principle. In this assay, clotting is initiated by a commercial tissue factor reagent, called thromboplastin. Plasma, thromboplastin, and calcium are mixed and the clotting time determined. The thromboplastin reagent contains phospholipid, so that all activities of the extrinsic and common pathway are measured. The PT depends on the concentration of prothrombin and factors V, X, and VII and fibrinogen. The PT will be prolonged when factor levels are low, and normal when factor levels are borderline or normal. Because three of the five factors measured by the PT are vitamin K–dependent (prothrombin and factors VII and X), this assay is useful in identifying vitamin K deficiency (usually associated with liver disease or oral anticoagulant therapy). The PT assay does not measure the intrinsic factors (VIII, IX, XI, contact factors) or factor XIII activity. Depending on the thromboplastin reagent used, the normal PT reference range may encompass 10 to 16 seconds.

Specimen. Citrated plasma obtained by clean venipuncture is used in the PT assay.

Procedure. The plasma sample is added to the thromboplastin reagent, which also contains calcium. The test is performed in duplicate and the clotting time average is reported.

Table 40-4 Coagulation Factors Measured by the PT and aPTT Assays

aPTT	PT	Both Tests
XII	VII	
HMW-K		
Prekallikrein		
XI		
IX		
VIII		
X	X	X
V	V	V
Prothrombin	Prothrombin	Prothrombin
Fibrinogen	Fibrinogen	Fibrinogen

Abbreviations: aPTT = activated partial thromboplastin time; PT = prothrombin time; HMW-K = high-molecular-weight kininogen.

Interpretation. The large number of commercial thromboplastins in use in this country and their variable sensitivity in the detection of vitamin K deficiency has led to renewed awareness of the pitfalls of comparing PT assay results using different thromboplastins. The use of the PT assay to monitor oral anticoagulant therapy is discussed in Chapter 48. In interpreting PT assay results for this purpose, the sensitivity of the reagent compared with the World Health Organization standard should be known. A prolongation of the PT usually indicates defective or decreased synthesis of the vitamin K–dependent clotting factors. The PT assay is also sensitive to a decrease in factor V and fibrinogen concentrations, which may occur in end-stage liver disease, or in disseminated intravascular coagulation. Another variable affecting the PT reference range is instrumentation used in the assay. If photo-optical instruments are used, and plasma samples are turbid or icteric, the optical density change induced by clotting may not be detected, and these instruments will record the highest value of which they are capable.

Shortened PT values may be due to poor quality venipuncture, resulting in an activated sample. If this etiologic factor is excluded, another cause of shortened PT values includes chronic disseminated intravascular coagulation (in vivo activation).

An inherited deficiency of one of the factors affecting the PT assay is uncommon. The PT may also be prolonged due to antibodies to prothrombin (seen in patients with autoantibodies associated with the lupus anticoagulant) or to factor V, or in patients with certain abnormal fibrinogens (dysfibrinogens).

Notes and Precautions. If a normal plasma sample is left at cold temperatures for several hours, the PT of that sample may shorten substantially. Contact (factor XII) activation of factor VII may be responsible for this phenomenon.

40.2 Activated Partial Thromboplastin Time

Purpose. The activated partial thromboplastin time (aPTT) assay is used to detect inherited and acquired factor deficiency of the intrinsic pathway, to screen for the lupus anticoagulant, and to monitor heparin therapy.

Principle. The aPTT is an assay of the intrinsic and common pathways. A platelet substitute (crude phospholipid), and a surface-activating agent such as micronized silica (to activate factor XII) are added to plasma. This achieves optimal contact activation. Calcium is then added and the clotting time is recorded. The aPTT assay measures all factors except factors VII and XIII (Table 40-4). Depending on the reagent used, the aPTT reference clotting times may encompass 25 to 45 seconds. Because platelet-poor plasma is used, the aPTT is not influenced by quantitative or qualitative abnormalities in platelets.

Specimen. Citrated plasma obtained by a clean venipuncture is used.

Procedure. Patient plasma specimen is mixed with an aPTT reagent (containing phospholipid and contact activator), followed by addition of calcium. The test is performed in duplicate and the average of the clotting times is reported.

Interpretation. The aPTT reference range depends on two major variables—the aPTT reagent and the instrumentation used. The aPTT is prolonged when one or more of the factors measured by the assay is deficient. If the period of contact activation is greater than 2 to 3 minutes, the aPTT may not detect prekallikrein deficiency.

It must be realized that many commercial aPTT reagents are insensitive in screening for factor deficiency; mild deficiency (eg, factor VIII level of 35%) will not be detected with most reagents. In addition, there will be reagent variability in detecting the lupus anticoagulant. When evaluating patients for the lupus anticoagulant, it is important to ensure that aPTT plasma samples are prepared such that they are platelet-poor. Heparin contamination must be considered in evaluation of unexplained prolonged PTT values, especially when these samples are obtained from patients in intensive care settings.

Specific inhibitors of clotting factors may also prolong the aPTT, the most common being factor VIII antibodies. Isolated prolonged aPTT values of unknown causes should be evaluated with a mixing study. The patient's plasma sample is mixed in equal volume with a normal plasma specimen, and the aPTT assay is run immediately (0 time) and 1 to 2 hours later. Correction of the prolonged aPTT value into the normal reference range with mixing at both intervals suggests factor deficiency as the cause of the prolonged aPTT value. Failure of the patient's prolonged aPTT value to correct suggests an inhibitor to coagulation; possibilities include heparin, the lupus anticoagulant, or an antibody to a specific coagulation protein. If the patient's sample displays a markedly prolonged thrombin time, but not reptilase time, heparin is present in the sample (discussed later). If the mixing study results at 0 and 1 to 2 hours are similarly prolonged, the lupus anticoagulant is suspected, and confirmatory tests for this antiphospholipid antibody can be performed (discussed later). If the mixing study results demonstrate time-dependent prolongation, typically seen with protein-antibody interactions, an antibody to a specific coagulation factor is suggested, and specific factor assays can then be performed.

Notes and Precautions. If plasma samples are turbid or icteric, the optical density change induced by clotting may not be detected, and photo-optical instruments will record the highest value of which they are capable. Similarly, if plasma samples have been activated, and fibrin formation occurs during the instrument's lag period, the maximal clotting time again will be printed. Whenever these maximal clotting time values are obtained on photo-optical instruments, the clotting assay should be repeated using a manual method.

Shortened aPTT values may be due to poor quality venipuncture, resulting in an activated sample. Excluding this etiologic factor, two other causes of shortened aPTT values are marked elevation in factor VIII levels or chronic disseminated intravascular coagulation (in vivo activation).

40.3 Thrombin Time

Purpose. The thrombin time is used to screen for abnormalities in the conversion of fibrinogen to fibrin. Common causes of a prolonged thrombin time include fibrinogen deficiency (quantitative or qualitative), heparin, and fibrin degradation products. Less commonly, certain paraproteins may inhibit fibrin monomer polymerization and prolong the thrombin time. Hyperfibrinogenemia may also prolong the thrombin time.

Principle. The addition of thrombin to plasma converts fibrinogen to fibrin, bypassing the intrinsic and extrinsic pathways. The time necessary for fibrinogen to clot is a function of fibrinogen concentration.

Procedure. In this test, thrombin (3 U/mL) is added to the patient's plasma sample and the clotting time measured.

Interpretation. A prolongation of more than 3 seconds over the control value is abnormal. Markedly long thrombin time values suggest the presence of heparin in the sample. The presence of heparin can be confirmed by using the reptilase time, which also measures the conversion of fibrinogen to fibrin, but is insensitive to heparin. Thus, a prolonged thrombin time and normal reptilase time indicate the presence of heparin.

Prolonged thrombin time values not due to heparin can be evaluated using assays for fibrinogen (functional and immuno-logic) and fibrin degradation products (discussed in Chapter 44).

Notes and Precautions. The concentration of thrombin used in this assay determines the reference range for this test, as well as sensitivity. High concentrations of thrombin will give shorter clotting times and decreased sensitivity.

40.4 Platelet Count

This screening test of hemostasis is performed routinely on almost all patients using particle counters as part of the routine complete blood count. The normal platelet count usually ranges from 150 to 440 x 10^3/mm^3 (150-440 x 10^9/L); bleeding disorders may be associated with either thrombocytopenia or thrombocytosis. A bone marrow examination is frequently helpful in evaluating these two disorders.

40.5 Bleeding Time

Purpose. The bleeding time should be used to screen patients for inherited platelet dysfunction (von Willebrand's disease, qualitative platelet abnormalities).

Principle. The bleeding time is the time (in minutes) that it takes for bleeding to cease from a small, superficial wound made under standardized conditions. The bleeding time is mainly affected by primary hemostatic mechanisms (platelet number and function), but is also affected by a variety of other conditions.

Procedure. The Ivy bleeding time is the preferred method. A blood pressure cuff is placed around the patient's upper arm and the pressure is raised to 40 mm Hg. Two small punctures are made along the volar surface of the patient's forearm. The drops of blood issuing from the bleeding points are absorbed at intervals of 30 seconds into two filter paper disks, one for each puncture wound, until bleeding ceases. The average of the times required for bleeding to stop from the puncture wounds is taken as the bleeding time.

Several modifications of this technique have been devised in attempts to standardize the skin puncture. Perhaps the best and least traumatic of these is a sterile disposable device (Simplate, General Diagnostics, Division of Warner-Lambert Pharmaceuticals Co, Morris Plains, NJ) that makes two uniform incisions 5 x 1 mm by means of spring-loaded blades contained in plastic housing. The bleeding time device is placed firmly on the volar surface of the forearm without pressure and positioned so that the incision will be parallel to the fold of the elbow, with care taken to avoid superficial veins, scars, and bruises; the blade is then released by depression of the triggering device. The normal bleeding time with this method of making the parallel incision is less than 9 minutes.

Interpretation. Older studies using the bleeding time indicated that this test might be an indicator of platelet function, and therefore, might be helpful in predicting bleeding in individual patients. More recent studies suggest that the bleeding time is determined not only by platelet function, but also by hematocrit, certain components of the coagulation mechanism, skin quality, and technique. There is no evidence that the bleeding time can predict bleeding, and there is no correlation between a skin template bleeding time and certain visceral bleeding times. Consequently, the test is recommended only to screen patients for inherited platelet dysfunction (von Willebrand's disease, qualitative platelet disorders). An abnormal bleeding time in patients with a history of lifelong bleeding justifies further hemostatic testing for platelet dysfunction. Some patients with inherited platelet dysfunction may have normal bleeding times. The postaspirin bleeding time may be helpful in further screening this latter group of patients. Aspirin (650 mg) is given and

Table 40-5   Aspirin-Containing Drugs*

Alka-Seltzer (extra strength)
Anacin (maximum strength)
Anodynos
APC
Arthritis pain formula
ASA
Ascriptin
  (regular or extra strength); A/D
Aspercin (extra)
Aspergum
Aspermin (extra)
Aspirbar
Aspirjen Jr
Aspirtab (maximum strength)
Azdone[†]
Azotal[†]
Bayer Aspirin (genuine; maximum;
  children's) delayed-release Enteric;
  extended-release 8-hour; plus buffered;
  plus extra strength buffered; therapy
Buffered (therapy)
Buff-A; Buff-A-Comp[†],
  Buff-A-Comp 3[†]
Buffaprin (extra)
Buffasal (maximum)
Bufferin (arthritis strength;
  extra strength; tri-buffered)
Buffex
Buffinol (extra)
Butalbital compound[†]
Cama arthritis pain reliever
Cope
Damason-P[†]
Darvon compound 65[†]
Doloral[†]
  (cold tablets for children)
Duradyne
Easprin[†]
Ecotrin (maximum)
Empirin; with codeine (2[†], 3[†], 4[†])
Epromate[†]
Equagesic[†]
Equazine[†]

Excedrin (extra strength)
Fiorinal[†]; with codeine[†]
Genprin
Isollyl improved*
Lanorinal[†]
Lorprin[†]
Lortab ASA[†]

Magnaprin (arthritis strength)
Maxiprin
Measurin
Meprogesic Q[†]
Midol
Momentum
Norgesic[†]; Forte[†]
Norwich; extra strength
Orphenagesic[†]; Forte[†]

PAC revised formula analgesic
Palagesic

Percodan[†]; Demi[†]
Presalin
Rid-A-Pain with codeine[†]

Robaxisal[†]
Roxiprin[†]
Salecto
Salocol
Sedalgesic inserts[†]
Sine-Off tablets
Soma compound[†]; with codeine[†]
St. Joseph's aspirin

Stanback powder (original formula)
Synalgos-DC[†]
Trigesic
Tri-Pain
Vanquish
Verin
Wesprin buffered
ZORprin[†]

*From Billups NF, ed. *American Drug Index 1994*. 38th ed. St Louis, Mo: Facts and Comparisons; 1994.
[†]Available through prescription only.

the bleeding time test is repeated 2 hours later. Some believe that the postaspirin bleeding time substantially increases the sensitivity of the bleeding time in detecting patients with abnormal platelet function. The postaspirin bleeding time may be helpful in that patients with equivocal bleeding histories with normal routine and postaspirin bleeding times are deemed inappropriate for laboratory testing for inherited platelet dysfunction.

Notes and Precautions. Antiplatelet drugs usually prolong skin bleeding times (but not necessarily visceral bleeding times). However, patients who are hemostatically normal will have bleeding times that usually stay within the normal reference range after aspirin ingestion. In contrast, patients with platelet dysfunction will demonstrate marked prolongation of their bleeding time after taking aspirin. Table 40-5 lists drug preparations containing aspirin.

The bleeding time test may leave two small scars, and the patient should be so informed. The bleeding time test should not be performed on patients with moderate thrombocytopenia (platelet count, <50 x $10^3/mm^3$ [50 x 10^9/L]). The postaspirin bleeding time test should not be performed on patients who are actively bleeding.

References

Broze GJ Jr. The role of tissue factor pathway inhibitor in a revised coagulation cascade. *Semin Hematol*. 1992;29:159-169.

Hougie C. Partial thromboplastin time (PTT) and activated partial thromboplastin time tests: one-stage prothrombin time. In: Williams WJ, Beutler E, Erslev AJ, Lichtman MA, eds. *Hematology*. 4th ed. New York, NY: McGraw-Hill; 1990: 1766-1770.

Rapaport SI. Hemostatic mechanisms. In: *Introduction to Hematology*. Philadelphia, Pa: JB Lippincott Co; 1987:432-469.

Rapaport SI. Screening evaluation of hemostasis. In: *Introduction to Hematology*. Philadelphia, Pa: JB Lippincott Co; 1987:470-482.

Rodgers RPC, Levin J. A critical reappraisal of the bleeding time. *Semin Thromb Hemost*. 1990;16:1-20.

Stuart MJ, Miller ML, Davey FR, Wolk JA. The post-aspirin bleeding time: a screening test for evaluating hemostatic disorders. *Br J Haematol*. 1979; 43:649-656.

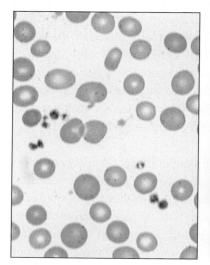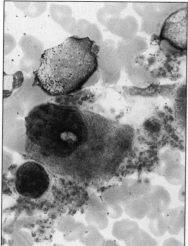

Image 40-1 Platelet and megakaryocyte morphology. The left panel is a Wright-stained peripheral blood smear showing approximately 10 platelets in the field (x50). The right panel is a Wright-stained bone marrow aspirate showing two megakaryocytes in the field (x50). The megakaryocytes shown are shedding platelets.

41

Thrombocytopenia

The typical clinical findings associated with thrombocytopenia include petechial hemorrhage, ecchymoses (bruises), and bleeding from mucous membranes (epistaxis, gum bleeding, menorrhagia).

Pathophysiology

The causes of thrombocytopenia are summarized in Table 41-1; thrombocytopenic disorders have been classified according to mechanism. Major mechanisms of thrombocytopenia include decreased marrow production, increased platelet destruction, and splenic sequestration. Occasionally, hemodilution occurs, resulting in thrombocytopenia.

Since splenic sequestration can usually be easily excluded by physical examination (palpable splenomegaly is almost always present), the typical evaluation for thrombocytopenia is to distinguish decreased platelet production from increased platelet destruction. If no obvious marrow insult can be identified (chemotherapeutic agents, ionizing radiation, toxic chemicals such as benzene, etc), a

Table 41-1   Causes of Thrombocytopenia

Failure of marrow production
    Reduced megakaryocytes
        Marrow infiltration with tumor, infection, or fibrosis
        Marrow aplasia (fatty replacement) due to drugs, chemicals, or radiation
        Congenital abnormalities (Wiskott-Aldrich syndrome,
          Fanconi's syndrome)
    Ineffective megakaryocytopoiesis
        Megaloblastic anemia
        Myelodysplasia
        Alcohol suppression
Increased platelet destruction
    Immune thrombocytopenia
        Autoantibody-mediated systemic lupus erythematosus, lymphomas,
          drugs, infections, idiopathic (ITP)
        Alloantibody-mediated posttransfusion purpura, fetal-maternal
          incompatibility
    Nonimmune thrombocytopenia
        Disseminated intravascular coagulation
        Thrombotic thrombocytopenic purpura
        Mechanical (prosthetic materials)
Splenic sequestration
Hemodilution

---

bone marrow examination is necessary to categorize the thrombocytopenia. If decreased megakaryocytes are present, the causative disorder should be identifiable, such as leukemia or solid tumor, infection (granuloma), fibrosis, or fatty infiltration as may be seen in marrow aplasia. Less commonly, an inherited disorder of megakaryocytopoiesis may be present.

If increased megakaryocytes are present, peripheral platelet destruction is suggested. This categorization mandates distinguishing possible immune vs nonimmune mechanisms by considering a variety of disorders, including disseminated intravascular coagulation (DIC), connective tissue diseases, lymphoproliferative disorders, infection, mechanical destruction, drugs, thrombotic thrombocytopenic purpura, and certain alloantibody-mediated thrombocytopenias. If consideration of the above-mentioned disorders associated with increased platelet destruction is nondiagnostic, then the patient is considered to have immune idiopathic thrombocytopenic purpura (ITP).

Antibody-mediated thrombocytopenia may be associated with autoantibodies or alloantibodies to platelets. Autoantibodies are found in patients with connective tissue or lymphoproliferative diseases. In these cases, antibodies are elicited, which react with target platelet antigens, including platelet membrane receptors such as glycoprotein Ib and the glycoprotein IIb-IIIa complex. Virtually any drug may be associated with immune thrombocytopenia, especially sulfa drugs, quinidine, and heparin. In many cases, the drug acts as a hapten, combining with a serum protein to form an immunogenic complex. Antibody formation is induced against the drug-hapten complex; the antibodies then cross-react with platelets. Certain drugs, such as thiazide diuretics, may cause thrombocytopenia by suppressing platelet production. Antibodies to platelets may develop after viral or bacterial infection, resulting in thrombocytopenia. Regardless of the mechanism, antibody-coated platelets are removed from the circulation by macrophages of the reticuloendothelial system.

In posttransfusion purpura, patients lacking the Pl^{A1} antigen receive blood products containing this antigen and develop alloantibody-mediated thrombocytopenia 7 to 10 days later. For unknown reasons, the alloantibody cross-reacts with the patient's own platelets as well, resulting in severe thrombocytopenia.

Neonatal thrombocytopenia may result from two mechanisms. Maternal platelet antibodies may cross the placenta to interact with fetal platelets. In this situation, the mother has underlying immune thrombocytopenia. Alternatively, fetal platelet antigens may immunize the mother to induce maternal platelet antibodies, similar to the situation of Rh hemolytic disease.

Clinical Aspects

Antecedent viral infections may occur in association with immune thrombocytopenia, especially in children. The acute form of immune thrombocytopenia may present with significant mucocutaneous (or visceral) hemorrhage, while chronic immune thrombocytopenia usually is more indolent with bruising only. Splenomegaly is usually absent in immune thrombocytopenia. Idiopathic thrombocytopenic purpura is a diagnosis of exclusion, and a search for potential underlying causes of thrombocytopenia is important, including drugs, connective tissue disease, lymphoproliferative disease, and human immunodeficiency virus (HIV) or other infections.

The inherited thrombocytopenic conditions are infrequent and include Fanconi's syndrome and thrombocytopenia with absence of radii, in which megakaryocytic hypoplasia is present. The Wiskott-Aldrich syndrome is another inherited disorder (X-linked) characterized by thrombocytopenia, recurrent infections, and eczema.

Approach to Diagnosis

The widespread use of automated blood counters makes the diagnosis of thrombocytopenia an easy matter. However, spurious thrombocytopenia may be observed, especially in blood specimens obtained from certain patients in whom ethylenediaminetetraacetic acid (EDTA) is used as the anticoagulant. A discrepancy is observed between the platelet count obtained using EDTA-anticoagulated blood and the platelet estimate on the peripheral smear, which reveals platelet clumping and/or platelet satellitism (platelets adherent to neutrophils). A correct automated platelet count can be obtained in these cases by using citrate or heparin as the anticoagulant.

In addition to confirming the automated platelet count, a survey of the blood smear may provide clues to underlying disorders that may be associated with thrombocytopenia (infection, leukemia). Figure 41-1 depicts an algorithm for evaluating patients with thrombocytopenia. If thrombocytopenia is confirmed on evaluation of the blood smear, and there is no obvious reason for the presence of thrombocytopenia, a bone marrow examination is mandatory. The presence or absence of megakaryocytes helps to categorize the thrombocytopenia (Figure 41-1). If megakaryocytes are increased or normal, the marrow is otherwise normal, and if splenomegaly is not present, specific disorders associated with platelet destruction should be evaluated. DIC should be excluded with a test for fibrinogen and D-dimer. Thrombotic thrombocytopenic purpura is a clinical diagnosis suggested by the presence of microangiopathic hemolysis, thrombocytopenia, absence of DIC,

Figure 41-1   Algorithm for evaluation of thrombocytopenia.

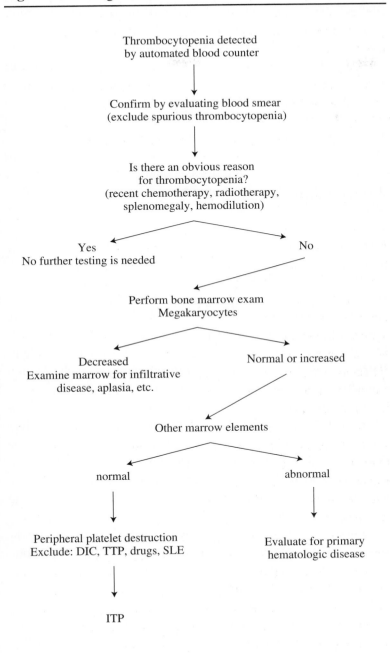

Thrombocytopenia detected
by automated blood counter

↓

Confirm by evaluating blood smear
(exclude spurious thrombocytopenia)

↓

Is there an obvious reason
for thrombocytopenia?
(recent chemotherapy, radiotherapy,
splenomegaly, hemodilution)

Yes ←   → No
No further testing is needed

↓

Perform bone marrow exam
Megakaryocytes

Decreased ←   → Normal or increased
Examine marrow for infiltrative
disease, aplasia, etc.

↓

Other marrow elements

normal ←   → abnormal

↓   ↓

Peripheral platelet destruction   Evaluate for primary
Exclude: DIC, TTP, drugs, SLE   hematologic disease

↓

ITP

Abbreviations: DIC = disseminated intravascular coagulation; TTP = thrombotic thrombocytopenic purpura; SLE = systemic lupus erythematosus; ITP = idiopathic thrombocytopenic purpura.

and other appropriate clinical findings (fever, neurologic abnormalities, renal dysfunction). A drug history is helpful given the large number of medications associated with immune thrombocytopenia. Tests for systemic lupus erythematosus (antinuclear antibodies, anti-double stranded DNA) may uncover a systemic autoimmune disorder. The utility of evaluating the bleeding time in thrombocytopenic patients is marginal.

Clinically important thrombocytopenia (in the absence of platelet dysfunction) does not occur until the platelet count falls below $100 \times 10^3/mm^3$ ($100 \times 10^9/L$), usually below $50 \times 10^3/mm^3$ ($50 \times 10^9/L$). Serious hemorrhage should not occur (again, in the absence of platelet dysfunction) unless the platelet count is under $20 \times 10^3/mm^3$ ($20 \times 10^9/L$).

Hematologic Findings

Peripheral Blood Smear Morphology. In immune thrombocytopenia, the peripheral blood smear is unremarkable except for decreased or absent platelets. If significant hemorrhage has occurred, evidence for iron deficiency may also be present. Atypical lymphocytes suggest a viral origin for thrombocytopenia, such as infectious mononucleosis or HIV infection. Left-shifted myeloid cells (bands, metamyelocytes) together with features of neutrophil toxicity (prominent granules, vacuoles, Döhle bodies) suggest the presence of bacterial infection. Very immature cells (myeloblasts, promyelocytes) indicate a leukemic process, while in aplastic anemia, neutropenia is present along with thrombocytopenia.

Fragmented red blood cells (schistocytes, helmet cells) indicate a microangiopathic hemolytic process (DIC, thrombotic thrombocytopenic purpura, hemolytic-uremic syndrome); these disorders are distinguished by results of coagulation tests for DIC and by the clinical picture. Oval macrocytes and hypersegmented neutrophils are seen in megaloblastic anemia (vitamin B_{12} or folic acid deficiency). Thrombocytopenia seen in association with spherocytes, polychromasia, and an elevated reticulocyte count indicate immune hemolysis and thrombocytopenia (Evan's syndrome).

Bone Marrow Examination. This test is necessary in evaluating most cases of thrombocytopenia to exclude a primary hematologic disorder or a systemic disorder affecting the bone marrow. Disorders involving the marrow will usually be apparent, while the marrow in immune thrombocytopenia will be normal, except for possibly increased megakaryocytes that may be more immature than those found in normal marrows. If the suspicion of marrow disease is low (ie, normal blood smear except for thrombocytopenia, no obvious systemic disease), a bone marrow aspirate without biopsy may be sufficient.

Other Laboratory Tests

41.1 Bleeding Time

The bleeding time will usually be prolonged in most cases of thrombocytopenia, and no useful clinical information will be gained from performing the test in this setting.

41.2 Prothrombin Time and Activated Partial Thromboplastin Time

These tests will be normal in immune thrombocytopenia, unless the patient has an additional disorder (liver disease, systemic lupus erythematosus with a lupus anticoagulant, etc). The prothrombin time and activated partial thromboplastin time, fibrinogen, and D-dimer should be evaluated in all patients with unexplained thrombocytopenia to exclude DIC.

41.3 Platelet Aggregation Studies

Platelet aggregation studies should not be routinely performed in evaluating thrombocytopenic disorders, unless an inherited disorder is suspected. For example, patients with Bernard-Soulier syndrome, an inherited qualitative disorder affecting the von

Willebrand's factor receptor, may have mild thrombocytopenia, and aggregometry will identify these patients. For the majority of patients with acquired thrombocytopenia, little additional clinically useful information will be gained with this test.

41.4 Test for Heparin-Induced Thrombocytopenia

Purpose. Thrombocytopenia may occur as a serious and diagnostically difficult complication of heparin therapy. Five to ten percent of patients may be affected, and a small portion of these have an associated arterial thrombosis. The thrombocytopenia that develops typically occurs 6 to 10 days after initiation of heparin therapy, but may occur after only 2 days in patients who have previously received heparin therapy.

Principle. Serum samples from patients with heparin-induced thrombocytopenia will initiate ^{14}C-serotonin release from labeled platelets at therapeutic concentrations of heparin, but not at high concentrations of heparin.

Specimen. Citrated whole blood is obtained from patients after the development of thrombocytopenia.

Procedure. Platelet-rich plasma is prepared and incubated with ^{14}C-serotonin, and the platelets are then washed. The platelet count is adjusted. Test serum is then mixed with one of two heparin concentrations (0.1 U/mL and 100 U/mL final concentration) and with an aliquot of ^{14}C-serotonin–labeled platelets. After incubation and mixing, EDTA is added to terminate the release reaction. The mixture is then centrifuged, and an aliquot of the supernatant is counted in a scintillation counter. The percentage of serotonin release can then be calculated from the values for background radioactivity, test sample release, and total radioactivity.

Interpretation. A positive test result occurs when there is over 20% release at 0.1 U/mL of heparin and less than 20% release at 100 U/mL of heparin.

Notes and Precautions. This test is not routinely offered by most laboratories because it involves isotopes and is tedious to perform. A recent report has described a mechanism for developing heparin-associated thrombocytopenia that involves complex formation between heparin and platelet factor-4, a platelet-specific α-granule protein. Antibodies to heparin-platelet factor-4 form immune complexes that react with platelet Fc receptors, leading to thrombocytopenia and platelet activation. An enzyme-linked immunosorbent assay (ELISA) was described to identify these patients (Visentin et al). It is likely that commercial equivalents of this ELISA will supplant the previous isotopic platelet aggregation method.

41.5 Test for Platelet-Associated Immunoglobulins

Purpose. This test is used to measure IgG and IgM bound to the patient's platelets (direct test) or present in patient's serum sample (indirect test). The direct test measures autoantibody on the surface of the platelet. It may be useful in distinguishing immune from nonimmune thrombocytopenia. The indirect assay is helpful in detecting the presence of alloantibodies, which may be found in posttransfusion purpura and also may be involved in drug-induced thrombocytopenia.

Principle. Monoclonal antibodies to antigenic determinants on IgG or IgM are obtained. These will bind to their target antigen in a 1:1 ratio, and the amount of ligand may be determined by detection of ^{125}I radiolabel previously attached to the monoclonal antibody. Patient platelets are used in the direct assay and are assayed for the amount of anti-IgG or anti-IgM bound. In the indirect assay, patient serum is first incubated with normal control platelets.

Specimen. The minimum sample required is 35 mL of whole blood collected in EDTA.

Procedure. The platelet count of the sample is determined, and platelet-rich plasma is prepared. A platelet pellet is isolated by centrifugation and then resuspended in buffer. The platelets are washed by the same procedure two more times. The platelets are recentrifuged, taken up in a small aliquot of buffer, and counted. A measured quantity of platelets is then mixed with ^{125}I–labeled anti-IgG (or anti-IgM) monoclonal antibody and incubated with mixing at 37°C. A measured quantity of these platelets is then layered over a phthalate oil support and microcentrifuged. The platelet pellet produced is then isolated and counted in a gamma counter.

The number of IgG (or IgM) molecules on each platelet can then be determined from the known quantities of the specific activity of the antibody, the molecular weight of the targeted immunoglobulin, the number of platelets, and Avogadro's number.

Interpretation. The results are reported as the number of immunoglobulin molecules per platelet. Significantly elevated levels may indicate involvement of an immunologic process. However, the clinical utility of this test is uncertain, since increased amounts of platelet-associated antibody is not specific for immune thrombocytopenia.

Notes and Precautions. A newer method uses flow cytometry to quantitate platelet-associated antibody; however, whether this method is superior to older methods is unproven. One advantage of the flow method is that isotopes are not required. Platelet antibody tests that measure IgG levels on individual platelet glycoproteins may prove to be more useful than currently used methods.

Course and Treatment

Childhood immune thrombocytopenia is usually a self-limited disorder, and most patients recover with no treatment. Adult immune thrombocytopenia virtually always requires treatment. Prednisone is usually the initial therapy (1 mg/kg daily); if no response occurs, or if thrombocytopenia recurs after prednisone dosage taper, splenectomy should be considered. Approximately 60% to 70% of patients will have a complete response (normal platelet count) after splenectomy. Refractory immune thrombocytopenia can be managed by immunosuppression. Intravenous immunoglobulin is the treatment of choice for emergent bleeding associated with immune thrombocytopenia. Following IgG therapy, patients will frequently respond to platelet transfusions.

The primary treatment of thrombocytopenia associated with decreased marrow production of platelets or ineffective megakaryocytopoiesis is platelet transfusion. Posttransfusion platelet counts should be obtained within 1 hour after transfusion to document efficacy of this expensive and potentially risky therapy. Patients with thrombocytopenia due to nonimmune platelet destruction (DIC, thrombotic thrombocytopenic purpura, etc) may not have significant responses to platelet transfusion until the underlying cause for thrombocytopenia has been treated.

References

Bithell TC. Thrombocytopenia: pathophysiology and classification. In: Lee GR, Bithell TC, Foerster J, Athens JW, Lukens JN, eds. *Wintrobe's Clinical Hematology*. Philadelphia, Pa: Lea & Febiger; 1993:1325-1328.

Kelton JG, Murphy WG, Lucarelli A, et al. A prospective comparison of four techniques for measuring platelet-associated IgG. *Br J Haematol.* 1989;71:97-105.

Visentin GP, et al. Antibodies from patients with heparin-induced thrombocytopenia/thrombosis are specific for platelet factor 4 complexed with heparin or bound to endothelial cells. *J Clin Invest.* 1994;93:81-88.

42

Qualitative Platelet Disorders and von Willebrand's Disease

Qualitative platelet disorders refer to the group of bleeding disorders in which platelet dysfunction is associated with a normal platelet count. These disorders are characterized clinically by petechiae and purpura, and can be inherited or acquired.

Pathophysiology of Primary Hemostasis

When platelets are exposed to damaged endothelium, they adhere to the exposed collagen of basement membrane and change their shape from smooth discs to spheres with pseudopods. They then secrete the contents of their granules, a process referred to as the "release reaction." Additional platelets then form aggregates on those platelets that have already adhered to the vessel wall; this constitutes the primary hemostatic plug and arrests bleeding. Shape change and release are induced readily in vitro by a variety of stimuli, and are reversible. Thrombin and adenosine diphosphate (ADP) are potent release and aggregation agents; the addition of relatively low concentrations of ADP to platelet-rich plasma induces primary aggregation of platelets, which is reversible, while the secretion from the platelets of ADP derived from dense bodies during the release reaction induces the secondary phase or irreversible aggregation. Arachidonic acid is formed from platelet phospholipids by the action of phospholipase A_2 whenever platelets are stimulated. Arachidonic acid, in turn, is converted by cyclo-oxygenase to labile endoperoxide precursors (PGG_2 and PGH_2), which, in turn, are converted by thromboxane synthetase to thromboxane A_2. Thromboxane A_2, which has a very short half-life, is a powerful platelet-aggregating agent and vasoconstrictor, and can induce the platelet release reaction. An important controlling mechanism for the release reaction is the concentration of cyclic adenosine monophosphate, which is derived from adenosine triphosphate by adenylate cyclase and is degraded by phosphodiesterase. Cyclic adenosine monophosphate activates a kinase that decreases the sensitivity of platelets to activating stimuli. Theophylline and dipyridamole (Persantine) inhibit phosphodiesterase, and prostacyclin stimulates adenylate cyclase. Both of these actions increase platelet cyclic adenosine monophosphate levels, thereby inhibiting the release reaction. Prostaglandin synthesis also occurs in endothelial cells with formation of arachidonic acid and labile endoperoxides, but there is no thromboxane synthetase in endothelial cells, and prostacyclin is formed instead of thromboxane A_2. Aspirin irreversibly acetylates and inactivates cyclo-oxygenase in the platelets, resulting in decreased synthesis of thromboxane A_2, with inhibition of the release reaction. In endothelial cells, however, decreased prostacyclin synthesis occurs, resulting in enhancement of the platelet release reaction. As endothelial cells, unlike platelets, can synthesize more cyclo-oxygenase, the aspirin effect is relatively short-lived, while the effect on platelets is as long as the life span of the affected platelet (9 to 10 days).

The mechanisms for platelet adhesion and aggregation involve plasma adhesion molecules such as von Willebrand's factor (vWf) and fibrinogen, as well as platelet receptors for these adhesion molecules, glycoprotein Ib and the glycoprotein IIb-IIIa complex, respectively. vWf is essential for normal platelet adhesion; fibrinogen is required for normal platelet aggregation. The fibrinogen receptor (glycoprotein IIb-IIIa) is deficient in the rare inherited qualitative platelet disorder, Glanzmann's thrombasthenia. The receptor for vWf (glycoprotein Ib) is deficient in an inherited platelet disorder known as Bernard-Soulier syndrome.

von Willebrand's disease (vWD) is the most common bleeding disorder and may affect up to 1% of the population; it is characterized by the deficiency or functional abnormality of vWf, the plasma protein essential for normal platelet function. vWf is a high-molecular-weight glycoprotein synthesized by endothelial cells and megakaryocytes, and is present in the α-granules of platelets and in the subendothelium. It circulates in the blood as a noncovalently linked complex with the procoagulant protein, factor VIII (also known as factor VIIIC), which is present in only trace amounts; vWf stabilizes factor VIII and plays an important role in the interaction of platelets with the injured vessel wall. Electrophoresis of normal plasma in agarose-containing sodium dodecyl sulfate, followed by incubation with ^{125}I–labeled antibody to vWf, reveals multiple bands with molecular weights ranging from 1×10^6 to 20×10^6, reflecting the presence of large circulating polymers of a single subunit protein (MW 230,000); this technique is known as multimeric analysis. Incubation of platelets with vWf and the antibiotic ristocetin results in platelet aggregation. It has been shown that the larger multimers of vWf are the most effective in this regard.

Clinical Findings

Most patients with inherited qualitative platelet disorders or vWD usually have a mild to moderate bleeding disorder, in which there is excessive bleeding from the smallest cuts or wounds, a prolonged bleeding time, mucous membrane bleeding, and easy bruising, which occurs after trivial trauma or apparently spontaneously. The ecchymoses are almost invariably superficial, and the deep-tissue hematoma and hemarthroses of severe hemophilia are rarely seen. These disorders are all transmitted in an autosomal manner, but there is an apparent predilection for women, because heavy menstrual bleeding focuses attention on the bleeding disorder. Normally, except in the rare severe cases, the easy bruising and excessive bleeding from cuts are not significant enough to cause patients of either sex to seek medical attention. Many of the cases are so mild that symptoms are manifested only when some precipitating factor, such as ingestion of aspirin or mild associated thrombocytopenia following an infection, is present. A careful history of recent medication use is essential, with special attention to aspirin or over-the-counter pain relievers containing aspirin. Patients frequently deny ingestion of aspirin or any medicines containing aspirin, yet on repeated questioning or after an abnormal result is obtained on platelet function testing, they recall taking an over-the-counter aspirin preparation (see Table 40-5).

Many other drugs, such as antihistamines, may interfere with platelet function; the most important of these are shown in Table 42-1. The thrombocytopenia that can accompany an infectious fever, such as infectious mononucleosis, may precipitate bleeding in a patient with a previously undiagnosed inherited qualitative platelet disorder or vWD. If, in such a case, the first platelet count is performed a few days after the bleeding episode, the reduction in the platelet count may seem insignificant. Subsequent platelet counts, however, will show a progressive increase, suggesting that moderate thrombocytopenia may have existed at the time that bleeding occurred.

Approach to Diagnosis

Figure 42-1 illustrates an algorithm for evaluating patients with suspected platelet-type bleeding disorders. Since patients with Bernard-Soulier syndrome and variant (type IIb) vWD may have mild thrombocytopenia, the presence of thrombocytopenia should not exclude such patients from consideration of disorders of platelet function. This scheme uses the Ivy bleeding time and postaspirin bleeding time as screening tests to justify extensive and expensive hemostatic testing. vWD is also suggested when a family history of bleeding compatible with an autosomal dominant disorder is found. Evaluation of vWD is considered initially because it is much more common than the inherited disorders of platelet dysfunction. The tests used to diagnose vWD are discussed below. Platelet aggregation studies should be reserved for patients in whom vWD has been excluded, and who have a potential inherited qualitative platelet disorder. Platelet aggregation studies are

Table 42-1   Drugs That Affect Platelet Function*

Anesthetics
    Cocaine (local)
    Procaine (local)
    Volatile general anesthetics
Antibiotics
    Ampicillin
    Carbenicillin
    Gentamicin
    Penicillin G
    Ticarcillin
Anticoagulants
    Dextran
    Heparin
Anti-inflammatory Agents and Analgesics
    Aspirin
    Colchicine
    Ibuprofen (Motrin)
    Indomethacin (Indocin)
    Naproxen (Naprosyn)
    Phenylbutazone (Butazolidin)
    Sulfinpyrazone (Anturane)
Cardiovascular Drugs (ie, vasodilators and antilipemic)
    Clofibrate
    Dipyridamole (Persantine)
    Nicotinic acid
    Papaverine (Myobid)
    Theophylline
Genitourinary Drugs
    Furosemide (Lasix)
    Nitrofurantoin (Furadantin)
Psychiatric Drugs
    Phenothiazines
    Tricyclic antidepressants; imipramine (Tofranil),
      Triavil, amitriptyline (Elavil)
Sympathetic Blocking Agents
    Phenoxybenzamine hydrochloride (Dibenzyline)
    Propranolol (Inderal)
Miscellaneous
    Antihistamines (diphenhydramine hydrochloride)
    Ethanol
    Glyceryl guaiacolate ether (cough suppressant)
    Hashish compounds
    Hydroxychloroquine sulfate
    Nitroprusside sodium

*Reprinted with permission from Triplett DA, Harms OS, Newhouse P, et al. *Platelet Function: Laboratory Evaluation and Clinical Application.* Chicago, Ill: ASCP Press; 1978.

rarely needed in the diagnosis of acquired disorders of platelet dysfunction (eg, uremia, myeloproliferative disorder, etc).

Qualitative Platelet Disorders

The inherited platelet disorders may be classified on the basis of findings on platelet aggregation tests (Tables 42-2 and 42-3; Figures 42-1 through 42-5). They fall into three main groups—Bernard-Soulier disease, Glanzmann's thrombasthenia, and thrombopathies. Bernard-Soulier disease is characterized by failure of the platelets to aggregate with ristocetin in the presence of normal plasma; aggregation is normal with ADP, epinephrine, collagen, and thrombin. The aggregation pattern in Bernard-Soulier disease is very similar to that of vWD (Figure 42-4). Moderate thrombocytopenia may be present, and the platelets tend to be very large. The basic defect is an abnormality of a membrane-specific glycoprotein, GPIb. Other similar conditions may have been termed "giant platelet syndromes." Bernard-Soulier disease is inherited in an autosomal recessive manner; it is very rare, and consanguinity is common among the parents of affected individuals. The hemorrhagic manifestations are severe.

Glanzmann's thrombasthenia is another very rare condition in which there is no aggregation with any concentration of ADP, epinephrine, or collagen (Figure 42-3); however, aggregation with ristocetin is normal. Clot retraction is poor or absent. The basic defect is an abnormality or absence of a platelet surface glycoprotein, GP IIb-IIIa. The platelets, while failing to aggregate, undergo most of the normal changes, including the release reaction when stimulated by collagen or thrombin. The platelets on the peripheral blood film are round and isolated, but are otherwise unremarkable. Like Bernard-Soulier disease, the condition is associated with severe bleeding manifestations and is inherited in an autosomal recessive manner.

The thrombopathies, characterized by abnormalities in the release reaction, are quite common, in contrast to Bernard-Soulier and Glanzmann's diseases. They can be divided into two subgroups—storage pool disease, in which there is a deficiency of the specialized pool of ADP, and defects in the mechanism responsible for the release of the storage pool contents. Both of these sub-

Figure 42-1 Algorithm for the diagnosis of qualitative platelet disorders or von Willebrand's disease (vWD).

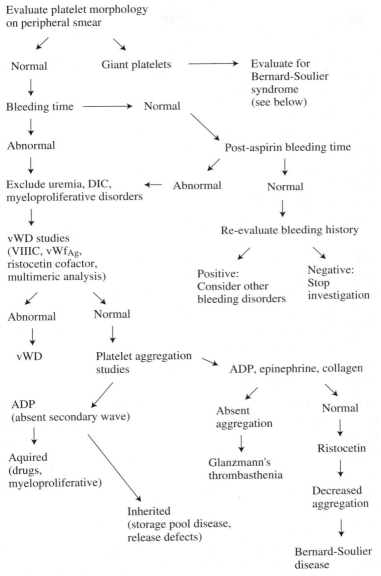

The algorithm uses the bleeding time and postaspirin bleeding time as screening tests.
Evaluation of vWD is considered first because it is much more common than the inherited qualitative platelet disorders.
Abbreviations: DIC = disseminated intravascular coagulation; vWf$_{Ag}$ = von Willebrand's factor antigen; and ADP = adenosine diphosphate.
Reprinted with permission from Rodgers GM. Common clinical bleeding disorders. In: Boldt DH, ed. *Update on Hemostasis*. New York, NY: Churchill Livingstone Inc; 1990:75-120.

Table 42-2 Inherited Qualitative Platelet Disorders: Platelet Aggregation Responses

| Disorders | ADP or Epinephrine | | Collagen | Ristocetin | Special Features |
	Primary	Secondary			
Bernard-Soulier disease	Normal	Normal	Normal	Absent	Large platelets seen on smear, clinically severe
von Willebrand's disease	Normal	Normal	Normal	Absent or decreased	Patient's platelets aggregate with ristocetin in presence of normal plasma
Glanzmann's thrombasthenia	Absent	Absent	Absent	Normal	Clot retraction poor or absent; clinically severe
Storage pool disease	Normal or decreased	Absent	Normal or decreased	Normal	Electron microscopy shows decreased or absent dense granules; platelet ATP:ADP ratio increased
Release defect (aspirin-like disorder)	Normal or decreased	Absent	Normal or decreased	Normal	Normal dense granules on electron microscopy
Intermediate type	Normal	Decreased	Normal or decreased	Normal	Bleeding time abnormal after aspirin ingestion; very mild

Abbreviations: ADP = adenosine diphosphate; ATP = adenosine triphosphate.

Figure 42-2 Platelet aggregation studies: normal tracing. Adenosine diphosphate (ADP) concentration was high (1 μg/mL). Note that the initial steep slope of the primary or reversible wave begins to flatten out and is rapidly followed by the steep slope of the secondary irreversible wave.

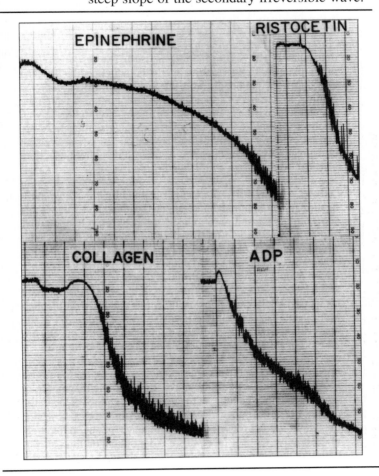

groups are characterized by the absence of a secondary wave of aggregation with epinephrine or ADP; aggregation with ristocetin is normal (Figure 42-5). Differentiation of the two subgroups requires special tests or procedures not usually available in most coagulation laboratories. In storage pool disease, dense granules are decreased, as seen with electron microscopy. In the second subgroup, the dense granules appear normal, but fail to release their constituents when the platelets are exposed to ADP, epinephrine, or collagen. This type is by far the most frequently encountered type of inherited qualitative abnormality of platelets, and the platelet defects closely resemble those seen after ingestion of aspirin. It has been pointed out recently that many patients with this condition have normal to borderline bleeding times, which are significantly prolonged after aspirin ingestion; this type of case has been referred to as intermediate syndrome of platelet dysfunction. For convenience, however, this condition may be considered a very mild type of release defect. Its importance lies in the fact that postoperative bleeding can be avoided in these patients by abstinence from drugs known to interfere with platelet function. The condition may not be recognized with routine screening tests for hemostasis.

Qualitative platelet abnormalities have been reported in patients with glycogen storage disease, type I, and Wilson's disease, as well as in some patients with inherited disorders of connective tissue, including Ehlers-Danlos and Marfan's syndromes (Table 42-3).

von Willebrand's disease

There are several variants of vWD. The great majority of cases exhibit a quantitative deficiency of vWf. The activity of this protein, as determined by ristocetin cofactor activity, is reduced in proportion to the protein (vWf antigen), as measured with immunologic methods, usually by Laurell immunoelectrophoresis. In addition, the factor VIII coagulant activity seen in these patients is reduced similar to the ristocetin cofactor activity and the vWf antigen. Multimeric analysis reveals all polymeric forms for vWf, but the intensity of the bands is decreased (Figure 42-6). This is by far the most frequently encountered type of vWD and is referred to as type I. The bleeding time is usually also prolonged. Asymptomatic or mild forms of this type of vWD are frequently found, in which the level of the vWf falls between 40% and 60%; in these patients, the bleeding time is usually normal. Another frequently encountered type is referred to as type IIA. In this form of the disease, a qualitative defect of vWf is seen, while the amount of protein synthesized may be normal. The defect appears to be a failure to form

Table 42-3   Inherited Conditions Associated With Decreased Platelet Aggregation*

Glanzmann's thrombasthenia
Essential athrombia
Storage pool defect (decreased content of ADP)
    Chédiak-Higashi syndrome
    Thrombocytopenia with absent radii (TAR syndrome)
    Wiskott-Aldrich syndrome
    Hermansky-Pudlak syndrome
Aspirin-like defect
    Cyclo-oxygenase deficiency
    Thromboxane synthetase deficiency
Inborn errors of metabolism
    Homocystinuria
    Wilson's disease
    Glycogen storage disease, type I
Connective tissue abnormalities
    Ehlers-Danlos syndrome (collagen[†])
    Pseudoxanthoma elasticum (collagen[†])
    Osteogenesis imperfecta (collagen[†])
    Marfan's syndrome
    Constitutional abnormality of collagen (patient's collagen only[†])
Afibrinogenemia
Bernard-Soulier disease (ristocetin[†])
von Willebrand's disease (ristocetin[†])
Gray platelet syndrome

*Reprinted with permission from Triplett DA, Harms CS, Newhouse P, et al. *Platelet Function: Laboratory Evaluation and Clinical Application.* Chicago, Ill: ASCP Press; 1978.
[†]The abnormal aggregation patterns are obtained only when this aggregation reagent is used.

---

the intermediate and large multimers, which is revealed on multimeric analysis (Figure 42-6) or, alternatively, on crossed immunoelectrophoresis. In type IIA, the bleeding time is usually prolonged, and the factor VIII level is decreased or normal. Other types of vWD appear to be less common. The recognition of type IIB is considered important because these patients may not respond to desmopressin (1-deamino-8-D-arginine vasopressin [DDAVP]). In this form of the disease, the bleeding time is prolonged, and vWf antigen is usually reduced, while the ristocetin cofactor activity is somewhat lower than that of the antigen. The diagnostic feature is that a concentration of ristocetin too low to induce aggregation in

Figure 42-3 Platelet aggregation studies: Glanzmann's thrombasthenia. Note absent aggregation with epineph-
rine, collagen, and adenosine diphosphate
(ADP), but normal aggregation with ristocetin.

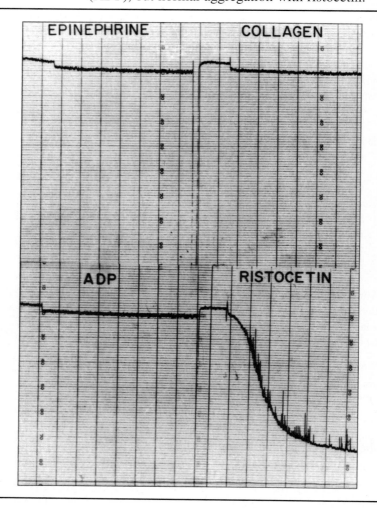

normal platelet-rich plasma will do so in the patient's platelet-rich
plasma. In this form of the disease, the largest multimers appear to
be lacking (Figure 42-6), and it resembles another very rare form
(pseudo-vWD or platelet-type vWD), in which there are abnormal
platelet receptors for vWf. The laboratory findings in type IIB and

Figure 42-4 Platelet aggregation studies: von Willebrand's disease (vWD). Note absent aggregation with ristocetin, but normal aggregation with epinephrine, collagen, and adenosine diphosphate (ADP). In milder cases, ristocetin aggregation is diminished but not absent. A similar pattern is seen in the inherited qualitative platelet disorder, Bernard-Soulier disease. Decreased ristocetin cofactor activity in vWD distinguishes it from Bernard-Soulier disease.

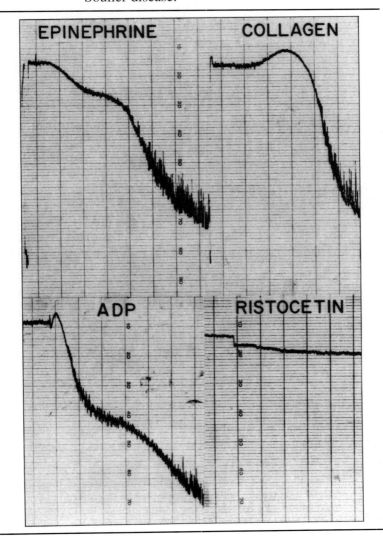

Figure 42-5 Platelet aggregation studies: storage pool disease. Note primary aggregation waves with epinephrine, collagen, and adenosine diphosphate (ADP), with absence of secondary waves. The response to ristocetin is normal. Similar tracings may be seen with aspirin ingestion or defects in the platelet release reaction (secretion).

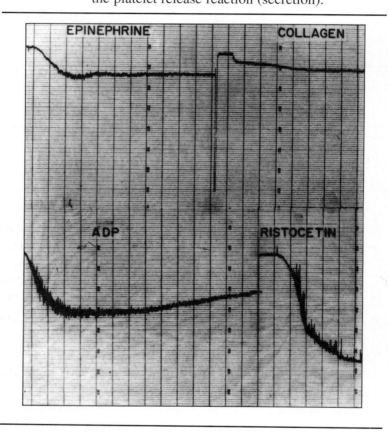

the platelet-type are similar, showing enhanced responsiveness of platelet-rich plasma to lower-than-normal concentrations of ristocetin. Direct binding of vWf to the patient's platelets with aggregation in the absence of another agonist, however, has been demonstrated in the platelet-type vWD. Patients with type III vWD have a severe bleeding disorder resembling hemophilia A. These

Table 42-4   Laboratory Features of von Willebrand's Disease*

	Type I	Type IIA	Type IIB	Type III	Platelet-Type
Bleeding time	I	I	I	I	I
Factor VIIIC activity	D	D or N	D or N	D	D or N
von Willebrand's factor antigen	D	N or D	N or D	D	D or N
Ristocetin cofactor activity	D	D	D or N	D	D
Ristocetin-induced platelet aggregation	D or N	D	I	D	I
Multimeric analysis	N	A	A	A	A

Abbreviations: I = increased; D = decreased; N = normal; A = abnormal.
*The bleeding time (or postaspirin bleeding time) is usually increased in all patients. Since patients with mild von Willebrand's disease may have borderline normal test results, repeated testing may be necessary to establish the diagnosis.

have very low levels of factor VIIIC, vWf antigen, and ristocetin cofactor activity. The laboratory features of vWD are summarized in Table 42-4.

Acquired forms of vWD have been reported. These disorders may result from development of an autoantibody against vWf appearing in a previously healthy individual without any apparent cause or in an individual with systemic lupus erythematosus. Acquired vWD may also occur in lymphoma or multiple myeloma due to the presence of an abnormal protein that in some way inhibits a hypothetical physiologic counterpart of ristocetin.

Qualitative abnormalities of platelets are encountered in the myeloproliferative disorders (especially essential thrombocytosis) and, to a lesser extent, in polycythemia vera and myelofibrosis with myeloid metaplasia. Mild abnormalities are found in uremia and cirrhosis. Certain acquired disorders of platelet function result from in vivo platelet activation, and result in an acquired storage pool defect (certain disorders associated with antiplatelet antibodies or immune complexes, disseminated intravascular coagulation, cardiopulmonary bypass, hairy cell leukemia) (Table 42-5). Evaluation of these disorders proceeds as follows:

Figure 42-6 Multimeric analysis of von Willebrand's factor. Plasma was obtained from a normal subject (N), and from patients with various types of von Willebrand's disease (I, IIA, IIB, III). Plasma was electrophoresed in an agarose gel, then von Willebrand's factor was identified using an immunoperoxidase method. The dark bands at the top of the gel (N) represent the high-molecular-weight multimers most important in platelet adhesion. Note the generalized decrease in band intensity characteristic of type I, loss of intermediate and high-molecular-weight multimers in type IIA, loss of only high-molecular-weight multimers in type IIB, and virtual absence of all multimers in type III. This photograph is taken from an idealized drawing.

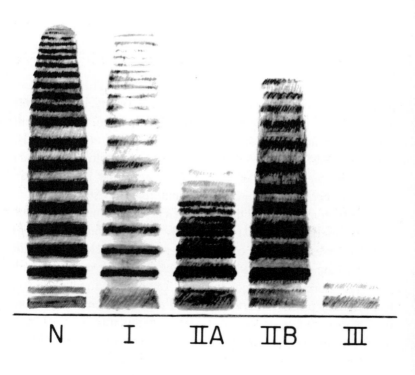

Table 42-5   Acquired Conditions Associated With Platelet Dysfunction

---

Myeloproliferative disorders
    Essential thrombocytosis
    Polycythemia vera
    Myelofibrosis
Lymphoproliferative disorders
    Waldenström's macroglobulinemia
    Myeloma
Other hematologic disorders
    Paroxysmal nocturnal hemoglobinuria
    Acute myeloid leukemia
    Sideroblastic anemia
    Immune thrombocytopenia
    Hairy cell leukemia
Cirrhosis
Uremia
Drug-induced
Disseminated intravascular coagulation
Cardiopulmonary bypass
Connective tissue disorders

---

1. Hematologic evaluation with particular attention to platelet number and morphology.

2. Screening tests for hemostasis, including the activated partial thromboplastin time (aPTT), prothrombin time (PT), bleeding time, and the platelet count. In general, a coagulation-type abnormality may be excluded if the aPTT and prothrombin time are normal. If results of one or both of these tests are prolonged, specific assays are performed (see Chapter 40). If the bleeding time test result is normal and a qualitative platelet abnormality is suspected, the test may be repeated 2 hours after ingestion of two aspirin (aspirin tolerance test), but this should be performed only when all other types of coagulopathies have been excluded.

3. vWD is evaluated by testing the three components of the von Willebrand's panel—factor VIII coagulant activity, vWf antigen, and ristocetin cofactor activity. Classification of vWD subtypes is performed using multimeric analysis.

4. Platelet aggregation tests, which are nonquantitative, are primarily used for the diagnosis of the qualitative platelet disorders. Less commonly, some patients with vWD will have a normal von Willebrand's panel, but will exhibit abnormal ristocetin-induced platelet aggregation. If ristocetin-induced platelet aggregation is abnormal and the aggregation patterns with ADP, collagen, epinephrine, and arachidonic acid are normal, the patient has vWD or, rarely, Bernard-Soulier disease. A ristocetin cofactor activity test is then performed, using the patient's plasma specimen and freshly washed or formalin-fixed normal platelets. This test gives a measure of the vWf activity in the plasma specimen. It is normal in Bernard-Soulier disease, because normal platelets are used in the test; the defect in Bernard-Soulier disease resides in the platelets, whereas the plasma is normal. This is the reverse of vWD, in which the plasma ristocetin cofactor activity is reduced.

Hematologic Findings

General features are usually unremarkable, and apart from the Bernard-Soulier syndrome in which giant platelets are seen, abnormal platelets are seen only rarely on the smear. On occasion, there may be hematologic features consistent with iron deficiency anemia.

Peripheral Blood Smear Morphology.   The number of platelets in the peripheral blood should be estimated, and the presence of any large platelets should be noted. Unless there has been significant bleeding, the red and white blood cells will be normal. A direct platelet count should be performed.

Bone Marrow Examination.   Characteristic changes in bone marrow are seen with acquired platelet defects secondary to myeloproliferative or myelodysplastic disorders, or in association with the dysproteinemias of lymphoproliferative disorders.

Other Laboratory Tests

42.1 Platelet Aggregation Test

Purpose.   Platelet aggregation tests are used to detect abnormalities in platelet function (Figures 42-2 through 42-5). Such defects, which may be inherited or may result from the ingestion of certain drugs, can be the cause of bleeding in certain patients.

Principle.   When an aggregating agent is added to a platelet-rich plasma specimen in the cuvette of an aggregometer, the initially turbid platelet-rich plasma specimen clears as platelets clump, permitting more light to pass through the plasma. The aggregometer is basically a photo-optical instrument, and the amount of light transmitted through the cuvette is recorded on a strip of recording chart.

Specimen.   A platelet-rich plasma specimen is prepared from whole blood anticoagulated with sodium citrate. The responsiveness of the platelets to aggregating agents is influenced by the time elapsing from collection, and the tests should be completed within 1 to 3 hours of collection. The temperature at which the platelet-rich plasma specimen is prepared, as well as the temperature at which the actual aggregation tests are carried out, have a significant influence on the rate and extent of aggregation. Platelets prepared at room temperature are more sensitive to ADP than are platelets stored at 37°C.

Procedure.   Platelet-rich plasma is obtained by the slow centrifugation of whole blood anticoagulated with sodium citrate; this procedure is carried out in plastic tubes at room temperature, and at no time should the plasma be cooled. The supernatant (platelet-rich plasma) is pipetted off and retained. The remaining portion of anticoagulated blood is recentrifuged at high speed to obtain a platelet-poor plasma specimen. The platelet-rich plasma specimen is then mixed with a platelet-poor plasma specimen to obtain a final platelet count of 250,000/mm³ (250 x 10⁹/L). The aggregation agents used are ADP, collagen suspensions (which may be obtained commercially or prepared by homogenizing tissue obtained on site), epinephrine, and ristocetin (Figures 42-2 through 42-5); some laboratories also use arachidonic acid or calcium ionophore. A blank value is obtained by using a platelet-poor plasma sample from the patient. The adjusted platelet-containing plasma sample is placed in the cuvette and warmed to 37°C, the aggregating agent is added, and the contents of the cuvette are stirred constantly by means of a small Teflon® stirring rod.

Interpretation. The results with each aggregation agent may be recorded as the slope of the curve, the absolute magnitude of the transmittance change, or the percentage change of the transmittance or of the optical density. In most laboratories, however, the results are not reported in a quantitative manner, but merely in descriptive terms, ie, normal vs abnormal aggregation, with a comment as to the type of abnormality. The results depend on the concentration of the aggregating agents, which should be stated in the report. With relatively low doses of ADP (1 µg/mL), two waves of aggregation are seen. The first, or primary, wave is induced by the ADP added to the patient's plasma, while the secondary wave is attributed to release of relatively large amounts of intrinsic ADP from the storage pool within the platelets (release reaction). With even lower concentrations of ADP (0.5 µg/mL), the release reaction does not occur, the platelets disaggregate, and only a primary wave is seen, while with relatively large doses of ADP a single broad wave is seen. A biphasic response is seen with epinephrine in up to 80% of healthy persons. However, 20% to 30% of healthy people will exhibit abnormal epinephrine aggregation. Because collagen acts by inducing release of ADP, a primary wave is not seen. In thrombasthenia, there is no aggregation with any concentration of ADP, epinephrine, or collagen, but aggregation is seen with ristocetin (Figure 42-3). In storage pool disease and in release defects (aspirin-catalyzed disorders), the secondary waves with ADP and epinephrine are absent (Figure 42-5), and aggregation with collagen is reduced or absent; ristocetin aggregation is normal.

More subtle changes may be clinically significant when ristocetin is used as the aggregating agent, and the slope should be compared with that of the control. A normal tracing with ristocetin does not exclude a moderate deficiency of vWf. Thus, when this disease is suspected, a quantitative ristocetin cofactor activity must be performed. In addition to the usual concentration of ristocetin, a lower concentration (0.5 mg/mL final concentration) should also be used in the platelet aggregation test to detect the rare type IIB, vWD. In this condition, aggregation occurs with the patient's platelet-rich plasma specimen and the lower concentration of ristocetin, while aggregation with the normal control platelet-rich plasma specimen and the low ristocetin concentration is not seen.

Notes and Precautions. Specimens left for more than 4 hours at room temperature may lose their ability to aggregate. Platelets stored at 0°C sometimes undergo spontaneous aggregation. Plasma should not be lipemic or icteric. Whenever an unexpectedly abnormal result is obtained, the test should be repeated on another specimen collected some days later.

42.2 von Willebrand Factor–Ristocetin Cofactor Activity Test

Purpose. This test is used to measure the biologic activity of the patient's vWf.

Principle. The ability of the patient's plasma specimen to aggregate normal platelets in the presence of ristocetin is compared with that of a normal pooled plasma specimen.

Specimen. Plasma specimens used for the aPTT or PT tests are satisfactory; the specimens may be stored for several weeks at -70°C without losing activity.

Procedure. A standard curve is prepared by making serial dilutions of plasma in saline. An aliquot of each is then added to a fixed amount of a saline suspension of washed platelets in the cuvette of an aggregometer. Ristocetin is then added and the slope of the wave determined (maximum change in light transmittance). By plotting slope against dilution of the plasma on log-log paper, a straight line is obtained. A dilution of the patient's plasma specimen is then tested, and the equivalent dilution of the normal plasma specimen that would give the same slope is read from the straight-line curve, eg, if a 1:5 dilution of the patient's plasma specimen gives the same slope as a 1:10 dilution of normal plasma specimen, the activity of vWf in the patient's plasma specimen is 50% of that of the normal control subject.

Interpretation. A decrease in vWf parameters in a patient with a lifelong history of bleeding is diagnostic of vWD. Acquired deficiencies caused by antibodies against vWf and certain paraproteins may also result in a decrease in vWf.

42.3 Laurell Immunoelectrophoresis Assay for von Willebrand's Factor Antigen

Purpose. The immunoelectrophoresis assay is used for the diagnosis of vWD. In this disease, vWf antigen is usually decreased.

Principle. A precipitating rabbit antibody is used to quantitate vWf. The immunoassay is usually performed using the Laurell technique, which is an electroimmunodiffusion method for the quantitation of proteins in which rocket-shaped anodic immunoprecipitates are formed. The height of the rocket is proportional to the concentration of vWf.

Specimen. The patient's plasma or serum sample may be used, but the former is preferable. Plasma sample collected for the aPTT or PT test is satisfactory.

Procedure.   The antibody is mixed with liquid agarose, which is then poured onto a plate and allowed to solidify by cooling. Holes are punched on one side of the plate, which is then placed in an electrophoresis chamber. Serial dilutions of normal pooled plasma (1:2, 1:4, 1:8, etc, in saline) are made to prepare the standard curve. The 1:2 and 1:4 dilutions of the plasma being tested are prepared and placed in the wells. Electrophoresis of the sample is then performed, and when the run is completed, the plate is examined. The rocket-shaped immunoprecipitates are sometimes hard to see, but the visibility can be increased by immersing the plates in tannic acid for a few minutes.

Interpretation.   A value below 40% is consistent with vWD, and values between 40% and 60% are borderline. vWf antigen and ristocetin cofactor activity are both increased by exercise, by hepatitis, by estrogen therapy, and during pregnancy. Patients with vWD and these conditions may have normal levels of vWf. Repeated testing may be necessary to diagnose vWD.

Notes and Precautions.   The determination of vWf antigen, often referred to as factor VIII–related antigen, should be distinguished from the determination of the factor VIII antigen. The latter is the antigen corresponding to the factor VIII coagulant protein, which is decreased in at least 90% of patients with hemophilia A. The test to determine factor VIII antigen is currently available in only a few laboratories.

42.4 von   Willebrand's   Factor   Multimeric Analysis

Purpose.   This test measures the qualitative aspects of vWf in a plasma specimen of patients with vWD.

Principle.   The patient's vWf is separated by gel electrophoresis and identified with immunologic methods. The patient's multimeric pattern is compared to that of normal patients.

Specimen.   Plasma specimens used for the aPTT and PT assays are satisfactory. Plasmas frozen at -70°C for several weeks may also be used.

Procedure.   An agarose gel is prepared (1% to 2%, FMC Bioproducts), and patient and normal plasma samples are electrophoresed. The electrophoresed plasma proteins are then transferred to nitrocellulose paper and incubated with an antibody to vWf. Immunodetection of multimers can be performed with an ^{125}I label on the antibody, followed by autoradiography, or with the avidin-biotin-peroxidase technique.

Interpretation.   Patients with type I vWD will have the full range of multimers, but reduced quantities; type IIA patients will be missing the intermediate and high-molecular-weight bands, while type IIB patients will be missing the highest-molecular-weight bands. Type III patients will show a virtual absence of all bands (see Figure 42-6).

Notes and Precautions.   This is a laborious technique for most laboratories, and this test is performed usually by coagulation reference laboratories.

References

Bennett JS, Shattil SJ. Congenital qualitative platelet disorders. In: Williams WJ, Beutler E, Erslev AJ, Lichtman MA, eds. *Hematology*. New York, NY: McGraw-Hill Publishing Inc; 1990:1407-1419.

Bennett JS. Platelet aggregation. In: Williams WJ, Beutler E, Erslev AJ, Lichtman MA, eds. *Hematology*. New York, NY: McGraw-Hill Publishing Inc; 1990: 1778-1781.

Zimmerman TS, Ruggeri ZM. von Willebrand's disease. *Hum Pathol*. 1987; 18:140-152.

43

Inherited Coagulation Disorders

Inherited coagulation disorders result from quantitative deficiency or qualitative abnormality of a clotting factor. Deficiency of factors VIII or IX (hemophilia A or B, respectively) constitute the vast majority of patients with inherited coagulation disorders.

Pathophysiology

When a small vessel is punctured or cut, a hemostatic plug formed from aggregated platelets seals the leak, and the plug is subsequently reinforced by fibrin. In conditions in which the formation of fibrin is abnormal, the hemostatic plug may be relatively weak and unstable, resulting in delayed bleeding, sometimes several days following the injury. Based on the degree of severity of symptoms for the same level of reduced activity, factors VIII and IX appear to be the two most important procoagulant factors required for normal hemostasis. Factor XI deficiency is either very mild or asymptomatic, while factors V, VII, or X deficiencies are intermediate in severity. Deficiencies of the contact factors are not associated with any clinically important hemostatic abnormalities, which may be explained by the presence of bypass mechanisms (see Chapter 40).

Clinical Findings

The characteristic clinical features of a bleeding disorder caused by an abnormality of a blood clotting factor (features that distinguish them from platelet disorders) are outlined in Table 40-2.

The great majority of inherited disorders of the coagulation type are relatively benign, and bleeding only occurs when the hemostatic mechanism is severely challenged. A history of easy bruising and excessive bleeding after minor surgery, such as tonsillectomy or tooth extraction, usually exists. Such bleeding is troublesome but rarely life-threatening. Hemarthroses are usually seen only in severe cases, but may occur in mild cases following joint injury. The clinical differentiation of a coagulation-type disorder from a platelet-type disorder may be difficult, but a history of bleeding from a wound or injury starting after an interval of several hours or days suggests a coagulation-type rather than a platelet-type disorder. The lifelong nature of the bleeding disorder is usually sufficient to permit categorization of the disorder as inherited rather than acquired. Acquired disorders of clotting are considered in Chapter 44.

Approach to Diagnosis

Hemarthroses in a male patient may be considered the hallmark of a severe coagulation disorder. If this is sex-linked, the patient has either hemophilia A or hemophilia B; exceptions to this rule are rare. All that is then needed to establish the diagnosis is a specific assay of factor VIII, and if the results are normal, an assay for factor IX. Petechiae or purpura are rare in a coagulation disorder and suggest either von Willebrand's disease or the coexistence of thrombocytopenia or a qualitative platelet disorder.

Evaluation of inherited coagulation disorders proceeds as follows:

1. Hematologic evaluation to exclude thrombocytopenia and anemia.

Table 43-1 PT and aPTT Profiles in Inherited Deficiencies of Clotting Factors

Factor	aPTT	PT
HMW-K, prekallikrein, XII, XI, IX, VIII	Increased	Normal
V, X, prothrombin hypofibrinogenemia	Increased	Increased
VII	Normal	Increased
Dysfibrinogenemia	Increased or normal	Increased or normal
XIII deficiency	Normal	Normal

Abbreviations: HMW-K = high-molecular-weight kininogen; PT = prothrombin time; aPTT = activated partial thromboplastin time.

2. Screening tests of coagulation, including activated partial thromboplastin time (aPTT) and prothrombin time (PT). The necessity for, and nature of, subsequent studies depend on the results of these tests (Tables 43-1 and 43-2). If the diagnosis of an inherited coagulation disorder is uncertain, bleeding disorders such as von Willebrand's disease or qualitative platelet dysfunction should be considered (Chapter 42).

3. An isolated prolonged PT suggests factor VII deficiency, which can be confirmed with a specific assay for factor VII.

4. An isolated prolonged aPTT in a patient with lifelong bleeding suggests deficiency of factors VIII, IX, or XI. von Willebrand's disease should also be considered, especially if the bleeding time is prolonged or if an autosomal dominant pattern of bleeding exists in the family history.

5. Since deficiency of factor XII, high-molecular-weight kininogen (HMW-K), or prekallikrein is not associated with excessive bleeding, their routine assay is not necessary to evaluate prolonged aPTT values in patients with bleeding disorders.

6. If both the aPTT and PT assays are prolonged, deficiency of prothrombin, fibrinogen, or factors V or X is possible. A prolonged thrombin time in such cases suggests hypofibrinogenemia or dysfibrinogenemia, and specific fibrinogen assays (functional and antigenic) will identify these patients. A normal thrombin time in such cases necessitates

Table 43-2   Use of aPTT, PT, and Bleeding Time Tests for
Screening for Inherited Bleeding Disorders

aPTT	PT	Bleeding Time	Further Tests to be Performed
Normal	Normal	Normal or increased	Platelet aggregation studies, vWD studies, factor XIII screen
Increased	Normal	Increased	VIIIC assay, vWf_{Ag}, ristocetin cofactor activity
Increased	Normal	Normal	VIIIC assay, if normal, IX, then XI; if VIII is low, perform vWf_{Ag} and ristocetin cofactor activity, exclude inhibitor
Increased	Increased	Normal or increased	Thrombin time, if normal, do V, X, and prothrombin assays; if thrombin time is prolonged, assay fibrinogen by functional and antigenic methods
Normal	Increased	Normal or increased	VII assay

Abbreviations: aPTT = activated partial thromboplastin time; PT = prothrombin time;
vWD = von Willebrand's disease; vWf = von Willebrand's factor; Ag = antigen;
VIIIC = factor VIII coagulant activity.

specific assays for factors V, X, and prothrombin to identify the deficient factor.

7. If the aPTT, PT, and thrombin time are normal, a test for clot
solubility in 5 mol/L of urea should be performed to exclude
factor XIII deficiency.

8. When the aPTT is prolonged and the PT is normal, the
aPTT should be repeated using a mixture of equal parts of
the patient's plasma and normal plasma. This test is called
an inhibitor screen (mixing study) and is useful to screen
for antibodies or other inhibitors (heparin). This test is,
however, relatively insensitive and nonspecific, and in all
patients with a known deficiency of factor VIII, a specific
test for the presence of an antibody against factor VIII
should be performed. In patients with other types of inherited deficiencies, the development of an antibody specifically directed against the deficient factor is rare.
Accordingly, unless there is some unusual circumstance,
such as failure to respond to treatment with the appropriate
concentrate, or when the aPTT inhibitor screen is positive,

Table 43-3 Distinguishing vWD From Hemophilia A

Characteristic	vWD	Hemophilia A
Inheritance	Autosomal dominant	Sex-linked recessive
Hemarthroses or joint damage	Rare	Present in most severe cases
Clinical severity	Usually mild and rarely dangerous or crippling	Mild to severe cases
Bleeding time	May be prolonged	Normal if performed correctly
Factor VIIIC level	Usually 6% to 50%	0% to 35%
vWf antigen	<50%	>50%
Ristocetin cofactor activity	Abnormal	Normal

Abbreviations: vWD = von Willebrand's disease; vWf = von Willebrand's factor; VIIIC = factor VIII coagulant activity.

a specific search for antibody is not a routine part of the evaluation of hereditary deficiencies of a clotting factor other than factor VIII.

9. In some patients with von Willebrand's disease, the bleeding time may be normal and the clinical and laboratory findings may mimic those seen in mild hemophilia (Table 43-3). It is therefore necessary to consider testing for von Willebrand's disease in all patients with decreased levels of factor VIII in whom there is no clear-cut sex-linked family history.

10. Patients with mild bleeding disorders may have normal results on screening studies. If vascular disorders are excluded (hereditary hemorrhagic telangiectasia), the following hemostatic disorders should be considered in these patients: von Willebrand's disease, carriers for factor VIII or IX deficiency, factor XI deficiency, dysfibrinogenemia, factor XIII deficiency, platelet dysfunction, and alpha$_2$-antiplasmin deficiency. It is important to remember that normal coagulation screening tests do not exclude a significant hemostatic defect.

Figure 43-1 summarizes one approach to evaluating isolated, prolonged aPTT values in patients with bleeding disorders.

Figure 43-1   An approach to the evaluation of a patient with bleeding and prolonged activated partial thromboplastin time (aPTT).*

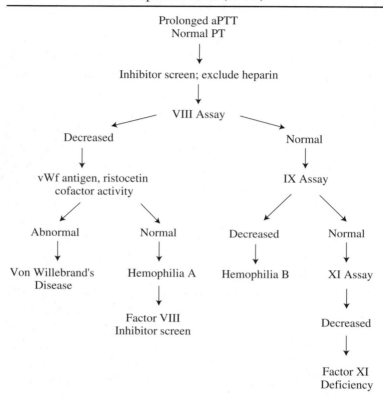

Abbreviation: PT = prothrombin time.
*This algorithm refers only to patients with clinical bleeding who are candidates for an inherited disorder, and who have prolonged aPTT values. Patients who have negative diagnostic studies as listed above should be further evaluated for lupus anticoagulants associated with platelet dysfunction, thrombocytopenia, or hypoprothrombinemia.

Hematologic Findings

Apart from the exclusion of anemia and thrombocytopenia, the morphology of the formed elements in the blood are usually unremarkable.

Blood Cell Measurements.   Blood counts and red blood cell morphology may be consistent with chronic blood loss.

Other Laboratory Tests

43.1 Assay for Factor VIII

Purpose. The determination of the factor VIII level is necessary for the diagnosis of hemophilia A and von Willebrand's disease. The level usually correlates well with clinical severity. Assays are also used for monitoring the response to therapy. Factor VIII is usually decreased in von Willebrand's disease in proportion to the level of von Willebrand's factor. While hemophilia A carriers also have decreased levels of factor VIII, their von Willebrand's factor antigen level is normal. Stress or pregnancy in hemophilia A carriers may cause the factor VIII to rise to normal, but the ratio of von Willebrand's factor antigen to factor VIII activity remains increased. Factor VIII deficiency must be considered in every patient who has a coagulopathy with a prolonged aPTT and a normal PT.

Principle. The ability of dilutions of a sample of patient plasma deficient in factor VIII to correct the prolonged aPTT of commercially deficient plasma is compared with that of normal pooled plasma. For example, if a 1:20 dilution of normal plasma shortens the clotting time of the deficient plasma to the same extent as a 1:5 dilution of the patient's plasma, the latter sample has 25% of normal activity.

Specimen. The plasma sample collected for the PT or aPTT assay is used. Factor VIII activity is fairly stable, and the test may be performed on a plasma sample frozen within 30 minutes of collection and stored at $-30°C$.

Procedure. The deficient plasma sample used is obtained from a patient known to have less than 1% factor VIII. It may be kept for several years if stored at $-70°C$. Dilutions of normal pooled plasma (1:5, 1:10, 1:20, 1:40, 1:80) and the patient's plasma sample (1:5, 1:10) in saline are prepared. One part of each dilution is added to one part of the deficient plasma, and an aPTT is performed in duplicate.

Interpretation.   The 1:5 dilution of the normal pooled plasma sample is arbitrarily taken as 100% activity, the 1:10 as 50%, the 1:20 as 25%, and so forth. A line of best fit is obtained on log-log paper when clotting times are plotted against percentage concentration of normal plasma. The normal plasma concentrations that would give the same clotting times as the 1:5 and 1:10 dilutions of the patient's plasma sample are determined from the graph. The percentage concentration obtained with the 1:5 dilution is the actual concentration of factor VIII in the patient's plasma sample, while the value obtained with the 1:10 dilution has to be multiplied by 2. The mean of the two values is reported. If the value with the 1:10 dilution is significantly higher than that of the 1:5 dilution, an inhibitor should be suspected, but the assay should be repeated to exclude an error in technique. The normal range for factors VIII and IX is approximately 60% to 150%.

Notes and Precautions.   The activity of factor VIII may be increased significantly by trace amounts of thrombin that may form if the blood is collected too slowly or if it is incompletely mixed with the anticoagulant. Factor VIII is also sometimes increased in low-grade disseminated intravascular coagulation, presumably owing to thrombin activation. Vigorous exercise for 5 minutes may double or even triple the level, which may remain high for several hours.

43.2 Assays for Other Factors Involved in Intrinsic Coagulation Only

Purpose.   Assays for other factors involved in the intrinsic pathway may reveal the cause of a prolonged aPTT not attributable to factor VIII.

Principle.   The principle is the same as that underlying the one-stage procedure for the factor VIII assay described previously. The relative ability of plasma to shorten prolonged aPTTs of commercially deficient plasma is compared with that of pooled normal plasma.

Procedure. The procedure is the same as that described for the assay of factor VIII, using the appropriate deficient plasma in place of factor VIII–deficient plasma. For the assay of prekallikrein, the preincubation period in the aPTT test after addition of contact activator should not exceed 3 minutes; longer incubation periods cause the aPTT of prekallikrein-deficient plasma to approach the normal value. Accordingly, certain automated instruments in which the preincubation period exceeds 3 minutes cannot be used. In the HMW-K assay, the 1:20 dilution of normal plasma may be as effective in shortening the aPTT of the HMW-K–deficient plasma as the 1:5 dilution. Therefore, in performing this assay, it is advisable to start at a 1:20 dilution and to continue up to a 1:640 dilution. The unknown is tested at 1:5 dilution up to a 1:20 dilution.

Interpretation. The normal range for these factors is approximately 60% to 150%.

Notes and Precautions. The deficient plasma may be obtained from a commercial source. Prekallikrein and HMW-K–deficient plasmas are rare, and accordingly, few coagulation laboratories are able to perform these assays, although they are technically quite simple. In most instances, however, a provisional diagnosis of these two deficiencies may be made by a process of exclusion. Thus, if the patient has a prolonged aPTT, normal PT, normal levels of the relevant intrinsic factors (factors VIII, IX, and XI), and a negative bleeding history, a deficiency of factor XII, prekallikrein or HMW-K should be considered. Prekallikrein-deficient plasma shortens progressively on incubation with kaolin (Celite), and may be normal after 8 minutes of preincubation, thereby distinguishing it from HMW-K deficiency or factor XII deficiency.

43.3 Assays for Prothrombin and Factors V, VII, and X

Purpose. Assays for prothrombin and factors V, VII, and X are performed to determine the specific cause(s) of a prolonged PT.

Principle. The principle is the same as that for the assays described previously, but the PT is used instead of the aPTT.

Specimen. Blood is collected in the same manner as for the factor VIII assay. The assay for factor V should be performed within 4 hours of collection because it is relatively labile. Assays for factor VII are best performed as soon as possible after collection because factor VII may increase in activity when the plasma is stored in the refrigerator (cold activation).

Procedure. The actual technique using plasma samples from patients deficient in prothrombin and factors V, VII, or X is very simple; however, these deficient states are very rare, and the deficient plasma samples are usually prepared artificially and are available commercially. For example, factor V–deficient plasma is prepared by aging plasma at 37°C. The assays are performed in the same manner as the assays for the intrinsic factors (eg, factor VIII) using the PT instead of the aPTT. The ability of the patient's plasma to shorten the prolonged PT of commercially deficient plasma is compared with that of normal plasma.

Interpretation. The normal range for prothrombin and for factors V, VII, and X is approximately 60% to 150%.

43.4 Inhibitor Screening Test

Purpose. The inhibitor screening test is used for detection of inhibitors of clotting, which are usually immunoglobulins or heparin-like substances.

Principle. The addition of plasma containing an inhibitor of a factor involved in intrinsic clotting prolongs the aPTT of normal plasma.

Specimen. The same plasma specimen used in the aPTT test is used.

Procedure. One part of the plasma being tested is incubated with an equal part of normal plasma. The aPTTs of the mixture are determined immediately and after incubation at 37°C for 1 to 2 hours.

Interpretation. When one part of plasma congenitally deficient in a clotting factor such as factor VIII is mixed with an equal part of normal plasma, the aPTT of the mixture should be normal. Failure of the aPTT to correct to within the normal reference range suggests the presence of an inhibitor. The two most common types of inhibitors encountered by the coagulation laboratory are, excluding heparin, the lupus anticoagulant (antiphospholipid antibody) and antibody to factor VIII. In many cases, these two possibilities can be distinguished using the inhibitor screening test at two incubation times. The lupus anticoagulant frequently exhibits immediate prolongation of the aPTT (0 time) with very similar values observed at the 1-hour incubation time. In contrast, antibodies to factor VIII exhibit time-dependence, with increasing aPTT values seen in the 1-hour sample.

An inhibitor (especially the lupus anticoagulant) may result in spuriously low values of the intrinsic factors. Consequently, inhibitor screening should be considered a routine procedure in evaluating an isolated prolonged aPTT value.

43.5 Factor VIII Antibody Screening Test

Purpose. Antibodies against factor VIII develop in up to 30% of patients with hemophilia A. The titer of antibody increases after transfusions of factor VIII concentrates, and their detection is important because the patient may become refractory to treatment. Factor VIII antibodies are an important cause of severe bleeding in previously healthy individuals; in patients with a background of immunologic disorder, such as systemic lupus erythematosus, rheumatoid arthritis, and penicillin sensitivity; and in women following parturition. An antibody to factor VIII should be considered in every patient found, during a preoperative workup, to have an inhibitor. While the vast majority of inhibitors are lupus-like (Chapter 44) and do not give rise to excessive bleeding, surgery in a patient with a factor VIII inhibitor is dangerous and may be fatal.

Principle. If a plasma specimen suspected of containing a factor VIII inhibitor is incubated with an equal volume of a normal plasma specimen, after a period of incubation the factor VIII concentration of the mixture will be significantly decreased below normal.

Specimen. Plasma specimen collected for the aPTT is used; the antibodies are remarkably stable and are present in both plasma and serum.

Procedure. One part of plasma from the patient is mixed with an equal volume of normal pooled plasma (used as the 100% standard). After incubation for 2 hours at 37°C, the mixture is diluted in a ratio of 1:5 in saline and assayed for factor VIII.

Interpretation. If the factor VIII concentration of the mixture is 35% or more, the patient does not have an inhibitor, or the inhibitor is too weak to be significant.

Notes and Precautions. To detect a low-titer inhibitor, it is advisable to obtain plasma specimens several days after, as well as before, replacement therapy.

43.6 Factor VIII Antibody Titer

Purpose. Serial dilutions of the plasma specimen containing the inhibitor are incubated with a normal plasma specimen for a specified period, and the residual factor VIII activity is determined. Factor VIII inhibitor titers are commonly expressed in Bethesda units, which are defined as the amount that, when incubated with normal plasma, neutralizes half of the factor VIII activity in 2 hours.

Specimen. Blood is collected as for the aPTT test or factor VIII assay.

Procedure. Serial dilutions in saline (1:2, 1:4, etc) of the plasma sample being tested are incubated with an equal volume of normal plasma for 2 hours at 37°C. The residual factor VIII in each of the incubation mixtures is determined. The inhibitor titer in Bethesda units is the reciprocal of the dilution of the test plasma sample that gives 50% inhibition; this may be determined by drawing a curve relating activity of residual factor VIII to the reciprocal of the dilution, or by a rough approximation made by inspection of the data.

Interpretation. A factor VIII antibody titer of up to 5 Bethesda units is considered a "low-titer" inhibitor, while a value greater than 5 Bethesda units is considered a "high-titer" inhibitor. The clinical importance of quantitating the titer of a factor VIII antibody is that it may determine therapy. Low-titer inhibitors can usually be overcome by infusion of factor VIII, while this therapy is less effective in high-titer inhibitor patients.

There is considerable heterogeneity between the factor VIII antibodies of different patients. The antibodies seen in nonhemophiliacs may differ strikingly from those seen in hemophiliac patients. For example, some of the antibodies seen in nonhemophiliacs may only neutralize 80% of the available factor VIII in normal plasma over a period of 12 hours, reaching a plateau, yet when the factor VIII concentration of the mixture is increased to 100% by addition of factor VIII concentrate, the level again falls to only 20%, indicating that the antibody was only partially neutralized. Moreover, if a factor VIII concentrate is given to a patient with a factor VIII antibody, the factor VIII level determined in the laboratory may not be a true reflection of the level at the time the plasma was withdrawn, as destruction occurs in vitro between the time of collection and actual performance of the assay. Other test systems are used to assay factor VIII antibodies, with different definitions of a unit. The results obtained using different test systems are in general poorly correlated; however, each method gives useful information with respect to the relative potency of the antibody in any one patient over time.

43.7 Alpha$_2$-Antiplasmin Determination

Purpose.   An alpha$_2$-antiplasmin determination is performed in patients with an acquired or inherited bleeding diathesis who have normal bleeding times, normal platelet function, and normal levels of the known coagulation factors.

Principle.   A known amount of plasmin is added to the patient's plasma specimen and, after a short interval, the amount of residual plasmin activity is measured. The method for determining the plasmin level is essentially the same as that used in the plasminogen assay, in which a fluorescent or chromogenic substrate is used (Chapter 47). The percentage of plasmin inhibited provides a measure of the alpha$_2$-antiplasmin level. The alpha$_2$-antiplasmin level may also be measured with immunologic methods.

Specimen.   Citrated plasma.

Procedure.   Aliquots of a standardized and stable preparation of human plasmin are added to the patient and control plasma samples and also to a saline control sample. After exactly 1 minute, the mixture containing the plasmin is then added to a fluorescent or chromogenic synthetic substrate as described for the plasminogen assay (Chapter 47). The residual plasmin is the difference between the values obtained for the plasma test sample and the control containing saline instead of plasma. A normal range has to be established for each laboratory and is usually 80% to 120%.

Interpretation.   Heterozygotes for inherited alpha$_2$-antiplasmin deficiency with levels between 25% and 60% of normal may bleed excessively following surgery. In acquired deficiencies, which are seen in liver disease and in thrombotic states, especially disseminated intravascular coagulation, plasminogen activity is depressed concomitantly.

Notes and Precautions. Alpha$_2$-antiplasmin levels cannot be determined in patients who are receiving fibrinolytic inhibitors (eg, epsilon aminocaproic acid [Amicar]).

Course and Treatment

The specific treatment for the bleeding of inherited coagulation disorders is to raise the level of deficient or defective protein above the minimum concentration believed adequate for normal hemostasis, ie, approximately 50% of the mean normal level for most factors. To achieve this level in a patient with a very low baseline value with plasma alone is virtually impossible; therefore, concentrated forms of clotting factors are necessary. Monoclonal-purified factor VIII and IX preparations are available; these products, in addition to being highly purified, appear to be sterile in terms of not transmitting viral infections. Concentrates to treat deficiencies of factors V, XI, or XIII are not yet available, so that fresh-frozen plasma is used for these patients. A solvent-treated plasma product is undergoing studies, and appears to offer safety from viral infection. The dosage schedules depend on the half-life of the factor being replaced, which is roughly 12 hours for factor VIII and 24 hours in the case of factor IX. Replacement therapy is indicated for life-threatening hemorrhages (eg, central nervous system or intraperitoneal bleeds), surgery, and the early treatment of hemarthroses and deep-tissue hematomas. Almost all patients with mild hemophilia A and many patients with von Willebrand's disease (with the exceptions that include the rare type IIB) respond well to the intravenous or subcutaneous administration of desmopressin, a synthetic analogue of vasopressin given in a dose of 0.3 µg/kg over a period of 15 to 30 minutes. This drug often induces increases of factor VIII and von Willebrand's factor, which may be as much as twofold or threefold above the basal level, often without any side effects. Thus, plasma or plasma concentrates are rarely required by these patients when they have minor bleeding. Epsilon aminocaproic acid (Amicar) or tranexamic acid are sometimes useful for minor bleeding episodes in the coagulation disorders and are very effective in the treatment of alpha$_2$-antiplasmin deficiency.

References

Giddings JC, Peake IR. The investigation of factor VIII deficiency. In: Thomson JM, ed. *Blood Coagulation and Haemostasis: A Practical Guide*. New York, NY: Churchill-Livingstone Inc; 1985:135-207.

Santoro SA. Laboratory evaluation of hemostatic disorders. In: Hoffman R, Benz EJ, Shattil SJ, Furie B, Cohen HJ, eds. *Hematology: Basic Principles and Practice*. New York, NY: Churchill-Livingstone Inc; 1991:1266-1276.

44

Acquired Coagulation Disorders

The most common causes of acquired deficiencies of clotting factors associated with hemorrhagic manifestations are decreased or abnormal synthesis of clotting factors caused by liver disease or disseminated intravascular coagulation (DIC); the latter is seen in many severe illnesses, including metastatic carcinoma and infectious diseases. Vitamin K deficiency is an important but now less common cause of a hemorrhagic diathesis. While lupus anticoagulants are encountered very frequently and result in apparent decreases in certain clotting factors, they are not associated with excessive bleeding. However, because lupus anticoagulants are associated with thrombosis and recurrent miscarriage, their laboratory identification is increasingly important. Antibodies against prothrombin and factors V, VIII, and XIII, although rare, may arise de novo in individuals with no previous hemorrhagic disorder, causing severe bleeding.

Pathophysiology

Liver Disease and Vitamin K Deficiency. The liver is the major site of synthesis of clotting factors, and a hemorrhagic diathesis can occur in severe hepatitis or cirrhosis. In these conditions, the vitamin K–dependent clotting factors (ie, prothrombin and factors VII, IX, and X) (see Chapter 40) are usually the first to be reduced, followed by factor V. Factor VIII is not synthesized by hepatic parenchymal cells, and levels of this protein are actually increased in liver disease (acute-phase response). Similarly, von Willebrand's factor, synthesized in vascular endothelial cells, is elevated in liver disease. In addition to altered coagulation protein levels, other hemostatic defects exist in liver disease, including decreased clearance of activated clotting factors and increased degradation products of fibrinogen and fibrin. Fibrin degradation products inhibit hemostasis by interfering with both platelet function and fibrin formation. Fibrinolysis may also be enhanced in liver disease.

Significant liver disease, with associated portal hypertension and splenomegaly, can result in mild thrombocytopenia. Hepatoma and cirrhosis have also been associated with synthesis of a qualitatively abnormal fibrinogen (dysfibrinogen).

From this description, it can be appreciated that the coagulopathy of liver disease is complex, affecting global hemostasis, including platelet number and function, coagulation, and fibrinolysis. These defects usually result in a bleeding tendency.

Vitamin K is essential for the normal synthesis of the vitamin K–dependent clotting factors. In its absence, the vitamin K–dependent factors do not bind calcium and, although synthesized in normal amounts, are inactive. Naturally occurring vitamin K is fat-soluble, and bile is essential for its absorption from the gastrointestinal tract. In any condition in which influx of bile into the gut is impeded, a hemorrhagic diathesis may ensue. The absorption of vitamin K occurs in the small intestine and may be deficient in such diseases of the intestinal wall as regional ileitis and nontropical sprue. Because bacterial flora play an important part in the synthesis of vitamin K in the gut, sterilization of the bowel resulting from the administration of antibiotics may also result in vitamin K deficiency.

Disseminated Intravascular Coagulation. The delicate hemostatic balance between the procoagulant factors and the natural inhibitors that is necessary for the maintenance of the fluidity of the blood may be disturbed in many disease states (Table 44-1).

Table 44-1   Causes of Disseminated Intravascular Coagulation

Release of tissue factor activity after necrosis or trauma
     Metastatic carcinoma (adenocarcinomas)
     Tissue injury, eg, brain tissue destruction, lung surgery
     Extensive burn
     Heat stroke
     Promyelocytic leukemia
Infections
     Gram-negative endotoxinemia
         Meningococcemia
         Septicemia
     Severe gram-positive septicemia
     Rocky Mountain spotted fever
     Viral infections
Obstetric disorders
     Concealed antepartum hemorrhage
     Amniotic fluid embolism
     Retained dead fetus
     Hypertonic saline abortion
Hemolytic transfusion reactions
Endothelial cell injury (vasculitis)
Giant hemangioma
Snake bites

This may result in the uncontrolled generation of thrombin in the blood, leading to formation of thrombi in the microcirculation, a process referred to as "DIC." This term is usually used to include a paradoxical hypocoagulable state that is the natural sequela of DIC and is attributable to the consumption of platelets, fibrinogen, and other procoagulant factors in the formation of the thrombi. The thrombi removal, essential for the survival of the patient, is accomplished by fibrinolysis, and this mechanism, although primarily protective, may in itself aggravate the bleeding tendency. The formation of thrombin is believed to be a sine qua non of DIC. Its presence is presumed by the recognition of the products of its action on fibrinogen and fibrin. These products include fibrinopeptides A and B, fibrin monomer, and D-dimer. While some of the fibrin monomers polymerize, forming fibrin, a proportion form soluble complexes with native fibrinogen and with the degradation products that result from the lysis of formed fibrin. The fibrinopeptides have half-lives of only a few minutes, which limits their usefulness as an index of DIC. On the other hand, the soluble fibrin monomer complexes remain in the circulation for several hours. Fibrinolysis occurs as a consequence of thrombin generation, and results in the formation of several fibrin degradation products, of which products D and E are the most stable and readily measured.

Fibrin is cross-linked by the action of factor XIIIa (transglutaminase). One major soluble degradation product is referred to as D-dimer. Specific monoclonal antibodies to these cross-linked domains are used to detect D-dimer; such antibodies do not react with fibrinogen or fibrinogen degradation products because they lack the specific covalent bonds. Fibrinogen degradation products appear when urokinase or streptokinase is infused intravenously to convert plasminogen into plasmin and dissolve thrombi. The plasmin may not be neutralized completely by alpha$_2$-antiplasmin and can degrade fibrinogen, factor V, and other plasma proteins. If the therapy is efficacious, the thrombus will lyse, and D-dimer will be found as well as fibrinogen degradation products derived from the action of the plasmin on fibrinogen.

One of the consequences of intravascular fibrin deposition is the fragmentation of red blood cells by strands of fibrin in the microcirculation, resulting in schistocytes or helmet cells. When associated with a significant hemolytic anemia, it is referred to as "microangiopathic hemolytic anemia." This is prominent in a group of conditions referred to as "thrombotic microangiopathies" characterized by hyaline microthrombi composed of fibrin and aggregated platelets in terminal arterioles and capillaries. The thrombotic microangiopathies include DIC, thrombotic thrombocytopenic purpura, and the hemolytic-uremic syndrome.

A common cause for many cases of DIC is tissue factor expression, either by tumor tissue (promyelocytic leukemia, adenocarcinoma), damaged normal tissue (obstetric emergencies, extensive burns), or induced by vascular endothelium (gram-negative sepsis). Initiation of contact activation is not usually an important mechanism for DIC.

Clinical Findings

The bleeding found in thrombocytopenia and functional disorders of the platelets is purpuric, while the bleeding manifestations of acquired deficiencies of coagulation factors are of the coagulation type (see Table 40-2). In DIC, however, features of both types of bleeding may be present.

Hemorrhagic disease of the newborn caused by deficiency of vitamin K has been virtually eliminated as a result of prophylactic vitamin K therapy. The bleeding typically occurs during the second to sixth day after delivery. Hemorrhagic disease of the newborn is an exaggeration of physiologic hypoprothrombinemia, a temporary state that reaches its maximum point of bleeding on the second or third day and usually returns to normal within 1 week. The onset of bleeding is usually abrupt, and the most common presenting symptoms include melena with hematemesis, umbilical bleeding, epistaxis, submucosal hemorrhages affecting the buccal cavity, and urethral and vaginal bleeding. The disease may also present as excessive bleeding at circumcision or persistent bleeding following a heel prick. Multiple ecchymoses may be found. Petechial hemorrhages are exceptional and suggest thrombocytopenia. Premature infants are particularly prone to excessive bleeding, as immaturity of the liver cells results in decreased synthesis of vitamin K–dependent factors, which is enhanced by vitamin K deficiency.

Approach to Diagnosis

DIC. If a patient with a severe illness, such as metastatic carcinoma or fulminant septicemia or viremia, develops purpuric manifestations, the likely cause is DIC (Table 44-1). Fibrinogen is an acute-phase reactant protein and in many of the conditions that can cause DIC, the fibrinogen level may be very high. A significant decrease in the concentration may therefore not be apparent from a single fibrinogen determination, as it may be normal or even high depending on the baseline level. Serial fibrinogen determinations to follow the course of the process should therefore be performed. Factor VIII is also an acute-phase reactant protein and its level may remain above normal in DIC despite a significant fall. Thrombin is believed to cause activation of factor VIII, and a high factor VIII level may also be attributed to this cause. Factor V activity is usually decreased but rarely sufficiently to raise the PT by more than 1 or 2 seconds. Milder depressions of the other factor levels such as factor XIII also occur, but these changes are of little or no diagnostic value.

Table 44-2   Acquired Coagulation Inhibitors

Type	Clinical Associations	Nature of Antibody
Specific antibodies against factor VIII	Previously healthy elderly persons; patients with autoimmune disorders; postpartum	IgG, monoclonal
Specific antibodies against factor V	Usually preceded by streptomycin administration; may develop after massive blood transfusion	IgG or IgM polyclonal
Specific antibodies to prothrombin	Usually associated with lupus anticoagulants	IgG
Specific antibodies against factor XIII or XIIIa	Therapy with isoniazid	IgG
Specific antibody against vWf	Myeloma; lymphoproliferative disorders; connective tissue disorders	IgG
Lupus anticoagulant	Procainamide, chlorpromazine, quinidine, lupus erythematosus, pregnancy, HIV infection, no apparent disease	Usually IgG, sometimes IgM, or both

Abbreviations: aPTT = activated partial thromboplastin time; PT = prothrombin time; vWf = von Willebrand's factor; HIV = human immunodeficiency virus; DRVVT = dilute Russell's viper venom time.

A falling platelet count is of considerable diagnostic and prognostic importance and suggests ongoing DIC. The parameter probably used most, however, is the presence of fibrin degradation products, and of these, the D-dimer appears to be the most specific. D-dimer is more helpful in diagnosing DIC than measurement of other fibrin (fibrinogen) degradation products, because the latter are elevated in both liver disease and DIC, while D-dimer is a specific marker for the presence of thrombin in blood (DIC). The presence of microangiopathic hemolytic anemia confirms the diagnosis of DIC.

Table 44-2 *Continued*

Clinical Findings and Course	Laboratory Findings
May be persistent, especially in elderly patients; life-threatening bleeding can occur	aPTT: increased; PT: normal; factor VIII: decreased
Bleeding tendency usually disappears in weeks or months	aPTT: increased; PT: increased; factor V: decreased
Bleeding tendency usually disappears in weeks	aPTT: increased; PT: increased; inhibitor screen: positive; prothrombin: decreased; factors V, VII, X: normal
Bleeding tendency usually disappears in weeks or months	aPTT: normal; PT: normal, clot soluble in 5 mol/L of urea
Mild bleeding tendency	Bleeding time: increased; ristocetin cofactor activity: decreased; factor VIII: normal or decreased
Bleeding tendency absent; patients may have thromboembolic events or recurrent abortions	aPTT: increased; PT: usually normal; inhibitor screen positive; DRVVT positive

Vitamin K Deficiency and Liver Disease.   The response of the prothrombin time (PT) to the parenteral administration of vitamin K in patients lacking vitamin K–dependent factors is useful in differentiating hepatocellular diseases from other forms of vitamin K deficiency (malnutrition, biliary disease, etc). The PT remains prolonged in hepatocellular disease, while it returns to normal in the other conditions unless some associated liver parenchymal damage is also present. In the case of a previously healthy individual in whom a bleeding diathesis has developed, a prolonged PT with otherwise normal liver function test results can often be attributed to ingestion of warfarin sodium (Coumadin).

Antibodies to Coagulation Factors. The development of a coagulation type of bleeding disorder in an individual with previously normal hemostasis is often manifested by deep-tissue hematoma and suggests an antibody specifically directed against factor VIII, factor V, or more rarely, one of the other clotting factors. Antibodies against specific factors are encountered far less frequently than the lupus anticoagulant (Table 44-2). This antibody results in a prolongation of the activated partial thromboplastin time (aPTT) and occasionally the PT. Patients with this nonspecific antibody rarely bleed excessively, even while undergoing major surgery. Because such an antibody was first found in a patient with systemic lupus erythematosus, it is referred to as the lupus anticoagulant, even though lupus erythematosus is now known to be a relatively rare cause. The lupus antibody may be seen in individuals who are taking certain drugs, such as quinidine, procainamide, and chlorpromazine, and after viral infections, such as human immunodeficiency virus (HIV), but is also commonly found in individuals in whom no causative factor can be determined. The VDRL test may give a false-positive result in these patients. The lupus anticoagulant probably comprises a heterogenous group of antibodies with different actions—IgG or IgM—that are believed to be targeted against negatively charged phospholipids. When the lupus anticoagulant results in a marked prolongation of the aPTT, the aPTT of an equal part of the patient's and control plasma usually exceeds that of the normal reference range. The coagulant activities of factors VIII, IX, XI, and XII appear reduced when assayed at a 1:5 dilution, but when assayed at higher dilutions, they usually, but not always, increase significantly. This phenomenon is attributed to "diluting out the inhibitor." Factor VIII usually appears to be reduced the least and factors XI and XII the most. Weak lupus anticoagulants that result in only a slight prolongation of the aPTT are difficult to diagnose. In these cases, mixing studies may demonstrate correction of the prolonged aPTT, and additional specific tests for the lupus anticoagulant may be necessary for diagnosis (DRVVT). Rarely, a lupus anticoagulant may be associated with a deficiency of prothrombin with normal levels of

Table 44-3   Use of Screening Tests in Acquired Bleeding Disorders

Disorder	Platelet Count	aPTT	PT
Thrombocytopenic purpura*	Decreased	Normal	Normal
Liver disease	Normal or decreased	Normal or increased	Increased
Vitamin K deficiency	Normal	Normal or increased	Increased
Factor VIII antibody	Normal	Increased	Normal
Lupus anticoagulant	Normal	Increased	Normal or increased
DIC†	Decreased	Normal or increased	Increased

Abbreviations: aPTT = activated partial thromboplastin time; PT = partial thromboplastin time; DIC = disseminated intravascular coagulation.
*See Chapter 41.
†Patients with low-grade, chronic DIC may have normal screening test results.

factors V, VII, and X. This is attributable to another auto-antibody that binds to but does not neutralize prothrombin, with rapid clearance in vivo of the antibody-prothrombin complex. Such patients may develop a bleeding tendency. A lupus anticoagulant can develop in a patient with a preexisting congenital or acquired coagulation abnormality and give rise to diagnostic problems.

A rare cause of an acquired hemorrhagic diathesis that can result in severe bleeding is the acquired deficiency of factor X seen in primary amyloidosis. Evaluation of the acquired coagulation disorders proceeds as follows:

1. Hematologic evaluation, with attention to platelet number, red blood cell morphology indicative of DIC, and white blood cell count and differential.

2. Screening tests for bleeding disorders, including platelet count, aPTT, and PT. This battery of tests is useful in differentiating the thrombocytopenic purpuras, and the acquired diathesis caused by inhibitors, liver disease, vitamin K deficiency, or DIC (Table 44-3).

3. In all instances in which the aPTT is significantly prolonged, it is now customary to perform inhibitor screening on a mix-

ture of equal parts of normal plasma and the patient's plasma (sometimes referred to as a "50:50 mix"). Failure of the addition of normal plasma to correct the prolonged aPTT is evidence of a circulating anticoagulant. This is in contrast to the finding in deficient states in which the aPTT value of the 50:50 mix with normal plasma rarely exceeds the aPTT reference range. Correction, however, does not necessarily exclude the presence of an inhibitor. This is particularly applicable when the aPTT of the patient's plasma alone is only a few seconds outside the upper limit of the normal range. If a plasma sample containing a potent lupus anticoagulant is diluted with a normal plasma sample to shorten the aPTT to approximately 40 seconds, it will often be difficult to demonstrate the presence of a lupus anticoagulant in the resulting plasma mixture based solely on a failure to correct. In this instance, a specific test for the lupus anticoagulant such as the DRVVT test may be helpful. In the case of some very slow-acting factor VIII inhibitors, correction may also be observed, particularly if the aPTT test is performed within a few minutes of preparing the 50:50 mix with normal plasma. However, the 1-hour incubation sample should indicate the presence of an antibody.

4. If an inhibitor is present or cannot be excluded on the basis of the aPTT of the 50:50 mix, and the PT is normal, the presence of an inhibitor directed against factor VIII must be excluded. One practice is to perform assays of factors VIII, IX, and XI routinely in all such cases in which the patient has clinical bleeding. If the factor VIII level appears higher than that of the other factors, a factor VIII inhibitor can be excluded, and the patient is considered to most likely have a lupus anticoagulant without further testing.

   On the other hand, if the factor VIII level is significantly decreased, equal to, or lower than that of the other factors, and does not appear to increase when tested at a higher dilution (eg, 1:20), a test for factor VIII inhibitor is performed (see Chapter 43). When both the aPTT and PT are prolonged, and neither is corrected in the 50:50 mix, a specific inhibitor against factor V should be considered. If the

PT prolongation, but not the aPTT, is corrected in the 50:50 mix, specific assays for prothrombin and factors VII, V, and X should be performed. If they are all normal, the cause of the PT prolongation may be an unusual type of lupus anticoagulant; if prothrombin is the only factor whose level is decreased, then an inhibitor against prothrombin should be considered. The diagnosis of a lupus anticoagulant should be confirmed using the DRVVT or the kaolin clotting time test.

5. Assay of D-dimer or fibrin monomer (using the protamine sulfate paracoagulation test) and also serial fibrinogen determinations, are useful if DIC is suspected.

6. Serial PT assays after vitamin K therapy will confirm vitamin K deficiency due to warfarin sodium ingestion or malnutrition, if the PT corrects.

Hematologic Findings

If platelets are absent or markedly reduced, the patient is evaluated for thrombocytopenic purpura (see Chapter 41). A moderate to severe reduction, however, is found in liver disease or DIC, and may be associated with schistocytes and spherocytes in the peripheral blood smear in the case of DIC.

Peripheral Blood Smear Morphology. A platelet count is performed, and the morphology of red blood cells (schistocytes, etc) is evaluated.

Other Laboratory Tests

44.1 The Protamine Plasma Paracoagulation Test

Purpose. This test detects fibrin monomer in plasma and is used for the diagnosis of DIC.

Principle. Soluble complexes of fibrin monomer with fibrin (fibrinogen) degradation products or fibrin dissociate on the addition of protamine sulfate, and the fibrin monomers then polymerize, forming a fibrin web.

Specimen. Platelet-poor plasma is used as collected for the aPTT test.

Procedure. Ten drops of plasma are placed in a small glass test tube warmed to 37°C; one drop of 1% protamine sulfate is then added and, after gentle shaking, incubated for 20 minutes.

Interpretation. Webs or strands of fibrin are considered an unequivocally positive result, while a finely granular, noncohesive precipitate is usually interpreted as a weakly positive result.

Notes and Precautions. False-positive results may be obtained if there is difficulty with venipuncture or delay in mixing the blood with anticoagulant because of the formation of small amounts of thrombin in vitro. A test should not be performed on oxalated or heparinized blood, but the administration of heparin to the patient does not interfere with the test.

44.2 Latex Particle Agglutination Tests for Fibrin or Fibrinogen Degradation Products; D-Dimer Test

Purpose. This test detects the presence of fibrin or fibrinogen degradation products (FDP) and is used in the diagnosis of DIC.

Principle. Antibodies to fibrin (fibrinogen) degradation products are bound to latex particles, which clump in the presence of the antigen. If an antiserum to highly purified fibrinogen fragments D and E is employed in the FDP test, a positive result is obtained with fibrinogen and fibrinogen degradation products as well as with fibrin degradation products. In another version of the test, a highly specific monoclonal antibody to D-dimer (a cross-linked fibrin degradation product) is used, and in this type of test (D-dimer test), positive results are obtained only with the D-dimer fragment.

Specimen. In the FDP test, only serum samples may be used. The blood specimen must be obtained by careful and clean venipuncture and placed in a special sample collection tube that contains soybean trypsin inhibitor and thrombin or reptilase. After formation of a clot, the tube is incubated at 37°C for approximately 30 minutes before separating the serum by centrifugation. For the D-dimer test, either plasma or serum samples may be used, but the former is preferred.

Procedure. In the D-dimer test, the undiluted plasma (or serum) sample, a 1:2 dilution in buffer, and a 1:4 dilution in buffer are added to the suspension of latex beads on a glass slide. The suspensions are rotated on the slides for a precise number of minutes. After this period, the slide is inspected for macroscopic agglutination. Known negative or positive controls are run with each test. The procedure is almost identical in the FDP test, except for the 1:5 and 1:20 dilutions of the serum in buffer that are used. In the FDP test, the normal serum level of degradation products derived from fibrinogen or fibrin is less than 10 μg/mL, and the reagents are so adjusted that a serum sample with less than this concentration will give no agglutination with either 1:5 or 1:20 dilutions of normal serum. In DIC, the level of FDP exceeds 10 μg/mL, and in acute cases may exceed 40 μg/mL. The normal plasma concentration of cross-linked FDP containing the D-dimer domain is less than 200 ng/mL, and the reagents for this test are adjusted to give negative readings with this concentration. The concentration of D-dimer can be assayed semiquantitatively by preparing serial dilutions of the specimen and determining the highest dilution titer that remains positive. Most patients with clinically significant DIC will have D-dimer values greater than 4 μg/mL.

Notes and Precautions. Degradation products of fibrinogen or fibrin may be incorporated into the clots formed in vitro during the preparation of the serum sample, thereby giving a normal (negative) result or a spuriously low value. As plasma may be used in the D-dimer test but not in the other type of test, this is a significant advantage. False-positive results may be seen with the FDP test in patients with dysfibrinogenemia in which residual fibrinogen remains in the serum. For all of these reasons, the D-dimer test is considered the better test. The D-dimer test cannot be used for monitoring fibrinolytic therapy (eg, streptokinase), in which it is desirable to assay fibrinogen degradation products as well as fibrin degradation products. Both types of tests may give positive results following surgical procedures or in patients with deep-vein thrombosis and pulmonary embolism. False-positive results can be seen with the D-dimer test in patients with rheumatoid factors (IgM molecules).

Since FDP are cleared by the liver, patients with liver disease will have elevated FDP levels. Consequently, the D-dimer assay will be a better test to distinguish DIC from the coagulopathy of liver disease.

44.3 Functional Fibrinogen Determination

Purpose. This test quantitates functional plasma fibrinogen levels, and is most commonly used in the diagnosis of DIC. Less commonly, the assay is used to diagnose inherited disorders of fibrinogen (dysfibrinogenemia, afibrinogenemia).

Principle. A thrombin time–based clotting assay is used. Thrombin directly cleaves fibrinogen to fibrin monomer; fibrin monomers then polymerize. The clotting time is inversely proportional to the amount of fibrinogen in the sample when read off a standard curve.

Specimen. Citrated plasma sample as collected for the PT or aPTT assay is used.

Procedure. A calibration curve is constructed using serial dilutions of a fibrinogen reference preparation. Serial dilutions of patient plasma are prepared. Thrombin is added, and clotting times measured in duplicate. Fibrinogen levels of the patient are determined from the standard curve.

Interpretation. The reference range for normal fibrinogen levels is 150 to 350 mg/dL (1.5-3.5 g/L). Fibrinogen is an acute-phase reactant with elevated levels occurring in liver disease and inflammatory diseases. Low levels are seen in end-stage liver disease, DIC, dysfibrinogenemias, and the inherited disorders, afibrinogenemia/hypofibrinogenemia.

Notes and Precautions. Large concentrations of heparin in the plasma sample or high levels of FDP may prolong the clotting time and falsely indicate low fibrinogen levels. When evaluating patients for dysfibrinogenemia, functional and antigenic fibrinogen levels should be tested on the same sample.

44.4 Confirmatory Test for the Lupus Anticoagulant

Purpose. The dilute Russell's viper venom time (DRVVT) test confirms the presence of the lupus anticoagulant in patients with positive findings on inhibitor screening or in patients with negative findings on inhibitor screening in whom the lupus anticoagulant is strongly suspected.

Principle. A modified PT assay is used in which clotting is initiated by a snake venom (Russell's viper venom) and dilute phospholipid. Russell's viper venom directly converts factor X to factor X_a. Factor X_a, factor V, and phospholipid convert prothrombin to thrombin. By diluting the Russell's viper venom and the phospholipid, the assay is able to better detect antiphospholipid antibodies inhibitory to coagulation (lupus anticoagulant).

Specimen. Platelet-poor plasma is used as collected for the aPTT assay. Since platelets can neutralize antiphospholipid antibodies in these plasma samples, it is critical that measures be taken to ensure a very low platelet count in the sample (<10 x 10^3/mm^3 [10 x 10^9/L].

Procedure. Normal or patient plasma samples are mixed with a source of phospholipid (eg, aPTT reagent) and the dilute Russell's viper venom reagent. Clotting times are then measured. If the patient's clotting time is prolonged, the clotting time test is repeated after mixing patient plasma sample with a normal pooled plasma sample. Our laboratory's DRVVT reference range is 26 to 35 seconds.

Interpretation. A prolonged DRVVT result in a plasma sample with a normal PT is suspicious for the lupus anticoagulant. A mixing study with a normal plasma sample that also results in a prolonged DRVVT would be diagnostic of the lupus anticoagulant.

Notes and Precautions. Obtaining platelet-poor plasma samples is important in maintaining sensitivity of this test. Samples with prolonged PT values will exhibit prolonged DRVVT values even in the absence of the lupus anticoagulant. For patients who have prolonged PT values and in whom the lupus anticoagulant is suspected, anticardiolipin antibodies may be a helpful surrogate test. Alternative confirmatory tests for the lupus anticoagulant include the kaolin clotting time test.

Course and Treatment

The treatment of DIC is directed at the primary cause. For patients with significant thrombocytopenia and hypofibrinogenemia, platelet transfusion and cryoprecipitate may be helpful. Patients who have DIC and primarily thrombotic symptoms may benefit from heparin therapy. New therapies are being developed to inhibit thrombin and other coagulation proteases important in DIC.

Patients with the coagulopathy of liver disease and clinical bleeding rarely respond to vitamin K therapy, because of significant hepatocellular damage; these patients may benefit transiently from fresh-frozen plasma. Other disorders associated with vitamin K deficiency (malnutrition, biliary obstruction, antibiotics, warfarin sodium ingestion) should reverse with vitamin K therapy.

Usually no treatment is required for the lupus anticoagulant, unless it is associated with thrombosis or recurrent miscarriage. In these cases, anticoagulant therapy or immunosuppression (steroids) may be helpful. Antibodies to specific coagulation factors (especially factor VIII) are best treated with immunosuppression (steroids plus cyclophosphamide), since major bleeding is common in these patients. Low-titer factor VIII antibodies may be overcome with excess factor VIII concentrate therapy.

References

Exner T, Burridge J, Power P, Rickard KA. An evaluation of currently available methods for plasma fibrinogen. *Am J Clin Pathol.* 1979;71:521-527.

Greenberg CS, Devine DV, McCrae KM. Measurement of plasma fibrin D-dimer levels with the use of a monoclonal antibody coupled to latex beads. *Am J Clin Pathol.* 1987;87:94-100.

Hougie C. Latex particle agglutination tests for fibrin or fibrinogen degradation products. In: Williams WJ, Beutler E, Erslev AJ, Lichtman MA, eds. *Hematology.* 4th ed. New York, NY: McGraw-Hill; 1990:1770-1773.

Rodgers GM. Common clinical bleeding disorders. In: Boldt DH, ed. *Contemporary Management in Internal Medicine: Update on Hemostasis. Volume 1, No. 2.* New York, NY: Churchill-Livingstone Inc; 1990:75-120.

Thiagarajan P, Pengo V, Shapiro SS. The use of the dilute Russell viper venom time for the diagnosis of lupus anticoagulants. *Blood.* 1986;68:869-874.

45

Laboratory Evaluation of the Patient With Bleeding

The previous chapters on inherited and acquired bleeding disorders discussed specific diseases and their laboratory tests. The purpose of this chapter is to synthesize this information into an approach to evaluate a patient with a bleeding disorder. Table 45-1 summarizes the profiles of hemostasis screening tests in patients with bleeding with a differential diagnosis for each profile. A major assumption in this chapter is that the patient with bleeding has a hemostatic disorder and not structural bleeding, ie, esophageal varices, surgical bleeding due to a lacerated blood vessel, etc. Structural bleeding should always be considered before embarking on a potentially expensive hemostasis evaluation.

The appropriate confirmatory tests are suggested by the differential diagnosis. For example, an isolated, prolonged prothrombin time (PT) is most commonly evaluated by liver function studies or by obtaining a history of warfarin use or malnutrition. An isolated, prolonged activated partial thromboplastin time (aPTT) should be evaluated by an inhibitor screen and assays for factors VIII, IX, and XI, if heparin contamination is excluded. For patients with prolonged PT and aPTT values in whom disseminated intravascular coagulation is suspected, fibrinogen and D-dimer values should be

Table 45-1 Profiles of Hemostasis Screening Tests in Patients With Bleeding Disorders*

PT	PTT	Platelet Count	Differential Diagnosis	
I	N	N	Common	Factor VII deficiency (early liver disease, early vitamin K deficiency, early warfarin therapy)
			Rare	Factor VII inhibitor, dysfibrinogenemia
N	I	N		Deficiency or inhibitor of factors VIII, IX, or XI; vWD, heparin, lupus inhibitor with qualitative platelet defect
I	I	N	Common	Vitamin K deficiency, liver disease, warfarin, heparin
			Rare	Deficiency or inhibitor of factors X, V, prothrombin, or fibrinogen; lupus inhibitor with hypoprothrombinemia; DIC
I	I	D		DIC, liver disease, heparin therapy with associated thrombocytopenia
N	N	D		Increased platelet destruction, decreased platelet production, splenomegaly, hemodilution
N	N	I		Myeloproliferative disorders
N	N	N	Common	Mild vWD, acquired qualitative platelet disorders (uremia)
			Rare	Inherited qualitative platelet disorders, vascular disorders, fibrinolytic disorders, factor XIII deficiency, autoerythrocyte sensitization, dysfibrinogenemia, mild factor deficiency (VIII, IX, XI)

Abbreviations: PT = prothrombin time; PTT = partial thromboplastin time; I = increased; D = decreased; N = normal; vWD = von Willebrand's disease; and DIC = disseminated intravascular coagulation.

*The differential diagnosis of hemostasis screening test results in patients with a history of bleeding is included. Consideration of patients with abnormal coagulation test results and negative bleeding histories is not included in this table. Modified from Rodgers GM. Common clinical bleeding disorders. In: Boldt DH, ed. *Update on Hemostasis.* New York, NY: Churchill Livingstone; 1990:75-120.

obtained. Patients with bleeding and normal findings on screening studies present a challenge because normal screening test results do not exclude mild factor deficiency, for example, carriers of factors VIII or IX deficiency, or mild factor XI deficiency. In addition, many patients with mild von Willebrand's disease will have normal findings on screening studies. These patients may require extensive investigation before a laboratory diagnosis is achieved.

References

Rodgers GM. Common clinical bleeding disorders. In: Boldt DH, ed. *Contemporary Management in Internal Medicine: Update on Hemostasis. Volume 1, No. 2.* New York, NY: Churchill-Livingstone; 1990:75-120.

Santoro SA. Laboratory evaluation of hemostatic disorders. In: Hoffman R, Benz EJ, Shattil SJ, Furie B, Cohen HJ, eds. *Hematology: Basic Principles and Practice.* New York, NY: Churchill-Livingstone; 1991:1266-1276.

46

Preoperative Hemostasis Screening

The use of screening coagulation tests in preoperative patients is controversial. Large amounts of money are routinely spent to obtain a low yield of positive results. On the other hand, the outcome of major surgery in a patient with an unknown hemostatic defect may be catastrophic. One sensible approach would be to balance the financial costs of preoperative testing with the extent of surgery to be done and with the amount of bleeding that can be safely tolerated. This approach places critical importance on obtaining a thorough hemostasis history. Patients scheduled for minor procedures (dental, skin biopsy) do not need routine screening tests if they have a negative history. Patients undergoing neurosurgery or procedures that may induce a hemostatic defect (cardiothoracic surgery with a bypass pump), or those with a positive bleeding history need a hemostasis evaluation by the laboratory. Table 46-1 summarizes the recommendations of Rapaport in evaluating preoperative patients.

Table 46-1 Guidelines for Preoperative Hemostasis Evaluation*

Level	Bleeding History	Surgical Procedure	Recommended Hemostasis Evaluation
I	Negative	Minor	None
II	Negative	Major	Platelet count, aPTT
III	Equivocal	Major, involving hemostatic impairment	PT, aPTT, platelet count, bleeding time, factor XIII assay, ECLT
IV	Positive	Major or minor	Level III tests; if negative, then factors VIII and IX assays, thrombin time, alpha$_2$ antiplasmin assay, postaspirin bleeding time

Abbreviations: aPTT = activated partial thromboplastin time; PT = prothrombin time; and ECLT = euglobulin clot lysis time, a screen for abnormal fibrinolysis

*Information in this table is based on the suggested preoperative guidelines for hemostasis testing by Rapaport. Based on the patient's bleeding history and the type of planned surgery, four levels are identified. Based on these levels of concern, recommendations are made as to the intensity of suggested hemostasis evaluation. Assay for factors VIII and IX are suggested in the level IV evaluation because most aPTT reagents are insensitive in detecting mild factor deficiency; factor levels of 20% to 30% may not be detected, and these patients would bleed with surgery. The thrombin time screens for dysfibrinogens, while the alpha$_2$-antiplasmin assay screens for deficiency of this fibrinolysis inhibitor.

Reference

Rapaport SI. Preoperative hemostatic evaluation: which tests, if any? *Blood*. 1983; 61:229-232.

PART
XIII

Thrombotic Disorders

47

Inherited Thrombotic Disorders

Thrombosis is defined as the formation of a blood clot in the circulatory system during life. Arterial thrombi, especially those in the smallest vessels, are composed predominantly of platelets, while fibrin is the predominant component of venous thrombi. Hypercoagulability, which is a much-abused term, should be used only to refer to changes in the blood that are associated with an abnormal tendency toward thrombosis; it should never be used to refer to conditions in which the clotting time is shortened or procoagulant factor levels are increased, unless these changes are known to be associated with an abnormal tendency toward thrombosis.

Pathophysiology

Hemostasis is a very complex process in which the vascular endothelial cell surface plays a pivotal role in maintaining the fluidity of the blood. The coagulation cascade is modulated by many regulatory mechanisms. Figure 47-1 summarizes the anticoagulant properties of endothelium. One example is the protein C pathway that consists of three plasma proteins—protein C, protein S, and activated protein C

Figure 47-1 Antithrombotic properties of the blood vessel wall. The major antithrombotic properties are depicted within boxes. Heparin-like glycosaminoglycans (GAG) present on the luminal surface catalyze inactivation of coagulation proteases, including thrombin, by antithrombin III (AT III). Complex formation of the endothelial cell membrane protein, thrombomodulin with thrombin generates activated protein C (APC). Binding of APC to endothelial cell–bound protein S in the presence of APC cofactor (factor V) promotes proteolysis of factors Va and VIIIa, resulting in inhibition of coagulation. Tissue-plasminogen activator (tPA) is secreted by endothelial cells to initiate fibrinolysis. Vascular endothelium also secretes two antiplatelet substances—prostacyclin (PGI$_2$) and nitric oxide (not shown).*

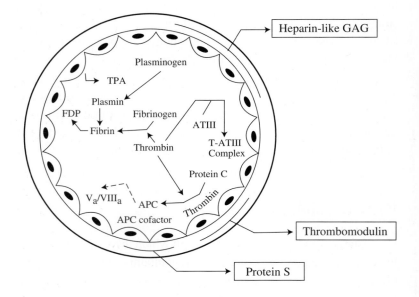

*Modified with permission from Rodgers GM. Hemostatic properties of normal and perturbed vascular cells. *FASEB J.* 1988;2:116-123.

(APC) cofactor. Proteins C and S are vitamin K–dependent proteins (Table 47-1). Neither protein C nor protein S has any apparent role in in vitro blood coagulation; however, they are potent anticoagulants. Protein C is converted to an active form (APC); this activation is mediated by a receptor, thrombomodulin, present on endothelial cell surfaces (Figure 47-1). Thrombomodulin forms a stoichiometric complex with thrombin on the endothelial cell surface, and this complex activates protein C, which in turn inactivates factors Va and VIIIa. Protein S binds to the endothelial cell surface providing a receptor for APC. Protein S circulates in the blood in a free form possessing anticoagulant activity and a form bound to C4b-binding protein, which has no anticoagulant activity. Another component of the protein C pathway was recently described, and is termed APC cofactor. The APC cofactor has recently been identified as the normal factor V molecule. A factor V mutation has recently been described that results in thrombosis due to inability of APC to degrade the abnormal factor Va molecule (APC cofactor deficiency, APC resistance). Both protein S and factor V promote activation of protein C.

Antithrombin III is another naturally occurring plasma protein with anticoagulant activity. Antithrombin III irreversibly binds to and inactivates certain activated clotting factors such as factor Xa and thrombin; this inactivation is catalyzed (enhanced) by heparin-like glycosaminoglycans on the endothelial cell surface (Figure 47-1) or by commercial heparin used therapeutically.

The formation of fibrin is essential in wound healing as well as hemostasis, but its removal, as soon as it has served its purpose, is equally important. This removal is accomplished by the fibrinolytic mechanism that, like the coagulation system, is composed of activators and inhibitors in delicate balance. Moreover, this system, which is part of the overall hemostatic mechanism, functions cooperatively with the coagulation system. Both may be triggered by the same mechanism, and the formation of fibrin greatly enhances activation of fibrinolysis.

Well-characterized components of the fibrinolytic system (Table 47-2) include the active serine protease plasmin, which is derived from the inactive zymogen, plasminogen; alpha$_2$-antiplasmin, an inhibitor that neutralizes free plasmin almost instantaneously; tissue-plasminogen activator (t-PA); and the major inhibitor of plasminogen activators, PAI-1.

Table 47-1   Features of Vitamin K–Dependent Anticoagulant Proteins

	Protein C	Protein S
Activation	Zymogen activated by thrombin-thrombomodulin complex	None required
Function	Inactivation of factors Va and VIIIa	Cofactor of APC; binds to C4b binding protein
Inactivation	APC inhibitor	Thrombin cleavage

Abbreviation: APC = activated protein C.

The fibrinolytic system may be initiated by the coagulation cascade or by tissue injury. As soon as fibrin is formed, it binds plasminogen, plasminogen activators, and alpha$_2$-antiplasmin. Plasminogen activation occurs in the fibrin clot, but any plasmin formed may be neutralized by alpha$_2$-antiplasmin, which is present in the clot at the equivalent molar concentration as the fibrin-bound plasminogen. Such is the state of equilibrium that when clots are formed in vitro, they do not lyse under normal conditions. In the circulation, however, plasminogen activators are released from the endothelial cell surface in contact with the clot and are absorbed onto the thrombus so that the equilibrium then favors fibrinolysis (Figure 47-1). In congenital or acquired states in which the activity of the fibrinolytic inhibitor alpha$_2$-antiplasmin is decreased, excessive clot lysis occurs at a site of injury, and the hemostatic plugs break down prematurely, resulting in bleeding.

Fibrin plays an integral role in the interplay between t-PA, plasminogen, and alpha$_2$-antiplasmin. Tissue-plasminogen activator has little effect on plasminogen in the absence of fibrin. The affinity of plasminogen for fibrin is attributable to lysine-rich binding sites and is inhibited by lysine, epsilon-aminocaproic acid, and tranexamic acid. Even a hundredfold increase of free t-PA activity such as occurs in good responders after strenuous exercise does not result in the presence of free plasmin in the blood. Kallikrein formed during the initial contact phase of blood coagulation converts precursor urinary plasminogen activator or urokinase (which is present in plasma) from a single chain form to a more active two-chain form.

Table 47-2   Components of the Fibrinolytic Mechanism

Protein	Site of Synthesis or Source	Comments
Plasminogen	Liver	Precursor of plasmin
t-PA	Endothelial cells	Most is inactivated by PAI-1; high concentrations released from endothelial cells by occlusion, exercise, epinephrine, etc
PAI-1	Endothelial cells, platelets	Inhibits t-PA
Alpha$_2$-antiplasmin	Liver	Potent inhibitor of plasmin

Abbreviations: t-PA = tissue-plasminogen activator; PAI-1 = plasminogen activator inhibitor 1.

Of the classic triad of Virchow (ie, risk factors predisposing to thrombosis—endothelial cell damage, stasis, and hypercoagulability), endothelial cell damage is by far the most important factor in arterial thrombosis. Because platelets adhere to damaged endothelium, thrombosis may be considered the natural sequela of arterial disease; by far, the most common cause of this is atherosclerosis. Thrombotic episodes, usually arterial and involving the smaller vessels, are frequent in the myeloproliferative disorders, especially in polycythemia vera and essential thrombocytosis when the platelet count is very high. The vessel wall regulates platelet activation and aggregation by secreting two mediators, prostacyclin (PGI$_2$) and nitric oxide. However, the clinical importance of these mediators in preventing arterial thrombosis in vivo is uncertain.

In contrast to arterial thrombosis in which underlying vascular disease is of major importance, stasis and hypercoagulability are critical factors in venous thrombosis. Thus, even in normal individuals, venous thrombosis in the lower extremity occurs with surprising frequency whenever the leg is immobilized for a number of hours, eg, during a long plane journey, but the fibrinolytic system almost always lyses the thrombi. Abnormalities or decreases in activity of the natural anticoagulants, protein C, protein S, antithrombin III, or the presence of a mutant factor V molecule (APC resistance) may be associated with an increased incidence of primarily venous thrombosis, while the therapeutic infusions of antifibrinolytic agents or activated clotting factors have resulted in massive venous thrombosis. This may explain why altering the equilibrium between procoagulants and anticoagulants by anticoagulant drugs is generally more useful in the treatment of venous than in arterial thrombosis.

Clinical Findings

The symptoms of arterial thrombosis or embolism are dependent on the size of the vessel, the state of the vessel wall, the degree and length of time of occlusion, adequacy of a collateral circulation, and the organ involved. If the thrombus or embolus occludes the retinal artery, permanent loss of sight may result; on the other hand, occlusion of a small branch of a renal artery may be asymptomatic. The consequences of venous thrombosis are, as a rule, not as severe as those of arterial thrombosis. Thus, thrombi in the lower calf veins are often asymptomatic. Because deep venous thrombosis is so frequently asymptomatic, a high index of suspicion is usually required for its recognition, and the differential diagnosis is, more often than not, difficult. The diagnosis is best established by objective testing, such as venography or ultrasonography.

Summary of the Inherited Thrombotic Disorders

Table 47-3 classifies the inherited thrombotic disorders, and briefly describes their prevalence, inheritance patterns, and clinical features. It can be seen that abnormalities of the protein C pathway (protein C, protein S, APC resistance) constitute at least half of all cases of inherited thrombosis. In general, the inherited disorders are transmitted in an autosomal dominant manner, and venous thromboembolism is the common clinical feature. The prevalence of abnormal fibrinolysis is uncertain because few studies have used optimal assay methods for t-PA and PAI-1. When optimal assays were used, abnormal fibrinolysis was observed in approximately 30% of cases. However, it has not been established whether the abnormal fibrinolysis is inherited. Consequently, the importance of inherited t-PA deficiency or excess PAI-1 activity is uncertain.

Table 47-3 A Summary of the Inherited Thrombotic Disorders*

Classification and Disorders	Inheritance	Estimated Prevalence (%)	Clinical Features
1. Deficiency or qualitative abnormalities of inhibitors to activated coagulation factors			
AT III deficiency	AD	1-5	Venous thromboembolism (usual and unusual sites), heparin resistance
Protein C deficiency	AD	5-6	Venous thromboembolism
Protein S deficiency	AD	5-6	Venous and arterial thromboembolism
APC cofactor deficiency (APC resistance)	AD	20-50	Venous and arterial thromboembolism
2. Impaired clot lysis			
Dysfibrinogenemia	AD	1-2	Venous thrombosis > arterial thrombosis
Plasminogen deficiency	AD, AR	1-2	Venous thromboembolism
t-PA deficiency	AD	?	Venous thromboembolism
Excess PAI-1 activity	AD	?	Venous thromboembolism and arterial thrombosis
3. Metabolic defect			
Homocystinuria	AR	?	Homozygous patients have arterial and venous thrombosis
			Heterozygous patients develop premature arterial thrombotic disease (coronary, cerebral)

Abbreviations: AT III = antithrombin III; APC = activated protein C; t-PA = tissue plasminogen activator; PAI-1 = plasminogen activator inhibitor 1; AD = autosomal dominant; AR = autosomal recessive.

*Prevalence data are estimated by pooling information from studies in which large groups of patients with thrombosis were screened for these disorders. Results are expressed in terms of a percentage that each disorder might constitute of the total patient population with inherited thrombosis. (Modified, with permission, from Rodgers GM, Chandler WL. Laboratory and clinical aspects of inherited thrombotic disorders. *Am J Hematol.* 1992;41:113-122.)

? = The prevalence of abnormal fibrinolysis is uncertain because few studies have used optimal assay methods for t-PA and PAI-1. The prevalence of homocystinuria in patients with inherited thrombosis is uncertain because this diagnosis has not been routinely considered.

Lastly, a metabolic disorder is associated with thrombosis: homocystinuria. The prevalence of homocystinuria in patients with inherited thrombosis is uncertain because this diagnosis has not been routinely considered. While pediatric patients present clinically with the homozygous defect, adult patients heterozygous for homocystinuria have primarily premature arterial disease. Heterozygous homocystinuria may account for a significant number of patients with premature vascular disease in the absence of traditional risk factors (tobacco use, hypertension, hyperlipidemia). It has been estimated that 1% to 2% of the general population has heterozygous homocystinuria.

Approach to Diagnosis

Obesity, diabetes, smoking, hyperlipidemia, and hypertension are associated with an increased risk of atherosclerosis as well as arterial and venous thrombosis. Venous thrombosis is particularly common after surgical procedures associated with tissue injury, after fractures of the neck or the femur, and in the postpartum period; in these conditions, immobilization of the lower limbs is also an important causative factor. Whenever one or more of these conditions is present, a special hematologic workup is rarely indicated. On the other hand, when a predisposing cause is absent, the venous thrombosis occurred at a very early age or at an unusual site (eg, axillary vein), there have been several episodes, or there is a family history of venous thrombosis, the possibility of an inherited or primary hypercoagulable state should be considered. Six key points to consider in the laboratory evaluation of these patients include:

1. The laboratory evaluation should be deferred until 2 to 3 months after the acute thrombotic event when the patient is clinically well and preferably has not been receiving anticoagulant therapy for 2 weeks. Thrombosis induces an acute phase response that may make interpretation of certain tests difficult. Optimal data will be obtained in the absence of anticoagulants, since these drugs alter levels of important factors to be assayed. If anticoagulants cannot be discontinued,

symptomatic family members who are not receiving antico-agulants can be tested.

2. The likelihood of obtaining positive results is increased if the patient population being evaluated is restricted to young patients with recurrent thrombosis or patients with a single event and a positive family history.

3. Functional assays are preferable to immunologic assays. Functional assays will detect patients with either quantitative deficiency of the protein or patients with qualitative abnormality of the protein.

4. Assay for components of the protein C pathway should be performed initially, since abnormalities of these components (protein C, protein S, APC resistance) comprise at least half of the patients with inherited thrombosis.

5. If fibrinolytic assays are to be performed, optimal assays are critical.

6. Consider heterozygous homocystinuria as a cause for thrombosis in middle-aged patients with premature vascular disease. These patients are evaluated by a methionine-loading test, usually assayed by the chemistry laboratory.

Establishing a specific diagnosis of inherited thrombosis is important, because it allows a single test to be performed on the patient's siblings and children who may also be at risk for thrombosis.

Strategy for Laboratory Evaluation of Inherited Thrombosis

Figure 47-2 summarizes one approach to the laboratory evaluation of these patients. Patients with arterial thrombosis should initially be evaluated by assays for PAI-1 or homocystinuria, depending on their age. In contrast, patients with venous thromboembolism are initially evaluated by assays of the protein C pathway (protein C, protein S, APC resistance); if these are normal, then less common causes of inherited thrombosis can be considered (antithrombin III deficiency, dysfibrinogenemia, abnormal fibrinolysis).

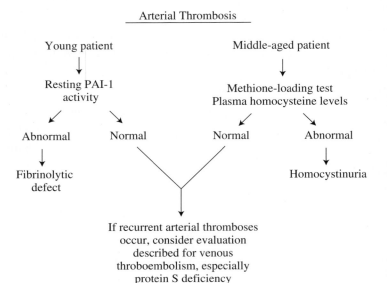

Arterial Thrombosis

Young patient
↓
Resting PAI-1
activity
↙ ↘
Abnormal   Normal

Fibrinolytic
defect

Middle-aged patient
↓
Methione-loading test
Plasma homocysteine levels
↙ ↘
Normal   Abnormal
↓
Homocystinuria

If recurrent arterial thromboses
occur, consider evaluation
described for venous
throboembolism, especially
protein S deficiency

Figure 47-2 A suggested algorithm for evaluation of patients with inherited thrombosis. In this approach, patients with an appropriate personal and family history are tested at a time distant from the acute thrombotic event, preferably at a time when they are not taking anticoagulants. Patients with venous thromboembolism who have negative findings on protein C studies, activated protein C (APC) resistance, protein S, antithrombin III (AT III), and dysfibrinogenemia should be considered for fibrinolytic testing. Samples for plasminogen activator inhibitor 1 (PAI-1) and tissue plasminogen activator activities should be obtained and assayed at appropriate research centers. With recent reports indicating that APC resistance is very common in the population with inherited thrombosis, consideration should be given to assaying for this disorder initially in the evaluation. (Modified with permission from Rodgers GM, Chandler WL. Laboratory and clinical aspects of inherited thrombotic disorders. *Am J Hematol.* 1991;41:113-122.)

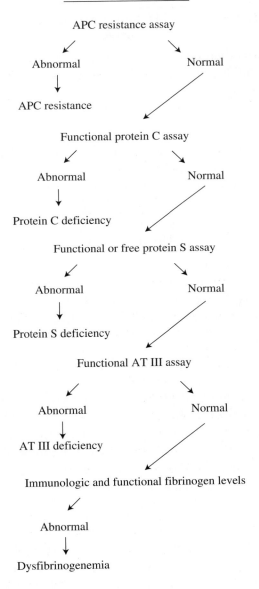

Venous Thromboembolism

APC resistance assay

Abnormal   Normal

APC resistance

Functional protein C assay

Abnormal   Normal

Protein C deficiency

Functional or free protein S assay

Abnormal   Normal

Protein S deficiency

Functional AT III assay

Abnormal   Normal

AT III deficiency

Immunologic and functional fibrinogen levels

Abnormal

Dysfibrinogenemia

Laboratory Tests

47.1 Antithrombin III Determination

Purpose. Antithrombin III determinations are usually performed to detect a hypercoagulable state associated with venous thrombotic episodes and may be useful in patients who appear to be resistant to heparin therapy.

Principle. A known amount of thrombin is added to the patient's plasma sample, and the residual thrombin activity is determined. Antithrombin III antigen levels may also be measured by the Laurell immunoelectrophoretic rocket technique or radial diffusion methods using specific antibodies. The functional assay is preferred.

Specimen. Citrated plasma is used in methods that use synthetic substrates. In the clotting assay methods, either citrated plasma or serum may be used, but plasma should be defibrinated.

Procedure. A known amount of thrombin is added to the plasma sample in the presence of heparin; after a timed interval, an aliquot is removed and added to a specific synthetic chromogenic or fluorescent thrombin substrate. In the chromogenic method, colored P-nitroaniline is liberated from the colorless substrate by the thrombin and measured spectrophotometrically; in the fluorescence method, a fluorescent compound is released and measured in a fluorometer.

Interpretation. The normal range appears to be a relatively narrow one (85% to 122% based on a normal pool). The level is slightly decreased by oral contraceptives; it is also decreased in the last trimester of pregnancy, but the levels rarely fall below 75% of normal. Such minor decreases may have no clinical relevance. Prolonged use of heparin can result in marked decreases in antithrombin III, whose level may also fall following a thrombotic event, especially in disseminated intravascular coagulation (DIC). Low values are also associated with liver disease. In the inherited deficiency states, the levels are usually in the 40% to 65% range. In approximately 10% of cases of antithrombin III deficiency, the antigen level may be normal, so that a functional measurement should be performed, at least initially, to exclude these variant types.

Notes and Precautions. Serum samples give values approximately 30% lower than plasma samples. Long-term warfarin therapy may increase plasma antithrombin III levels in certain patients. One disadvantage of functional antithrombin III assays is that the presence of heparin cofactor II in the plasma may result in overestimation of antithrombin III activity. Assays using bovine thrombin and lower heparin concentrations (3 U/mL) may minimize thrombin inhibition by heparin cofactor II. Assays based on inhibition of factor Xa (rather than thrombin) also yield more accurate results.

47.2 Protein C Determination

Purpose. This test is performed to detect hypercoagulable states associated with protein C deficiency. The functional assay can detect both quantitative and qualitative abnormalities in protein C.

Principle. Protein C in plasma is most commonly activated by a specific snake venom (Protac). The APC is then assayed by its ability to prolong the aPTT of normal plasma (clotting assay) or to cleave a specific synthetic substrate. Specific antibodies are available commercially, and antigenic determinations can be performed using Laurell immunoelectrophoresis or enzyme-linked immunosorbent assays.

Specimen. Citrated plasma sample is used.

Procedure. The protein C in the plasma sample is activated directly with Protac. The APC is then assayed either by a clotting method or an amidolytic assay using a chromogenic substrate.

Interpretation. The normal range in adults is 78% to 232%; however, the normal range is age-dependent for younger patients. The level is reduced in hepatocellular disease, and even a moderate disturbance of liver function may reduce the level to as low as 30%. Heterozygotes have levels of 30% to 65%. Homozygotes are born with DIC (neonatal purpura fulminans) with protein C levels less than 5% of normal; their parents are heterozygotes. A normal antigenic level does not exclude heterozygosity because there are rare variants in which there is synthesis of an abnormal protein. As protein C is a vitamin K–dependent protein with a very short half-life, it is depressed early during oral anticoagulant therapy. The ratio of protein C activity to protein C antigen is reduced by warfarin therapy even in the absence of an inherited abnormality of protein C. The protein C level is reduced in DIC and is lower in serum than plasma. Newborn infants have physiologically low levels of protein C that rise slowly during postnatal life; the levels are even lower in premature infants.

Protein C can be assayed in patients receiving stable oral anticoagulation; however, identification of protein C deficiency in patients who are receiving warfarin therapy requires comparison of these patient's laboratory values with that of patients receiving warfarin who do not have protein C deficiency. Most commonly, ratios of protein C activity to prothrombin activity are compared.

Notes and Precautions. Disadvantages of the Protac functional protein C assay include inability of chromogenic substrate assays to measure all functional aspects of protein C activity in patients receiving oral anticoagulants. Clot-based functional protein C assays have the advantage of measuring complete biologic functions of APC. Clotting assays are hampered by acute elevations in plasma factor VIII activity, which result in falsely low protein C values, and by heparin treatment. Therapeutic heparin levels do not affect the functional chromogenic substrate assay.

47.3 Protein S Determination

Purpose. Protein S acts as a cofactor for APC. Protein S deficiency should be considered in patients evaluated for an inherited disorder of thrombosis.

Specimen. Citrated plasma.

Principle. Immunologic methods are currently used, and the Laurell method is the immunologic technique used in most laboratories. A functional assay has just been introduced, which includes use of the aPTT assay with activated factor V as a substrate for APC. Protein S–deficient plasma is mixed with a reference or test plasma sample. APC and factor Va are added prior to recalcification. The normal range for the functional assay in adults is 62% to 125%.

Interpretation. Heterozygotes with levels between 30% and 60% of the normal range may have recurrent venous thrombotic episodes. The functional protein S assay detects quantitative deficiency and qualitative abnormality of protein S.

Notes and Precautions. The functional protein S assay is sensitive to APC resistance. Spuriously low protein S values may be obtained in patients with APC resistance.

47.4 APC Cofactor Determination (APC Resistance Assay)

Purpose. APC cofactor is necessary for normal APC activity. Deficiency of APC cofactor appears to be the major cause of inherited venous thrombosis; this disorder is also called APC resistance. APC cofactor has been identified as factor V.

Specimen. Citrated plasma.

Principle. aPTT assays are performed with and without APC. Reference range values are determined with a normal population.

Interpretation. Affected patients have APC-dependent aPTT prolongations less than the mean minus 2 SDs of the normal population.

Notes and Precautions. Since patients with APC resistance may have spuriously low functional protein S levels, APC resistance should be considered in protein S–deficient patients who were diagnosed with a functional assay. Because APC resistance appears to be the most common cause of inherited thrombosis, this disorder should be evaluated initially. A polymerase chain reaction based assay has been described that will detect most patients with APC resistance.

47.5 Plasminogen Determination

Purpose. In addition to identifying inherited plasminogen deficiency, this test is also used to distinguish inherited from acquired deficiencies of alpha$_2$-antiplasmin; in the former, plasminogen is normal, but in acquired states (eg, liver disease, DIC), plasminogen and alpha$_2$-antiplasmin are reduced in parallel.

Principle. Plasminogen is converted to its active form, plasmin, by addition of an activator; the plasmin is then assayed by the release of a colored marker or fluorescent molecule from a small synthetic peptide substrate. Specific antibodies are available commercially, and immunologic assays can be used.

Specimen. Citrated plasma.

Procedure. Streptokinase is usually added to the plasma sample, converting inactive plasminogen to plasmin. The plasmin is then assayed by removing an aliquot and adding a small synthetic peptide substrate bound either to a fluorescent molecule or to a *P*-nitroanilide compound. The release of fluorescence is measured by a fluorometer, while the release of the colored *P*-nitroanilide compound from the colorless substrate is followed by measurement of optical density at 405 nm in a spectrophotometer.

Interpretation. The normal plasminogen level is 2.4 to 4.4 CTA (Committee on Thrombolytic Agents) units/mL. Striking decreases are found in primary and secondary fibrinolysis (disseminated intravascular coagulation). Plasminogen levels are decreased in liver disease and may be very low or absent following treatment with t-PA, urokinase, or streptokinase.

Notes and Precautions. The test cannot be performed on patients who have received fibrinolytic inhibitors (eg, epsilon aminocaproic acid or Amicar) or on specimens containing these types of inhibitors. Antigenic assays give higher values than functional methods, probably because of the action of natural inhibitors in the latter. Several different substrates such as fibrin or casein may be used, but these have been almost completely replaced in routine coagulation laboratories by methods using synthetic chromogenic or fluorescent substrates.

Methods to measure alpha$_2$-antiplasmin levels are described in the chapter on inherited bleeding disorders (Chapter 43).

47.6 Tissue-Plasminogen Activator Determination

Purpose. Fibrinolytic disorders may constitute a common cause for inherited thrombosis. Assays for t-PA need to take into consideration sample collection and timing issues necessary for optimal results.

Principle. Functional assays for t-PA use a plasminogen-chromogenic substrate assay. Total t-PA antigen (free t-PA and t-PA complexed with PAI-1) is measured using an enzyme-linked immunosorbent assay.

Specimen. Activity of t-PA is unstable in normal plasma. For optimal measurements, citrated blood must be immediately acidified and the red blood cells rapidly removed. Acidification prevents neutralization of t-PA by PAI-1, and prevents PAI-1 from interfering in the assay. To measure t-PA antigen levels, citrated plasma can be used. Since there is diurnal variation in fibrinolysis, samples should be obtained between 8:00 and 9:00 AM. Some investigators recommend obtaining postvenous occlusion samples to optimally distinguish normal individuals from patients with abnormal fibrinolysis.

Procedure. Citrated blood must be acidified with 0.5 M acetate buffer, pH 4.2 (0.5 mL blood:0.25 mL acetate buffer), mixed, then centrifuged. The acidified plasma is immediately collected. For the assay, acidified plasma is incubated with plasminogen, cyanogen-bromide cleaved fibrinogen fragments, and a chromogenic substrate for plasmin. The change in absorbance at 405 nm is proportional to the t-PA activity in the sample; a standard curve is prepared using purified one-chain t-PA.

Interpretation. Low t-PA levels indicate diminished fibrinolysis and may represent a risk factor for thrombosis. Elevated t-PA levels have been associated with excessive fibrinolysis and a bleeding tendency.

Notes and Precautions. As mentioned before, optimal results require attention to sample collection and timing. Otherwise, it may be difficult to correctly classify patients who may have abnormal findings on fibrinolysis assays. A recent literature survey by Prins and Hirsh evaluated the evidence for an association between venous thromboembolism and abnormal fibrinolysis. The authors concluded that the published evidence does not prove an association between abnormal fibrinolysis and thrombosis except in the postoperative setting. Therefore, the association between abnormal fibrinolysis and inherited thrombosis remains unestablished.

47.7 Plasminogen Activator Inhibitor-1 Determination

Purpose. Elevated levels of PAI-1 have been linked to recurrent thrombosis, and abnormal fibrinolysis has been suggested as a common cause for thrombosis.

Principle. PAI-1 activity is measured using a back-titration method with t-PA. PAI-1 antigen levels can be measured using an enzyme-linked immunosorbent assay.

Specimen. PAI-1 activity and antigen levels can be measured in citrated plasma. Acidification of plasma is not necessary. Some investigators suggest obtaining postvenous occlusion samples to optimally distinguish normal individuals from patients with abnormal fibrinolysis.

Procedure. PAI-1 activity is measured by using multiple dilutions of citrated plasma to which a standard amount of purified one-chain t-PA is added. After incubation, the plasma samples are acidified (to inhibit alpha$_2$-plasmin inhibitor), and residual t-PA activity is measured as described previously using the chromogenic substrate assay.

Interpretation. Elevated PAI-1 levels may be associated with thrombosis.

Notes and Precautions. Sample collection and timing are important variables in fibrinolysis assays. Since an association between inherited thrombosis and abnormal fibrinolysis has not been conclusively demonstrated, the routine use of these assays in evaluating patients for inherited thrombosis is not recommended.

References

Chandler WL, Trimble SL, Loo SC, Mornin D. Effect of PAI-1 levels on the molar concentrations of active tissue plasminogen activator (t-PA) and the t-PA/PAI-1 complex in plasma. *Blood.* 1990;76:930-937.

Comp PC. Measurement of the natural anticoagulant protein S: how and when. *Am J Clin Pathol.* 1991;92:242-243.

Hirsh J. Congenital antithrombin III deficiency: incidence and clinical features. *Am J Med.* 1989;87(suppl 3B):34-38.

Marlar RA, Adock DM. Clinical evaluation of protein C: a comparative review of antigenic and functional assays. *Hum Pathol.* 1989;20:1040-1047.

Nguyen G, Horellou MH, Kruithof EKO, Conard J, Samama MM. Residual plasminogen activator inhibitor activity after venous stasis as a criterion for hypofibrinolysis: a study in 83 patients with confirmed deep vein thrombosis. *Blood.* 1988;72:601-605.

Prins MH, Hirsh J. A critical review of the evidence supporting a relationship between impaired fibrinolytic activity and venous thromboembolism. *Arch Intern Med.* 1991;151:1721-1731.

Rodgers GM, Chandler WL. Laboratory and clinical aspects of inherited thrombotic disorders. *Am J Hematol.* 1992;41:113-122.

Svensson PJ, Dahlback B. Resistance to activated protein C as a basis for venous thrombosis. *N Engl J Med.* 1994;330:517-522.

PART
XIV

Anticoagulant Therapy

48

Laboratory Monitoring of Anticoagulant and Fibrinolytic Therapy

Anticoagulant therapy is designed to inhibit the formation of thrombi and to prevent the extension and propagation of formed thrombi. The goal of fibrinolytic therapy is to dissolve or lyse a recent thrombus. Antiplatelet therapy is a form of anticoagulant therapy aimed at reducing the ability of platelets to adhere to one another (aggregate) or to adhere to the damaged endothelium and thereby inhibit thrombosis.

Pathophysiology

Endothelial cell damage is by far the most important factor in arterial thrombosis. As this damage is almost always induced by atherosclerosis, measures designed to reverse or halt this process may be considered antithrombotic. Platelets adhere to the damaged endothelial cell lining, forming the foundation for a thrombus; moreover, platelets can form aggregates in the circulation that may be large enough to block a small artery. In venous thrombosis, in contrast to arterial thrombosis, endothelial cell damage is not an essential component. Stasis, by impeding the removal of activated coagulation proteases by the flowing blood from the site of the thrombus, is relatively more important. Thus, immobilization of the lower limb, particularly in bedridden patients or following surgery or delivery, may precipitate venous thrombosis.

The oral anticoagulants comprise derivatives of coumarin and include warfarin (Coumadin) and a closely related compound used in Europe, phenindione (Dindevan). They inhibit the synthesis of vitamin K–dependent proteins by the liver. The vitamin K–dependent proteins involved in coagulation are the procoagulants, prothrombin and factors VII, IX, and X, and the anticoagulants, proteins C and S. The normal biosynthesis of these proteins requires vitamin K. In the absence of vitamin K, an inactive molecule is synthesized. Vitamin K is essential for a post-translational event in which certain glutamic acid residues are carboxylated. As the half-lives of the various vitamin K–dependent factors differ, they decrease at different rates. Factor VII and protein C have half-lives of less than 10 hours and are the first to decrease with therapy and to reappear on cessation of drug therapy, while prothrombin has the longest half-life (3 days) and is the last to decrease and reappear.

The other type of anticoagulant widely used is heparin, a heterogenous substance consisting of glycosaminoglycans of widely varying but high average molecular weight. Several low-molecular-weight heparins are also now available. Heparin, which is negatively-charged, binds to antithrombin III and sterically modifies this molecule so that its ability to bind to and inactivate thrombin and factors IXa and Xa are greatly enhanced; it is rapidly neutralized by protamine sulfate, which is positively charged. Heparin is usually administered intravenously and may be administered subcutaneously, but not intramuscularly.

In contrast to anticoagulant therapy with either oral anticoagulants or heparin, fibrinolytic agents have a relatively rapid action. Treatment with fibrinolytic agents, which include urinary-plasminogen activator (u-PA) or urokinase, streptokinase, and tissue-plasminogen activator (t-PA), may result in bleeding from sites at which venipuncture was performed some days earlier, indicating dissolution of the hemostatic plugs and the effectiveness of these agents.

When the degree of anticoagulation with oral anticoagulants exceeds a level considered toxic, hematuria is almost invariable, and purpura is a frequent complication. Similarly, a patient receiving heparin is likely to bleed from an open wound. Despite the hemorrhagic complications associated with these drugs, their efficacy in preventing or treating thrombotic disease is well established, and these drugs are among the most commonly used in treating hospitalized patients.

Clinical Indications

Heparin is currently used for the prophylaxis and treatment of venous thromboembolism, unstable angina, acute myocardial infarction, and chronic disseminated intravascular coagulation. Heparin is also used in hemodialysis, cardiac bypass surgery, and to maintain catheter patency. Warfarin is used in the treatment and prophylaxis of venous thromboembolism, and the prevention of systemic embolism in the settings for tissue heart valves, mechanical heart valves, acute myocardial infarction, and atrial fibrillation.

Common indications for fibrinolytic therapy include acute myocardial infarction, massive venous thrombosis or pulmonary embolism, peripheral arterial thromboembolism, and restoration of catheter patency.

Methods of Administration

Anticoagulant therapy in patients with acute venous thrombosis initially consists of administration of heparin. Heparin is best given intravenously, starting with a bolus of 5,000 or 10,000 units followed by a constant infusion of at least 1,300 units/hour. After therapeutic anticoagulation with heparin has been achieved (preferably within the first 24 hours), oral warfarin is started, usually at dosages of 5 to 10 mg/day. There should be at least a 5-day overlap period of heparin and warfarin, so that the patient remains anticoagulated until attaining therapeutic vitamin K deficiency with warfarin. When heparin is used prophylactically, the usual regimen is 5,000 units, given subcutaneously, every 8 to 12 hours.

Fibrinolytic agents are administered intravenously. Streptokinase and urokinase are given in bolus form, followed by continuous infusion over 12 to 72 hours, while t-PA is given in a shorter intravenous infusion.

Laboratory Monitoring

With increasing use of anticoagulant drugs in treatment of thrombotic disease, accurate laboratory methods to monitor anticoagulant intensity is an important issue. Recognition of laboratory variables that may result in inaccurate laboratory monitoring has led to attempts to standardize these assays.

Monitoring Heparin Therapy. The effect of heparin can be monitored by a variety of assays, but the standard method used is the activated partial thromboplastin time (aPTT) test. Heparin should be given in doses sufficient to prolong the aPTT to 1.5 to 2.5 times the mean laboratory control aPTT (mean of the therapeutic range). This recommendation assumes that the aPTT reagent will be responsive to heparin such that plasma heparin levels of 0.2 to 0.4 U/mL (measured by protamine titration) or 0.35 to 0.7 U/mL as measured by anti–factor Xa activity, result in the aPTT being prolonged in the suggested range. However, since aPTT reagents may vary widely in terms of heparin responsiveness, each laboratory should establish its own therapeutic range, so that it corresponds to the plasma heparin levels stated above.

The timing and type of sample collected for monitoring heparin therapy is important. The aPTT should be checked 4 to 6 hours after heparin bolus or after a change in infusion rate, so that steady-state levels are being measured. Samples drawn from indwelling lines may give nonrepresentative results. If prophylactic subcutaneous heparin or low-molecular-weight heparin is being used, laboratory monitoring is not necessary.

Monitoring Warfarin Therapy. All patients receiving warfarin (or other oral anticoagulants) should be monitored using the prothrombin time (PT) assay. Only recently has there been any measure of agreement as to an efficacious or therapeutic range at which the PT should be maintained because of the absence of a uniform or standard way of performing the one-stage PT test (see Chapter 40). The reason for this is that different tissue extracts or so-called "tissue thromboplastins" can give quite different PT values with different pathologic plasma samples, although the normal control times may be the same. Even extracts prepared by the same method from the same tissue do not always give identical results with a pathologic plasma, although the differences are minimized. In general, human brain extracts, now rarely used, give longer clotting times than rabbit brain extracts. When the test was first devised by Armand Quick, it was believed to measure prothrombin specifically, provided the concentration of fibrinogen was above a certain critical level, and the results were often recorded as a percentage of prothrombin activity. With the subsequent discovery of factors V, VII, and X, which, with prothrombin, are also measured by the test, this method of reporting became invalid. In addition, in the past, laboratories used a variety of reporting methods to quantify oral anticoagulation intensity. These differences in assays and reporting methods resulted in inadequate anticoagulation or excessive anticoagulation with adverse consequences.

A recent advance has been the adoption of a World Health Organization (WHO) international reference thromboplastin preparation. Each new batch of thromboplastin can be calibrated against the primary WHO reference material by using each batch to determine the PTs of plasma samples from different patients whose conditions have been stabilized with long-term oral anticoagulant therapy. The unknown preparation of thromboplastin will be found to give PT values that are the same as, longer (higher ratios), or shorter (lower ratios) than those obtained with the standard thromboplastin, but a consistent and reproducible pattern will be obtained. These results are used to calculate the relative sensitivity of the unknown preparation compared to the standard (International Sensitivity Index, ISI). Figure 48-1 illustrates how ISI values are derived. From this value, an International Normalized Ratio (INR), defined as the PT ratio that would have been obtained if the WHO international reference thromboplastin had been used, can be determined for any ratio obtained with the unknown thromboplastin (INR = [PT ratio]^{ISI}) (Figure 48-2).

The calibration should be performed by the manufacturer on each new lot of thromboplastin, and a table enabling conversion to the equivalent INR should be included in the product insert. The laboratory report should always state the PT value in seconds, as well as the PT ratio and the INR. Only then can a result be interpreted by a physician at another institution without having to first consult the pathologist performing the test. In the past, many physi-

Figure 48-1 Derivation of an International Sensitivity Index (ISI) value for a thromboplastin preparation. Log prothrombin time (PT) values are determined using a reference thromboplastin reagent and the commercial laboratory thromboplastin reagent. Patients receiving stable oral anticoagulants are tested, as are a group of normal volunteers. The best-fit line is determined, and the slope of this line multiplied by the ISI of the reference thromboplastin reagent is the ISI value for the commercial thromboplastin reagent.

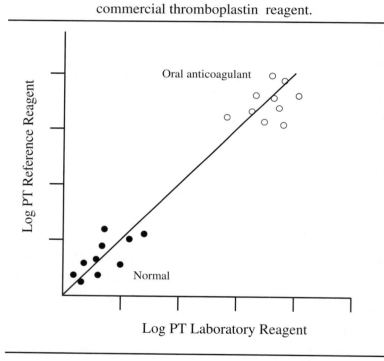

cians strived to maintain the PT ratio at 2, but with some reagents, this represented an excessive degree of anticoagulation and resulted in a relatively high incidence of hemorrhagic manifestations, while with other reagents, this ratio provided relatively little protection against thrombosis. Table 48–1 summarizes the guidelines issued by a consensus conference (American College of Chest Physicians-National Heart Lung and Blood Institute, October

Figure 48-2 Relationship between the prothrombin time (PT) ratio and the International Normalized Ratio (INR) for thromboplastin reagents over a range of International Sensitivity Index (ISI) values. The example shown is for a PT ratio of 1.3 to 1.5 for a thromboplastin preparation with an ISI value of 2.3. From the formula, INR = PT ratio^{ISI}, the INR is calculated as $1.3^{2.3}$ to $1.5^{2.3}$, or 1.83 to 2.54.*

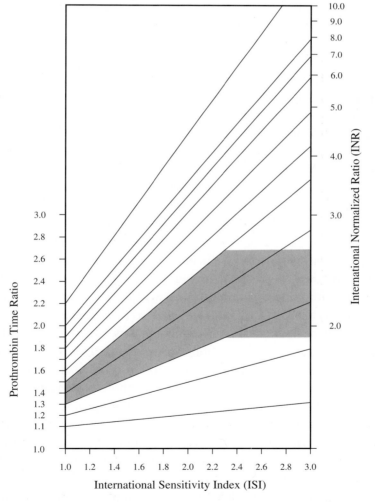

*Reprinted, with permission, from Hirsh J. Oral anticoagulant drugs. *N Engl J Med.* 1991;324: 1865-1875.

Table 48-1 Recommended Therapeutic Range for Warfarin Therapy*

Indication	International Normalized Ratio (INR)
Treatment of venous thrombosis	
Treatment of pulmonary embolism	
Prevention of systemic embolism	
Tissue heart valves	2.0-3.0 (low intensity)
Acute myocardial infarction	
Atrial fibrillation	
Recurrent embolism	
Mechanical heart valves	2.5-3.5 (high intensity)

*From a consensus conference report published in *Chest.* 1992;102(suppl):312S-326S.

1992); the therapeutic ranges in terms of INR are shown. PT ratios are less useful since the ISI values of thromboplastins used in the United States still differ dramatically. It can be seen that with the exception of treating prosthetic (metal) heart valves or patients with recurrent embolism, standard warfarin therapy is targeted at an INR of 2.0 to 3.0.

With more widespread use, difficulties in using the INR format have been reported. Manufacturers of thromboplastin reagents do not provide ISI values derived for all instrument-reagent combinations. Consequently, the thromboplastin ISI package insert will not be accurate for all laboratories. Less sensitive thromboplastins (higher ISI values) will yield INR results with greater variability than will more sensitive thromboplastins (lower ISI values) because determination of PT results using less sensitive thromboplastins is associated with higher coefficients of variation. More optimal INR values will be obtained if the coagulation laboratory uses a sensitive thromboplastin (ISI of 1.0 to 1.5), and if the laboratory ensures that the ISI value is correct either by calibrating the reagent, or by using a thromboplastin whose ISI is appropriate for the laboratory's instrumentation. Many manufacturers now provide sensitive thromboplastins, and recombinant thromboplastins with ISI values of 1.0 are also available.

Many drugs or medical conditions inhibit or enhance the effect of oral anticoagulants. Recent ingestion of such a drug or

Table 48-2 Drugs and Medical Conditions Affecting the Potency of Warfarin

Drugs	Conditions
Increased	
Antibiotics	Age
Aspirin	Liver disease
Cimetidine	Malabsorption
Allopurinol	Congestive heart failure
	Malnutrition
Decreased	
Barbiturates	Excess dietary vitamin K
Vitamin K	Nephrotic syndrome

one of these illnesses should be suspected whenever the PT changes unexpectedly in a patient whose condition was previously stabilized (Table 48-2). In an individual in whom dietary vitamin K intake is marginal, sterilization of the gut by an antibiotic can result in increased sensitivity to oral anticoagulants; this is perhaps the most common adverse interaction that occurs with warfarin.

Monitoring Fibrinolytic Therapy. The systemic intravenous infusion of streptokinase has been used for at least three decades to dissolve arterial or venous clots. Streptokinase, however, is a bacterial product derived from streptococci and, as many individuals have significant titers of antistreptokinase antibodies as a result of a previous streptococcal infection, this complicates therapy and may also result in severe side effects. Until recently, urokinase and t-PA were derived only from human sources and were scarce and very expensive; however, these drugs are now available as recombinant products. Fibrinolytic drugs can be administered systemically to treat venous thromboembolism or myocardial infarction, or infused locally to lyse catheter clots. Local infusions do not require routine laboratory monitoring. However, when these agents are used systemically, it is useful to ensure that a "lytic effect" is achieved. This is especially true for streptokinase therapy, because some patients may have neutralizing antibodies to this bacterial antigen. The lytic state is most easily monitored using the thrombin time assay; prolongation of the thrombin time to values between two to five times over baseline indicates the presence of the lytic state. Since there is no correlation between efficacy of therapy and changes in coagulation or fibrinolytic assays, no additional testing is necessary if an appropriate increase in the thrombin time occurs. For patients with myocardial infarction who receive short-term infusion of t-PA, laboratory monitoring may not be necessary. If the patient is receiving concomitant heparin therapy, the thrombin time will not be a useful test, and the reptilase test or fibrinogen assays should be considered as assays to monitor the lytic state.

Aspirin Therapy. Aspirin is now used extensively to treat arterial thromboembolic disease and to prevent occlusion of arterial grafts and formation of thrombi on prosthetic heart valves. It reduces thromboxane production for the lifetime of the platelet, thereby decreasing platelet aggregation. On the other hand, it also diminishes the production of prostacyclin by the endothelium, albeit for a relatively shorter time, thereby enhancing aggregation. Extensive studies have been performed to evaluate the possibility that low-dose aspirin therapy might be used selectively to inhibit platelet thromboxane synthesis without affecting vascular prostacyclin formation. In recent clinical trials, the daily dose has varied from as low as 80 mg ("baby aspirin") to as high as 650 mg. Antiplatelet therapy is not monitored by laboratory testing.

Laboratory Tests

48.1 Heparin Level

Purpose. It is occasionally necessary to determine plasma heparin levels to monitor heparin anticoagulation in patients in whom the aPTT is not a reliable assay (lupus anticoagulant).

Principle. The ability of dilutions of the patient's plasma to inhibit factor Xa is compared to that of standard concentrations of heparin in normal pooled plasma.

Specimen. Citrated plasma collected during stable heparin infusion is appropriate. Blood specimens should not be drawn from indwelling catheters.

Procedure. The manual (fibrometer) method to assay heparin levels is tedious. Dilutions of heparin are made in saline and normal pooled plasma. Calcium, the aPTT reagent, and factor Xa are added and clotting times measured. Control and patient plasma standard curves are constructed, and a best-fit line is drawn. Plasma heparin levels are determined from these curves.

Interpretation. The therapeutic heparin level by the assay is 0.35 to 0.7 U/mL. The heparin used to construct laboratory standard curves should be the same brand as that being assayed for in the sample.

Notes and Precautions. Automated methods to measure heparin levels are available from a variety of manufacturers. In these methods, a chromogenic substrate assay is used to quantitate inhibition of bovine factor Xa by heparin-antithrombin III.

References

Hirsh J. Oral anticoagulant drugs. *N Engl J Med.* 1991;324:1865-1875.

Hirsh J, Dalen JE, Deykin D, Poller L. Oral anticoagulants: mechanism of action, clinical effectiveness, and optimal therapeutic range. *Chest.* 1992; 102(suppl):312S-326S.

Hirsh J, Poller L. The international normalized ratio: a guide to understanding and correcting its problems. *Arch Intern Med.* 1994;154:282-288.

Hirsh J. Heparin. *N Engl J Med.* 1991;324:1565-1574.

Shojania AM, Tetreault J, Turnbull G. The variations between heparin sensitivity of different lots of activated partial thromboplastin time reagent produced by the same manufacturer. *Am J Clin Pathol.* 1988;89:19-23.

APPENDIX

Hematology Reference Values

Table 1   Hematology Reference Values in Adults for Common Tests[*]

Test	Men	
	Conventional Units	SI Units
Hemoglobin	13-18 g/dL	130-180 g/L
Hematocrit	40%-52%	0.40-0.52
Red blood cell count	4.4-5.9 x 10^6/mm^3	4.4-5.9 x 10^{12}/L
White blood cell count	3.8-10.6 x 10^3/mm^3	3.8-10.6 x10^9/L
MCV	80-100 μm^3	80-100 fL
MCH	26-34 pg	26-34 pg
MCHC	32-36 g/dL	320-360 g/L
Platelet count	150-440 x 10^3/mm^3	150-440 x 10^9/L
Reticulocyte count	0.8%-2.5%	0.008-0.025
Reticulocyte count	18,000-158,000/mm^3	18-158 x 10^9/L
Sedimentation rate[†]	0-10 mm/h	0-10 mm/h
Zeta sedimentation rate	40-52	40-52

Abbreviations: MCV = mean corpuscular volume; MCH = mean corpuscular hemoglobin
MCHC = mean corpuscular hemoglobin concentration.
[*]Modified from: Wintrobe MM. *Clinical Hematology*. 8th ed. Philadelphia, Pa: Lea & Febiger; 1984
Henry JB. *Clinical Diagnosis and Management by Laboratory Methods*. 17th ed. Philadelphia, Pa:
WB Saunders Co; 1984. Miale JB. *Laboratory Medicine: Hematology*. 6th ed. St Louis, Mo: CV
Mosby; 1982. Williams WJ, Beutler E, Erslev AJ, Lichtman MA. *Hematology*. 3rd ed. New York,
NY: McGraw-Hill Book Co; 1983.
[†]May be age dependent, according to method.

Women	
Conventional Units	SI Units
12-16 g/dL	120-160 g/L
35%-47%	0.35-0.47
3.8-5.2 x 10^6/mm^3	3.8-5.2 x 10^{12}/L
3.6-11.0 x 10^3/mm^3	3.6-11.0 x 10^9/L
80-100 μm^3	80-100 fL
26-34 pg	26-34 pg
32-36 g/dL	320-360 g/L
150-440 x 10^3/mm^3	150-440 x 10^9/L
0.8%-4.0%	0.008-0.04
18,000-158,000/mm^3	18-158 x 10^9/L
0-20 mm/h	0-20 mm/h
40-52	40-52

Table 2 Automated Hematology Reference Values in Normal Men at 4,500 ft[*]

Test	Coulter S+ STKR (80 Men)	
	Mean	Central 95% Range
White blood cells (x 10^3/mm^3)	6.6	3.5-9.8
Platelets (x 10^3/mm^3)	280	147-412
Red blood cells (x 10^6/mm^3)	5.4	4.76-6.04
Hemoglobin (g/dL)	16.4	14.7-18.1
Hematocrit (%)	48.7	43.7-53.6
MCV (μm^3)	90.3	83.3-97.2
MCH (pg)	30.5	28.1-32.9
MCHC (g/dL)	33.8	33.0-34.6
RDW	12.4	11.5-13.4
Mean platelet volume	8.4	6.8-10.0

Abbreviations: MCV = mean corpuscular volume; MCH = mean corpuscular hemoglobin; MCHC = mean corpuscular hemoglobin concentration; RDW = red cell distribution width.

[*]Data are based on measurements from healthy male medical students, age range 23-31 years, at an altitude of 4,500 ft. From *Wintrobe's Clinical Hematology*. 9th ed. Philadelphia, Pa: Lea & Febiger; 1993.

Table 3 Effect of Altitude on VPRC in Normal Men[*]

Altitude			
Feet	Meters	No. of Subjects	VPRC (L/L)
0	0	721	0.47
4,400	1,340	744	0.495
7,457	2,280	100	0.51
12,240	3,740	40	0.54
14,900	4,540	32	0.61
17,800	5,430	10	0.69

Abbreviation: VPRC = volume packed red cells.

[*]Mean values in males. From *Wintrobe's Clinical Hematology*. 9th ed. Philadelphia, Pa: Lea & Febiger; 1993.

Technicon HI (64 Men)	
Mean	Central 95% Range
6.7	4.4-8.2
285	147-422
5.54	4.87-6.20
16.2	14.6-17.8
48.7	43.6-53.8
88	80.9-95.2
29.3	27.0-31.7
33.3	32.1-34.6
12.8	12.0-13.6
8.9	7.6-10.2

Table 4   Manual White Blood Cell Differential Count, Reference Values in Adults

Cell Type	Conventional Units	
	Relative	Absolute Counts
Segmented neutrophils	50%-70%	2,400-7,560/mm^3
Bands	2%-6%	96-648/mm^3
Lymphocytes	20%-44%	960-4,752/mm^3
Monocytes	2%-9%	96-972/mm^3
Eosinophils	0%-4%	0-432/mm^3
Basophils	0%-2%	0-216/mm^3

Table 5   Automated Leukocyte Differential Counts, Reference Values in Normal Male Adults[*]

	Coulter S+ STKR (80 Men)	
Percentage	Mean	Central 95% Range
Lymphocytes	36.1	22.3-49.9
Monocytes	4.1	0.7-7.5
Granulocytes	59.7	45.5-74.0
Neutrophils	—	—
Eosinophils	—	—
Basophils	—	—
LUC	—	—
Absolute Numbers		
Lymphocytes (x 10^3/mm^3)	2.4	1.2-3.5
Monocytes (x 10^3/mm^3)	0.3	0.0-0.5
Granulocytes (x 10^3/mm^3)	4.0	1.4-6.6
Neutrophils (x 10^3/mm^3)	—	—
Eosinophils (x 10^3/mm^3)	—	—
Basophils (x 10^3/mm^3)	—	—
LUC (x 10^3/mm^3)	—	—

Abbreviation: LUC = large unstained cells.

[*]Data are based on measurements from healthy male medical students, age range 23-31 years, at an altitude of 4,500 ft. From *Wintrobe's Clinical Hematology.* 9th ed. Philadelphia, Pa: Lea & Febiger; 1993.

SI Units	
Relative	Absolute Counts
0.5-0.7	2.40-7.56 x 10^9/L
0.02-0.06	0.10-0.65 x 10^9/L
0.2-0.44	0.96-4.75 x 10^9/L
0.02-0.09	0.10-0.97 x 10^9/L
0.0-0.04	0.00-0.43 x 10^9/L
0.0-0.02	0.00-0.22 x 10^9L

Technicon HI (64 Men)	
Mean	Central 95% Range
31.3	18.3-44.2
5.5	2.6-8.5
—	—
58.8	45.5-73.1
1.9	0.0-4.4
0.7	0.2-1.2
1.8	0.0-4.9
2.06	0.9-3.22
0.37	0.12-0.62
—	—
4.01	1.31-6.71
0.13	0.00-0.30
0.05	0.01-0.09
0.12	0.00-0.31

Table 6 Hematologic Reference Ranges in Racial and Ethnic Subgroups (2.5th to 97.5th Percentiles) in Men*

	Range	
	White	Black
Test		
	(n = 181)	(n = 172)
WBCs (x $10^3/mm^3$)	3.7-10.4	3.5-9.6
RBCs (x $10^6/mm^3$)	4.3-5.8	4.0-5.8
Hemoglobin (g/dL)	13.0-17.3	11.9-16.7
MCHC (g/dL)	32.4-35.4	32.1-35.2
Platelets (x $10^3/mm^3$)	176-372	167-408
MPV (μm^3)	7.7-11.2	7.5-12.4
Hematocrit (%)	38-49	36-48
MCV (μm^3)	81.6-96.6	71.8-99.8
MCH (pg)	27.2-33.4	23.3-33.9
RDW (%)	11.9-14.3	12.1-16.2
Three-part differential cell count		
	(n = 106)	(n = 114)
Lymphocytes (x $10^3/mm^3$)	1.26-3.05	1.20-3.17
Monocytes (x $10^3/mm^3$)	0.13-0.66	0.14-0.77
Granulocytes (x $10^3/mm^3$)	1.78-7.72	1.49-6.56
Manual differential cell count		
	(n = 80)	(n = 72)
Segmented neutrophils (x $10^3/mm^3$)	1.51-7.00	1.11-6.70
Band cells (x $10^3/mm^3$)	0.00-0.07	0.00-0.07
Lymphocytes (x $10^3/mm^3$)	0.65-2.80	0.97-3.30
Monocytes (x $10^3/mm^3$)	0.00-0.51	0.02-0.83
Eosinophils (x $10^3/mm^3$)	0.00-0.42	0.00-0.47
Basophils (x $10^3/mm^3$)	0.00-0.16	0.00-0.16

Abbreviations: MCHC = mean corpuscular hemoglobin concentration; MPV = mean platelet volume; MCV = mean cell volume; MCH = mean corpuscular hemoglobin; RDW = red cell distribution width.

*From Saxena S, Wong ET. Heterogeneity of common hematologic parameters among racial, ethnic and gender subgroups. *Arch Pathol Lab Med*. 1990;114:715-719.

	Range	
Latino	Asian

Latino	Asian
(n = 141)	(n = 72)
4.1-11.5	3.4-11.5
4.4-5.6	4.0-6.2
13.7-17.0	12.5-17.0
32.5-35.6	32.1-35.3
176-397	223-422
7.4-11.3	7.4-10.9
40-50	36-50
82.0-96.5	67.3-96.3
26.7-33.2	21.6-33.4
12.1-14.7	11.8-14.6
(n = 101)	(n = 46)
1.12-3.36	1.03-3.38
0.14-0.68	0.08-0.77
2.41-8.33	1.51-7.26
(n = 48)	(n = 43)
2.40-7.59	2.02-5.50
0.00-0.21	0.00-0.06
0.94-4.22	0.90-3.50
0.00-0.68	0.00-0.53
0.00-0.80	0.00-0.32
0.00-0.17	0-0.14

Table 7 Hematologic Reference Ranges in Racial and Ethnic Subgroups (2.5th to 97th Percentiles) in Women[*]

Test	Range White (n = 482)	Black (n = 525)
WBCs (x 10^3/mm^3)	3.8-10.6	3.4-11.2
RBCs (x 10^6/mm^3)	3.8-5.0	3.6-5.3
Hemoglobin (g/dL)	11.4-15.5	10.6-14.9
MCHC (g/dL)	32.7-35.3	31.9-35.0
Platelets (x 10^3/mm^3)	188-438	193-485
MPV (μm^3)	7.7-11.5	7.7-11.6
Hematocrit (%)	34-45	31-44
MCV (μm^3)	78.0-98.0	72.9-97.5
MCH (pg)	25.9-33.8	23.7-33.1
RDW (%)	11.7-15.2	12.0-17.3
Three-part differential cell count	(n = 284)	(n = 375)
Lymphocytes (x 10^3/mm^3)	1.14-3.19	1.28-3.29
Monocytes (x 10^3/mm^3)	0.10-0.74	0.10-0.67
Granulocytes (x 10^3/mm^3)	2.03-7.46	1.43-7.68
Manual differential cell count	(n = 216)	(n = 175)
Segmented neutrophils (x 10^3/mm^3)	2.023-7.33	1.50-8.14
Band cells (x 10^3/mm^3)	0.00-0.13	0.00-0.09
Lymphocytes (x10^3/mm^3)	1.01-3.38	1.05-3.48
Monocytes (x 10^3/mm^3)	0.00-0.82	0.02-0.72
Eosinophils (x 10^3/mm^3)	0.00-0.52	0.00-0.46
Basophils (x10^3/mm^3)	0.00-0.16	0.00-0.20

Abbreviations: MCHC = mean corpuscular hemoglobin concentration; MPV = mean platelet volume; MCV = mean cell volume; MCH = mean corpuscular hemoglobin; RDW = red cell distribution width.

[*]From Saxena S, Wong ET. Heterogeneity of common hematologic parameters among racial, ethnic and gender subgroups. *Arch Pathol Lab Med.* 1990;114:715-719.

Range	
Latina	Asian
(n = 394)	(n =175)
4.1-11.8	3.5-9.7
3.7-5.1	3.7-5.4
10.3-15.1	11.3-15.0
32.0-35.3	32.2-35.5
198-460	193-417
7.8-11.5	7.6-11.1
31-44	33-44
69.6-95.8	72.4-97.0
22.3-33.0	22.1-33.8
11.9-16.4	11.6-16.6
(n = 295)	(n = 130)
1.07-3.44	0.94-2.75
0.11-0.67	0.09-0.51
2.19-8.24	1.93-6.13
(n = 114)	(n = 50)
1.85-7.57	1.60-7.33
0.00-0.13	0.00-0.11
0.89-3.73	1.24-2.59
0.06-0.66	0.00-0.65
0.00-0.50	0.00-0.49
0.00-0.15	0.00-0.16

Table 8 Red Blood Cell Values at Various Ages: Mean and Lower Limit of Normal (-2 SD)[*],[†]

Age	Hemoglobin (g/dL)		Hematocrit (%)	
	Mean	−2 SD	Mean	−2 SD
Birth (cord blood)	16.5	13.5	51	42
1-3 Days (capillary)	18.5	14.5	56	45
1 Week	17.5	13.5	54	42
2 Weeks	16.5	12.5	51	39
1 Month	14.0	10.0	43	31
2 Months	11.5	9.0	35	28
3-6 Months	11.5	9.5	35	29
0.5-2 Years	12.0	10.5	36	33
2-6 Years	12.5	11.5	37	34
6-12 Years	13.5	11.5	40	35
12-18 Years				
Female	14.0	12.0	41	36
Male	14.5	13.0	43	37
18-49 Years				
Female	14.0	12.0	41	36
Male	15.5	13.5	47	41

[*]From *Wintrobe's Clinical Hematology*. 9th ed. Philadelphia, Pa: Lea & Febiger; 1993.

[†]These data were compiled from several sources. Emphasis is on recent studies employing electronic counters and on the selection of populations that are likely to exclude individuals with iron deficiency. The mean ±2 SD can be expected to include 95% of the observations in a normal population. (From Dallman PR. In: Rudolph A, ed. *Pediatrics*. 16th ed. East Norwalk, Conn:

Table 9 Hematology Reference Values During the First Month of Life in the Term Infant[*]

Value	Cord Blood	Day 1
Hemoglobin (g/dL)	16.8	18.4
Hematocrit (%)	53	58
RBCs (x 10^6/mm^3)	5.25	5.8
MCV (μm^3)	107	108
MCH (pg)	34	35
MCHC (g/dL)	31.7	32.5
Reticulocytes (%)	3-7	3-7
Nucleated RBCs (x 10^3/mm^3)	500	200
Platelets (x 10^3/mm^3)	290	192

Abbreviations: MCV = mean corpuscular volume; MCH = mean corpuscular hemoglobin; MCHC = mean corpuscular hemoglobin concentration.

[*]From Oski F, Naiman JL. *Hematologic Problems in the Newborn*. 2nd ed. Philadelphia, Pa: WB Saunders Co; 1972.

RBCs (x 10^6/mm³)		MCV (µm³)		MCH (pg)		MCHC (g/dL)	
Mean	−2 SD	Mean	−2 SD	Mean	−2 SD	Mean	−2 SD
4.7	3.9	108	98	34	31	33	30
5.3	4.0	108	95	34	31	33	29
5.1	3.9	107	88	34	28	33	28
4.9	3.6	105	86	34	28	33	28
4.2	3.0	104	85	34	28	33	29
3.8	2.7	96	77	30	26	33	29
3.8	3.1	91	74	30	25	33	30
4.5	3.7	78	70	27	23	33	30
4.6	3.9	81	75	27	24	34	31
4.6	4.0	86	77	29	25	34	31
4.6	4.1	90	78	30	25	34	31
4.9	4.5	88	78	30	25	34	31
4.6	4.0	90	80	30	26	34	31
5.2	4.5	90	80	30	26	34	31

Appleton-Century-Crofts; 1977. Lubin BH. Reference values in infancy and childhood. In: Nathan DG, Oski FA, eds. *Hematology of Infancy and Childhood*. 3rd ed. Philadelphia, Pa: WB Saunders Co; 1987.)

Day 3	Day 7	Day 14	Day 28
17.8	17.0	16.8	15.6
55	54	52	45
5.6	5.2	5.1	4.7
99	98	96	91
33	32.5	31.5	31
33	33	33	32
1-3	0-1	0-1	0-1
0-5	0	0	0
213	248	252	240

Table 10 Leukocyte Counts and Differential Counts: Reference Values in Children*†

Age	Total Leukocytes		Neutrophils		
	Mean	(Range)	Mean	(Range)	%
Birth	18.1	(9.0-30.0)	11	(6.0-26.0)	61
12 Hours	22.8	(13.0-38.0)	15.5	(6.0-28.0)	68
24 Hours	18.9	(9.4-34.0)	11.5	(5.0-21.0)	61
1 Week	12.2	(5.0-21.0)	5.5	(1.5-10.0)	45
2 Weeks	11.4	(5.0-20.0)	4.5	(1.0-9.5)	40
1 Month	10.8	(5.0-19.5)	3.8	(1.0-9.0)	35
Months	11.9	(6.0-17.5)	3.8	(1.0-8.5)	32
1 Year	11.4	(6.0-17.5)	3.5	(1.5-8.5)	31
2 Years	10.6	(6.0-17.0)	3.5	(1.5-8.5)	33
4 Years	9.1	(5.5-15.5)	3.8	(1.5-8.5)	42
6 Years	8.5	(5.0-14.5)	4.3	(1.5-8.0)	51
8 Years	8.3	(4.5-13.5)	4.4	(1.5-8.0)	53
10 Years	8.1	(4.5-13.5)	4.4	(1.8-8.0)	54
16 Years	7.8	(4.5-13.0)	4.4	(1.8-8.0)	57
21 Years	7.4	(4.5-11.0)	4.4	(1.8-7.7)	59

*From *Wintrobe's Clinical Hematology.* 9th ed. Philadelphia, Pa: Lea & Febiger; 1993.

†These data were compiled from several sources. Emphasis is on recent studies employing electronic counters and on the selection of populations that are likely to exclude individuals with iron deficiency.   The mean ±2 SD can be expected to include 95% of the observations in a normal population. (From Dallman PR. In: Rudolph A, ed. *Pediatrics.* 16th ed. East Norwalk, Conn: Appleton-Century-Crofts; 1977. Lubin BH. Reference values in infancy and childhood. In: Nathan DG, Oski FA, eds. *Hematology of Infancy and Childhood.* 3rd ed. Philadelphia, Pa: WB Saunders Co; 1987.)

Table 11 Hematology Reference Values in Adults for Ancillary Tests*

Test	Men	
	Conventional Units	SI Units
Serum iron	70-201 µg/dL	12.7-35.9 µmol/L
Total iron-binding capacity	253-435 µg/dL	45.2-77.7 µmol/L
Ferritin	20-250 ng/mL	20-250 µg/L
Serum B_{12}	200-1,000 pg/mL	150-750 pmol/
Serum folate	2-10 ng/mL	4-22 nmol/L
Red cell folate	140-960 ng/mL	550-2,200 nmol/L
Hemoglobin A_2	1.5%-3.5%	0.015-0.035
Hemoglobin F	<2%	<0.02
<2%	<0.02	

*Modified from: Wintrobe MM. *Clinical Hematology.* 8th ed. Philadelphia, Pa: Lea & Febiger; 1984. Henry JB. *Clinical Diagnosis and Management by Laboratory Methods.* 17th ed. Philadelphia, Pa: WB Saunders Co; 1984. Miale JB. *Laboratory Medicine: Hematology.* 6th ed. St Louis, Mo: CV Mosby; 1982. Williams WJ, Beutler E, Erslev AJ, Lichtman MA. *Hematology.* 3rd ed. New York, NY: McGraw-Hill Book Co; 1983.

Lymphocytes			Monocytes		Eosinophils	
Mean	(Range)	%	Mean	%	Mean	%
5.5	(2.0-11.0)	31	1.1	6	0.4	2
5.5	(2.0-11.0)	24	1.2	5	0.5	2
5.8	(2.0-11.5)	31	1.1	6	0.5	2
5	(2.0-17.0)	41	1.1	9	0.5	4
5.5	(2.0-17.0)	48	1	9	0.4	3
6	(2.5-16.5)	56	0.7	7	0.3	6
7.3	(4.0-13.5)	61	0.6	5	0.3	3
7	(4.0-10.5)	61	0.6	5	0.3	3
6.3	(3.0-9.5)	59	0.5	5	0.3	3
4.5	(2.0-8.0)	50	0.5	5	0.3	3
3.5	(1.5-7.0)	42	0.4	5	0.2	3
3.3	(1.5-6.8)	39	0.4	4	0.2	2
3.1	(1.5-6.5)	38	0.4	4	0.2	2
2.8	(1.2-5.2)	35	0.4	5	0.2	3
2.5	(1.0-4.8)	34	0.3	4	0.2	3

Women	
Conventional Units	SI Units
62-173 µg/dL	11-30 µmol/L
253-435 µg/dL	45.2-77.7 µmol/L
10-200 ng/mL	10-200 µg/L
200-1,000 pg/mL	150-750 pmol/L
2-10 ng/mL	4-22 nmol/L
140-960 ng/mL	550-2,200 nmol/L
1.5%-3.5%	0.015-0.035

Table 12   Age-Related Coagulation Reference Values[*]

	Age	
Coagulation test	5 d	90 d
Fibrinogen (g/L)	1.62-4.62	1.5-3.79
Prothrombin (U/mL)	0.33-0.93	0.45-1.05
Factor V (U/mL)	0.45-1.45	0.48-1.32
Factor VII (U/mL)	0.35-1.43	0.39-1.43
Factor VIII (U/mL)	0.5-1.54	0.5-1.25
Factor IX (U/mL)	0.15-0.91	0.21-1.13
Factor X (U/mL)	0.19-0.79	0.35-1.07
Factor XI (U/mL)	0.23-0.87	0.41-0.97
Factor XII (U/mL)	0.11-0.83	0.25-1.09
HMWK (U/mL)	0.16-1.32	0.3-1.46
Prekallikrein (U/mL)	0.2-0.76	0.41-1.05
vWf antigen[†] (U/mL)	0.5-2.54	0.5-2.06
Ristocetin cofactor (U/mL)	—	—
Antithrombin III (U/mL)	0.41-0.93	0.73-1.21
Protein C (U/mL)	0.2-0.64	0.28-0.80
Protein S[†] (U/mL)	0.22-0.78	0.54-1.18
Plasminogen (U/mL)	—	—
TPA (ng/mL)	—	—
PAI (U/mL)	—	—
α_2-Antiplasmin (U/mL)	—	—

Abbreviations: HMWK = high molecular weight kininogen; vWf = von Willebrand's factor; TPA = tissue plasminogen activator; PAI = plasminogen activator inhibitor.

[*]Prothrombin time and partial thromboplastin time values are not shown due to dependence of these values on reagent selection. Adult values represent those of the University of Utah Medical Center Hemostasis and Thrombosis Laboratory. Pediatric values are for healthy full-term infants (from Andrew M, et al. Maturation of the hemostatic system during childhood. *Blood.* 1992;80:1998; and Andrew M, et al. Development of the hemostatic system in the neonate and young infant. *Am J Pediatr Hematol Oncol.* 1990;12:95).

[†]Results are based on antigenic assays. All other results are based on functional assays. The adult fibrinolysis tests (TPA, PAI) are based on reference range values drawn between 7 and 9 AM.

[‡]Adult α_2-antiplasmin values are listed in terms of mg/dL.

1-5 y	6-10 y	11-16 y	Adult
1.7-4.05	1.57-4.0	1.54-4.48	1.5-3.50
0.71-1.16	0.67-1.07	0.61-1.04	0.79-1.31
0.79-1.27	0.63-1.16	0.55-0.99	0.62-1.39
0.55-1.16	0.52-1.2	0.58-1.15	0.50-1.29
0.59-1.42	0.58-1.32	0.53-1.31	0.50-1.50
0.47-1.04	0.63-0.89	0.59-1.22	0.65-1.50
0.58-1.16	0.55-1.01	0.5-1.17	0.77-1.31
0.56-1.5	0.52-1.2	0.5-0.97	0.65-1.50
0.64-1.29	0.6-1.4	0.34-1.37	0.50-1.50
0.64-1.32	0.6-1.3	0.63-1.19	0.60-1.46
0.65-1.3	0.66-1.31	0.53-1.45	0.60-1.46
0.6-1.2	0.44-1.44	0.46-1.53	0.43-1.50
—	—	—	0.52-1.60
0.82-1.39	0.9-1.31	0.77-1.32	0.85-1.22
0.4-0.92	0.45-0.93	0.55-1.11	0.78-2.32
0.54-1.18	0.41-1.14	0.52-0.92	0.62-1.25
0.78-1.18	0.75-1.08	0.68-1.03	0.74-1.24
1.0-4.5[†]	1.0-5.0[†]	1.0-4.0[†]	3.0-12.0
1.0-10.0	2.0-12.0	2.0-10.0	2.0-15.0
0.93-1.17	0.89-1.10	0.78-1.18	4.4-8.5 mg/dL[‡]

Table 13   Differential Counts of Bone Marrow Aspirates From 12 Healthy Men[*]

Cell Type	Mean (%)	Observed Range (%)	95% Confidence Limits (%)
Neutrophilic series (total)	53.6	49.2-65.0	33.6-73.6
Myeloblasts	0.9	0.2-1.5	0.1-1.7
Promyelocytes	3.3	2.1-4.1	1.9-4.7
Myelocytes	12.7	8.2-15.7	8.5-16.9
Metamyelocytes	15.9	9.6-24.6	7.1-24.7
Band	12.4	9.5-15.3	9.4-15.4
Segmented	7.4	6.0-12.0	3.8-11.0
Eosinophilic series (total)	3.1	1.2-5.3	1.1-5.2
Myelocytes	0.8	0.2-1.3	0.2-1.4
Metamyelocytes	1.2	0.4-2.2	0.2-2.2
Band	0.9	0.2-2.4	0-2.7
Segmented	0.5	0-1.3	0-1.1
Basophilic and mast cells	0.1	0-0.2	—
Erythrocytic series (total)	25.6	18.4-33.8	15.0-36.2
Pronormoblasts	0.6	0.2-1.3	0.1-1.1
Basophilic	1.4	0.5-2.4	0.4-2.4
Polychromatophilic	21.6	17.9-29.2	13.1-30.1
Orthochromatic	2.0	0.4-4.6	0.3-3.7
Lymphocytes	16.2	11.1-23.2	8.6-23.8
Plasma cells	1.3	0.4-3.9	0-3.5
Monocytes	0.3	0-0.8	0-0.6
Megakaryocytes	0.1	0-0.4	—
Reticulum cells	0.3	0-0.9	0-0.8
Myeloid:Erythroid ratio	2.3	1.5-3.3	1.1-3.5

[*]From Wintrobe MM. *Clinical Hematology.* 8th ed. Philadelphia, Pa: Lea & Febiger; 1984.

INDEX

Numbers in *italics* refer to pages on which Tables or Figures appear. Numbers in **boldface** refer to pages on which Tests appear.

iron metabolism in, 26
with liver disease, 48-50
pathophysiology of, 40-41, *42*
peripheral blood smear morphology in, 42, 44
with renal disease, 46-47
serum ferritin quantitation in, 45-46
serum iron quantitation in, *32,* 44
stainable bone marrow iron in, *32*
total iron-binding capacity in, *32, 45*
transferrin saturation in, 45
treatment of, 46-51
Anesthetics, *318, 661*
Angiocentric lymphoma, *524,* 541
Angioimmunoblastic lymphadenopathy, *63, 330, 337, 581*
Angioimmunoblastic T-cell lymphoma, *524,* 540-541
Angiotensin-converting enzyme test, 338
Anisocytosis, 4-5, 9, *161*
Anisopoikilocytosis, 64, *372*
Antibiotics, *753*
Antibody
to coagulation factors, 704-707
drug-induced immune hemolysis, 196-199, *198*
Antibody identification, **178-179**
in extrinsic hemolytic anemia, 175, 178-179
in transfusion reaction, 178-179
Antibody-induced hemolytic anemia, *172*
Antibody testing. *See* Antibody identification; Antibody titers; Antinuclear antibody test; Epstein-Barr virus serologic tests; Factor VIII antibody screening test; Factor VIII antibody titer; Heterophil antibody test; Maternal antibody screening/identification; Platelet-associated immunoglobulins test; Red blood cell eluates; Serum antibody detection; Serum antibody screening; Serum immunoglobulin quantitation

Antibody titers
for mycoplasma, **220**
in autoimmune hemolytic anemia, 220
for viruses, **220**
in autoimmune hemolytic anemia, 220
Anti-C antibodies, 176, 179, 184, 190
Anticoagulant therapy
administration of, 747
clinical indications for, 747
goal of, 745
heparin level in, 754-755
monitoring of, 748-753
pathophysiology of, 745-747
prothrombin time test in, 634-636
Anticonvulsants, *58, 76*
Anti-D antibodies, 189
Anti-Duffy antibodies, 176
Anti-E antibodies, 176, 179, 184, 190
Anti-Fy^a antibodies, 179
Antiglobulin testing. *See* Direct antiglobulin test
Antihistamine, *661*
Anti-I antibodies, 215, 217
Anti-Jk^a antibodies, 176, 179
Anti-Jk^b antibodies, 176, 179
Anti-Kell antibodies, 176, 179, 184, 190
Anti-Kidd antibodies, 176, 179
Anti-Lewis antibodies, 179, 189
Antilymphocyte globulin, *318,* 319
Anti-M antibodies, 179
Antinuclear antibody test, **221**
in autoimmune hemolytic anemia, 221
Anti-P1 antibodies, 179
Antiphospholipid antibody. *See* Lupus anticoagulant
Antiplatelet therapy, 643, 745, 754
Anti-S antibodies, 176
Antithrombin III (AT III), *724,* 725
Antithrombin III (AT III) deficiency, *727, 729, 733,* 734-735
Antithrombin III (AT III) determination, **734-735**
reference values for, *772-773*
in thrombotic disorders, *733,* 734-735

Antituberculosis drug, *76*
Anturane. *See* Sulfinpyrazone
APC cofactor, 723-725, *724*
APC cofactor deficiency, 725, 727-728, *729, 731, 733,* 737
APC cofactor determination, **737-738**
   reference values for, *772-773*
   in thrombotic disorders, *733,* 737-738
APC inhibitor, 726
APC resistance. *See* APC cofactor deficiency
Aplastic anemia
   acquired, *54-55,* 56-57, *58,* 59-61
   approach to diagnosis of, 11, *12,* 58-59
   blood cell measurements in, *10, 55,* 59
   bone marrow examination in, *55,* 60, *67*
   characteristics of, 53-56, *54-55*
   clinical findings in, *54,* 58
   constitutional, *54,* 59
   course of, 61-62
   cytogenetic studies in, 61
   fetal hemoglobin quantitation in, 60-61
   hematologic findings in, 59-60
   neutropenia in, *262*
   pathophysiology of, 56-57, *58*
   peripheral blood smear morphology in, 59-60
   red cell i antigen test in, 61
   treatment of, 61-62
aPTT. *See* Activated partial thromboplastin time
Arsenic poisoning, 357, *368*
Arterial oxygen saturation, **462**
   in polycythemia, 458, 462, *464*
Arterial thrombosis, 727-728, 730, *732,* 745
L-Asparaginase, 430
Aspirin, *271,* 658, 660, *661, 753. See also* Post-aspirin bleeding time
   as antiplatelet therapy, 754
   drugs containing, *642*
Asynchronous acute lymphoblastic leukemia, 425-426
Ataxia telangiectasia, 411, *519*

Atherosclerosis, 727, 745
AT III. *See* Antithrombin III
ATLL. *See* Adult T-cell leukemia/lymphoma
Atypical chronic myelogenous leukemia, 485
Atypical myeloproliferative syndrome, 450
Auer rods, 381, 384-385, 387, *398, 404-405*
Autoantibody, 171, 196. *See also* Autoimmune hemolytic anemia
   cold-type, *172*
   warm-type, *172*
Autoerythrocyte sensitization, *716*
Autoimmune disorder
   granulocyte functional defects in, *271*
   lymphadenopathy in, *330*
   neutropenia in, 260, *261-262, 267*
Autoimmune hemolytic anemia (AIHA)
   acid hemolysis test in, 218
   antibody titers for mycoplasma and viruses in, 220
   antinuclear antibody test in, 221
   approach to diagnosis of, 11, *13,* 211-212
   blood cell measurements in, *10,* 212-213
   bone marrow examination in, 213
   in chronic lymphocytic leukemia, 492, 498
   clinical findings in, *208,* 210-211
   cold agglutinin titer in, 212, 216-217
   cold-type, 207-216, *208-210, 212,* 218-220, 222
   complement activation in, 209, *209*
   course of, 222
   definition of, 207
   direct antiglobulin test in, *209,* 212-214
   diseases associated with, 209, *210*
   Donath-Landsteiner test in, 212, 217-218
   hematologic findings in, 211-213
   immunoglobulin G-mediated, 173
   occult lymphoma in, 221

osmotic fragility test in, 116, *209,* 220

pathophysiology of, 207-209

peripheral blood smear morphology in, *209,* 213

primary, 209

red cell eluates in, 216

secondary, 209

serum antibody detection in, 214-215

serum complement measurement in, *209,* 219

serum haptoglobin quantitation in, 219

with spherocytosis, 116, 126

sucrose hemolysis test in, 166

treatment of, 222

warm-type, 198, 202-208, *208-210,* 210, 212-214, 216, 220-222

Automated hematology, 4-5, *760-761*

Azotemia, 47

B

Babesiosis, 173

Bacterial overgrowth disorder, 85

Band 4.1, 109-110

Band neutrophils, 227-228, 230

Banti's syndrome, *347*

Barbiturates, *753*

Basophil(s), 245

Basophilia

approach to diagnosis of, 247-248

blood cell measurements in, 248

bone marrow examination in, 248

clinical findings in, 247

course of, 248-249

definition of, 245

hematologic findings in, 248

pathophysiology of, 246-247

peripheral blood smear morphology in, 248

treatment of, 248-249

Basophilic stippling, *6-7*

B cell(s), monoclonal antibodies against, *324*

B-cell acute lymphoblastic leukemia, *423,* 424, *425-426,* 428

B-cell chronic lymphocytic leukemia (B-CLL), *524,* 527-529, *534-535*

B-cell lymphoblastic lymphoma (B-LBL), *524,* 525

B-cell lymphoma, 522, *524,* 525-527, *526-529*

B-cell precursor acute lymphoblastic leukemia, 424-425, *423,* 428, 430

B-cell prolymphocytic leukemia (B-PLL), *524,* 527-529

B-cell small lymphocytic lymphoma (B-SLL), *524,* 527-529, *534-535*

bcl-1 gene, 530, *535, 558,* 563

bcl-2 gene, 531, *535, 558,* 563, *575,* 588

bcr-abl fusion gene, 476, 481-482, 485

Benzene, *58, 94, 172, 445, 519*

Benzidine, 104

Bernard-Soulier disease, 651-652, 659-662, *663-664, 667, 669,* 674

β_2-microglobulin

in multiple myeloma, 605

in non-Hodgkin's lymphoma, 564

Beta-thalassemia, *16, 26,* 141, *142,* 145-146, 154, *155,* 158-159

Beta-thalassemia major, 141, 145

Beta-thalassemia minor, 141, 145, *160*

Bilirubin, 95

in amniotic fluid, 192-193

Bilirubin testing. *See* Indirect bilirubin test; Serum bilirubin test

Biliverdin, 95

Biliverdin reductase, 95

Biopsy. *See* Lymph node biopsy; Tissue biopsy

Bipedal lymphangiography, 552

Bite cells, *6-7,* 132

Blasts, *361*

B-LBL. *See* B-cell lymphoblastic lymphoma

Bleeding disorders

acquired. *See* Acquired coagulation disorders

activated partial thromboplastin time in, 637-639, 715, *716*

in acute myeloid leukemia, 397-399
approach to diagnosis of, 631-633
bleeding time test in, 640-643
clinical findings in, 631-633, *633*
coagulation type, 631-633, *634*
history in, 631
inherited. *See* Inherited coagulation
  disorders
laboratory evaluation of, 715-717,
  716
laboratory screening tests in, 634
platelet count in, *635,* 640, 715, *716*
platelet-vascular type, 631-633, *634*
postaspirin bleeding time in, 641-
  643
prothrombin time test in, 634-637,
  636, 715, *716*
reptilase time in, 639-640
structural bleeding vs, 715
thrombin time in, 639-640
Bleeding time test, **640-643**
  in bleeding disorders, 640-643
  in hemophilia, *635*
  in inherited coagulation disorders,
    684
  postoperative, *720*
  in qualitative platelet disorders,
    640-641, 660
  in thrombocytopenia, *635,* 651
  in vitamin K deficiency, *635*
  in von Willebrand's disease, *635,*
    640-641, 660, *671,* 673
Blind loop syndrome, *74*
Blood antigens, associated with
  alloantibodies, *172*
Blood cell counter
  impedance counter, 4
  light scatter counter, 4
Blood cell measurements
  in accelerated erythrocyte turnover,
    100
  in acute lymphoblastic leukemia,
    414
  in acute myeloid leukemia, 379-
    380
  in anemia, 9, *10*
  in anemia of chronic disease, *10,*
    43-44
  in aplastic anemia, *10, 55, 59*

in autoimmune hemolytic anemia,
  10, 212-213
in basophilia, 248
in bone marrow replacement disorders, 64
in chronic lymphocytic leukemia,
  493-495
in chronic myelogenous leukemia,
  476-477
in cold agglutinin disease, *10*
in drug-related hemolytic anemia,
  200
in eosinophilia, 241
in erythrocyte membrane defect,
  10, 112
in extrinsic hemolytic anemia, 176
in folate deficiency, *10*
in glucose-6-phosphate dehydrogenase deficiency, 132-133
in granulocyte functional defects,
  275
in hemoglobinopathy, *10,* 100
in hemoglobin synthesis disorders,
  147
in hemolytic disease of the newborn, 186-187
in hereditary nonspherocytic
  hemolytic anemia, 123
in Hodgkin's disease, 584-585
in hypersplenism, 348
in hypochromic anemia, 29
in hypoplastic anemia, *55, 59*
in infectious mononucleosis, 309
in inherited coagulation disorders,
  686
in iron deficiency anemia, *10,* 29
in leukocytic disorders of abnormal
  morphology, 287
in lymphadenopathy, 331-332
in lymphocytopenia, 321-322
in lymphocytosis, 297, 299-300
in megaloblastic anemia, 77-78
in monoclonal gammopathy of
  undetermined significance, 614
in monocytosis, 254-255, *257*
in multiple myeloma, 597
in myelodysplastic syndromes, *10,*
  357-358
in myelofibrosis with myeloid
  metaplasia, 443-445

in neutropenia, 264
in neutrophilia, 229-230
in non-Hodgkin's lymphoma, 550
in paroxysmal nocturnal hemoglobinuria, 100, 165
in polycythemia, 460
in sickle cell anemia, *10*
in thalassemia, *10, 29*
in vitamin B$_{12}$ deficiency, *10*
Blood coagulation. *See also* Bleeding
disorders; Hemostasis
extrinsic pathway of, *628,* 629-630
intrinsic pathway of, *628,* 630
mechanisms of, 625-626, *628, 632*
physiology and biochemistry of,
626-631
reference values for in, *772-773*
Blood coagulation inhibitor, 638
Blood coagulation testing. *See*
Activated partial thromboplastin
time; Bleeding time test;
Prothrombin time test;
Thrombin time
Blood group determination, **187-188**
in hemolytic disease of the newborn, 187-188
Blood smear morphology. *See*
Peripheral blood smear morphology
Blood vessel, antithrombotic properties of, *724*
Blood viscosity, 463
Bloom syndrome, 377
Bone marrow aplasia, *646*
Bone marrow cell culture studies, in
myelodysplastic syndromes,
366
Bone marrow discordance, 551
Bone marrow examination, **19-21.** *See
also* Stainable bone marrow
iron
in accelerated erythrocyte turnover,
97, 101
in acute lymphoblastic leukemia,
413-415, *434*
in acute myeloid leukemia, 379-
382
in amyloidosis, 619
in anemia, 19-21

in anemia of chronic disease, 43-44
in aplastic anemia, *55,* 60, *67*
in autoimmune hemolytic anemia,
213
in basophilia, 248
in bone marrow replacement disorders, 64
in cancer, 21
in chronic lymphocytic leukemia,
493, 495, *508*
in chronic myelogenous leukemia,
477-478, *488*
in congenital dyserythropoietic
anemia, 65
in drug-related hemolytic anemia,
200
in eosinophilia, 241
in erythrocyte membrane defect,
113
in essential thrombocythemia, 471,
471
in extrinsic hemolytic anemia, 176
in granulocyte functional defects,
275
in hairy cell leukemia, 502
in hemoglobin synthesis disorders,
148
in Hodgkin's disease, 584-586
in hypersplenism, 349
in hypochromic anemia, 29
in hypoplastic anemia, *55,* 60
indications for, *21*
in iron deficiency anemia, 29
in leukocytic disorders of abnormal morphology, 287
in lymphadenopathy, 332-333
in lymphocytopenia, 321-322
in lymphocytosis, 300
in lymphoma, 21, *21*
in megaloblastic anemia, 78-79
in monoclonal gammopathy of
undetermined significance, 615
in monocytosis, 255
in multiple myeloma, 598-599,
611-612
in myelodysplastic syndromes,
358, *359, 374*
in myelofibrosis with myeloid
metaplasia, 444, 446, *451-452*

Chronic myelogenous leukemia
(CML)
accelerated phase in, 483-485
approach to diagnosis of, *459, 469,*
476-477
atypical, 485
basophilia in, 245-248
blast crisis in, 483-485, *488*
blood cell measurements in, 476-
477
bone marrow examination in, 477-
478, *488*
characteristics of, *484*
clinical findings in, *9,* 476
course of, 483
cytogenetic studies in, 447, 477,
479-481, *487*
definition of, 475
eosinophilia in, *239,* 241
hematologic findings in, 477-478
leukocyte alkaline phosphatase in,
232-233, *233,* 446, 472, 476,
478-479, *480*
leukocytic disorders of abnormal
morphology in, *284,* 285
molecular diagnostic studies in,
481-482
monocytosis in, 252, *253,* 254
myelofibrosis in, 441, *442, 443*
neutrophilia vs, *231*
pathophysiology of, 475-476
peripheral blood smear morphology
in, 476-477, *487*
polymerase chain reaction in, 482
Southern blot hybridization in,
481-482
terminal deoxynucleotidyl transferase in, 483
thrombocytosis in, *468*
treatment of, 483
Chronic myeloid leukemia, juvenile,
365-366
Chronic myelomonocytic leukemia
(CMML), 356, *361,* 362-363,
369, *369, 373-374*
monocytosis in, 252, *253,* 254,
257
in transformation (CMML-T), 360,
361, 363, 369

Chronic myelosclerosis. *See*
Myelofibrosis with myeloid
metaplasia
Chronic obstructive pulmonary dis-
ease, 454, *455*
Cigarette smoking. *See* Smoking
Cimetidine, *753*
Cirrhosis, 50, 347-348, *347,* 671, *673,*
698
CLL. *See* Chronic lymphocytic
leukemia
Clofibrate, *661*
CML. *See* Chronic myelogenous
leukemia
CMML. *See* Chronic myelomonocytic
leukemia
CMML-T. *See* Chronic myelomono-
cytic leukemia, in transformation
CMV infection. *See* Cytomegalovirus
infection
c-myc gene, 546, 563-564
Coagulation. *See* Blood coagulation
Coagulation disorders. *See* Bleeding
disorders
acquired. *See* Acquired coagulation disorders
inherited. *See* Inherited coagulation disorders
Cocaine, *661*
Coccidioplasmosis, *330*
Codocytes. *See* Target cells
Colchicine, *74, 284,* 285, *661*
Cold agglutinin(s), 11, 172, 210-211,
218
interference with direct antiglobulin test, 106
Cold agglutinin disease (CAD), *10,*
211, *212,* 216-217, 222, 619
Cold agglutinin titer, **216-217**
in accelerated erythrocyte turnover,
100
in autoimmune hemolytic anemia,
212, 216-217
Cold-type autoantibody, *172*
Cold-type autoimmune hemolytic anemia, 207-216, *208-210, 212,*
218-220, 222
Colitis, *13*

Elliptocytes, *6-7*, 110, 112, *118*
Elliptocytosis, 11
    hereditary. *See* Hereditary ellipto-
        cytosis; Erythrocyte membrane
        defect, hereditary
Embden-Meyerhof pathway. *See*
    Glycolytic pathway
Embryonal rhabdomyosarcoma, 430
Endocrine disorder
    anemia in, 47-48
    basophilia in, *246, 247*
    bone marrow failure in, *63*
Enzyme-linked immunosorbent assay
    (ELISA), 334
Eosinophil(s), 237
Eosinophilia
    in acute lymphoblastic leukemia,
        417
    approach to diagnosis of, 240
    blood cell measurements in, 241
    bone marrow examination in, 241
    clinical findings in, 239-240
    course of, 242
    definition of, 237
    hematologic findings in, 241
    nasal, 242
    pathophysiology of, 238-239
    peripheral blood smear morphology
        in, 241, *244*
    reactive, 237, *238*
    treatment of, 242
Eosinophilia-myalgia syndrome, 237,
    240
Epinephrine, *226,* 228, *271*
Epipodophyllotoxin, 363
Epsilon aminocaproic acid (Amicar),
    695-696, 739
Epstein-Barr virus infection, 57, *58,*
    210, 211, *519,* 588. *See also*
    Infectious mononucleosis
Epstein-Barr virus serologic tests,
    312-313, *313*
    in infectious mononucleosis, 307,
        312-313, *313*
Erythremic myelosis, 389
Erythroblast(s), 389, *408*
Erythroblastopenia. *See* Transient ery-
    throblastopenia of childhood
Erythroblastosis fetalis, 186

Erythrocyte(s). *See also* Red blood
    cell(s)
    monoclonal antibodies against,
        324
Erythrocyte disorders. *See* Accelerated
    erythrocyte turnover;
    Erythrocyte membrane defect,
    hereditary; Hereditary nonsphe-
    rocytic hemolytic anemia;
    Hexose monophosphate shunt
    disorders
Erythrocyte membrane defect, heredi-
    tary
    approach to diagnosis of, 111-112
    blood cell measurements in, 112
    bone marrow examination in, 113
    clinical findings in, 110-111
    course of, 116
    direct antiglobulin test in, 112
    glycolysis in, 112
    hematologic findings in, 112-113
    hexose monophosphate shunt in,
        112
    osmotic fragility test in, 112-116,
        114-115
    paroxysmal nocturnal hemoglobin-
        uria, 163-168
    pathophysiology of, 109-110
    peripheral blood smear morpholo-
        gy in, 112-113, *118*
    treatment of, 116
Erythrocyte sedimentation rate (ESR)
    in lymphadenopathy, 331, 333
    reference values for, *758-759*
Erythrocytosis. *See also* Polycythemia
    definition of, 453
    primary. *See* Polycythemia vera
    relative, 454-455, 457-458, *459,*
        460-461, *464,* 465
    secondary, 454-458, *457, 459,* 460,
        464, 465
    stress. *See* Erythrocytosis, relative
    types of, 453-455, *455*
Erythroleukemia (M6), *382-383,* 389,
    392, 394, *395, 399-400, 408*
Erythromelalgia, 456
Erythropoiesis
    decreased, 40, 47
    ineffective, 65

goal of, 745
monitoring of, 753-754
pathophysiology of, 745-747
Fibrinopeptide A, 699
Fibrinopeptide B, 699
Fine needle aspiration (FNA), of
lymph nodes, **553-554**
in lymphadenopathy, 336
in non-Hodgkin's lymphoma, 549,
553-554
Fixative, 549, 555
Flow cytometry, in immunophenotyping, 422, 496, *497,* 554
Fludarabine, 500
Fluid overload, 47, *49*
Fluorescent screening test
for glucose-6-phosphate dehydrogenase, **133-134**
for pyruvate kinase deficiency,
123-125
FNA. *See* Fine needle aspiration
Folate
biochemistry of, *72*
characteristics of, 69-70, *70*
physiology of, *71*
Folate deficiency. *See also*
Megaloblastic anemia
in alcoholism, *49*
approach to diagnosis of, 11, *12*
blood cell measurements in, *10*
differential diagnosis of, *368*
leukocytic disorders of abnormal
morphology in, *284,* 285
mechanisms of, 75, *76*
sequence in development of, *73,*
75
Folate testing. *See* Red blood cell
folate quantitation; Serum
folate quantitation
Follicle center lymphoma, *524,* 531-
532, *534-535,* 550-551, 563-
564, 566, *574-575*
diffuse, predominantly small cell,
524, 532
follicular, *569*
mixed small and large cell, *524,*
531-532
predominantly large cell, *524,* 531-
532

predominantly small cell, *524,*
531-532
Follicular lymphoma, 518, 563
Fragmentation hemolysis, 11, *16*
Free erythrocyte protoporphyrin
(FEP), **35-37**
in anemia of chronic disease, 35-
37, 46
in iron deficiency anemia, 35-37
in hypochromic anemia, 27
in sideroblastic anemia, 35-37
"Full marrow, empty blood syndrome,"
348
Functional fibrinogen determination,
710-711
in acquired coagulation disorders,
710-711
reference values for, *772-773*
Furadantin. *See* Nitrofurantoin
Furosemide (Lasix), *661*

G

G6PD. *See* Glucose-6-phosphate
dehydrogenase
Gallstones, pigment, 96, 111, 122
Gamma-glutamylcysteine synthetase
assay, 138
Gamma-glutamylcysteine synthetase
deficiency, 128, *129,* 137
Ganciclovir, 301
Gastrin test, in megaloblastic anemia,
80-81, 84-85
Gastritis, 84, 533
Gastrointestinal cancer, *7,* 26, 37, *210*
Gaucher's disease, 35, *347, 445*
Gene rearrangement studies
in acute lymphoblastic leukemia,
422
in acute myeloid leukemia, 397
in Hodgkin's disease, 588-589
in non-Hodgkin's lymphoma, 559,
562
Genitourinary cancer, 26, 37
Gentamicin, *661*
γ heavy chain disease, 609
Giant hemangioma, *699*
Giant lymph node hyperplasia. *See*
Castleman's disease

blood cell measurements in, 275
bone marrow examination in, 275
clinical findings in, 273
constitutional, *271*
course of, 278
hematologic findings in, 275
myeloperoxidase stain in, 274,
276-277
neutrophil function tests in, 277-278
nitroblue tetrazolium dye test in,
274-276
pathophysiology of, 269-273
peripheral blood smear morphology
in, 275
treatment of, 278
Granulocyte-macrophage colony-stimulating factor, 368
Granulocyte-monocyte colony-stimulating factor, 227, 246, 252-253
Granulocytic sarcoma, 379, 387, *392,
554, 560, 575*
Granulocytopenia, *378*
Granulocytosis, 476
Granulopoiesis, 226-228
Gray platelet syndrome, *667*

H
Hairy cell leukemia (HCL), 501-503,
502, 510-511, 524, 673
Ham's test. *See* Acid hemolysis test
Hand mirror red blood cells, 349
Haptoglobin, 95, 104-105
Haptoglobin testing. *See* Serum hapto-
globin quantitation
Hashimoto's thyroiditis, *519,* 533
Hashish, *661*
HCL. *See* Hairy cell leukemia
HDN. *See* Hemolytic disease of the
newborn
Heart
in anemia, *9*
in megaloblastic anemia, 87
polycythemia in heart disease, 454,
455
posttransplantation lymphoprolif-
erative disorders, 545-546
Heart valve, prosthetic, *7, 94*
Heat stroke, *699*

Heavy chain disease, 595, *596-597,*
601, 608-609
Heinz body, 128, 132, 148, 196
Heinz body test, **204-205**
in accelerated erythrocyte turnover,
100
in drug-related hemolytic anemia,
199, 204-205
in glucose-6-phosphate dehydrogenase deficiency, 199, 204-205
in hemoglobin synthesis disorders,
158, *161*
Helmet cells. *See* Schistocytes
Hemangioblastoma, *455, 457*
Hematocrit, reference values for, *758-
761, 768-769*
Hematogones, 429, *430, 437*
Hematology, automated, 4-5, *760-761*
Hematology reference values, *758-774*
Hematopoiesis
in AIDS, 50
extramedullary, 442, *443,* 446-448
ineffective. *See* Myelodysplastic
syndromes
Hematopoietic neoplasms
eosinophilia in, 238, *239*
red cell aplasia in, *57*
Hematuria, *98, 107,* 181, 746
Heme metabolism, 26, *26,* 95
Hemochromatosis, 22, 35, 50, *347*
Hemodialysis, 47, 182
Hemodilution, *49, 646*
Hemoglobin
drug-induced oxidation of, 195-
196
reference values for, *758-761, 768-
769*
unstable, *123,* 131, *142, 149,* 156-
157, 196, 199, 204
Hemoglobin A, 139, *140*
Hemoglobin A_2, 139, *140*
Hemoglobin A_2 quantitation
in accelerated erythrocyte turnover,
100
with chromatography, **154-155**
in hemoglobin synthesis disorders,
154-155
reference values for, *770-771*
Hemoglobin Bart's, 144

Heparin therapy, 637-639, 647, *661,*
    711, *716,* 725, 746
  administration of, 747
  heparin level, **754-755**
  indications for, 747
  monitoring of, 748
  resistance to, 734-735
Hepatitis, 50, *295,* 296, 299-302, 679,
    698
  aplastic anemia and, 57, *58,* 59
Hepatoma, 698
Hepatomegaly
  in extrinsic hemolytic anemia, 174
  in hemolytic anemia, 96, 99-100
  in Hodgkin's disease, 578
Hepatosplenomegaly, in apoplastic/
    hypoplastic anemia, 59
Herbicide, *519*
Hereditary elliptocytosis. *See also*
    Erythrocyte membrane defect,
    hereditary
  accelerated erythrocyte turnover
    in, *94*
  peripheral blood smear morphology
    in, *7*
Hereditary hemochromatosis, 22
Hereditary nonspherocytic hemolytic
    anemia (HNSHA)
  approach to diagnosis of, 122-123
  blood cell measurements in, 123
  clinical findings in, 120-122
  course of, 126
  defects associated with, *123*
  direct antiglobulin test in, 122
  fluorescent screening for pyruvate
    kinase deficiency in, 123-125
  hematologic findings in, 123
  hemoglobin electrophoresis in, 122
  isopropanol stability test in, 122-
    123, 126
  osmotic fragility test in, 122, 126
  pathophysiology of, 119-120
  peripheral blood smear morphology
    in, 123
  red cell enzyme assays in, 125-126
  sucrose hemolysis test in, 122
  treatment of, 126
Hereditary persistence of fetal hemo-
    globin (HPFH), 192

acid elution test for fetal hemoglo-
    bin in red cells in, 156
  alkali denaturation test for fetal
    hemoglobin in, 153-154
Hereditary spherocytosis. *See also*
    Erythrocyte membrane defect,
    hereditary
  accelerated erythrocyte turnover
    in, *94*
  approach to diagnosis of, *15*
  blood cell measurements in, *10*
  hypersplenism in, *347,* 349, 351
  peripheral blood smear morphology
    in, *7*
Hereditary stomatocytosis, *7*
Hermansky-Pudlak syndrome, *667*
Herpes virus infection, *565*
Heterophil antibody test, **311-312**
  in infectious mononucleosis, 297,
    298, 306-308, *308,* 311-312,
    334
Hexokinase, *121*
Hexokinase deficiency, *122*
Hexose monophosphate shunt, 112,
    120, *121, 123,* 127-128, *128*
Hexose monophosphate shunt disor-
    ders, 127-138
Hiatal hernia, *13*
High altitude
  adaptation to, 454, *455*
  effect on volume of packed red
    cells, *760*
High-grade B-cell lymphoma, Burkitt-
    like, *524,* 536-537
High-molecular weight kallikrein
    assay
  in inherited coagulation disorders,
    688-689
  reference values for, *772-773*
High-molecular weight kallikrein
    deficiency, 630, *636,* 683, *683,*
    689
Histiocytosis X, *330, 337*
Histoplasmosis, *330,* 334, 338
HIV infection. *See* Human immunod-
    eficiency virus infection
HNSHA. *See* Hereditary nonsphero-
    cytic hemolytic anemia
Hodgkin's cells, 579

Hodgkin's disease
    approach to diagnosis of, 582-584
    autoimmune hemolytic anemia in,
        210
    blood cell measurements in, 584-
        585
    bone marrow examination in, 584-
        586
    bone scan in, 586
    classification of, 517, 578-582,
        579
    clinical findings in, 578
    computed tomography in, 586
    course of, 589-590
    cytogenetic studies in, 589
    definition of, 577
    differential diagnosis of, 537, 581
    eosinophilia in, 238
    Epstein-Barr virus in, 588
    gene rearrangement studies in,
        588-589
    hematologic findings in, 584-586
    histopathologic features of, 583
    immunophenotyping in, 537, 560-
        561, 587-588, 588-589
    incidence of, 578
    kidney function studies in, 584
    laparotomy in, 584, 587
    leukocyte alkaline phosphatase in,
        480
    liver function studies in, 584
    lymphadenopathy in, 330
    lymphangiogram in, 586
    lymph node biopsy in, 583, 586
    lymphocyte depletion, 525, 578,
        579, 581-582, 581, 583
    lymphocyte predominance, 525,
        577-578, 579, 580, 581, 583,
        584, 588-589, 588, 591
    lymphocyte predominant mixed
        cellularity, 580
    lymphocyte-rich classical, 525,
        580
    lymphocytopenia in, 318
    mixed cellularity, 525, 577-578,
        579, 580-581, 581, 583, 588,
        588, 591
    monocytosis in, 251, 252
    myelofibrosis in, 443, 445

    nodular sclerosis, 525, 579, 581,
        582, 583, 584, 588, 588, 592
    non-Hodgkin's lymphoma vs, 520
    pathophysiology of, 577-578
    peripheral blood smear morphology
        in, 585
    polymerase chain reaction in, 589
    radiologic studies in, 584, 586
    Southern blot analysis in, 589
    staging of, 583-584, 583-585
    treatment of, 589-590
    unclassifiable, 525
Homocystinuria, 667, 729, 730-731,
        732
Homologous restriction factor, 163-
        164, 168
Howell-Jolly body, 6-7, 149
HTLV. See Human T-cell leukemia
        virus
Human herpesvirus-6 infection, 295,
        296, 298
Human immunodeficiency virus
        (HIV) infection. See also AIDS
    coagulation disorders in, 702, 704
    granulocyte functional defects in,
        271, 274
    lymphadenopathy in, 330, 330,
        334-335
    lymphocytosis in, 295, 296, 298
    thrombocytopenia in, 650
    treatment of, 301, 325
Human T-cell leukemia virus-1
        (HTLV-1), 504, 519
Hydronephrosis, 454, 457
Hydrops fetalis, 144, 145, 184, 192
Hydroxychloroquine sulfate, 661
Hydroxyurea therapy, 464, 473, 483
Hyperbilirubinemia, 101-103
Hypercalcemia, 606
Hypercoagulability, 723
Hyperdiploidy, in acute lymphoblastic
        leukemia, 426, 426-427
Hypereosinophilic syndrome, idio-
        pathic, 239, 240-241, 244
Hyperfibrinogenemia, 639
Hypergranular promyelocytic
        leukemia (M3), 382-383, 385-
        386, 392, 395, 395-396, 397,
        398, 399, 400, 405-406

Hyperimmunoglobulin E syndrome, *271*
Hyperproliferative anemia, 10
Hypersensitivity reaction, 245, 247
Hypersplenism
    approach to diagnosis of, 347-348
    blood cell measurements in, 348
    bone marrow examination in, 349
    chromium-51 red cell studies in,
        348-351
    clinical findings in, 346-347
    course of, 351-352
    definition of, 345
    hematologic findings in, 348-349
    neutropenia in, 260, *261-262*
    pathophysiology of, 345-346, *347*
    peripheral blood smear morphology
        in, 348-349
    treatment of, 351-352
Hypertension, portal, *49, 50*
Hyperviscosity syndrome, 607-608
Hypochromic anemia. *See also* Iron
        deficiency anemia
    approach to diagnosis of, 27-28
    blood cell measurements in, 29
    bone marrow examination in, 29
    causes of, *26*
    clinical findings in, 27
    course of, 36-37
    free erythrocyte protoporphyrin in,
        27
    globin chain synthetic ratio in, 28
    hematologic findings in, 28-29, *30*
    hemoglobin electrophoresis in, 28
    pathophysiology of, 25-27
    peripheral blood smear morphology
        in, 27, 29, *31*
    serum iron test in, 27
    stainable bone marrow iron in, 28
    test selection in, 36
    total iron-binding capacity in, 27
    treatment of, 36-37
Hypochromic cells, *6-7*
Hypodiploidy, in acute lymphoblastic
        leukemia, 426, *426-427*
Hypofibrinogenemia, *683*
Hypogammaglobulinemia, 492, 498,
        600, 604
Hypophosphatemia, *480*

Hypoplastic anemia
    approach to diagnosis of, 58-59
    blood cell measurements in, *55,* 59
    bone marrow examination in, *55,* 60
    characteristics of, 53-56, *54-55*
    clinical findings in, *54,* 58
    course of, 61-62
    cytogenetic studies in, 61
    differential diagnosis of, *430*
    fetal hemoglobin quantitation in,
        60-61
    hematologic findings in, 59-60
    pathophysiology of, 56-57, *58*
    peripheral blood smear morphology
        in, 59-60
    red cell i antigen test in, 61
    treatment of, 61-62
Hypoproliferative anemia, 10
Hypothyroidism, *9,* 47-48
Hypoxemia, 462

I
Ibuprofen (Motrin), *661*
Idiopathic thrombocytopenic purpura
        (ITP), *480,* 646-648, *646*
Ie antigen, *172*
Ig. *See* Immunoglobulin
IL. *See* Interleukin
IM. *See* Infectious mononucleosis
Imipramine (Tofranil), *661*
Immune complex, toxic, *172,* 196-
        198, 202-203
Immune hemolysis
    blood specimen collection in, 200
    drug-induced, 196-199, *198*
Immune thrombocytopenia, 646-648,
        646, 653-655, *673*
Immune thrombocytopenic purpura,
        252
Immunoblast(s), *316, 340, 534, 571*
Immunoblastic lymphoma, 518, 566
Immunocytoma, *524,* 530, *534*
Immunodeficiency, *238*
Immunoelectrophoresis. *See* Laurell
        immunoelectrophoresis assay;
        Serum protein immunoelec-
        trophoresis; Urine protein
        immunoelectrophoresis

Infectious mononucleosis-like syndromes, 294, *295,* 296-297, 299-300
Inflammatory disease
anemia in, 39, *41*
autoimmune hemolytic anemia in, *210*
basophilia in, *246*
haptoglobin levels in, 105
neutrophilia in, *226*
serum ferritin quantitation in, 35
thrombocytosis in, *468*
Influenza, *58,* 245, *318,* 319
Inherited coagulation disorders
activated partial thromboplastin time in, 683-684, *683-684, 686*
alpha$_2$-antiplasmin determination in, 694-695
approach to diagnosis of, 682-686, *683-686*
bleeding time test in, *684*
blood cell measurements in, 686
clinical findings in, 682
course of, 695-696
factor V assay in, 689-690
factor VII assay in, 689-690
factor VIII antibody in, 684
factor VIII antibody screening test in, 691-692
factor VIII antibody titer in, 692-694
factor VIII assay in, 687-688
factor X assay in, 689-690
hematologic findings in, 686
high-molecular weight kallikrein assay in, 688-689
inhibitor screening test in, 684, 690-691
laboratory evaluation of, 715-717, *716*
pathophysiology of, 681-682
prekallikrein assay in, 688-689
prothrombin assay in, 689-690
prothrombin time test in, 683-684, *683-684*
thrombin time test in, 684
treatment of, 695-696
Inhibitor of plasminogen activators. *See* PAI-1

Inhibitor screening test, **690-691**
in acquired coagulation disorders, *703,* 705-706
in inherited coagulation disorders, 684, 690-691
Inosine triphosphatase deficiency, 126
Insecticides, *58*
Interferon-alpha, 483, 500, 607
Interferon therapy, 464, 503
Interleukin-1 (IL-1), 40-41, *42,* 47, 328
Interleukin-2 (IL-2), *271,* 500
Interleukin-3 (IL-3), 238, 241, 246
Interleukin-4 (IL-4), 246
Interleukin-5 (IL-5), 238, 246
Interleukin-6 (IL-6), 356
Interleukin therapy, 237
Intermediate syndrome of platelet dysfunction, 666
International Lymphoma Study Group, classification of lymphoma, 522, *523-524, 526-529*
Intestinal T-cell lymphoma, *524,* 541-542
Intrauterine transfusion therapy, 193
Intravascular hemolysis, 95, 103-104
Intrinsic factor, 74-75, *74*
Intrinsic factor antibodies, in megaloblastic anemia, *80-81,* 84
In vitro bone marrow cell culture studies, in myelodysplastic syndromes, 366
Iron deficiency anemia
in adult, 26
in alcoholism, *49*
anemia of chronic disease vs, *17,* 46
approach to diagnosis of, 13-14, *16,* 27-28
blood cell measurements in, *10,* 29
bone marrow examination in, 29
in child, 26
clinical findings in, *9,* 27
course of, 36-37
free erythrocyte protoporphyrin in, 35-37
hematologic findings in, 28-29
peripheral blood smear morphology in, *7,* 29, *31, 38*
serum ferritin quantitation in, 34-35

NK cell, *524,* 539
T-cell, *524,* 539
Large granular lymphocytosis. *See*
    Large granular lymphocyte
    leukemia
Lasix. *See* Furosemide
Latex particle agglutination test, for
    fibrin(ogen) degradation prod-
    ucts, 708-710
Laurell immunoelectrophoresis assay
    for von Willebrand's factor
    antigen, **678-679**
L-dopa, *210*
Lead poisoning, *7, 15,* 35, *368*
Leiomyoma, uterine, *455, 457*
Lepore syndrome, 146
Leprosy, *337*
Leptocytes, *6-7*
Leptomeningeal leukemia, *378,* 387
Leptospirosis, *226*
Leucovorin, 83
Leukemia. *See also* specific types of
    leukemia
    approach to diagnosis of, *15*
Leukemic infiltrate, *378*
Leukemoid reaction, *480*
Leukocyte adhesion deficiency, *271,*
    275
Leukocyte alkaline phosphatase
    (LAP), 227, **232-233**
    abnormal, conditions associated
        with, *480*
    in chronic myelogenous leukemia,
        232-233, *233,* 446, 472, 476,
        478-479, *480*
    in essential thrombocythemia, 472,
        480
    in Hodgkin's disease, *480*
    in myelofibrosis with myeloid
        metaplasia, 447
    in neutrophilia, 229, 232-233, *233*
    in paroxysmal nocturnal hemoglo-
        binuria, 168
    in polycythemia, *464*
Leukocyte counts, *770-771*
Leukocyte differential counts, *762-*
    763, 770-771
Leukocytic disorders of abnormal
    morphology

acquired, *284*
approach to diagnosis of, 286-287
blood cell measurements in, 287
bone marrow examination in, 287
clinical findings in, 286
course of, 288
cytogenetic studies in, 288
hematologic findings in, 287
hereditary, *282-283*
pathophysiology of, 285-286
peripheral blood smear morphology
    in, 287, *289*
treatment of, 288
Leukocytosis, *230*
Leukoerythroblastic leukemia. *See*
    Myelofibrosis with myeloid
    metaplasia
Leukoerythroblastic picture, in
    myelofibrosis with myeloid
    metaplasia, 445, *451*
Leukoerythroblastosis, *15, 21,* 349, *445*
Lewis antigen, *172*
LGL leukemia. *See* Large granular
    lymphocyte leukemia
L&H cells, 580, *591*
Light chain restriction, 559
Listeriosis, 251
Lithium, *226, 233*
Liver biopsy, in non-Hodgkin's lym-
    phoma, 549
Liver disease
    anemia in, *9,* 48-50
    antithrombin III in, 735
    coagulopathy in, *716*
    approach to diagnosis of, 703-704,
        705
    functional fibrinogen determina-
        tion in, 710-711
    pathophysiology of, 697-698
    treatment of, 713
    diagnosis of, *12*
    haptoglobin levels in, 105
    hypersplenism in, 349
    plasminogen in, 739
    protein C in, 736
    prothrombin time assay in, 636
    warfarin therapy in, *753*
Liver function tests, **552**
    in Hodgkin's disease, 584

in non-Hodgkin's lymphoma, 552
Löffler's pneumonia, 242
Lower extremity lymphangiogram, 586
Lukes and Butler classification, of Hodgkin's disease, 578-582, *579*
Lung disease, polycythemia in, 454
Lupus anticoagulant, 637-638, 691, 697, *702-703,* 704-707, *705,* 713, *716*
  confirmatory test for, **711-712**
Lymphadenitis, postvaccinal, *330*
Lymphadenopathy. *See also* Lymphoma
  in acute lymphoblastic leukemia, 412
  in anemia, *9*
  angioimmunoblastic, *63*
  in apoplastic/hypoplastic anemia, 59
  approach to diagnosis of, 331-332
  blood cell measurements in, 331-332
  bone marrow examination in, 332-333
  causes of, *330*
  chest roentgenogram in, 332, 338
  in chronic lymphocytic leukemia, 493
  clinical findings in, 330-331, *332*
  course of, 338
  definition of, 329
  dermatopathic, *565*
  erythrocyte sedimentation rate in, 331, 333
  hematologic findings in, 332-333
  in hemolytic anemia, 96
  in infectious mononucleosis, 306
  lymph node biopsy in, 332, 335-336, *337-338, 340-342*
  pathophysiology of, 329-330
  peripheral blood smear morphology in, 332-333
  serologic tests for infectious agents in, 332-335
  serum calcium in, 332, 338
  treatment of, 338
  tuberculin skin test in, 332, 338

Lymphangiogram, *337*
  bipedal, 552
  in Hodgkin's disease, 586
Lymph node
  fine needle aspiration of, 553-554
  pseudonodules in, 499
Lymph node biopsy, **335-336,** *337-338, 340-342*
  in benign vs malignant disease, *338*
  in Castleman's disease, *342*
  in child, 543
  in chronic lymphocytic leukemia, 499, *509*
  in Hodgkin's disease, 583, 586
  in infectious mononucleosis, *340*
  in Kikuchi-Fujimoto lymphadenitis, *341*
  in lymphadenopathy, 332, 335-336, *337-338, 340-342*
  in myelofibrosis with myeloid metaplasia, 447-448
  in non-Hodgkin's lymphoma, 548-549, *548*
  patterns observed in lymphadenopathy, 337, *337*
  in toxoplasmosis, *341*
Lymphoblast(s), 413-415, *434-436*
Lymphoblastic lymphoma, 551-552, 554, 566
  in child, 544, *544, 546, 573*
  differential diagnosis of, *537*
  T-precursor, *524,* 537-538
Lymphocyte(s)
  age-related reference values for, 293, *294*
  reactive disorders of
    approach to diagnosis of, 297-299, *298*
    blood cell measurements in, 297, 299-300
    bone marrow examination in, 300
    causes of, *295*
    clinical findings in, 295-296
    course of, 301-302
    culture of infectious agents in, 301
    definition of, 293

hematologic findings in, 299-
300
pathophysiology of, 293-295,
295
peripheral blood smear morphology in, 297, 300, *304*
serologic tests for infectious
agents in, *298,* 301
treatment of, 301-302
Lymphocyte testing. *See*
Immunophenotyping
Lymphocytopenia
approach to diagnosis of, 321
blood cell measurements in, 321-
322
bone marrow examination in, 321-
322
causes of, *318*
clinical findings in, 320-321
course of, 325
definition of, 317
hematologic findings in, 321-322
immunoglobulin quantitation in,
321-323
immunophenotyping in, 321, 323-
325, *324*
pathophysiology of, 317-320
treatment of, 325
Lymphocytosis. *See also* Chronic
lymphocytic leukemia;
Lymphocytes, reactive disorders of
differential diagnosis of, *430*
infectious, 296, 300
large granular. *See* Large granular
lymphocyte leukemia
Lymphogranuloma venereum, *330,*
334, *337*
Lymphoid nodule, benign, 551
Lymphoma. *See also* specific types of
lymphoma
accelerated erythrocyte turnover
in, *94*
anemia in, *41*
approach to diagnosis of, *15*
bone marrow examination in, 21,
21
bone marrow failure in, 63, *63*
clinical findings in, *9*

diseases simulating, 565, *565*
eosinophilia in, *238*
extranodal, 519
folate deficiency in, *76*
occult
in autoimmune hemolytic anemia, 221
evaluation of, **221**
thrombocytopenia in, *646*
unclassifiable, *525*
von Willebrand's disease in, 671
Lymphoma cells, circulating, 349
Lymphoplasmacytoid lymphoma, *524,*
530, *534-535*
Lymphoproliferative disorders
coagulation disorders in, *702*
posttransplantation, *519,* 545-546,
564
Lymphoproliferative syndrome, X-
linked, *519*
Lysosomal granule, 227

M

Macrocytes, *6-7, 89*
Macrocytic anemia, *10*
classification of, 11-12, *12-13*
without increased reticulocyte
response, *13*
Macrocytosis, *149*
masked, 5
Macroglobulinemia, Waldenström's.
See Waldenström's macroglob-
ulinemia
Macrophages, *324*
Malaria, *94,* 131, *172,* 173-174, 182,
347
Malignant histiocytosis, 252, *253*
Malignant lymphoma. *See*
Lymphoma; specific types of
lymphoma
Mantle cell lymphoma, 498, *524,* 530-
531, *534-535,* 563-564, *568*
Marfan's syndrome, 666, *667*
Marginal zone B-cell lymphoma, *524,*
532-533, *534-535*
MALT type, *519, 524,* 532-533,
569-570
nodal monocytoid, *524,* 533, *570*

undifferentiated, 450
Myelosclerosis
acute, 449-450
chronic. *See* Myelofibrosis with
myeloid metaplasia
Myobid. *See* Papaverine
Myocardial infarction, 753-754
Myoglobinuria, *98, 107*

N

Nalidixic acid, *131, 197*
Naphthalene, *131, 197*
Naprosyn. *See* Naproxen
Naproxen (Naprosyn), *661*
National Cancer Institute, staging for
lymphoma, 520, *521*
Natural killer (NK) cell(s), monoclonal
antibodies against, *324*
Natural killer (NK) cell lymphoma,
524, 537-543
NBT dye test. *See* Nitroblue tetrazolium dye test
Neonatal purpura fulminans, 736
Neoplastic disease. *See also* Cancer
anemia in, 39, *41, 43*
autoimmune hemolytic anemia in,
210
basophilia in, 245-248, *246*
eosinophilia in, 237-238, *238-239*
folate deficiency in, *76*
hypersplenism in, *347,* 349
lymphocytopenia in, *318*
monocytosis in, 252, *252,* 254-255
myelofibrosis in, *443*
polycythemia in, *455, 457*
thrombocytosis in, *468*
Nephrotic syndrome, *753*
Neuroblastoma, 429
Neurofibromatosis, 377
Neutropenia
approach to diagnosis of, 262-264
autoimmune, *267*
blood cell measurements in, 264
bone marrow examination in, 264,
267
causes of, 260, *261*
age-related, *262*

clinical findings in, 261-262
course of, 265
definition of, 259-260
hematologic findings in, 264
hereditary, 260
pathophysiology of, 260-261, *263*
peripheral blood smear morphology
in, 263-264
refractory, 363
treatment of, 265
Neutrophil(s), 259
demargination of, 228
hypersegmentation of, 78, *89,* 281,
284
hyposegmentation of, 281
Neutrophil actin deficiency, *271*
Neutrophil adhesion molecules, 270
Neutrophil defects. *See* Granulocyte
functional defects; Leukocytic
disorders of abnormal morphology
Neutrophil function tests, 277-278
Neutrophilia
approach to diagnosis of, 229
at birth, 225
blood cell measurements in, 229-
230
bone marrow examination in, 231-
232
chronic myelogenous leukemia vs,
231
clinical findings in, 228
course of, 234
cytogenetic studies in, 234
definition of, 225
hematologic findings in, 229-232
leukocyte alkaline phosphatase test
in, 229, 232-233, *233*
pathophysiology of, 226-228
peripheral blood smear morphology
in, 230-231, *230, 235*
reactive, 225-226, *226*
treatment of, 234
Newborn. *See* Hemolytic disease of
the newborn
NHL. *See* Non-Hodgkin's lymphoma
Nicotinic acid, *661*
Niemann-Pick disease, *347*
Nitric oxide, *724,* 727

Petechiae, 657
Phenindione (Dindevan), 746
Phenothiazine, *661*
Phenoxybenzamine hydrochloride (Dibenzyline), *661*
Phenylbutazone (Butazolidin), *58, 661*
Phenytoin, *330, 519, 565*
Pheochromocytoma, *457*
Philadelphia chromosome, 417, 428, 447, 475, 479-481, 485, *487.* See also Chronic myelogenous leukemia
Phlebotomy, in polycythemia, 463-465
Phosphofructokinase, *121*
Phosphofructokinase deficiency, *122*
6-Phosphogluconate dehydrogenase, 133, 135
Phosphoglycerate kinase deficiency, 120-121, *122*
Pigment gallstones, 96, 111, 122
Pigment testing. See Serum pigments
Plasma cell(s), *324*, 598-599, *611*
Plasma cell dyscrasias, 595
    classification of, *596*
    monoclonal immunoglobulins in, *597*
Plasma cell myeloma, *445, 480. See also* Multiple myeloma
Plasmacytoma, *524*
Plasma hemoglobin quantitation, **103-104**
    in accelerated erythrocyte turnover, *97*, 103-104
    in extrinsic hemolytic anemia, 175, 180-181
Plasma volume, decreased, 11, 454-455, *455*, 457-458, 465
Plasmin, 725-726
Plasminogen, 631, 725-726, *727*
Plasminogen activator inhibitor-1. *See* PAI-1
Plasminogen deficiency, *729*, 738-739
Plasminogen determination, **738-739**
    reference values for, *772-773*
    in thrombotic disorders, 738-739
Platelet(s). *See also* Hemostasis
    activation of, 627
    adhesion of, 657-658
    aggregation of, 657-659, 754

in coagulation, 627
drugs that affect function of, 660, *661*
increased destruction of, 646, *646*
production of, 626, *644*
release reaction of, 657-658
secretory granules of, 626
Platelet aggregation studies, **675-677**
    in Bernard-Soulier disease, *669*
    in essential thrombocythemia, 472
    in Glanzmann's thrombasthenia, *668,* 676
    in myelofibrosis with myeloid metaplasia, 447
    normal tracing in, *665*
    in platelet release reaction defects, 676
    in polycythemia, 463, *464*
    in qualitative platelet disorders, 660, 662, *664,* 675-677
    in storage pool disease, *670,* 676
    in thrombocytopenia, 651-652
    in von Willebrand's disease, *664, 669,* 675-677
Platelet-associated immunoglobulins test, **653-654**
    in thrombocytopenia, 653-654
Platelet count
    in acquired coagulation disorders, *705*
    in bleeding disorders, *635*, 640, 715, *716*
    postoperative, *720*
    reference values for, *758-761, 768-769*
Platelet disorders, 631-633, *634. See also* Qualitative platelet disorders; Thrombocytopenia
    postaspirin bleeding time in, 643
Platelet factor 4, 653
Platelet release reaction defects, 662-666, *663-664, 670,* 676
Platelet transfusion, 655
Pleural effusion, in non-Hodgkin's lymphoma, 552
PLL. *See* Prolymphocytic leukemia
PML-RARα fusion gene, 386, 397
PNH. *See* Paroxysmal nocturnal hemoglobinuria

in Waldenström's macroglobulinemia, 608
Serum protein immunoelectrophoresis,
602-603
in amyloidosis, 618
in multiple myeloma, 596-597,
600-603
in Waldenström's macroglobulinemia, 608
Serum sickness, *330*
Serum uric acid test
in acute myeloid leukemia, 399
in essential thrombocythemia, 472
in myelofibrosis with myeloid
metaplasia, 447
in non-Hodgkin's lymphoma, 565
in polycythemia, 456, *464*
Serum viscosity test
in multiple myeloma, 606
in Waldenström's macroglobulinemia, 608
Serum vitamin B$_{12}$ quantitation, **79-82**
in megaloblastic anemia, 79-82,
80-81, 85
reference values for, *770-771*
Severe combined immunodeficiency
disease (SCID), 317-318, *318,*
320, 323, 325
Sézary cells, 505, *513, 573*
Sézary syndrome, *502,* 505, *513, 524,*
539-540, *573*
Shwachman-Diamond syndrome, 53,
54-55
Sickle beta-thalassemia disease, 141-
143, *142,* 151
Sickle cell(s), *6-7, 149*
Sickle cell anemia, 140, 142, 151,
158, *161*
blood cell measurements in, *10*
granulocyte functional defects in,
271
peripheral blood smear morphology
in, *7*
Sickle cell disease. *See* Sickle cell
anemia
Sickle cell test, **151-152**
in hemoglobin synthesis disorders,
146, 151-152
Sickle cell trait, 140, 142, *150,* 151-153

Sideroblast(s), 32-33, *361*
ringed, 27, 29, 33, *38, 49,* 50, 101,
374. See also Refractory anemia, with ringed sideroblasts
Sideroblastic anemia
acquired idiopathic, *26,* 27
acquired toxic, *26,* 27
approach to diagnosis of, *15-16*
bone marrow examination in, 29
drug-related, 37
free erythrocyte protoporphyrin in,
35-37
hematologic findings in, 28-29
hereditary, *26, 27,* 37
peripheral blood smear morphology
in, *7,* 29, *31*
platelet dysfunction in, *673*
serum ferritin quantitation in, 35
serum iron quantitation in, *32*
stainable bone marrow iron in, *32*
total iron-binding capacity in, *32*
treatment of, 37
Silicone, *330*
Simplate, 641
Sinus histiocytosis with massive lymphadenopathy, *330, 337,* 565
Sjögren's syndrome, *330,* 334, *519,*
533
SLE. *See* Systemic lupus erythematosus
SLL. *See* Small lymphocytic lymphoma
Small cell tumor, metastatic, *430,*
430-431
Small cleaved cell leukemia (SCCL),
502, 503-504, *511*
Small lymphocytic lymphoma (SLL),
518, 550, 564, 566, *568, 581*
B-cell, *524,* 527-529, *534-535*
Smallpox, 245
Smoking
lymphocytosis and, 295-296, *295,*
300
neutrophilia in, *226*
Snake bite, *699*
Solubility test for hemoglobin S, **152-
153**
in hemoglobin synthesis disorders,
146, 152-153

Thromboxane synthetase deficiency, *667*
Thymic carcinoma, *210*
Thymidine synthesis, 86
Thymocytes, *324*
Thymoma, 56, *57,* 59
Thyrotoxicosis, *226*
TIBC. *See* Total iron-binding capacity
Ticarcillin, *661*
Tissue biopsy
  in amyloidosis, 618
  in Hodgkin's disease, 586
Tissue factor, 629-630
Tissue-plasminogen activator (t-PA), 631, *724, 725-726, 727*
Tissue-plasminogen activator (t-PA) deficiency, 728, *729,* 739-740
Tissue-plasminogen activator (t-PA) determination, **739-740**
  reference values for, *772-773*
  in thrombotic disorders, 739-740
Tissue-plasminogen factor (t-PA) therapy, 746-747, 753-754
Tissue thromboplastin, 748
TNT. *See* Trinitrotoluene
Tofranil. *See* Imipramine
Total bilirubin, 102
Total iron-binding capacity (TIBC), **30-32**
  in anemia of chronic disease, *32,* 45
  in hypochromic anemia, 27
  in iron deficiency anemia, 30-31, *32*
  in megaloblastic anemia, *80-81*
  reference values for, *770-771*
  in sideroblastic anemia, *32*
  in thalassemia, *32*
Total lactic dehydrogenase, in accelerated erythrocyte turnover, *97,* 107-108
Toxic granulation, *230,* 231
Toxin, *226, 443*
Toxoplasmosis, *226, 295, 298,* 330, *330, 333-335, 337, 341, 565*
t-PA. *See* Tissue-plasminogen activator
Tranexamic acid, 696
Transcobalamin deficiency, *74,* 82
Transferrin, 95
Transferrin saturation test, **30, 45**
  in anemia of chronic disease, 45

  in hemochromatosis, 22
Transferrin testing. *See* Total iron-binding capacity; Transferrin saturation test
Transfusion reaction
  alloantibodies in, 174
  antibody identification in, 178-179
  approach to diagnosis of, 174-175
  course of, 182
  direct antiglobulin test in, 179-180
  disseminated intravascular coagulation in, *699*
  hematologic findings in, 175-176
  serum antibody screening in, 176-177
  serum haptoglobin quantitation in, 180
  treatment of, 182
  urine hemoglobin test in, 181
Transfusion therapy
  in acquired coagulation disorders, 712
  in anemia, 22
  in autoimmune hemolytic anemia, 222
  in hypochromic anemia, 37
  in inherited coagulation disorders, 695
  intrauterine, 193
  in megaloblastic anemia, 87
  pyruvate kinase testing after, 125
  in thalassemia, 159
Transient erythroblastopenia of childhood, *54-55,* 56, 60-61
Transient stress lymphocytosis, 294, *295,* 296, 299-300
Transplant rejection, *457*
TRAP stain. *See* Tartrate-resistant acid phosphatase stain
Travel history, 174, 240
Trephine biopsy, 390, 415
Triavil, *661*
Trichinosis, 242
Tricyclic antidepressants, *661*
Trinitrotoluene (TNT), *131, 197*
Triosephosphate isomerase deficiency, 120, *122*
Trisomy 3, *535*
Trisomy 8, 365, *367*